S. Hombach-Klonisch, T. Klonisch, J. Peeler

Sobotta

Clinical Atlas of Human Anatomy

To Thomas, Susanne and Tobias

I am grateful to my husband Thomas who has encouraged me to engage in this atlas and supported me throughout all steps – thanks for all the discussions we had. Thank you to my lovely children Susanne and Tobias who have always been supportive and interested in my work. They have provided insight and motivation from a learner's perspective.

SHK

To Elisabeth and Karl-Heinz

I am forever grateful to my parents for their essential support which allowed me to chase my dreams. They have been there when it mattered most to provide encouragement and inspiration. All of this wouldn't have been possible without your strong determination and passion. You will always be with us.

TK

To Ang, Madi and Lauryn

You girls are my rock ... my foundation! The things that I have been able to accomplish in life are because of your unwavering love and support. I am so grateful to be a part of your amazing lives.

JP

To the Faculty and Staff of the Department of Human Anatomy and Cell Science at the University of Manitoba

Thank you for your ongoing support, encouragement, and collegiality. During the ongoing development of our curricula in the health professions each of you has played an important role and influenced the thinking that led to the development of this clinical atlas.

To our Students

This book is for you. Thank you for asking those tough questions ... saying I don't understand ... or seeking another example or explanation. Your insight, observations, enquiry, and inquisitive nature fuels our passion for teaching, and served as a driving force in the creation of this clinical atlas. We hope that this book will aid you to learn and apply your understanding of human anatomy in a clinically relevant manner.

To Their Teachers

We hope that this book serves as a valuable resource for you and your students. The Clinical Atlas of Human Anatomy is intended to support you in educating students of the different health science about human anatomy in a clinically relevant manner.

Sabine Hombach-Klonisch, Thomas Klonisch, Jason Peeler (eds.)

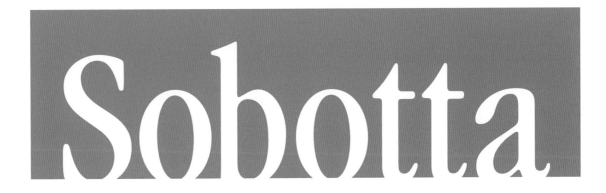

Clinical Atlas of Human Anatomy

1st edition

Based on the work by
Prof. Dr. Friedrich Paulsen, Erlangen, Germany
Prof. Dr. Jens Waschke, Munich, Germany

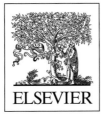

ELSEVIER

ELSEVIER

Hackerbrücke 6, 80335 Munich, Germany

All business correspondence should be made with:
books.cs.muc@elsevier.com

ISBN   978-0-7020-5273-6
e-ISBN   978-0-7020-5279-8

19 20 21 22 23   5 4 3 2 1

Content Strategist: Benjamin Rempe, Rainer Simader, Dr. Katja Weimann

Content Project Management: Dr. Andrea Beilmann, Sibylle Hartl

Production Management: Dr. Andrea Beilmann, Sibylle Hartl

Copy Editor: Sonja Hammer, Schwarzenbruck, Germany

Layout: Nicola Kerber, Olching, Germany

Composed by: abavo GmbH, Buchloe, Germany

Printed and bound by: Drukarnia Dimograf Sp. z o. o., Bielsko-Biała, Poland

Cover Design: Stefan Hilden, hilden_design, Munich, Germany; Spiesz Design, Neu-Ulm, Germany

More Information at **elsevierhealth.com**

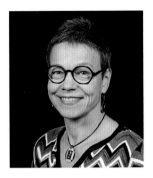

Dr. Sabine Hombach-Klonisch

Dr. med. habil., Certified Anatomist

Dr. Sabine Hombach-Klonisch is an Associate Professor in the Department of Human Anatomy and Cell Science of the Max Rady College of Medicine at the University of Manitoba. Teaching clinically relevant anatomy and clinical case-based anatomy learning are the main teaching focus of Dr. Hombach at the Medical Faculty of the University of Manitoba. Since her appointment in 2004, Dr. Hombach has been nominated annually for teaching awards by the Manitoba Medical Student Association.

Dr. Hombach graduated from Medical School at the Justus-Liebig University Giessen in 1991 and completed her doctoral thesis in 1994 under the supervision of Prof. Werner Seeger, Department of Medicine. Following a career break to attend to her two young children, she worked as a sessional lecturer at the Department of Anatomy and Cell Biology of the University of Halle-Wittenberg in 1997 and was awarded a post-doctoral fellowship by the province of Sax-

ony-Anhalt from 1998–2000. Thereafter, she joined the Department of Anatomy and Cell Biology faculty as an Assistant Professor. In 2003, Dr. Hombach successfully completed her accreditation as anatomist with the German Society of Anatomists and received accreditation by the Medical Association of Saxony-Anhalt. Dr. Hombach completed her habilitation in 2004 under the guidance of Prof. Bernd Fischer at the Medical Faculty of the Martin Luther University of Halle-Wittenberg, before accepting a position as Assistant Professor at the Department of Human Anatomy and Cell Science, Faculty of Medicine, at the University of Manitoba, Winnipeg, MB, Canada where, in 2012, Dr. Hombach was promoted to tenured Associate Professor.

Dr. Hombach has been the recipient of the Merck European Thyroid von Basedow Research Prize by the German Endocrine Society in 2002 and received the Murray L. Barr Young Investigator Award by the Canadian Association for Anatomy, Neurobiology and Cell Biology in 2009. For the last six years, Dr. Hombach has held the role as Section Head of Gross Anatomy at the Department of Human Anatomy and Cell Science. As a medically trained anatomist, Dr. Hombach emphasizes the importance of clinical anatomy as a foundation of clinical practise. Her committed efforts to constantly adapt anatomy teaching to the changing needs of students was recognized at several annual teaching award ceremonies and resulted in her receiving the 2016–2017 teaching award for "Best Small Group Teaching, Mentorship, Innovation and Inspiration" by the Manitoba Medical Student Association.

Her main research interests are in the field of Cancer Research with a focus on brain cancer and metastatic breast cancer to the brain. Her research team employs unique cell and animal models and patient-derived human tumor cells and tissues to study the molecular mechanisms that cause treatment failures and regulate cancer cell metastasis. Dr. Hombach holds national research funding and her productive lab continues to publish their results in international scientific journals with focus on cancer and cell biology.

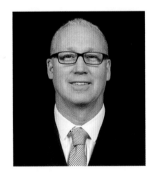

Dr. Jason Peeler

BPE, MSc, PhD (Manitoba), Certified Athletic Therapist – CAT(C)

Dr. Peeler is an Associate Professor in the Department of Human Anatomy and Cell Science of the Max Rady College of Medicine at the University of Manitoba. Born and raised in Winnipeg, Manitoba, his educational background includes undergraduate and graduate degrees in Kinesiology, with a major in the field of Athletic Therapy. Dr. Peeler's PhD training was completed in the Department of Hu-

man Anatomy and Cell Science at the University of Manitoba, where his studies bridged the fields of musculoskeletal anatomy and rehabilitation. He possesses a wealth of experience in musculoskeletal injury assessment and rehabilitation, and has worked as a Certified Athletic Therapist in Canadian high performance sport since 1992.

Dr. Peeler has more than 25 years of experience as a clinical educator in the field musculoskeletal anatomy. His academic background and clinical experiences have allowed him to develop a unique and diverse teaching skill-set. He currently serves as the musculoskeletal course director for the Max Rady College of Medicine, as well as teaches gross and clinically applied musculoskeletal anatomy across a broad spectrum of undergraduate, graduate, and post-graduate health science programs including Physical Therapy, Occupational Therapy, Respiratory Therapy, Pharmacy, Dentistry, Kinesiology, Biomedical Engineering, Physician's Assistant, and medical residency programs in Physical Medicine and Orthopaedics.

Dr. Peeler's research expertise lies in the areas of applied musculoskeletal anatomy and clinical orthopaedics and rehabilitation, with an emphasis on validity and reliability testing of musculoskeletal assessment and intervention/rehabilitation techniques that are designed to enhance patient care and musculoskeletal function. His unique combination of experiences as a sports medicine clinician and PhD anatomist have assisted him to develop a research agenda that is focused on bridging the gap between anatomical structure and biomechanical function.

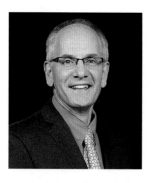

Dr. Thomas Klonisch
Dr. med. habil., Certified Anatomist

Dr. Klonisch is a Full Professor and Head of the Department of Human Anatomy and Cell Science (HACS). He teaches gross anatomy, histology and small group sessions and heads the Body Donation program at the University of Manitoba. Dr. Klonisch has initiated and contributed to restructuring initiatives of several anatomy teaching courses. During his tenure as department head, HACS has undergone major expansions and renovations of teaching and research space. The gross anatomy laboratory and morgue facilities have undergone a complete renovation to provide advanced state-of-the-art support for the extensive departmental anatomy teaching programs that serve the specific needs of undergraduate and graduate students, residents, and clinicians at the Colleges of Medicine, Dentistry, Medical Rehabilitation Sciences, Pharmacy, and Nursing and students at Bio-Engineering and the Arts.

Dr. Klonisch studied Human Medicine at the Ruhr University of Bochum and Justus Liebig University (JLU) Giessen and completed his doctoral thesis at the Institute of Biochemistry at JLU in 1991 under the guidance of Prof. Stefan Stirm. He completed a practical year of medical training in Medical Microbiology, University of Mainz, Germany, and thereafter joined the Institute of Medical Microbiology as Assistant Professor. In 1991, Dr. Klonisch was awarded a Feodor Lynen Fellowship from the Alexander von Humboldt Foundation, Bonn, Germany, to join the Microbiology department at the University of Guelph, Ontario, Canada, from 1991–1992. Thereafter, he continued his research as a postdoctoral fellow at the Ontario Veterinary College, Guelph, Ontario, before joining the Department. of Immunology, University College London, London, UK, as a senior research fellow from 1994–1996. In 1996, he was appointed at the Department of Anatomy and Cell Biology, Martin Luther University of Halle-Wittenberg, Germany, where he received his national accreditation as anatomist (1999) and completed his habilitation (2000) under the guidance of Prof. Bernd Fischer. Throughout this time, he taught anatomy to students of different health professions and continued his active nationally funded research program. In 2004, he was appointed Full Professor and Head at the Department of Human Anatomy and Cell Science, Faculty of Medicine, University of Manitoba, Winnipeg, Canada, where he is currently nearing the end of his third term as department head.

Dr. Klonisch is a cancer biologist and his research focuses is on human brain tumors and the role cell plasticity in cancer stem/progenitor cells has on treatment responses in brain tumor patients. His nationally funded, interdisciplinary and collaborative cancer research program explores molecular and cellular mechanisms that promote tumor cell tissue invasion and survival mechanisms in response to radio- and chemotherapy. The Klonisch lab has established patient-derived brain tumor cell and blood resources and cell/tissue based proteomics to study dynamic changes to the brain tumor micro-environment during treatment. Dr. Klonisch founded the Brain Tumor Research Alliance Manitoba (BTRAM) which serves as a scientific exchange forum for brain tumor researchers and was a co-founding member of the Regenerative Medicine Program at the University of Manitoba. He is also the director of the Histomorphology and Ultrastructural Imaging platform at the Faculty of Health Sciences which provides research services in histology and microscopy to researchers in Manitoba.

Preface

The Department of Human Anatomy and Cell Science (HACS) at the University of Manitoba has a strong history of publishing educational materials. Inspired by Dr. J.C.B. Grant (HACS chairperson from 1919–1930) and his foundational work Grant's Atlas of Anatomy, HACS has been the academic home for several renowned anatomists who have created important anatomy learning resources that continue to inspire generations of students across North America and the world. Among them are Dr. T.V.N. (Vid) Persaud (Professor Emeritus at the University of Manitoba, former HACS chairperson from 1977–1993), Dr. Keith L. Moore (Professor Emeritus at the University of Toronto, former HACS chairperson from 1965–1976), and Dr. J. Eduard Bruni (HACS faculty member and neuroanatomist [retired]). The members of the Anatomy Department at the University of Manitoba, Winnipeg, have always sought out novel approaches to support and encourage learning of human anatomy in a clinically relevant and applied manner. This new *Sobotta – Clinical Atlas of Human Anatomy* hopes to carry on with this tradition.

The atlas utilizes a regional approach for learning human anatomy. This integrates core concepts of anatomical structure and function with modernized methods of diagnostic imaging, cross-sectional anatomy, illustrations of real world functions and examples on how anatomical knowledge informs clinical reasoning. The organization and anatomical concepts presented are based on a "block" approach to teaching that is common within medical curricula in North America. This curricular model is designed to integrate human anatomy instruction into clinical teaching to provide students with greater clinical context and discipline-specific examples that highlight and re-inforce the importance of human anatomy a foundation of clinical knowledge. Based on a functional and regional approach to teaching anatomy, this Clinical Atlas of Human Anatomy integrates clinically relevant surface anatomy with the structure and function of the regional organ systems and associates motion with the respective musculoskeletal elements of movement. This atlas provides key anatomical landmarks that can be used for physical examination and employs diagnostic imaging as well as selected "Structure/Function" and "Clinical Remarks" to associate spatial and functional anatomical concepts with pathologies.

This clinical anatomy atlas features a total of 1892 images with 331 new images, including examples of daily activities to highlight muscle function, surface anatomy, diagnostic imaging, plus comprehensive tables to support learners.

The target audience for this clinical atlas is the health professions trainee – this includes students enrolled in programs such as medicine, dentistry, physician assistants, rehabilitation sciences (i.e. physical therapy, occupational therapy, respiratory therapy, athletic training/therapy, massage therapy), pharmacy, nursing, and kinesiology or the movement sciences. As such, each of the chapters uses an integrated approach to deliver detailed anatomical images in conjunction with clinically relevant surface anatomy, diagnostic imaging, cross-sectional anatomy, and functional images which depict some aspect of human body function. The "Clinical Remarks" and "Structure/Function" sections also provide important and easily identifiable clinical examples and anatomical detail which serves to reinforce application of anatomical knowledge. Furthermore, these vignettes are meant to assist the student to gain a better understanding of how the different anatomical structures contribute to specific body functions and pathologies. Finally, the anatomical images are accompanied by descriptive text and summary tables which serve to highlight the central concepts associated with each specific image that is depicted on each page.

Contributors

Dr. Noam Ze'ev Millo, MD, FRCPC
Assistant Professor
Department of Radiology
Section Head, Ultrasound
Max Rady College of Medicine, University of Manitoba, Canada

Meredith Brownlee, BSc, DMD, MDS (OMFR), FRCD(C), Dip. ABOMR
Assistant Professor
Division Head of Oral and Maxillofacial Radiology
Dental Diagnostic and Surgical Sciences, College of Dentistry
Rady Faculty of Health Sciences
University of Manitoba, Winnipeg, MB, Canada

Hugo Bergen, Ph.D.
Associate Professor
Department of Human Anatomy and Cell Science
Max Rady College of Medicine
Rady Faculty of Health Sciences
University of Manitoba, Winnipeg, MB, Canada

Acknowledgments

A special thank you to each of the following PhD anatomists who helped to mold the approach and influenced the thinking which resulted in the development of the musculoskeletal (MSK) chapters of this clinical atlas: Dr. Judy Anderson, Professor Emeritus and Former Head – Department of Biological Sciences, University of Manitoba; Dr. Juliette (Archie) Cooper, Professor Emeritus and Former Director – College of Rehabilitative Sciences, University of Manitoba; Dr. Mark Garrett, Senior instructor – College of Rehabilitative Science, University of Manitoba; Dr. Jeffrey Leiter, Albrechtsen Research Chair – Pan Am Clinic Foundation, Winnipeg, Manitoba; Dr. Vid Persaud, Professor Emeritus and Former Head – Department of Human Anatomy and Cell Science, University of Manitoba; Dr. James Thliveris, Professor Emeritus and Former Head – Department of Human Anatomy and Cell Science, University of Manitoba; and Dr. Mark G. Torchia, embryologist and Vice-Provost (Teaching and Learning) and Executive Director (Centre for the Advancement of Teaching and Learning) – University of Manitoba. Whether it be discussing the intricacies of MSK anatomy structure and function as it relates to rehabilitation, surgery or a potential research project; talking about the MSK anatomy curriculum or curricular design; or simply teaching MSK anatomy labs alongside of you to one of the various medical or health science programs at the University of Manitoba. Please know that the creation of this Clinical Atlas of Human Anatomy would not have been possible without your wisdom and insight. You are all amazing anatomists!!

We thank our colleagues in the Department of Human Anatomy and Cell Science for their insightful ideas and the numerous discussions on the structure of our anatomy teaching. We are grateful to our clinical colleagues who provided positive and constructive feedback on our teaching concepts and who value the anatomy education we provide to our students in the health professions.

In our pursuit of knowledge, we have been blessed to be students of exceptional teachers, researchers, and clinicians who continue to inspire us. Their examples have taught us to be passionate about discovery and innovation and to be enthusiastic teachers. We are indebted and grateful to Prof. Dr. Cuong Hoang-Vu, Department of General, Visceral and Vascular Surgery, Martin-Luther-University of Halle-Wittenberg, Faculty of Medicine, Germany; Prof. Dr. Sucharit Bhakdi, Professor Emeritus and Former Chair of the Institute of Medical Microbiology and Hygiene, University of Mainz, Germany; Prof. Dr. Werner Seeger, Director of the University Medical Clinic, Justus-Liebig-University Giessen, Germany; the late Dr. David G. Porter, Professor and Former Chair of the Department of Biomedical Sciences, Ontario Veterinary College, Guelph, Ontario, Canada and the late Prof. Dr. Hanns-Gotthard Lasch, Former Chair of the University Medical Clinic, Justus-Liebig-University Giessen, Germany.

Color Chart

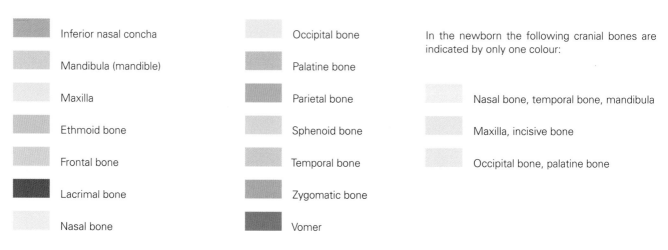

Inferior nasal concha	Occipital bone	In the newborn the following cranial bones are indicated by only one colour:	
Mandibula (mandible)	Palatine bone		
Maxilla	Parietal bone		Nasal bone, temporal bone, mandibula
Ethmoid bone	Sphenoid bone		Maxilla, incisive bone
Frontal bone	Temporal bone		Occipital bone, palatine bone
Lacrimal bone	Zygomatic bone		
Nasal bone	Vomer		

Picture Credits

Reference to the source for each figure in this work is given at the end of each caption in square brackets. All figures and graphics without a reference © Elsevier GmbH, Munich, Germany.

The editors sincerely thank all clinical colleagues that made ultrasound, computed tomographic and magnetic resonance images as well as endoscopic and intraoperative pictures available.

E247-09 Moore K. L., Persaud T., Torchia M. G.: The Developing Human – Clinically Oriented Embryology. 9th ed., Elsevier/Saunders, 2013

E273 Mir M. A.: Atlas of Clinical Diagnosis. 2nd ed., Elsevier/Saunders, 2003

E282 Kanski, J.: Clinical Ophthalmology: A Systematic Approach. 5th ed., Butterworth-Heinemann, 2003

E288 Forbes C. D., Jackson W. F.: Colour Atlas and Text Book of Clinical Medicine. 3rd ed., Elsevier/Mosby, 2003

E329 Pretorius E. S., Solomon J. A.: Radiology Secrets Plus. 3rd ed., Elsevier/Mosby, 2011

E336 LaFleur Brooks, M.: Exploring Medical Language – A Student-Directed Approach. 7th ed., Elsevier/Mosby, 2008

E339 Asensio, J., Trunkey, D.: Current Therapy of Trauma and Surgical Critical Care. 1st ed., Elsevier/Mosby, 2008

E347 Moore K. L, Persaud T.: The Developing Human – Clinically Oriented Embryology. 8th ed., Elsevier/Saunders, 2007

E355 Goldman, L., Ausiello, D., Arend, W.: Cecil Medicine. 23rd ed., Elsevier/Saunders, 2008

E372 McQuillen Martensen K.: Radiographic Image Analysis. 2nd ed., Elsevier/Saunders, 2006

E373 Swain J., Bus K.: Diagnostic Imaging for Physical Therapists. 1st ed., Elsevier/Saunders, 2008

E377 Eisenberg R., Johnson N.: Comprehensive Radiographic Pathology. 5th ed., Elsevier/Mosby, 2012

E380 Eiff M. P., Hatch R. L.: Fracture Management for Primary Care. 3rd ed., Elsevier/Saunders, 2012

E382 Coughlin, M.: Surgery of The Foot And Ankle, 2-Volume Set. 8th ed., Elsevier/Mosby, 2007

E393 Adam A., Dixon A. K.: Grainger & Allison's Diagnostic Radiology – A Textbook of Medical Imaging. 5th ed., Elsevier/Churchill Livingstone, 2008

E402 Drake R. L. et al.: Gray's Anatomy for Students. 1st ed., Elsevier/Churchill Livingstone, 2005

E404 Herring J. A.: Tachdijan's Pediatric Orthopaedics. 4th ed., Elsevier/Saunders, 2008

E422 Weston W., Lane A., Morelli J.: Color Textbook of Pediatric Dermatology. 4th ed., Elsevier/Mosby, 2007

E458 Kelley L. L., Petersen C.: Sectional Anatomy for Imaging Professionals. 2nd ed., Elsevier/Mosby, 2007

E460 Drake R. L. et al.: Gray's Atlas of Anatomy. 1st ed., Elsevier/Churchill Livingstone, 2008

E467 Marchiori D.: Clinical Imaging – With Skeletal, Chest and Abdomen Pattern Differentials. 2nd ed., Elsevier/Mosby, 2005

E475 Baren J. M. et al.: Pediatric Emergency Medicine. 1st ed., Elsevier/Saunders, 2008

E513-002 Herring, W.: Learning Radiology – Recognizing the Basics. 2nd ed., Elsevier/Saunders, 2012

E528 Wetmore R.: Pediatric Otolaryngology – The Requisites in Pediatrics. 1st ed., Elsevier/Mosby, 2007

E530 Frank E., Long B., Smith B.: Merrill's Atlas of Radiographic Positioning and Procedures. 12th ed., Elsevier/Mosby, 2012

E538 Skarin A.: Atlas of Diagnostic Oncology 4th ed., Elsevier/Mosby, 2010

E545 Shiland B.: Mastering Healthcare Terminology. 2nd ed., Elsevier/Mosby, 2006

E563 Evans R.: Illustrated Orthopedic Physical Assessment. 3rd ed., Elsevier/Mosby, 2009

E567 Lewis S.: Medical-Surgical Nursing in Canada – Assessment and Management of Clinical Problems. 1st ed., Elsevier/Mosby, 2006

E580 Drake R. L. et al.: Gray's Anatomy for Students. 2nd ed., Elsevier/Churchill Livingstone, 2010

E602 Adams J. et al.: Emergency Medicine. 1st ed., Elsevier/Saunders, 2008

E603 Yeo C.: Shackelford's Surgery of the Alimentary Tract. 6th ed., Elsevier/Saunders, 2007

E607-002 Muscolino J.: Kinesiology – The Skeletal System and Muscle Function. 2nd ed., Elsevier/Mosby, 2011

E625 Myers E.: Operative Otolaryngology – Head and Neck Surgery. 2nd ed., Elsevier/Saunders, 2008

E684 Herrick A. L. et al.: Orthopaedics and Rheumatology in Focus. 1st ed., Elsevier/Churchill Livingstone, 2010

E708 Marx J., Hockberger R., Walls R.: Rosen's Emergency Medicine – Concepts and Clinical Practice. 7th ed., Elsevier/Mosby, 2010

E748 Seidel H. M. et al.: Mosby's Guide to Physical Examination. 7th ed., Elsevier/Mosby, 2010

E754 Murray S. S., McKinney E. S.: Foundations of Maternal–Newborn Nursing. 4th ed., Elsevier/Saunders, 2006

E761 Fuller G., Manford M.: Neurology – An Illustrated Colour Text. 3rd ed., Elsevier/Churchill Livingstone, 2010

E813 Green N., Swiontkowski M.: Skeletal Trauma in Children. 4th ed., Elsevier/Saunders, 2009

E838 Mitchell B., Sharma R.: Embryology – An Illustrated Color Text. 2nd ed., Elsevier/Churchill Livingstone 2009

E867 Winn R.: Youmans Neurological Surgery, 4-Vol. Set. 6th ed., Elsevier/Saunders, 2011

E871 Som P. M., Curtin H. D.: Head and Neck Imaging. 5th ed., Elsevier/Mosby, 2011

E877 Sinnatamby C. S.: Last's Anatomy – Regional and Applied. 12th ed., Elsevier/Churchill Livingstone, 2012

E890 Frontera W., Micheli L., Herrin, S.: Clinical Sports Medicine – Medical Management and Rehabilitation. 1st ed., Elsevier/Saunders, 2006

E908-003 Corne J., Pointon K.: Chest X-ray Made Easy. 3rd ed., Elsevier/Churchill Livingstone, 2010

E943 Kanski J.: Clinical Ophthalmology – A Systematic Approach. 6th ed., Butterworth-Heinemann, 2007

E955 Liu G., Volpe N., Galetta S.: Neuro-Ophthalmology – Diagnosis and Management. 2nd ed., Elsevier/Saunders, 2010

E969 Weissman B. N.: Imaging of Arthritis and Metabolic Bone Disease. 1st ed., Elsevier/Saunders, 2009

E988 Wilson S. F., Giddens J. F.: Health Assessment for Nursing Practice. 4th ed., Elsevier/Mosby, 2008

E989 Magee D. J.: Orthopedic Physical Assessment. 5th ed., Elsevier/Saunders, 2008

E990 Moy R., Fincher E.: Procedures in Cosmetic Dermatology: Advanced Face Lifting, 1st ed. Elsevier/Elsevier/Saunders 2006

E993 Auerbach P. S.: Wilderness Medicine. 6th ed., Elsevier/Mosby, 2010

F217-003 Damian D. L. et al.: A Plethora of Protein. In: The American Journal of Medicine 2010, 123, p904–906

F264-003 Hartman R. P., Kawashima A., King B. F.: Evaluation of renal causes of hypertension. In: Radiol Clin North Am 2003, 41/5, p909–929

F264-004 Hwang S.: Imaging of Lymphoma of the Musculoskeletal System. In: Radiologic Clinics of North America 2008, 46, p75–93

F274-002 Hession W. G., et al.: Epidural steroid injections. In: Seminars in Roentgenology 2004, 39/1, p7–23

F276-005 Frost A., Robinson C.: The painful shoulder. In: Surgery (Oxford) 2006, 24, p363–367

F276-006 Marsh H.: Brain tumours. In: Surgery (Oxford) 2007, 25, p526–529

F276-007 Hobbs C., Watkinson J.: Thyroidectomy. In: Surgery (Oxford) 2007, 25, p474–478

F282 Goshtasby P., Miremadi R., Warwar R.: Retrobulbar Hematoma After Third Molar Extraction. In: Journal of Oral and Maxillofacial Surgery 2010, 68, p461–464

F371-003 Medow J., Trost G., Sandin J.: Surgical management of cervical myelopathy. In: The Spine Journal 2006, 6/6, p233–241

F589   Strauss R., Burgoyne C.: Diagnostic Imaging and Sleep Medicine. In: Dental Clinics 2008, 52/4, p891–915

F654   Hockenberry M., Wilson D.: Wong's Nursing Care of Infants and Children. 9th ed., Elsevier/Mosby, 2011

F698-002   Meltzer C. C. et al.: Serotonin in Aging, Late-Life Depression, and Alzheimer's Disease – The Emerging Role of Functional Imaging. In: Neuropsychopharmacology 1998, 18, p407–430

F903-004   Williams S. K., Eisholt F. I.: Concomitant Cervical and Lumbar Stenosis. In: Seminars in Spine Surgery 2007, 19/3, p165–176

F905-002   Saragaglia D., Pison A., Rubens-Duval B.: Acute and old ruptures of the extensor apparatus of the knee in adults (excluding knee replacement). In: Orthopaedics & Traumatology: Surgery & Research 2013, 99/1, pS67–S76

G042   Gates P.: Clinical Neurology. 1st ed., Elsevier/Churchill Livingstone, 2010

G052   Rakel R., Rakel D.: Textbook of Family Medicine. 8th ed., Elsevier/Saunders, 2012

G056   Hochberg M., Silman A., Smolen J., Weinblat, M., Weisman M.: Rheumatology. 5th ed., Elsevier/Mosby, 2011

G123   DeLee J. C., Drez D., Miller M. D.: DeLee & Drez's Orthopaedic Sports Medicine. 2nd ed., Elsevier/Saunders, 2003

G130   Pagana K.: Mosby's Manual of Diagnostic and Laboratory Tests. 3rd ed., Elsevier/Mosby, 2006

G159   Forbes, A. et al.: Atlas of Clinical Gastroenterology. 3rd ed., Elsevier/Mosby, 2004

G169   Miller F., Rubesin S.: The Teaching Files: Gastrointestinal. 1st ed., Elsevier/Saunders, 2010

G198   Mettler, F.: Essentials of Radiology. 3rd ed., Elsevier/Saunders, 2014

G199   Salvo, S.: Massage Therapy – Principles and Practice. 4th ed., Elsevier/Saunders, 2012

G210   Standring S.: Gray's Anatomy – The Anatomical Basis of Clinical Practice. 40th ed., Elsevier/Churchill Livingstone, 2008

G211   Ellenbogen R. G., Abdulrauf S. I.: Principles of Neurological Surgery. 3rd ed., Elsevier, 2012

G217   Waldman S., Bloch J.: Physical Diagnosis of Pain – An Atlas of Signs and Symptoms. 2nd ed., Elsevier/Saunders, 2010

G302   McCance, K. L. et al.: Pathophysiology – The Biologic Basis for Disease in Adults and Children. 6th ed., Elsevier/Mosby, 2010

G305   Hardy M., Snaith B.: Musculoskeletal Trauma – A Guide to Assessment and Diagnosis. 1st ed., Elsevier/Churchill Livingstone, 2011

G366   Callaway, W. J.: Mosby's Comprehensive Review of Radiography – The Complete Study Guide and Career Planner. 4th ed., Elsevier/Mosby, 2006

G425   Chang J., Neligan P.: Plastic Surgery: Volume 6: Hand and Upper Limb, Elsevier/Saunders 2013

G435   Perkin G. D. et al.: Atlas of Clinical Neurology. 3rd ed., Elsevier/Saunders, 2011

G460   Chintamani: Lewis's Medical-Surgical Nursing. 1st ed., Elsevier/Mosby, 2011

G463   DeLee J. C., Drez D.: DeLee & Drez's Orthopaedic Sports Medicine. 3rd ed., Elsevier/Saunders, 2010

G465   Tang J. et al.: Tendon Surgery of the Hand. 1st ed., Elsevier/Saunders, 2012

G493   Miller M., Sanders T.: Presentation, Imaging and Treatment of Common Musculoskeletal Conditions. 1st ed., Elsevier/Saunders, 2012

G533   Long B., Frank E., Ehrlich R.: Radiography Essentials for Limited Practice. 3rd ed., Elsevier/Saunders, 2009

G550   Zitelli B., McIntire S., Nowalk A.: Zitelli and Davis' Atlas of Pediatric Physical Diagnosis. 6th ed., Elsevier/Saunders, 2012

G568   Applegate E. J.: The Sectional Anatomy Learning System – Concepts. 3rd ed., Elsevier/Saunders, 2009

G570   Wein A., Kavoussi L., Novick A. C.: Campbell-Walsh Urology, 4-Vol. Set. 10th ed., Elsevier/Saunders, 2012

G645   Douglas G., Nicol F., Robertson C.: Macleod's Clinical Examination. 13th ed., Elsevier/Churchill Livingstone, 2013

G704   Hagen-Ansert S. L.: Textbook of Diagnostic Sonography. 7th ed., Elsevier/Mosby, 2012

G716   Pagorek S. et al.: Physical Rehabilitation of the Injured Athlete. 4th ed., Elsevier/Saunders 2011

G717   Milla S., Bixby S.: The Teaching Files – Pediatrics. 1st ed., Elsevier/Saunders, 2010

G718   Soto J., Lucey B.: Emergency Radiology – The Requisites. 1st ed., Elsevier/Mosby, 2009

G719   Thompson S. R., Zlotolow D. A.: Handbook of Splinting and Casting. 1st ed., Elsevier/Mosby, 2012

G720   Slutsky, David J.: Principles and Practice of Wrist Surgery. 1st ed., Elsevier/Saunders, 2010

G721   Canale S. T., Beaty J.: Campbell's Operative Orthopaedics, Vol.1. 11th ed., Elsevier/Mosby, 2008

G723   Rosenfeld, J. V.: Practical Management of Head and Neck Injury. 1st ed., Elsevier/Churchill Livingstone, 2012

G724   Broder J.: Diagnostic Imaging for the Emergency Physician. 1st ed., Elsevier/Saunders, 2011

G725   Waldmann S., Campbell R.: Imaging of Pain. 1st ed., Elsevier/Saunders, 2011

G728   Sahrmann, S.: Movement System Impairment Syndromes of the Extremities, Cervical and Thoracic Spines. 1st ed., Elsevier/Mosby, 2010

G729   Browner B. D., Fuller R. P.: Musculoskeletal Emergencies. 1st ed., Elsevier/Saunders, 2013

G730   Brown D. L. et al.: Atlas of Regional Anesthesia. 4th ed., Elsevier/Saunders, 2010

G731   Miller M., Hart J., MacKnight J.: Essential Orthopaedics. 1st ed., Elsevier/Saunders, 2009

G739   Cupett M., Walsh K.: General Medical Conditions in the Athlete. 2nd ed., Elsevier/Mosby, 2011

G740   Spaeth G. et. al.: Ophthalmic Surgery – Principles and Practice. 4th ed., Elsevier/Saunders, 2011

G741   Azizzadeh B. et al.: Master Techniques in Rhinoplasty. 1st ed., Elsevier/Saunders, 2011

G742   Ryan S., McNicholas M., Eustace S.: Anatomy for Diagnostic Imaging. 3rd ed., Elsevier/Saunders, 2011

G743   Payne-James J., Byard R. W.: Encyclopedia of Forensic and Legal Medicine. 2nd ed., Elsevier, 2015

G744   Weir J. et al.: Imaging Atlas of Human Anatomy. 4th ed., Elsevier/Mosby, 2011

G745   Anderson M. W., Fox M. G.: Sectional Anatomy by MRI and CT. 4th ed., Elsevier, 2017

G746   Shaw R. W., Luesley D., Monga, A.: Gynaecology. 4th ed., Elsevier/Churchill Livingstone, 2011

G748   Debry C., Mondain M., Reyt E.: ORL. 2nd ed., Elsevier/Masson, 2011

G749   Le Roux P., Winn H., Newell D.: Management of cerebral aneurysms. 1st ed., Elsevier/Saunders 2004

H043-001   Mutoh K. et al.: Possible induction of systemic lupus erythematosus by zonisamide. In: Pediatric Neurology, 2001, 25/4, p340–343

H060-001   Bilreiro, C., Bahia, C., & Oliveira e Castro, M.: Longitudinal stress fracture of the femur. In: European Journal of Radiology Open, 2016, 3, p31–34

H061-001   Dodds, S. D. et al.: Radiofrequency probe treatment for subfailure ligament injury: a biomechanical study of rabbit ACL. In: Clinical Biomechanics, 2004, 19/2, p175–183

H062-001   Sener, R. N.: Diffusion MRI: apparent diffusion coefficient (ADC) values in the normal brain. In: Computerized Medical Imaging and Graphics, 2001, 25/4, p299

H063-001   Heller et al.: Spontaneous brachial plexus hemorrhage – case report. In: Surgical Neurology, 2000, 53/4, p356–359

H064-001   Philipson, M., Wallwork, N.: Traumatic dislocation of the sternoclavicular joint. In: Orthopaedics and Trauma, 2012, 26/6, p380–384

H080   Kaiho, Y.: Retroperitoneoscopic Transureteroureterostomy with Cutaneous Ureterostomy to Salvage Failed Ileal Conduit Urinary Diversion. In: European Urology, 2009, 59/5, p875–878

H081   Yang, Bora: A Case of Recurrent In-Stent Restenosis with Abundant Proteoglycan Component. In: Korean Circulation Journal, 2003, 33/9, p827–831

H082-001   Sasaki, C.T., Jassin B.: Cancer of the pharynx and larynx. In: The American Journal of Medicine 2001, 111/8, p118–123

H083-001   Tavares E., Martins R.: Vocal evaluation in teachers with or without symptoms. In: Journal of Voice, 2007, 21/4, p407–414

H084-001 Custodio C. et al.: Neuromuscular Complications of Cancer and Cancer Treatments. In: Physical Medicine & Rehablititation Clinics of North America, 2008, 19, p27–45

J787 Colourbox.de

K340 Biederbick & Rumpf GbR, Adelsdorf, Germany

K383 Cornelia Krieger, Hamburg, Germany

L106 Henriette Rintelen, Velbert, Germany

L107 Michael Budowick, Munich, Germany

L126 Dr. med. Katja Dalkowski, Erlangen, Germany

L127 Jörg Mair, Munich, Germany

L141 Stefan Elsberger, Planegg, Germany

L231 Stefan Dangl, Munich, Germany

L238 Sonja Klebe, Löhne, Germany

L240 Horst Ruß, Munich, Germany

L266 Stephan Winkler, Munich, Germany

L271 Matthias Korff, Munich, Germany

L275 Martin Hoffmann, Neu-Ulm, Germany

L280 Johannes Habla, Munich, Germany

L284 Marie Davidis, Munich, Germany

L285 Anne-Kathrin Hermanns, Maastricht, The Netherlands

M467 Prof. Dr. med. Gain, Krankenhaus Barmherzige Brüder, Regensburg, Germany

M500 Prof. Dr. med. Günter Kauffmann, Heidelberg, Germany

M614 Prof. Dr. med. Wolfgang Rüther, Hamburg, Germany

P310 Prof. Dr. med. Friedrich Paulsen, Erlangen, Germany

P489 Dr. Jason Peeler, PhD, Department of Human Anatomy and Cell Science, University of Manitoba, Winnipeg, Canada

P496 Dr. med. Saadettin Sel, Universitätsklinik und Poliklinik für Augenheilkunde, Halle (Saale), Germany

P497 Prof. Robin Jarvis Brownlie, University of Manitoba, Winnipeg, Canada

P498 Prof. Dr. med. P. L. Pereira, SLK-Kliniken Heilbronn, Klinik für Radiologie, Germany

R104-05 Renz-Polster H., Krautzig S., Braun J.: Basislehrbuch Innere Medizin. 5. A., Elsevier/Urban & Fischer, 2013

R132 Classen M., Diehl V., Kochsiek K.: Innere Medizin. 5. A., Urban & Fischer, 2003

R170-3 Welsch U., Deller T.: Sobotta Lehrbuch Histologie. 3. A., Elsevier/Urban & Fischer, 2010

R170-4 Welsch U., Kummer W.: Sobotta Lehrbuch Histologie. 4. A., Elsevier/Urban & Fischer, 2014

R235 Böcker W., Denk H., Heitz P. U., Moch H.: Pathologie. 4. A., Urban & Fischer, 2008

R252 Welsch, U.: Sobotta Atlas Histologie – Zytologie, Histologie, Mikroskopische Anatomie. 7. A., Urban & Fischer, 2005

R316-007 Wicke, L.: Atlas der Röntgenanatomie. 7. A., Urban & Fischer, 2005

R333 Scharf H.-P., Rüter A.: Orthopädie und Unfallchirurgie. 2. A., Elsevier/Urban & Fischer, 2011

R363 Trepel M.: Neuroanatomie, 4. A., Elsevier/Urban & Fischer, 2008

R382 Gutermuth L., Gerstdorfer M.: Schockraum-Management – Organisation und Patientenversorgung. 1. A., Elsevier/Urban & Fischer, 2009

R388 Weinschenk S.: Handbuch Neuraltherapie. 1. A., Elsevier/Urban & Fischer, 2010

R389 Gröne B.: Schlucken und Schluckstörungen – Eine Einführung. 1. A., Elsevier/Urban & Fischer, 2009

S002-8 Prof. Dr. med. Herbert Lippert, Neustadt, Germany

S008-3 Kauffmann G. W., Moser E., Sauer R.: Radiologie. 3. A., Elsevier/Urban & Fischer, 2006

S010-17 Benninghoff A., Drenckhahn D.: Anatomie, Band 1. 17. A., Elsevier/Urban & Fischer, 2008

S130-5 Speckmann E.-J., Hescheler J., Köhling R.: Physiologie. 5. A., Elsevier/Urban & Fischer, 2008

T127 Prof. Dr. Dr. Peter Scriba, Munich, Germany

T620 Dr. med. Berit Jordan, Prof. Dr. med. Stephan Zierz, Universitätsklinik und Poliklinik für Neurologie, Halle (Saale), Germany

T719 Prof. Dr. med. Norbert Kleinsasser, Klinik und Poliklinik für Hals-, Nasen- und Ohrenkrankheiten, plastische und ästhetische Operationen, Universität Würzburg, Germany

T720 PD Dr. med. Hannes Kutta, Klinik und Poliklinik für Hals-, Nasen- und Ohrenheilkunde, Universitätsklinikum Hamburg-Eppendorf, Germany

T786 Dr. med. Stefanie Lescher, Prof. Dr. med. Joachim Berkefeldt, Neuroradiologie, Universitätsklinikum der Goethe-Universität Frankfurt, Germany

T824 Klinikum Dritter Orden, Munich, Germany

T898 Prof. Dr. med. Udo Jonas, Urologie, Medizinische Hochschule Hannover, Germany

T901 Dr. Meyer, Gastroenterologie und Hepatologie, Medizinische Hochschule Hannover, Germany

T908 Prof. Dr. med. Georg F. W. Scheumann, Klinik für Viszeral- und Transplantationschirurgie, Medizinische Hochschule Hannover, Germany

T913 Prof. Dr. med. Schumacher, Radiologie, Abt. Neuroradiologie, Universität Freiburg, Germany

T975 Dr. Noam Millo, Department of Radiology, Health Sciences Centre, University of Manitoba, Winnipeg, Canada

X338 The Visible Human Project®, U.S. National Library of Medicine, Bethesda, USA

Table of Content

1 General Anatomy

Surface Anatomy 3
Anatomical Regions 4
Anatomical Terminology 5
Anatomical Planes 6
Axes of Movement 7
Basic Movements of the Upper Extremity 8
Basic Movements of the Lower Extremity 9
Basic Movements of Head, Neck and Trunk 10
Anatomical Systems 11
Musculoskeletal System 12
Types of Bones 13
Bone Ossification 14
Structure of Bones 15
Types of Joints 16
Synovial Joints 17
Types of Cartilage 18
Types of Muscle 19
Skeletal Muscle – Structure 20
Skeletal Muscle – Architecture 21
Connective Tissue 22
Tendons and Ligaments 23
Integumentary System 24
Hair 25
Nails 26
Cardiorespiratory System 27
Arteries 28
Veins 29
Lymphatic System 30
Digestive System 31
Endocrine System 32
Reproductive System 33
Urinary System 34
Nervous System – Organization 35
Central Nervous System 36
Peripheral Nervous System 37

2 Back and Spine

Surface Anatomy of the Back 41
Organization of the Spine 42
Curvatures of the Spine 43
Vertebrae – Basic Features 44
Vertebrae – Foramina 45
Vertebral Column – Segmental Motion 47
Intervertebral Discs 48
Facet Joints 49
Vertebral Ligaments 50
Cervical Spine 53
Cervical Vertebrae – Distinguishing Features 55
Occiput (C0) and Atlas (C1) 56
Axis (C2) 57
Atlanto-occipital and Atlantoaxial Joints 58
Cervical Spine – Ligaments 59
Cervical Spine – Movements 60
Anterior Muscles of the Cervical Region – Superficial 61
Anterior Muscles of the Cervical Region – Deep 62
Posterior Muscles of the Cervical Region – Superficial 63
Posterior Muscles of the Cervical Region – Deep 64
Thoracic Spine 65
Thoracic Vertebrae – Distinguishing Features 66
Lumbar Spine 67
Lumbar Vertebrae – Distinguishing Features 69
Thoracolumbar Movements 70
Muscles of the Back – Superficial and Intermediate 71
Muscles of the Back – Intermediate 72
Muscles of the Back – Deep 73
Sacrum 74
Coccyx 76
Abdominal Muscles 77
Anterior Abdominal Wall 78
Posterior Abdominal Wall 80
Vessels of the Vertebral Column 81

3 Upper Extremity

Surface Anatomy of the Shoulder Region and
Upper Trunk 86
Surface Anatomy
of the Arm, Forearm, Wrist and Hand 87
Overview of Bones 88
Shoulder Girdle 89
Clavicle 90
Scapula 91
Proximal Humerus 92
Sternoclavicular Joint 94
Acromioclavicular Joint 95
Glenohumeral Joint 96
Shoulder Movements 99
Scapulohumeral Movement 100
Muscles of the Anterior Shoulder 101
Muscles of the Posterior Shoulder – Superficial and
Deep 102
Muscles of the Shoulder – Rotator Cuff 104
Axilla 105
Innervation of the Shoulder – Brachial Plexus 106
Arteries of the Shoulder 107
Neurovascular Structures of the Arm 108
Surface Anatomy of the Arm and Elbow 109
Bones of the Elbow Joint 110
Elbow Joint and Ligaments 111
Elbow Joint Alignment 112
Elbow Joint Movements 113
Muscles of the Anterior Arm – Biceps Region 114
Muscles of the Posterior Arm – Triceps Region 115
Cubital Fossa 116
Neurovascular Structures of the Elbow Region 117
Surface Anatomy of the Forearm, Wrist and Hand ... 118
Bones of the Forearm, Wrist and Hand 119
Ulna 120
Radius 121
Bones of Wrist and Hand 122
Wrist Joints 123
Wrist Ligaments 124
Wrist Movements 125
Joints and Ligaments of the Fingers 126

Finger and Thumb Movements 127
Muscles of the Forearm – An Overview 128
Muscles of the Anterior Forearm – Superficial and
Deep 129
Muscles of the Posterior Forearm – Superficial and
Deep 131
Neurovascular Structures of Forearm 133
Flexor Retinaculum and Carpal Tunnel 134
Extensor Retinaculum 135
Muscles of the Hand – Thenar Region 136
Muscles of the Hand – Hypothenar Region 137
Muscles of the Hand – Central Compartment 138
Neurovascular Structures of the Wrist and Hand 139
Arterial Arches of the Hand 140
Brachial Plexus of Nerves 141
Brachial Plexus – Supraclavicular Branches 142
Brachial Plexus – Infraclavicular Branches of the
Posterior Cord 143
Brachial Plexus – Infraclavicular Branches of the
Lateral and Medial Cord 145
Sensory Innervation – Cutaneous Nerves and
Dermatomes 147
Arteries 149
Veins and Lymphatic Nodes/Vessels 150

4 Lower Extremity

Surface Anatomy – Overview 156
Surface Anatomy of the Pelvis and Thigh 157
Pelvic Girdle 158
Hip Bone – Os coxae 159
Joints and Ligaments of the Pelvis 160
Pelvic Foramina 161
Femur 162
Hip Joint 163
Hip Joint – Functional Anatomy 165
Hip Joint Movements 166
Muscles of the Posterior Hip 167
Muscles of the Posterior Hip – Deep 168
Muscles of the Anterior Hip 169
Muscles of the Anterior Hip – Deep 170
Muscles of the Anterior Thigh – Quadriceps 171
Muscles of the Medial Thigh – Groin 172
Muscles of the Posterior Thigh – Hamstrings 173
Neurovascular Structures – Gluteal Region and
Posterior Thigh 174
Neurovascular Structures – Anterior and Medial Thigh ... 175
Surface Anatomy of the Knee 176
Knee joint 177
Bones of the Knee 178
Knee Joint Movements 180
Knee – Functional Anatomy 181
Collateral Ligaments of the Knee 182
Cruciate Ligaments of the Knee 183
Menisci of the Knee 184
Patella 185
Patellofemoral Joint 186
Knee Bursae 187
Popliteal Region of the Knee 188
Neurovascular Structures of the Knee 189
Surface Anatomy of the Lower Leg, Ankle and Foot 190
Bones of the Lower Leg 191
Tibia 192
Fibula 193
Bones of the Foot 194
Ankle Movements 196
Ankle – Talocrural Joint 197
Ankle – Subtalar Joint 198
Ankle Ligaments 199
Joints of the Foot 200
Muscular Compartments of the Lower Leg 201
Muscles of the Anterior Compartment 202
Muscles of the Lateral Compartment 203
Muscles of the Posterior Compartment – Superficial and
Deep 204
Retinacula and Tendinous Sheaths 206
Muscles of the Foot – Dorsum 207
Muscles of the Foot – 1st and 2nd Plantar Layers 208
Muscles of the Foot – 3rd and 4th Plantar Layers 209
Arches of the Foot 210
Gait 211
Neurovascular Structures of the Lower Leg,
Ankle and Foot 212
Lumbosacral Plexus of Nerves 214
Lumbar Plexus – Motor Innervation 215
Sacral Plexus – Motor Innervation 216
Sensory Innervation – Cutaneous Nerves 217
Sensory Innervation – Dermatomes 218
Arteries 219
Veins 221
Lymphatic Vessels 222

5 Thorax

Surface Anatomy 225
Cutaneous Innervation 229
Mammary Gland 230
Mammary Gland – Blood Supply 231
Ribs and Costovertebral Joints 234
Intercostal Muscles 235
Diaphragm 236
Muscles of Respiration 238
Thoracic Wall 239
Pleural Cavities 242
Lungs 245
Mediastinum 250
Surface Projection of the Heart 254
Pericardium 255
Heart 257
Cardiac Valves 261
Great Vessels and Heart 264
Coronary Arteries 266
Cardiac Veins 269
Conducting System of the Heart 270
Innervation of the Heart 272
Prenatal and Postnatal Blood Circulation 273
Superior Mediastinum 274
Posterior Mediastinum 278

6 Abdomen

Surface Anatomy 283
Cutaneous Innervation 284
Abdominal Wall 285
Inguinal Region 291

Abdominal Peritoneal Cavity 297
Esophagus 306
Stomach 310
Small Intestines – Duodenum 317
Small Intestines – Jejunum and Ileum 319
Large Intestines – Colon 321
Large Intestines – Cecum and Appendix vermiformis 322
Intestines 323
Arteries of Abdominal Viscera 329
Liver 330
Gall Bladder and Bile Ducts 339
Pancreas 342
Spleen 346
Kidneys and Ureters 347
Suprarenal (Adrenal) Gland 357
Kidney, Ureter and Suprarenal Gland 358
Branches of the Abdominal Aorta 359
Autonomic Innervation of Abdominal Viscera 360
Lymphatic Drainage Pathways in the Abdomen 361

7 Pelvis

Surface Anatomy 364
Male and Female Pelvis 365
Pelvic Floor 367
Pelvic Viscera – Overview 369
Rectum and Anal Canal 371
Urinary Bladder 376
Male Urethra 378
Female Urethra 379
Male Pelvic Viscera 380
Female Pelvic Viscera 385
Male Genitalia 397
Perineum 405
Female Perineum 406
Male Perineum 413
Ischioanal Fossa 416
Perineal Spaces 417
Pelvic Arteries 419
Pelvic Veins 420
Pelvic Nerves 421

8 Head

Surface Anatomy 425
Skull 426
Facial Muscles 439
Neurovascular Supply 442
Nose and Nasal Cavity 448
Paranal Sinuses 452
Neurovascular Supply to the Nasal Cavity 454
Oral Cavity 455
Bones of the Oral Cavity 456
Temporomandibular Joint 458
Muscles of Mastication 460
Dentition and Gingiva 461
Dentition 462
Hard Palate 464
Neurovascular Supply to the Teeth 465
Mucosa and Innervation of the Tongue 467
Muscles of the Tongue 468
Neurovascular Supply of the Tongue 470

Tonsils 471
Soft Palate 472
Hyoid Bone and Floor of Oral Cavity 473
Floor of Mouth 474
Salivary Glands 475
Innervation of Glands of the Head 479

9 Eye

Surface Anatomy 482
Eyelids 483
Bones of the Orbit 484
Anterior Orbit 486
Periorbital Blood Supply 487
Lacrimal Gland and Innervation 488
Lacrimal Apparatus 489
Extraocular Muscles 490
Innervation of Extraocular Muscles 491
Neurovascular Structures in the Orbit 492
Orbital Levels and Content 493
Eyeball and Blood Supply 495
Iris and Ciliary Body 496
Pupillary Reflexes 497
Ocular Fundus 498
Retina and Central Visual Pathway 499

10 Ear

Surface Anatomy 502
External Acoustic Meatus 503
Temporal Bone 504
Middle Ear – Tympanic Membrane 505
Middle Ear – Auditory Ossicles 506
Middle Ear – Pharyngotympanic Tube 507
Middle Ear – Neighboring Structures 508
Middle Ear – Blood Supply and Innervation 509
Inner Ear – Petrous Part of Temporal Bone 510
Inner Ear – Bony and Membranous Labyrinth 511
Inner Ear – Cochlea 512
Inner Ear – Mechanoelectrical Conduction 513
Central Auditory Pathways 514
Inner Ear – Vestibular Labyrinth 515
Central Vestibular Pathways 516

11 Neck

Surface Anatomy of the Neck 519
Triangles of the Neck 520
Cervical Fascia 521
Retropharyngeal Space 522
Anterior and Posterior Cervical Region – Superficial Layer 523
Anterior and Posterior Cervical Region – Vessels and Nerves 524
Anterior and Posterior Cervical Region – Deep Layer 525
Cervical Plexus 526
Subclavian and Vertebral Arteries 527
Anterior Cervical Region – Surface Anatomy and Superficial Layer 528
Anterior Cervical Region – Neurovascular Structures 529
Pharyngeal Spaces 530
Pharyngeal Muscles 532

Pharyngeal Neurovascular Structures and
Parapharyngeal Space 533
Swallowing (Deglutition) 535
Larynx and Laryngeal Cartilages 536
Laryngeal Cartilages 537
Laryngeal Cartilages and Vocal Cords 539
Laryngeal Muscles 540
Laryngoscopy 541
Endotracheal Procedures 542
Laryngeal Spaces 543
Laryngeal Neurovascular Structures 544
Development of the Thyroid Gland 545
Thyroid Gland 546
Neurovascular Structures of the Thyroid Gland 547
Topography of the Thyroid Gland 548
Parathyroid Glands 549
Lymphatic Drainage of the Neck 550
Superior Thoracic Aperture 551

12 Neuroanatomy

Major Parts of the Brain and Orientation 556
Structure of the Brain 557
Meninges of the Brain 558
Arterial Blood Supply to the Meninges of the Brain 559
Venous Sinuses 560
Venous Sinuses and Diploic Veins 561
Venous Drainage of the Brain 562
Arterial Blood Supply of the Brain 563
Internal Carotid Artery 564
Circle of WILLIS 565
Cerebral and Cerebellar Arteries 566
Cerebral Arteries 567
Vascular Territories of Cerebral and Cerebellar Arteries .. 568
Meninges of the Spinal Cord 569
Arterial Blood Supply of the Spinal Cord 570
Spinal Cord within the Vertebral Canal 571
Ventricular System 572

Blood-Brain/CSF-Barrier and Circumventricular Organs ... 575
Cranial Nerves – Overview 576
Cranial Nerves – Topography and Fiber Qualities 577
Cranial Nerves – Location of Cranial Nerve Nuclei
in the Brainstem 578
Cranial Nerves – Summary of Nuclei of
Cranial Nerves 579
Cranial Nerves – Sensory and Parasympathetic
Ganglia 580
Fila olfactoria [CN I] 582
[CN III], [CN IV], [CN VI] 583
Trigeminal Nerve [CN V] 585
Ophthalmic Branch [CN V/1] 587
Maxillary Branch [CN V/2] 588
Mandibular Branch [CN V/3] 589
Facial Nerve [CN VII] 590
Glossopharyngeal Nerve [CN IX] 594
Vagus Nerve [CN X] 597
Special Senses: Sensory System of Tongue and Taste 600
Spinal Accessory Nerve [CN XI] 601
Hypoglossal Nerve [CN XII] 602
Autonomic Nervous System – General Principles 603
Autonomic Outflow and Target Organs 604
Sympathetic Outflow 605
Relationship of Sympathetic Outflow with
Spinal Nerves 606
Autonomic Nervous System – HORNER's Syndrome 607
Spinal Cord – Segments and Nomenclature 608
Spinal Cord – Function 609
Spinal Nerves 610
Spinal Cord – Reflexes 612
Spinal Cord – Segmental Organization 613
Spinal Cord – Sensory Pathways 616
Spinal Cord – Motor Pathways 618
Spinal Cord Lesions 619

Index 621

General Anatomy

Surface Anatomy 3

Anatomical Regions 4

Anatomical Terminology 5

Anatomical Planes 6

Axes of Movement 7

Basic Movements of
the Upper Extremity 8

Basic Movements of
the Lower Extremity 9

Basic Movements of Head,
Neck and Trunk 10

Anatomical Systems 11

Musculoskeletal System 12

Types of Bones 13

Bone Ossification 14

Structure of Bones 15

Types of Joints 16

Synovial Joints 17

Types of Cartilage 18

Types of Muscle 19

Skeletal Muscle – Structure 20

Skeletal Muscle – Architecture 21

Connective Tissue 22

Tendons and Ligaments 23

Integumentary System 24

Hair 25

Nails 26

Cardiorespiratory System 27

Arteries 28

Veins 29

Lymphatic System 30

Digestive System 31

Endocrine System 32

Reproductive System 33

Urinary System 34

Nervous System – Organization 35

Central Nervous System 36

Peripheral Nervous System 37

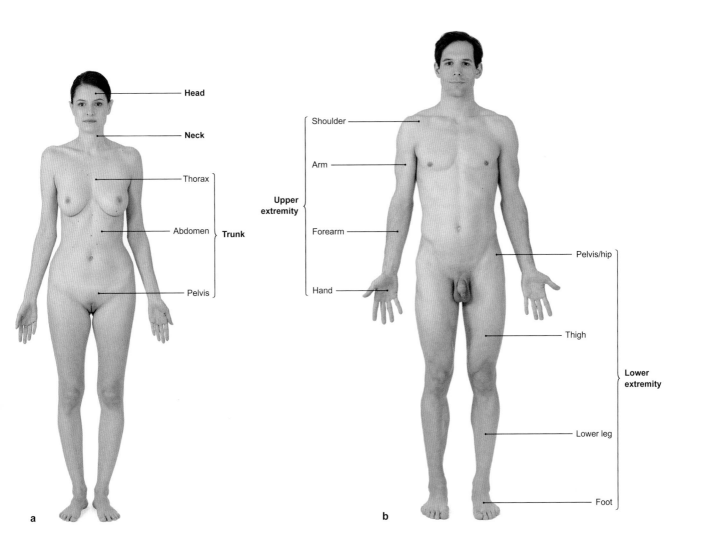

Fig. 1.1a and b Surface anatomy of Female (a) and Male (b); anterior views. [K340]

The term 'anatomical position' is used to describe a reference position in which the body is standing in an upright posture, with the head and body directly facing the observer; the feet are flat on the ground, and directed forward; the arms are located alongside the trunk, with the palm of each hand facing forward. The anatomical position serves as a reference point when describing movements or anatomical landmarks in relation to one another (i.e. the hand is positioned distal to the shoulder).

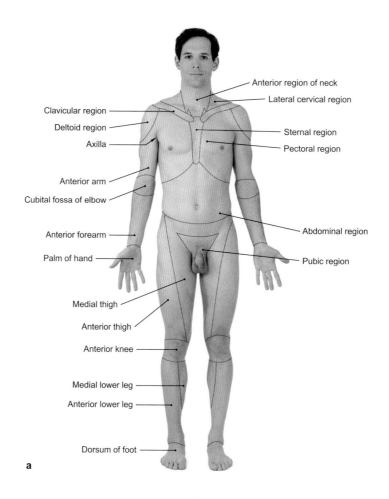

Anterior region of neck
Lateral cervical region
Clavicular region
Deltoid region
Axilla
Sternal region
Pectoral region
Anterior arm
Cubital fossa of elbow
Abdominal region
Anterior forearm
Palm of hand
Pubic region
Medial thigh
Anterior thigh
Anterior knee
Medial lower leg
Anterior lower leg
Dorsum of foot

a

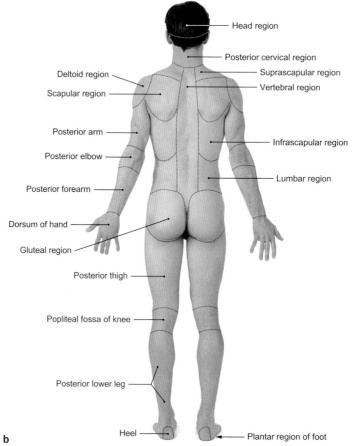

Head region
Posterior cervical region
Suprascapular region
Deltoid region
Vertebral region
Scapular region
Posterior arm
Infrascapular region
Posterior elbow
Lumbar region
Posterior forearm
Dorsum of hand
Gluteal region
Posterior thigh
Popliteal fossa of knee
Posterior lower leg
Heel
Plantar region of foot

b

Fig. 1.2a and b Anatomical regions; anterior **(a)** and posterior **(b)** views. [K340]

The body surface is divided into regions for better description and orientation.

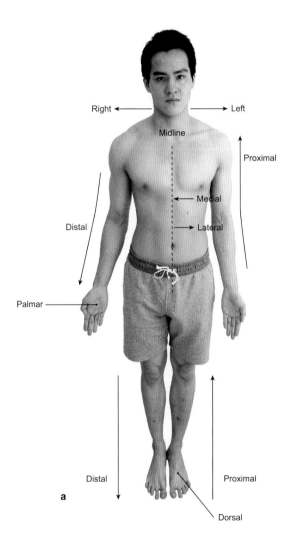

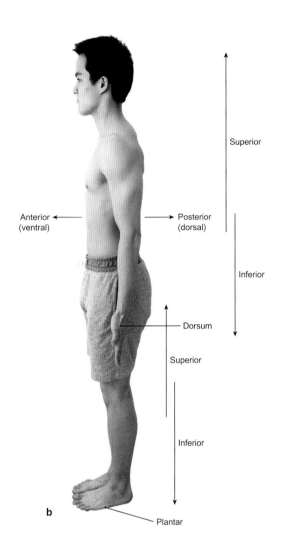

Fig. 1.3a and b Anatomical terminology; anterior **(a)** and lateral **(b)** views. [L271]

1. **Superior/inferior:** toward the head/toward the foot; sometimes referred to as cranial/caudal.
2. **Anterior/posterior:** front/back; sometimes referred to as ventral/dorsal.
3. **Medial/lateral:** toward the midline/away from the midline.
4. **Proximal/distal:** closer to/farther from the center of the body.
5. **Superficial/deep:** close(r) to the surface/deep(er) to the surface.
6. **Plantar/dorsal:** the sole of the foot/the top of the foot.
7. **Palmar/dorsum:** the palm of the hand/the back of the hand.

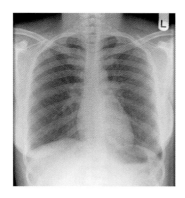

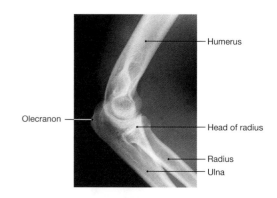

Fig. 1.4 Anterior/posterior (A/P) radiograph of the chest; frontal plane. [E908-003]

Fig. 1.5 Lateral radiograph of the elbow; sagittal plane.

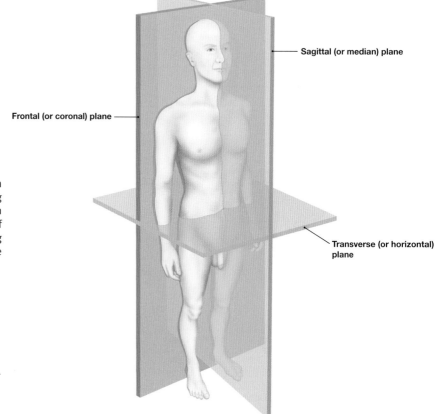

Fig. 1.6 Anatomical planes. [L127]

An **anatomical plane** is a definitional term used to provide orientation when observing the human body as a whole or in parts. Each plane is best illustrated by a colored sheet of glass that passes through the body, dividing it into two sections. In human anatomy there are three basic planes.

1. The **frontal (or coronal) plane** passes through the body from left to right and divides it into an anterior and a posterior portion.
2. The **sagittal (or median) plane** passes through the body from front to back and divides it into left and right.
3. The **transverse (or horizontal) plane** passes through the body as a cross-sectional plane, dividing it into a superior and an inferior portion.

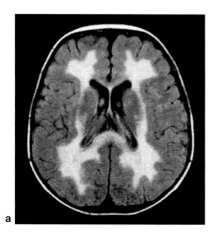

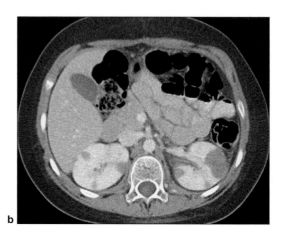

Fig. 1.7a and b Cross-sectional image in the transverse (horizontal) plane of MRI of the brain (a) and CT image of the abdomen (b).

a [H062-001], b [G717]

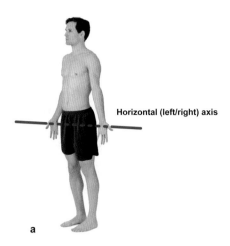

Horizontal (left/right) axis

a

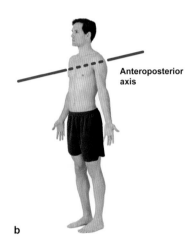

Anteroposterior axis

b

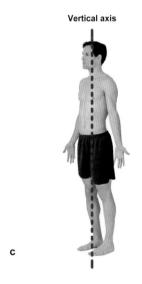

Vertical axis

c

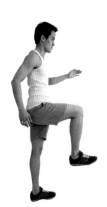

Fig. 1.9 Hip flexion and extension. [L271]
Hip flexion and extension movements occur about a horizontal axis.

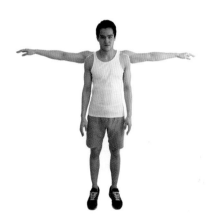

Fig. 1.10 Shoulder abduction and adduction. [L271]
Shoulder abduction and adduction movements occur about an anteroposterior axis.

Fig. 1.8a to c Anatomical axes. [K340]
Movements of the human body are described as occurring about three primary axes of rotation. As a general rule, each axis of rotation bisects or runs perpendicular to one of the three anatomical planes:
a Horizontal (left/right) axis: bisects the sagittal plane, rotation occurs about a line that runs through the body in a left to right direction, e.g. hip flexion/extension, knee flexion/extension.
b Anteroposterior axis: runs perpendicular to the frontal plane, rotation occurs about a line that runs through the body from the front to back, e.g. shoulder abduction/adduction.
c Vertical axis: bisects the horizontal plane, rotation occurs about a line that runs through the body from the head to the toes, e.g. neck rotation to the left or right.

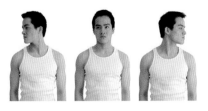

Fig. 1.11 Neck rotation. [L271]
Neck rotational movements occur about a vertical axis.

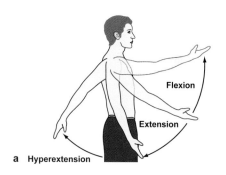
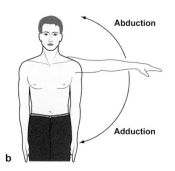
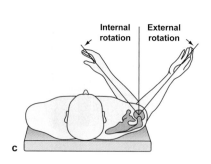

Fig. 1.12a to c Basic movements of the shoulder. [L126]
The shoulder is a multiaxial ball-and-socket joint that moves about three planes:
a Flexion movements typically involve a decrease in the joint angle at the shoulder. **Extension** movements involve an increase in the joint angle at the shoulder.

b Abduction involves moving the arm away from the midline. **Adduction** involves moving the arm towards the midline of the body.
c Rotational movements of the shoulder involve rotating the arm either towards the midline **(internal or medial rotation)** or away from the midline **(or external or lateral rotation)**.

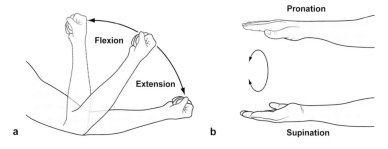

Fig. 1.13a and b Movements about the elbow and forearm. [L126]
a The elbow is a uniaxial hinge joint that is only able to perform **flexion** and **extension** movements.
b Pronation movements of the forearm occur below the elbow (at the radio-ulnar joint) and involve turning the palm downwards (palm faces posterior in the anatomical position), while **supination** movements involve rotating the palm upwards (palm faces anterior in the anatomical position).

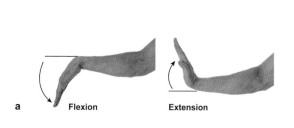
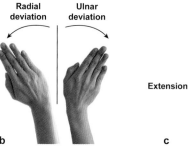
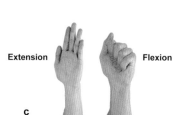

Fig. 1.14a to d Movements of wrist, hand and fingers. [L271]
a The wrist joint is capable of **flexion** and **extension** movements as well as performing
b radial deviation (moving the hand towards the radial side of the forearm) and **ulnar deviation** (moving the hand towards the ulnar side of the forearm).
c Many joints in the hand can perform **flexion** and **extension** movements.
d Abduction (movements away from the middle finger) and **adduction** (movements towards the middle finger) occur at the knuckles (metacarpophalangeal joints) of the hand.

Structure/Function

APLEY's Movements
Functional movements such as reaching over your head or behind your back to scratch between your shoulder blades are examples of combined movements of the upper extremity. They require a simultaneous multiaxial motion (often of more than one joint) in order to be effectively performed;
a Flexion, abduction and external rotation of the shoulder, along with elbow flexion and supination;
b extension, adduction and internal rotation of the shoulder, along with elbow flexion and pronation.
[L271]

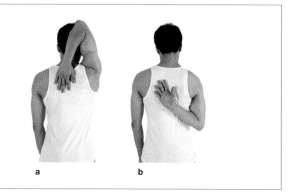

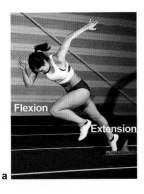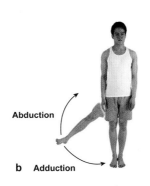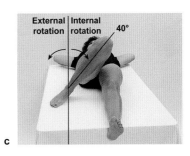

Fig. 1.15a to c Hip movements. a [J787], b [L271], c [E988]
Human locomotion is bipedal and primarily occurs in the sagittal plane.
a When walking or running, the lead hip **flexes** (resulting in a decrease in hip joint angle), while the trail hip **extends** (resulting in an increase in hip joint angle).

b Hip abduction (movement away from the midline) and **adduction** (movement towards the midline) occur in the frontal plane.
c Hip internal (medial) rotation occurs when the leg is rotated so that the foot is positioned lateral to the knee; **external (lateral) rotation** occurs when the leg is rotated so that the foot is positioned medial to the knee.

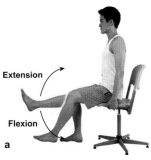

Fig. 1.16a and b Movements at the knee joint. a [L271], b [L126]
a The knee is a modified type of hinge joint, the basic movements of which are **flexion and extension**.

b When the knee is positioned in flexion, the joint is also capable of moving into **internal (medial) rotation** (forefoot rotates towards the midline) and **external (lateral) rotation** (forefoot rotates away from the midline of the body).

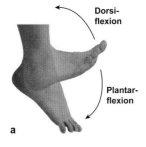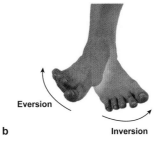

Fig. 1.17a and b Movements at the ankle. [L271]
Movements of the ankle occur about two anatomical planes.
a Plantar-flexion (pointing foot downward) and **dorsi-flexion** (pulling foot upward) movements occur about the sagittal plane.

b Inversion (rolling sole of foot inward) and **eversion** (rolling sole of foot outward) movements occur about the frontal plane.

Structure/Function

Open vs. closed kinetic chain movements
1. **Open kinetic chain movements** are described as movements of the body that occur about a single joint or limb segment (e.g. knee extension in a sitting position) and occur independent of movements at other joints (knee moves independent of ankle and hip joints).
2. **Closed kinetic chain movements** are described as movements of the body that involve the simultaneous motion at more than 1 joint or segment, and creates a 'linked' movement pattern (e.g. standing up from a sitting position – in order for the knee to extend, the ankle and hip joints must also

move). Closed chain movements are sometimes referred to as 'functional movements' because they replicate how the body moves during normal activities of daily living. [L231]

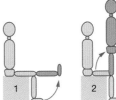

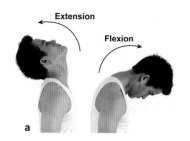
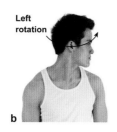
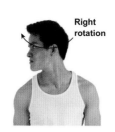
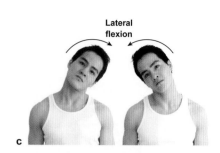

Fig. 1.18a to c Neck movements. [L271]
The neck (cervical region) is capable of moving about 3 planes.
a Flexion and **extension** movements are best visualized in the saggital plane.

b Rotational movements of the neck towards the left and right can occur about a vertical axis of rotation.
c Lateral flexion movements of the neck towards the left and right are best visualized in the frontal plane.

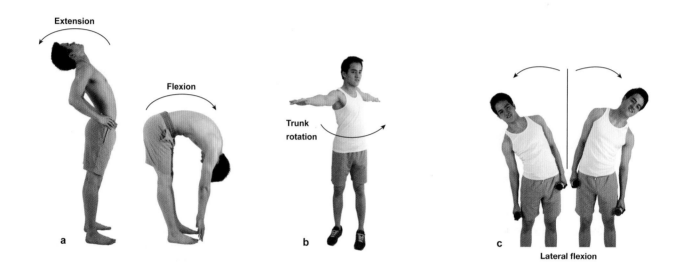

Fig. 1.19a to c Trunk movements. [L271]
The trunk is capable of moving in all 3 planes.
a Flexion and **extension** movements are best visualized in the saggital plane.

b Rotational movements of the trunk towards the left and right occur about a vertical axis.
c Lateral flexion movements of the trunk towards the left and right are best visualized in the frontal plane.

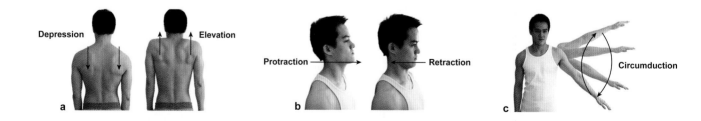

Fig. 1.20a to c Additional anatomical movements. [L271]
a Elevation and depression movements of the scapula on the trunk.
b Protraction and retraction movements of the lower jaw on the face.

c Circumduction movements of the upper or lower extremity are an example of a combined movement (i.e. a movement that occurs through multiple planes and involve multiple movements).

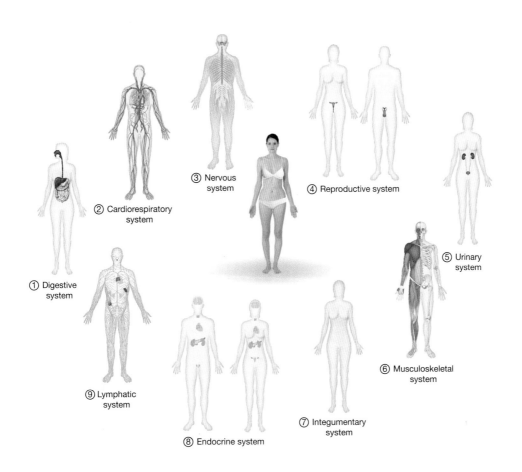

Fig. 1.21 Anatomical systems. [L275]
The human body is comprised of nine distinct anatomical systems each of which carries out specific functions necessary for normal everyday living. If one system is damaged, the human body may become unstable. This can lead to dysfunction, and ultimately to death. A clear understanding of the relationship between each system's structure (anatomy) and function (physiology) is required in order to fully appreciate the complexity of the human body.

System	Basic Structures*	Basic Functions*
① Digestive	Oral cavity, esophagus, stomach, small intestine, large intestine, anus, liver, pancreas, salivary glands, teeth, tongue	Digestion and resorption of food
② Cardiorespiratory	Heart, blood vessels (arteries, veins and capillaries), blood, lungs, nasal cavity, trachea, bronchi	Blood flow and pressure; circulate nutrients throughout the body; O_2/CO_2 gas exchange
③ Nervous	Brain, spinal cord, cranial and peripheral nerves, nerve endings and receptors	Controls and coordinates all body functions (conscious and unconscious)
④ Reproductive	Male: testes, epididymis, accessory sex organs Female: uterus, ovaries, FALLOPIAN tubes, accessory sex organs	Male: formation of sperm and semen; Female: formation of germ cells (eggs) and bearing the fetus during development
⑤ Urinary	Kidneys, ureters, urinary bladder, urethra	Production and excretion of urine
⑥ Musculoskeletal	Skeletal muscles, tendons, bones, joints, ligaments, and cartilage	Forms, supports, stabilizes and powers movement of the body; stores minerals/chemicals; aids in red blood cell production
⑦ Integumentary	Skin, hair, nails, and exocrine sweat glands	Retain body fluids, protection against disease, elimination of waste products, and regulation of body temperature
⑧ Endocrine	Endocrine glands: pituitary gland, thyroid gland, parathyroid glands, adrenal glands, pancreas (endocrine part); Male: testes (endocrine part); Female: ovary (endocrine part), liver (endocrine part)	Production and secretion of hormones and chemical substances that regulate the activities of cells and organs
⑨ Lymphatic	Lymph nodes and lymphatic vessels, central lymphoid tissue, peripheral lymphoid organs, lymphocytes	Drainage and protection, immunoprotection

* This is not an exhaustive list of all structures and functions.

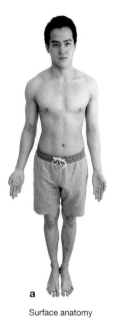

a

Surface anatomy

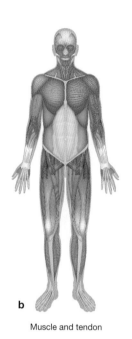

b

Muscle and tendon

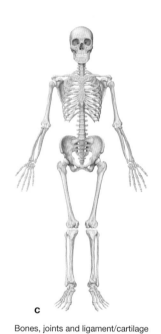

c

Bones, joints and ligament/cartilage

Fig. 1.22a to c Musculoskeletal system; anterior view. a [L271], b [L275], c [L127]

The musculoskeletal (MSK) system (also sometimes referred to as the locomotor system) is a complex system comprised of bones, muscles, tendons, joints, ligaments, cartilage, and other types of connective tissue which function to support, stabilize, and move the human body. Key components of the MSK system include:

1. **Bone:** 'mineralized' connective tissue that functions to support, protect, move, and act as a storage depot for key minerals and immature red blood cells.
2. **Muscle:** striated skeletal muscle that attaches to bone via tendons, and functions to power joint movements.

3. **Tendon:** dense fibrous connective tissue which connects muscle to bone.
4. **Joint:** facilitates movements of the body. Joints are typically reinforced by the following:
   - **Ligaments:** dense connective tissue that connects bone to bone across a joint, in order to enhance joint stability.
   - **Cartilage:** specialized connective tissue which functions to enhance joint stability, acts as a shock absorber, and ensures smooth joint motion, preventing the ends of bones from rubbing directly on one another.

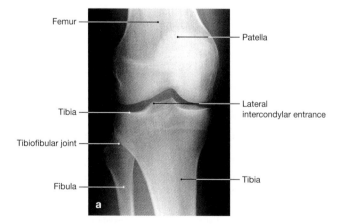

Femur

Patella

Tibia

Lateral intercondylar entrance

Tibiofibular joint

Fibula

Tibia

a

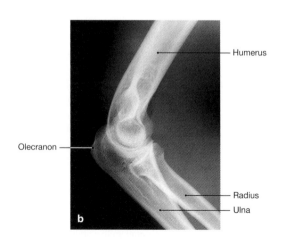

Humerus

Olecranon

Radius

Ulna

b

Fig. 1.23a and b Conventional radiograph (X-ray); A/P view of the knee **(a)** and lateral view of the elbow **(b).**

Radiographic imaging (radiology) is one of the most frequent and cost-efficient imaging methods used within the medical sciences for viewing structures of the musculoskeletal system (most commonly bone). Radiographic images are produced by transmitting

X-rays through a patient, with the image being formed based on which rays pass through (and are detected) versus those that are absorbed or scattered in the patient (and thus are not detected). Radiographic imaging is frequently used to diagnoze bony abnormalities of the upper and lower extremities as well as the trunk and spine.

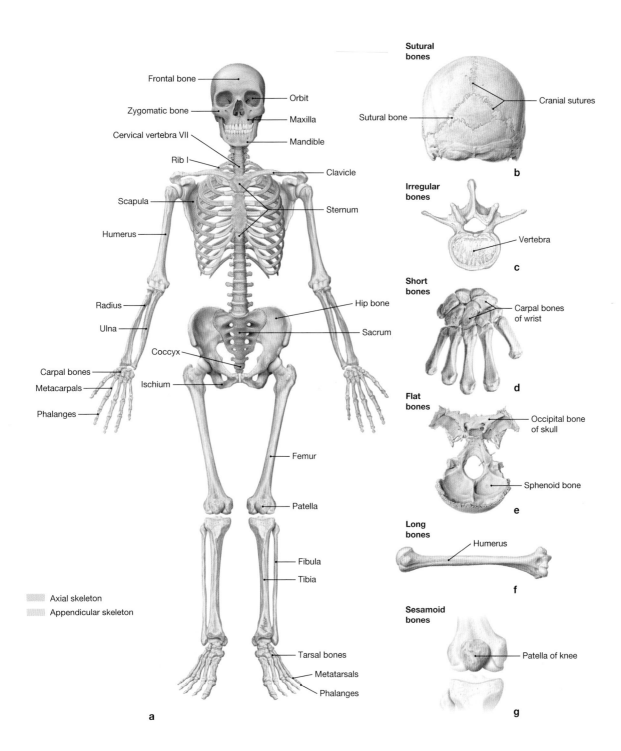

Fig. 1.24a to g Human skeleton (a), types of bones (b–g); anterior view. [L127]

a The adult human skeleton is comprised of 206 bones, which can be divided into 1. axial bones (blue color), and 2. appendicular bones (tan color).

These bones can be grouped (according to their specific shape and structure) into one of six types:

b Sutural bones: classified by their location rather than shape, e.g. small bones which form the sutural joints of the skull.

c Irregular bones: because of their complicated shape (typically as a result of specialized function) they cannot be grouped into one of the other categories, e.g. vertebrae, mandible.

d Short bones: have approximately equal length and width, e.g. carpal bones of the hand and tarsal bones of the feet.

e Flat bones: with their thin flat structure they provide a broad attachment area for muscles/tendons/ligaments, e.g. ribs, sternum, scapula, pelvis, bones of the skull.

f Long bones: have a length that is greater than width, and consist of a shaft and ending, e.g. femur and humerus.

g Sesamoid bones: are embedded in tendons in regions underlying considerable friction, tension, or physical stress, e.g. patella.

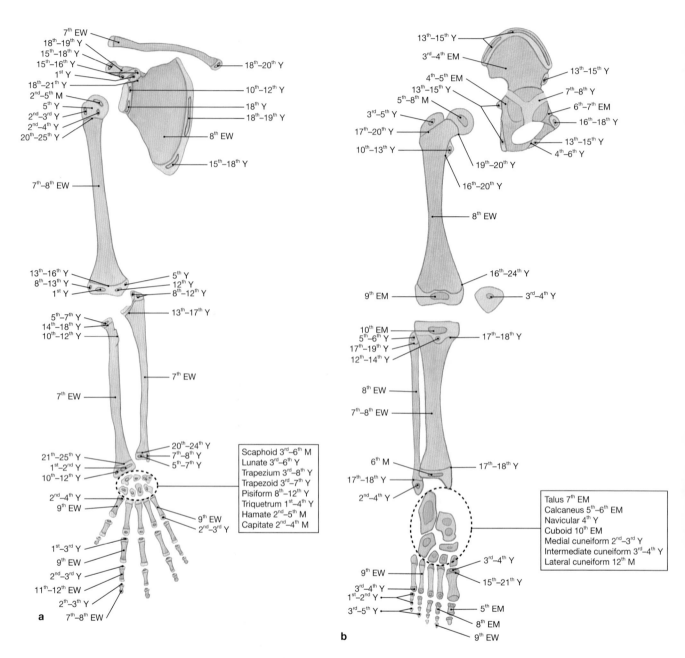

EW = embryonic week; EM = embryonic month; M = month of life; Y = year of life

Fig. 1.25a and b Skeletal ossification of the upper (a) and lower (b) extremities. Locations of the major sites of epiphysial and apophysial ossification, and the chronological sequence of the formation of these ossification centers.

The timing at which bone nucleation sites appear provides a clue to the stage of skeletal development and thus, an individual's skeletal and chronological age. Ossification centers formed around the shaft (diaphysis) of the cartilage model during the fetal period (diaphysial ossification) are distinguished from ossification centers which form during the second half of the fetal period and in the first years of life within the cartilaginous epi- and apophyses (epi- and apophysial ossification). No further increase in body height occurs once the cartilaginous epiphysial gaps ossify and disappear (synostosis). Thereafter, isolated bone nuclei are no longer visible on X-ray images.

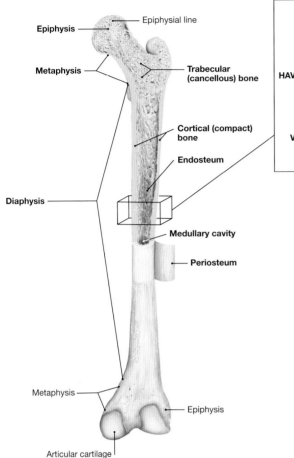

Epiphysis
Epiphysial line
Metaphysis
Trabecular (cancellous) bone
Cortical (compact) bone
Endosteum
Diaphysis
Medullary cavity
Periosteum
Metaphysis
Epiphysis
Articular cartilage

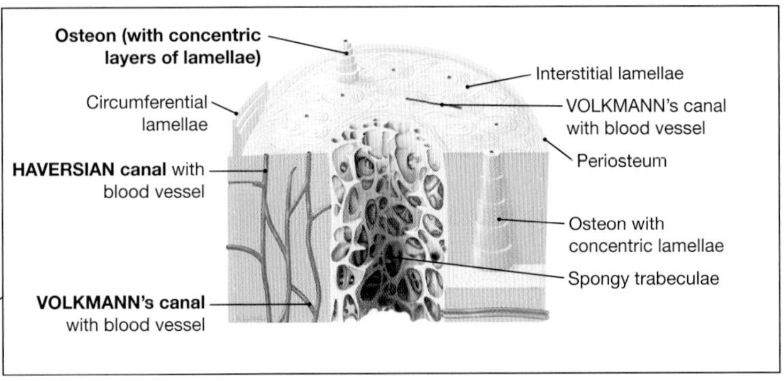

Fig. 1.27 Microstructure of a long bone. [L266]
The basic building block of bone is the **osteon** (or HAVERSIAN system) which consists of concentric layers (**lamellae**) of mineralized connective tissue surrounding a central canal that contains blood vessels and nerve fibers. This central canal is called a **HAVERSIAN canal**. Along the edge of each lamellar layer are small cavities known as **lacunae**, that each contain one bone cell called an **osteocyte**. Radiating from each lacuna are numerous tiny canals called **canaliculi**. They function to connect the lacunae of adjacent lamellae, ultimately reaching a HAVERSIAN canal. **VOLKMANN's canals** run at bisecting angles to each HAVERSIAN canal and function to create anastomosing vessels between adjacent HAVERSIAN capillaries, as well as to connect the HAVERSIAN system with the periosteal layer on the outside of the bone. A typical osteon is approximately 200 micrometers in diameter, meaning that all aspects of bone are never more than 100 micrometers from a central blood supply.

Fig. 1.26 Anatomical features of a long bone (femur). [L266]
Bone is mainly composed of two different types of tissue:
1. **Cortical or compact bone:** forms the hard outer shell of bone and consists of a very hard network of bony tissue arranged in concentric layers.
2. **Trabecular or cancellous bone** (sometimes referred to as spongy bone): bone tissue located beneath the compact bone that consists of a meshwork of bony pillars which form a framework of interconnecting spaces containing bone marrow.
The **epiphysis** is the rounded region at the end of a long bone that is covered by articular cartilage and facilitates smooth articulation

of the bone as part of a joint. The **metaphysis** is the wide portion of a bone between the epiphysis and diaphysis, and is the region that contains the epiphysial growth plate (region where bone elongation occurs).
The **diaphysis** is the main section or shaft of the bone, and is primarily composed of compact bone. This region comprises the **medullary cavity** containing yellow (adults) and red (infants) marrow. The medullary cavity is lined with a thin layer of connective tissue called the **endosteum**. The diaphysis is covered by **periosteum**, a protective layer of fibrous connective tissue.

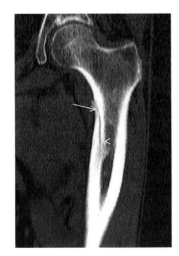

Fig. 1.28 Computed tomography; CT scan of the right femur that demonstrates a lesion through the proximal aspect of the leg (with no soft tissue involvement). [H060-001]
CT imaging is frequently used to diagnose complex injuries to bone. It was developed by Sir Godfrey HOUNSFIELD in the 1970s and has undergone constant refinement since its development.

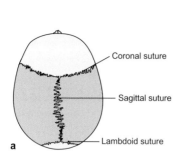

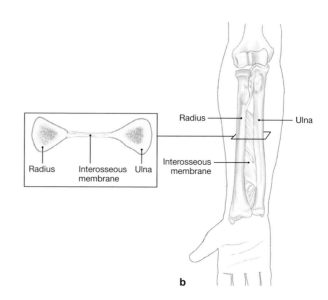

Fig. 1.29a and b Fibrous joints; sutural joints (a) and syndesmosis (b). a [L126], b [E607-002]

Fibrous joints are located between cranial bones **(sutural joints)** and between the tibia and the fibula of the lower leg or the radius and ulna bones of the forearm **(syndesmosis type joint).**

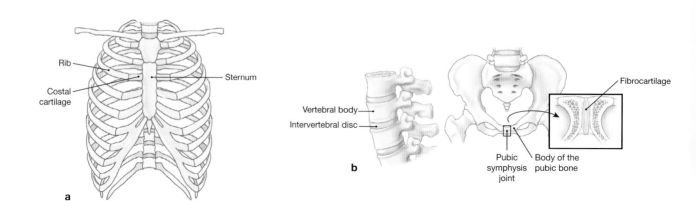

Fig. 1.30a and b Cartilaginous joints; synchondrosis (a) and symphysis (b). [E607-002]

Cartilaginous joints connect bones through hyaline cartilage **(synchondrosis,** e.g. connection between ribs and sternum) or fibrocartilage **(symphysis,** e.g. pubic symphysis).

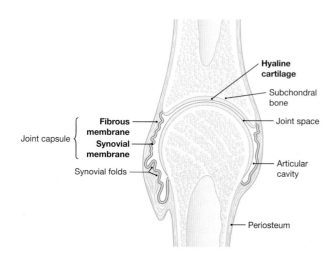

Fig. 1.31 Synovial joints. [L126]

Synovial joints are built for mobility. They are formed by **hyaline cartilage** which covers the ends of the subchondral bone, and a joint capsule that encloses the articular cavity. The joint capsule consists of an outer **fibrous membrane** and an inner synovial membrane. The **synovial membrane** secretes synovial fluid into the articular cavity which acts as 'lubricant' for movement. Synovial joints allow movements in:

- one plane – uniaxial,
- two planes – biaxial, or
- three planes – multiaxial.

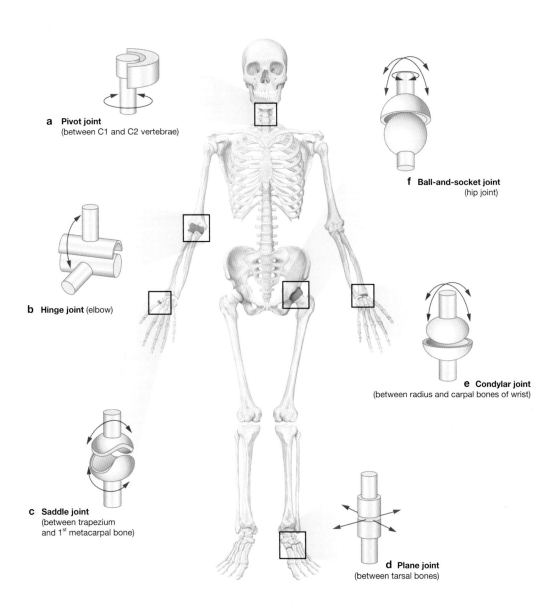

a **Pivot joint**
(between C1 and C2 vertebrae)

f **Ball-and-socket joint**
(hip joint)

b **Hinge joint** (elbow)

e **Condylar joint**
(between radius and carpal bones of wrist)

c **Saddle joint**
(between trapezium
and 1st metacarpal bone)

d **Plane joint**
(between tarsal bones)

Fig. 1.32a to f Types of synovial joints. [L127]
In order for the human body to effectively move, the various synovial joints about the body are structured differently in order to facilitate uniaxial, biaxial, and multiaxial movements. The body contains six types of synovial joints:
a **Pivot joint:** uniaxial joint, permits only rotational movements
b **Hinge joint:** uniaxial joint, permits flexion and extension movements

c **Saddle joint:** 'specialized' biaxial joint, permits flexion, extension, abduction, adduction, as well as restricted rotational movements
d **Plane joint:** permits subtle gliding movements of the joint in various directions
e **Condylar or ellipsoid joint:** biaxial joint, permits flexion, extension, abduction, adduction movements
f **Ball-and-socket joint:** multiaxial joint, permits movements of flexion, extension, abduction, adduction, and internal or external rotation.

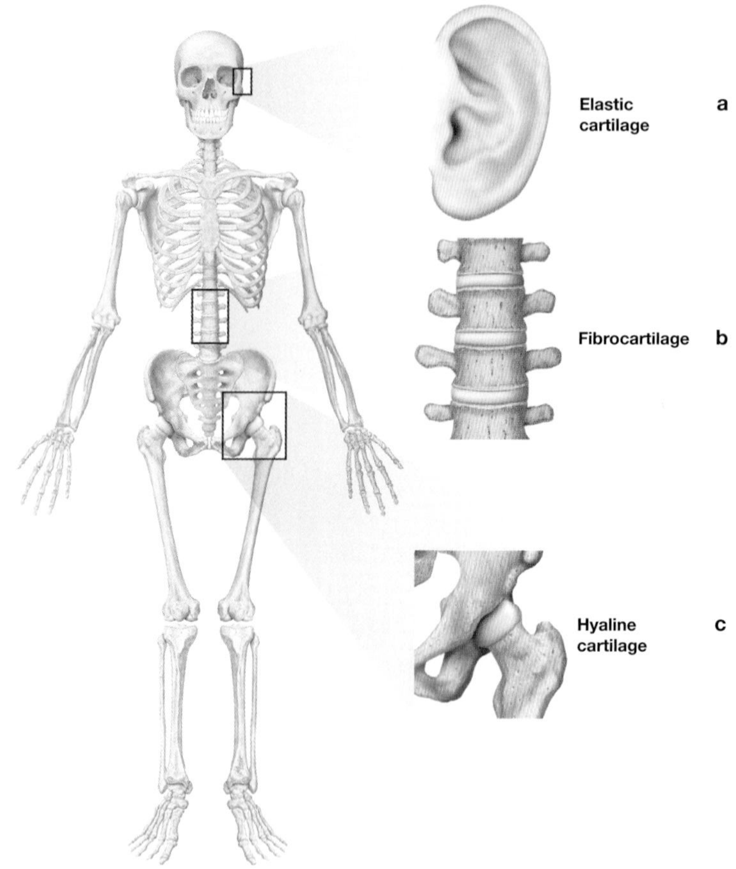

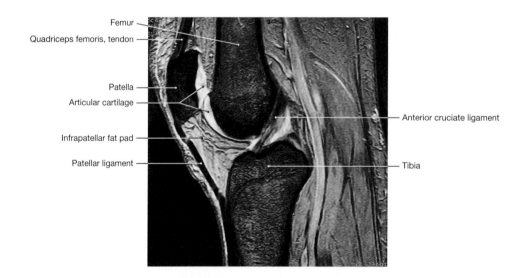

Elastic **a**
cartilage

Fibrocartilage **b**

Hyaline **c**
cartilage

Fig. 1.33a to c Types of cartilage. [L127]
Cartilage is a flexible but strong supportive connective tissue. Unlike bone and all other types of connective tissue, cartilage is avascular. For this reason, cartilage does not possess the regenerative capacity of bone or other connective tissues. Within the human body, there are three types of cartilage (from top to bottom):
a Elastic cartilage: involved in the formation of the outer ear, EUSTACHIAN tube, and epiglottis.

b Fibrocartilage: flexible and tough form of cartilage that serves as a shock absorber within the spine, knee and shoulder regions.
c Hyaline cartilage: most abundant type of cartilage in body; as a supportive tissue it can be found in the nose, ears, trachea, larynx, and smaller respiratory tubes. As articular cartilage, it covers the ends of long bones as part of synovial joints in order to ensure smooth articulation during joint movements. Degeneration of hyaline cartilage within a synovial joint is referred to as arthritis.

Femur
Quadriceps femoris, tendon

Patella
Articular cartilage

Infrapatellar fat pad

Patellar ligament

Anterior cruciate ligament

Tibia

Fig. 1.34 Sagittal magnetic resonance imaging (MRI) of a knee (T2-weighted). [R316-007]
Magnetic resonance imaging (MRI) is frequently used to diagnose cartilaginous lesions in the human body. During a MRI examination, a patient is exposed to a powerful magnetic field. Alterations in pulse frequency and scanning parameters result in T1-weighted (fluids: dark, fat: bright; e.g. joint effusion, dark) and T2-weighted images (fluids: bright, fat: gray; e.g. the infrapatellar fat pad between patella and tibia). Thus, T-weighted images can be used to emphasize particular tissue compartments.

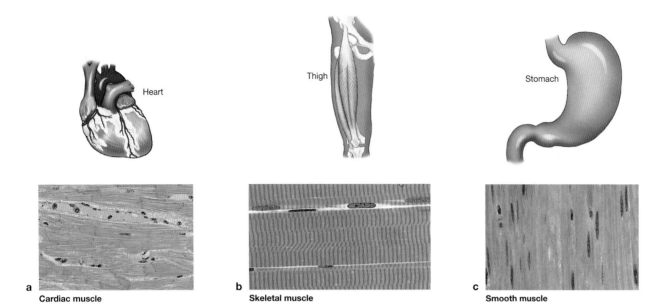

a **Cardiac muscle**

b **Skeletal muscle**

c **Smooth muscle**

Fig. 1.35a to c Types of muscle. [E336]
Three types of muscles are present in the human body.
a Cardiac muscle: involuntary striated muscle that is only found in the heart; basic building block is the sarcomere. Cardiac muscle cells connect at branching, irregular angles to intercalated discs.

b Skeletal muscle: voluntary muscle that connects to bone and powers movement of the human body; striated in appearance; the parallel arrangement of sarcomeres facilitates contraction (shortening) and relaxation (lengthening) of a muscle.

c Smooth muscle: fibers are spindle shaped, under involuntary control, and primarily found in the walls of hollow organs (except the heart) and structures such as the esophagus, stomach, intestines, bronchi, blood vessels, urethra, bladder, and uterus.

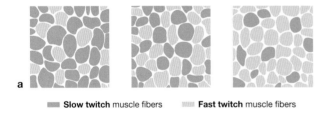

a

■ **Slow twitch** muscle fibers   ▨ **Fast twitch** muscle fibers

Types of Muscle Fibers	
Slow twitch or type I	**Fast twitch or type II**
Contract slowly	Contract quickly
Make ATP as needed by aerobic metabolism	Capable of rapidly breaking down ATP
Many mitochondria	Little or no mitochrondria
Well supplied with blood vessels	Well supplied with blood vessels
Store very little glycogen	Store a lot of glycogen
Red muscle	White muscle
Used for endurance activities	Used for brief high-intensity activities
	Capable of anaerobic metabolism

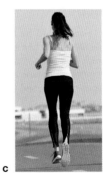

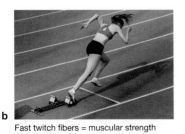

b
Fast twitch fibers = muscular strength

c
Slow twitch fibers = muscular endurance

Fig. 1.36a to c Skeletal muscles. a [L231], b, c [J787]
Skeletal muscles primarily consist of two types of muscle fibers: fast twitch and slow twitch **(a).** The proportion of each fiber type within a skeletal muscle is influenced by both genetic (i.e. hereditary) and environmental (i.e. how the muscle is used) factors. Some muscles are comprised of predominately slow twitch fibers, some have equal proportions of slow and fast fibres, while others are comprised mostly of fast twitch fibers. **b** Fast twitch fibers (also identified as type II fibers) use little or no oxygen during contraction, are highly fatigable, and are required for forceful muscle contraction. **c** Slow twitch fibers (also identified as type I fibers) need oxygen during contraction, are considered to be non fatigable, and are required for repetitive muscle contraction.

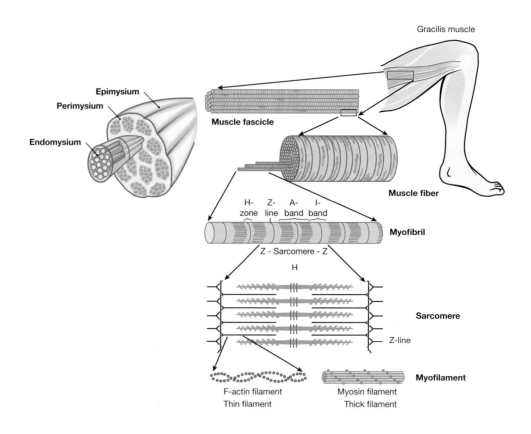

Fig. 1.37 Skeletal muscle structure. [L126]
All skeletal muscles within the human body display the same organization. Each individual **sarcomere** is formed by groups of **myo-
filaments** which are comprised of contractile proteins (actin and
myosin filaments). Groups of sarcomeres are linked together in
series (end to end) and in a parallel manner (side by side) to form a
myofibril. Groups of myofibrils are surrounded by connective tissue called **endomysium** to form a **muscle fiber**. Groups of muscle
fibers are surrounded by **perimysium** to form a **muscle bundle or
fascicle**. Finally, groups of fascicles are surrounded by **epimysium**
to form a skeletal muscle (e.g. gracilis muscle).

Structure/Function

Muscle contraction is controlled by the ability of each sarcomere to change its overall length (via a process described as the
sliding filament theory). Three types of muscle contractions are
normally used when performing typical activities of daily living.
These contraction types can be used to stabilize the body or to
power motion:
1. **Concentric contraction:** muscle shortens under load and diminishes the joint angle
2. **Eccentric contraction:** muscle lengthens under load and increases the joint angle
3. **Isometric contraction:** muscle contracts with no change in
   length, the joint position remains unchanged.
[L126]

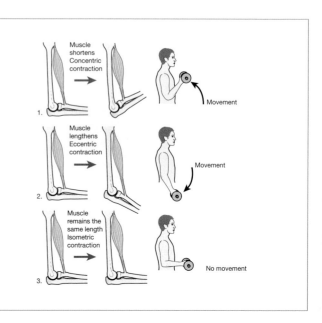

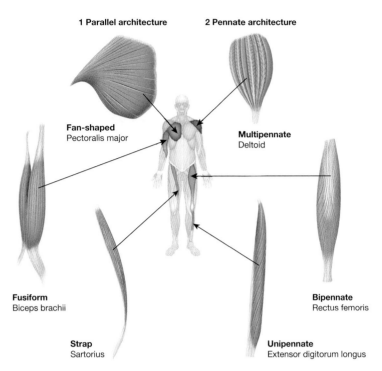

Fig. 1.38 Muscle architecture. [L275]
The fiber arrangement or 'architecture' of a muscle will have a significant bearing on its function. Muscles which converge at multiple angles to a central tendinous attachment (e.g. deltoid and pectoralis major) are built to develop tremendous force with little change in length, while muscles that demonstrate a parallel arrangement in muscle fibers (e.g. hamstrings, and tibialis anterior) may have difficulty developing large force, but lengthen very easily. In general, there are 2 types of muscle architecture:
1. Parallel – which can be subclassified into strap, fan-shaped, and fusiform fiber arrangements.
2. Pennate – which can be subclassified into uni, bi, and multi-pennate fiber arrangements.

Structure/Function

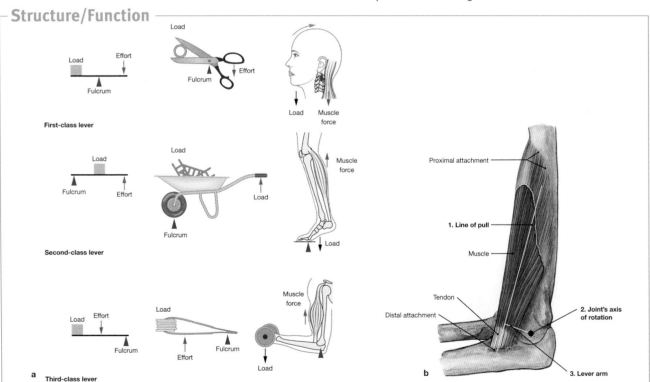

Muscle levers (a) and organization principle of skeletal muscles (b).
a The musculoskeletal system uses several types of levers to create effective and efficient movement. In simple terms, a joint (where two or more bones join together) forms an axis (or fulcrum), and the muscles crossing the joint apply a force to move the load or provide resistance. Levers are typically labeled as **first class, second class,** or **third class.** All three types are found in the body, but most levers in the human body are third class.

b The amount of force a muscle can generate along its **line of pull** (1) through the **joint's axis of rotation** (2) is dependent on the length of the **lever arm** (3). The length of the lever arm will vary depending on the position of the joint. The longer the lever arm, the less force is required from the muscle to create joint movement. a [L231]

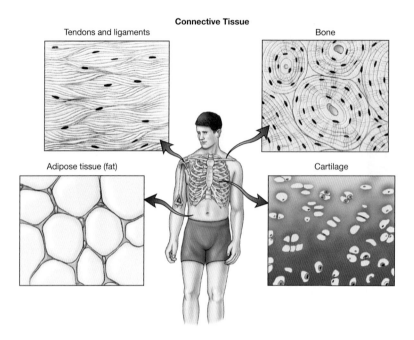

Fig. 1.39 Types of connective tissue. [G199]
Connective tissue is the most widespread and abundant type of tissue found within the human body. It functions to **support, anchor** and **connect** various parts of the body. All connective tissue (except for blood and lymphatics) consists of the same three basic components: fibers (collagen and elastin), ground substance, and cells (fibroblasts, macrophages, adipocytes, etc.). It can be generally classified into two main categories:

1. **Connective tissue proper:** surrounds all organs and body cavities, connecting one part with another, or separating one group of cells from another. Examples include adipose tissue (**fat**), loose connective tissue (fascia), and dense regular tissue (**tendons and ligaments**).
2. **Specialized connective tissue:** includes **cartilage and bone,** which form the skeletal framework of the body.

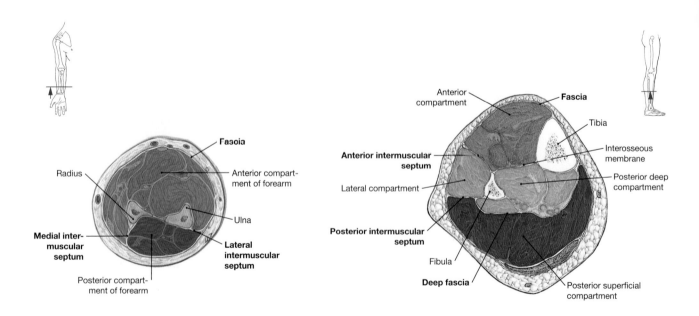

Fig. 1.40a and b Fascia of forearm and lower leg.
Fascia forms a band or sheet of connective tissue beneath the skin that attaches, stabilizes, encloses or separates muscles and organs from one another. The muscles of the forearm **(a)** and of the lower leg **(b)** are separated into distinct muscular compartments by strong and thick fascia that are called an **intermuscular septum.** This structural architecture within the body supports separate and distinct functions of the muscles of a specific compartment (e.g. forearm compartments: muscles of the anterior compartment perform flexion and pronation movements; muscles of the posterior compartment perform extension and supination movements), and serves to create pathways between the muscular compartments that facilitate passage of key neurovascular structures.

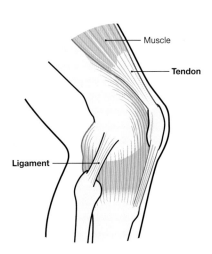

Fig. 1.41 Tendons and ligaments function. [L126]
Tendons, ligaments and the joint capsule each closely surround, connect and stabilize joints of the musculoskeletal system. While passive (they do not actively produce joint motion), each structure plays an essential role in controlling/guiding joint movements. **Ligaments and the joint capsule** both connect bone to bone, function to stabilize and guide joint motion, preventing abnormal or excessive movements. **Tendons** connect muscle to bone and transmit tensile loads to the bone when a muscle contracts – thereby creating joint motion.

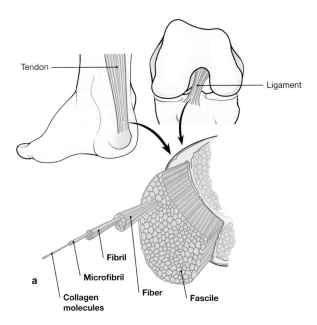

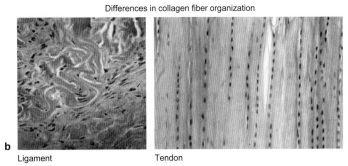

Differences in collagen fiber organization

Fig. 1.42a and b Tendons and ligaments organization. a [L126], b left [G716], b right [H061-001]
a Tendons and ligaments show a similar construction pattern. They are composed of dense regular connective tissue, with collagen fibers being the primary building block. Microscopically, both are made up of **collagen molecules** which are synthesized by fibroblasts, and embedded in an extracellular matrix to form a parallel arrangement of **microfibrils,** and then **fibrils.** The fibrils aggregate to form **collagen fibers,** which in turn group together to form densely packed **collagen bundles or fascicles** that are arranged in parallel patterns around points of stress/tension.
b Tendons demonstrate uniform patterns of collagen organization around stress; collagen organization in ligaments is more varied.

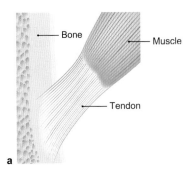

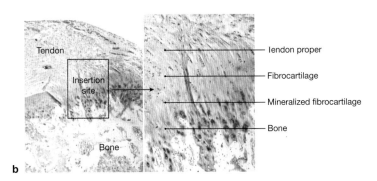

Fig. 1.43a and b Tendon insertion to bone. a [L275], b [G465]
a A tendon (or ligament) connects to a bone via an osseous junction. This represents a gradual transition in the structure and function of the tendon (or ligament) into solid bone. There are four transitional zones.

b The first zone is composed only of the tendon (or ligament) tissue, and in the second zone the tendon tissue has changed into fibrocartilage with chondrocyte-like cells. In the third zone, the fibrocartilage becomes mineralized, and in the final zone the tissue is now fully transitioned to bone.

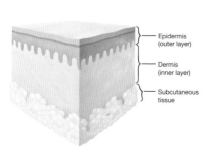

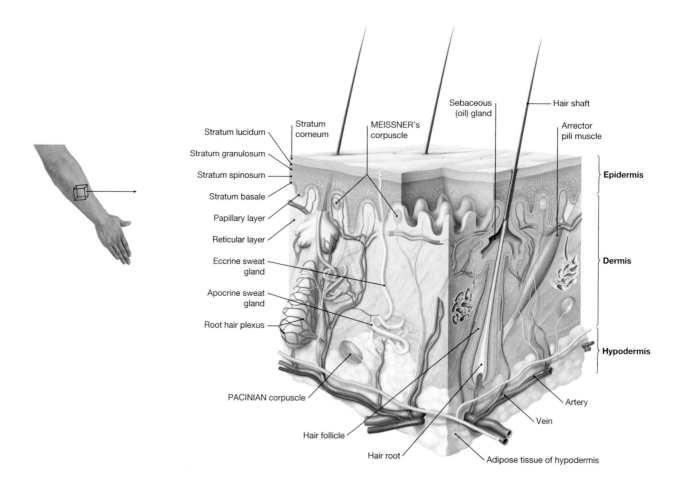

Fig. 1.44 Functions of the integumentary system. [L271], [L275]
The integumentary system is an organ system consisting of the skin, hair, nails, and exocrine glands. It functions to waterproof, cushion, and protect the deeper tissues, excrete wastes, and regulate temperature, and is interspersed with sensory receptors to detect pain, sensation, pressure, and temperature. The skin is composed of the **epidermis** and underlying **dermis** (fibro-elastic connective tissue with capillary plexus, specialized receptors, nerves, immune cells, melatonin-producing cells, sweat glands, hair follicles, sebaceous glands, smooth muscle cells; thickness varies depending on the body region). Beneath the dermis lies the **hypoder-**mis (subcutaneous fat tissue). While the skin is only a few millimeters thick, it is by far the largest organ in the body. In an adult, skin accounts for approximately 10 to 15% of the total body weight, and has a surface area of approximately 20 square feet. As the body's outer covering the skin forms a barrier to protect the body from chemicals, disease, UV light, and physical damage. Hair and nails extend from the skin to reinforce the skin and protect it from environmental damage. The exocrine glands of the integumentary system produce sweat, oil, and wax to cool, protect, and moisturize the skin's surface.

Clinical Remarks

A **blister** may form when the skin has been damaged by friction, rubbing, heat, cold or chemical exposure. Fluid collects between the epidermal (outermost) and dermal layer of skin. This fluid serves as a cushion, helping to protect the dermal layer (and its associated structures) from further damage. Less intensive or aggressive rubbing over long periods of time may cause a **callus** to form (instead of a blister).

[L275], [E422], [J787]

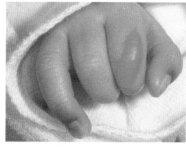

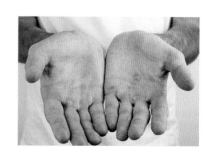

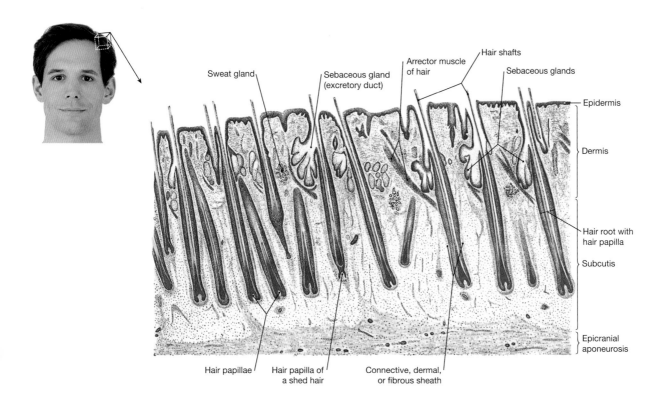

Fig. 1.45 Hair; longitudinal section through the human scalp. [K340], [R252]

Hair protects the skin from UV-light as well as cold, and serves to convey sensations of touch. It is the product of keratinization of the epidermis, and originates from invaginations of the epidermis which form follicles that contain mitotically active cells (matrix cells) at the base. Matrix cells differentiate to become keratinized cells which form the shaft of the hair. Postnatally, we distinguish two types of hair:

1. **Vellus hair** (fluffy hair) is soft, short, thin, largely without pigmentation, and does not contain a medulla (follicles are located in the dermis); vellus hair covers most of the body in children and women.
2. **Terminal hair** (long hair) is firm, long, thick, pigmented, and contains a medulla (follicles reach into the subcutis); it constitutes the hair of the head, eyebrows, pubic region, armpits, and beard (in men). The body distribution of terminal hair differs vastly across ethnic groups.

Fig. 1.46 Structure of a hair follicle; longitudinal section. [L141, R170-3]

Hair originates from hair follicles which are cylindrical invaginations of the epidermis into the dermis or subcutis. The follicular body consists of a **hair bulb** and the **hair papilla.** Each hair follicle receives a tuft of blood vessels to sustain its growth and is associated with a **sebaceous gland** (hair-sebaceous gland unit) and a smooth muscle (**arrector muscle of hair**). The latter is responsible for the erection of the hair (sympathetic activation) by indenting the epidermis to form small pits (goose bumps). Genetic predisposition and pigmentation (melanin content) determine the hair color. Once the production of melanin ceases, the hair turns from gray to white.

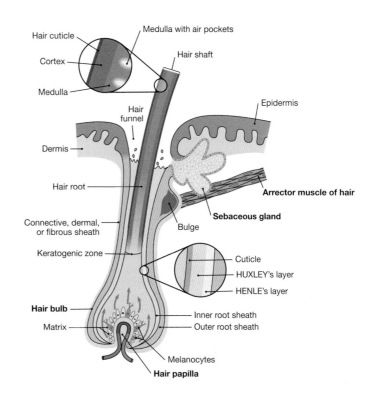

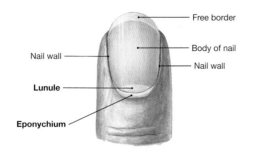

Fig. 1.47 Distal finger phalanx with nail.
The nail is a convex-shaped, translucent keratin plate on the upper side of the distal phalanx of the finger and toe. It serves to protect the tips of the fingers and toes and supports the grasping function of the fingers. The nail is embedded into cutaneous slits (nail wall) and its lateral margin is covered by the cutaneous nail wall or fold on both sides of the nail. The epithelial layer extending from the nail wall at the base of the nail onto the dorsal nail plate is called **eponychium**. The nail plate is anchored here to the nail bed, and the skin beneath the nail plate.

Fig. 1.48 Distal finger phalanx; nail partially removed.
The epithelium located beneath the free border of the nail at the tips of the phalanges is called **hyponychium** (also known as 'quick'). Beneath the epithelial hyponychium lies the fibrous base of the nail bed which is tightly connected with the periosteum of the distal phalanx. The proximal hyponychium forms the nail matrix which generates the nail plate. The **lunule** is the visible part of the nail matrix.

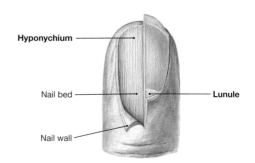

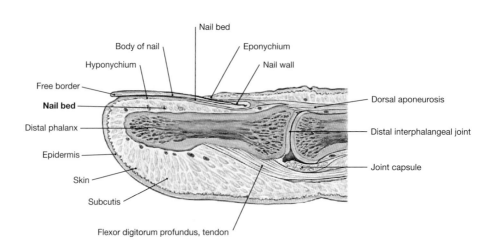

Fig. 1.49 Distal finger phalanx; phalanx distalis; sagittal section.
The **nail bed** comprises the region between the nail and the distal phalanx. It consists of epithelium (hyponychium and nail matrix) and the underlying dermis.

Clinical Remarks

White spots on nails are due to defective fusion of the nail plate with the nail bed. Changes in light reflection at these points cause the nail plate to appear milky-white. This lack of fusion may occur as a result of physical trauma, certain medications, or may be linked to various diseases. Brittle nails signal lack of biotin (vitamin H). Biotin is required for the formation of keratin, the main component of the nail plate. Numerous systemic diseases are associated with nail changes. Psoriasis leads to the formation of small pits, oily spots and sometimes crumbly nails up to a complete nail dystrophy.   [E382]

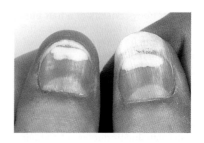

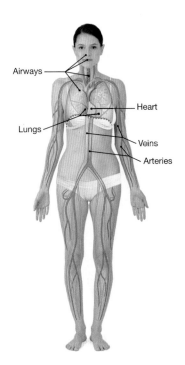

Airways

Heart

Lungs

Veins

Arteries

Fig. 1.50 Cardiorespiratory system. [K340, L126]
The cardiorespiratory system is comprised of the heart and blood vessels (arteries and veins), which work with the respiratory system of the lungs and airways. These body systems carry oxygen to the muscles and organs, and remove waste products, including carbon dioxide.

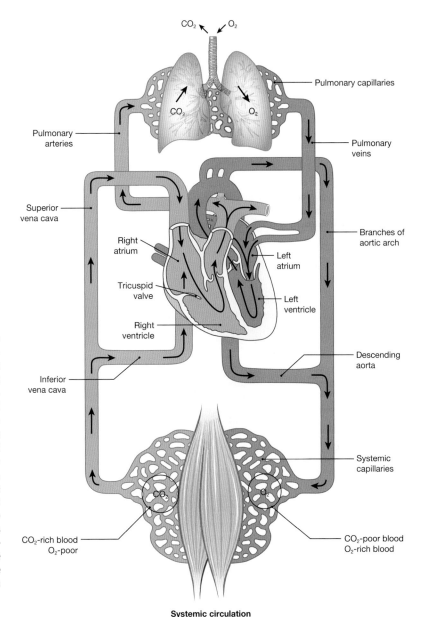

CO_2 O_2

Pulmonary capillaries

CO_2 O_2

Pulmonary arteries

Pulmonary veins

Superior vena cava

Branches of aortic arch

Right atrium

Left atrium

Tricuspid valve

Left ventricle

Right ventricle

Descending aorta

Inferior vena cava

Systemic capillaries

CO_2 O_2

CO_2-rich blood O_2-poor

CO_2-poor blood O_2-rich blood

Systemic circulation

Fig. 1.51 Cardiorespiratory system; schematic drawing. [L126]
The cardiorespiratory system works to keep the human body both oxygenated and free of waste products. As oxygen enters the lungs from the air, it flows into the alveolar sacs – small air chambers within the lungs. From there, individual oxygen molecules continue to the bloodstream through small arteries within the alveolar sacs. This newly oxygenated blood moves into the left atrium and ventricle of the heart through the pulmonary veins. The blood circulates throughout the body via the aorta, eventually traveling through every organ in the body. Cells receive oxygen from the arterial blood, and the deoxygenated blood returns to the heart through the venous system, carrying carbon dioxide and other waste products. The deoxygenated blood enters the right atrium and ventricle of the heart via the venae cavae, where it returns to the alveoli of the lungs to exchange its carbon dioxide and waste products for fresh oxygen. This carbon dioxide then exits the body upon exhalation.

Fig. 1.52 Radiograph (X-ray) of the thorax; A/P view.
[R316-007]
Simple radiographic images of the thorax are among those most frequently ordered. With a patient standing upright, the X-rays pass through the thorax in a posterior-anterior (P/A) direction (patient faces radiographic film). In the lying position, the X-rays pass through the patient in an anterior-posterior (A/P) direction. A good radiographic image of the thorax will display the major bronchi and blood vessels of the lungs, the cardiomediastinal contour, the diaphragm, the ribs, and the peripheral soft tissue.

Tracheal bifurcation, carina of trachea

Trachea

Aortic arch

Superior vena cava

Right main bronchus

Left pulmonary artery

Pulmonary trunk

Pulmonary vein

Right pulmonary artery

Pulmonary vein

Right atrium

Left main bronchus

Pulmonary vein

Left auricle

Inferior vena cava

Pulmonary vein

Diaphragm, (right dome)

Left ventricle

Fig. 1.53 Arteries of the systemic circulation.
The function of arteries is to transport blood from the heart to the periphery of the body or into the lungs. The arterial system can be divided into

1. **Systemic arteries** – which carry oxygenated blood from the heart to the whole body, and
2. **Pulmonary arteries** – which carry deoxygenated blood from the heart to the lungs.

Arteries can be described as either an elastic type (e.g. aorta, arteries close to the heart) or a muscular type (most of the arteries, e.g. brachial and femoral artery). Arteries have a higher blood pressure than other parts of the circulatory system. The pressure in arteries varies during the cardiac cycle. It is highest when the heart contracts and lowest when the heart relaxes. This variation in pressure creates a **pulse.**

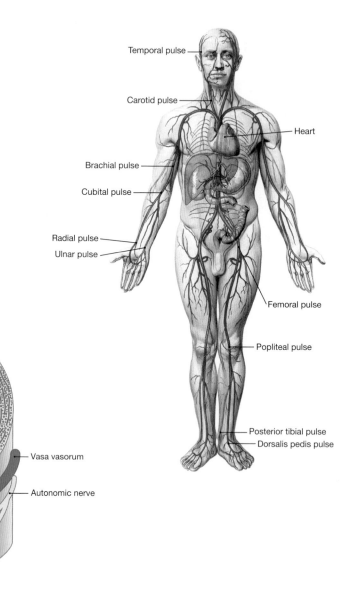

Fig. 1.54 Arterial structure. [L107, R170-4]
The microscopic structure of arteries is different from that of veins. The outermost layer of an artery is known as the **tunica externa** and is comprised of dense connective tissue made of collagen. Inside this layer is the **tunica media,** which contains smooth muscle and elastic tissue. The innermost layer of an artery is in direct contact with the flow of blood and is referred to as the **tunica intima.** This layer is composed primarily of endothelial cells. The hollow tube through which the blood flows is called the **lumen.**

Fig. 1.55 3-D CT angiography; scan of different structures of the abdomen and pelvis (volume-rendering technique, VRT) derived from multidetector CT sections. [R316-007]
Modern computed tomography technology (e.g. 64-lines volume spiral multilayer CT) provides new dimensions and indications for CT diagnostics and guarantees minimal dosage exposure for patients. CT angiography is based on the same multilayer CT technology. In a blood vessel, the region of interest is scanned during fast intravenous injection of an iodine-containing substance to increase contrast of the structure. The resulting sectional images of branching vessels are then assembled by a computer to generate a 3-D image of the region.

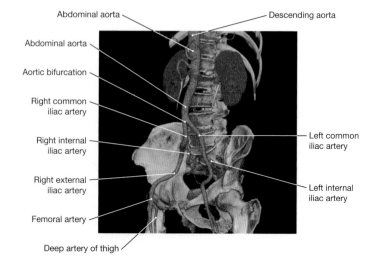

Fig.1.56 Veins of the systemic circulation.

Veins transport blood from the periphery of the body back to the heart. They expand easily and function as reservoirs. The veins of the systemic circulation transport deoxygenated blood, those of the lung circulation transport oxygenated blood. Most veins are concomitant veins, meaning they run in parallel with corresponding arteries. Compared to the arteries, their course is variable and the blood pressure is significantly lower. Veins, capillaries, and venoles are part of the low pressure system of blood circulation. Most of the time, veins transport blood against gravitational force. Thus, larger veins of the extremities and the lower neck region possess valves (venous valves) to support the venous blood flow back to the heart. Apart from the valves, muscles and the arterial pulse (only when venous valves are present) also affect the venous blood flow.

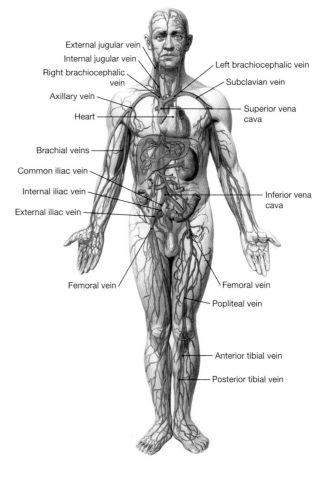

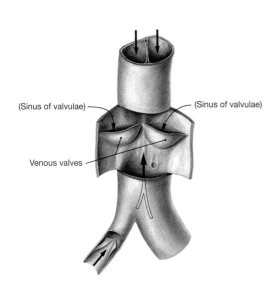

Fig.1.57 Function of venous valves.

Arrows pointing upwards indicate the direction of venous blood flow. When blood accumulates (arrows pointing downwards) the valves close.

Most parts of the body contain a superficial venous system in the subcutaneous fat which communicates with a deeper venous system running parallel to the arteries (both systems are separated by venous valves so that blood can only travel unidirectionally from the superficial to the deep veins).

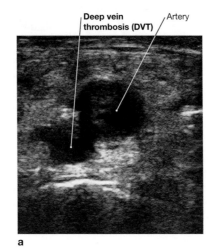

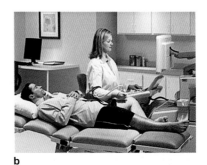

Fig.1.58a and b Ultrasonographic image of a deep vein thrombosis. a [E708], b [G704]

Deep vein thrombosis (DVT) occurs when a blood clot (thrombus) forms in one or more of the deep veins in the body. Deep vein thrombosis can cause leg pain or swelling, but may occur without any symptoms. A DVT is a serious condition in which blood clots in a vein can break loose, travel through the bloodstream and lodge in the lungs, blocking blood flow, and resulting in a pulmonary embolism.

a   b

Fig. 1.59 The lymphatic system.

The lymphatic system plays an important role in immune responses and resorption of lipids. Lymph capillaries (located in the periphery of the body) collect interstitial or lymph fluid and transport it via **lymphatic vessels** to lymph nodes. **Lymph nodes** are responsible for the collection and filtration of a particular region of the body (eg. axillary lymph nodes). Finally, the lymph is transported from the regional lymph nodes to two major lymphatic ducts which drain into the venous blood of systemic circulation. The **thoracic duct** drains into the left venous angle (located between left internal jugular vein and left subclavian vein), the **right lymphatic duct** drains into the right venous angle (located between right internal jugular vein and right subclavian vein). In addition to the lymphatic vessels and lymph nodes, the lymphoid tissue also includes lymphatic organs (thymus, bone marrow, spleen, tonsils, mucosa-associated lymphoid tissue [MALT]).

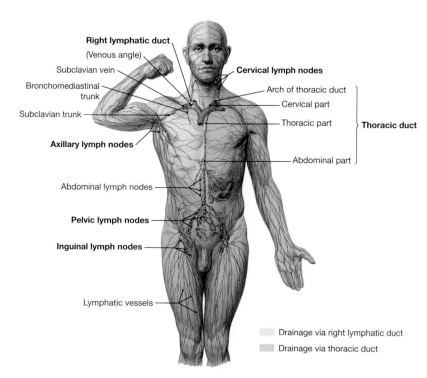

Fig. 1.60 Lymph nodes; schematic cross-section. [L127]

This cross-section of a representative lymph node shows in- and outgoing (afferent and efferent) lymphatic vessels, blood supply, and compartmentalization of the lymph node into **B region (secondary follicle), T region (paracortical zone)** with postcapillary or high endothelial venules, follicular and interdigitating dendritic cells, medullary sinus, intermediate sinus, and subcapsular or cortical sinus (with cellular composition shown).

* Reticular cells lining the sinus wall also reside within the sinus.

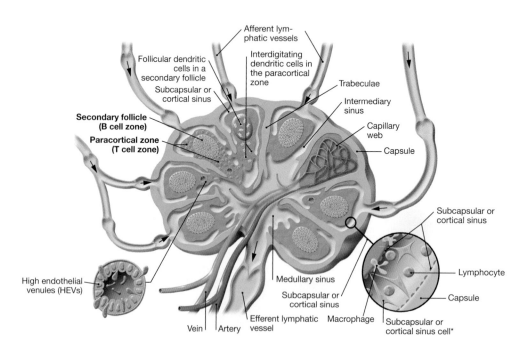

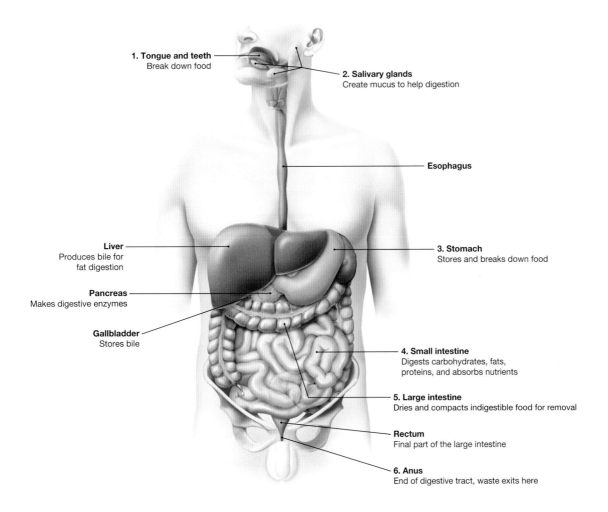

1. Tongue and teeth
Break down food

2. Salivary glands
Create mucus to help digestion

Esophagus

Liver
Produces bile for
fat digestion

3. Stomach
Stores and breaks down food

Pancreas
Makes digestive enzymes

Gallbladder
Stores bile

4. Small intestine
Digests carbohydrates, fats,
proteins, and absorbs nutrients

5. Large intestine
Dries and compacts indigestible food for removal

Rectum
Final part of the large intestine

6. Anus
End of digestive tract, waste exits here

Fig. 1.61 Main components and basic functions of the digestive system. [L275]
The drawing illustrates the major regions and organs of the digestive system together with their primary functions. The digestive system is responsible for the conversion of food into energy and basic nutrients to feed the entire body. Numbers 1 to 6 show the sequence of events in the digestive tract after eating a meal.

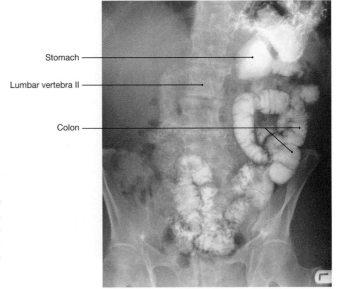

Stomach

Lumbar vertebra II

Colon

Fig. 1.62 Conventional radiograph (X-ray); fluoroscopy after barium swallow test. [E402]
Fluoroscopy is a special application of X-ray imaging. Hollow organs and intestinal loops of the digestive system are poor in contrast, and in order to be visualized radiographically, they need to be filled with a substance that absorbs X-rays to increase contrast. A frequently used substance to increase contrast of the gastrointestinal tract is the insoluble, non-toxic, high density salt barium sulfate.

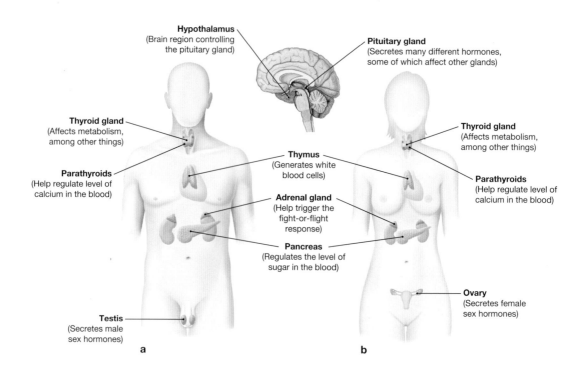

a   b

Fig. 1.63a and b Organs and basic functions of the male (a) and female (b) endocrine system. [L275]

The endocrine system is comprised of a collection of glands that produce and secrete hormones into the bloodstream to affect the activity of another part of the body (target site). The major glands of the endocrine system are the hypothalamus, pituitary gland, thyroid, parathyroids, thymus, adrenal gland, pancreas, and the reproductive organs (ovaries in females and testicles in males). Overall, the endocrine system has five main functions:

1. Regulation of metabolism
2. Maintaining salt, water, and nutrient balances in the blood
3. Control of responses to stress
4. Regulation of growth, development, and reproduction
5. Production of hormones.

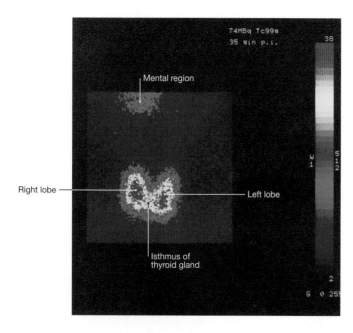

Fig. 1.64 Scintigraphy; scan of the thyroid gland of the neck. [R316-007]

Scintigraphy is a diagnostic test in nuclear medicine with radioisotopes (that emit radiation) which are attached to drugs. After injection of the drug they travel to a specific target organ or tissue, and the radiation that is emitted by the radioisotopes is captured by external detectors in the form of gamma rays (a form of electromagnetic rays). These gamma rays can be visualized by gamma cameras as a two-dimensional image (bone scan) or as a three-dimensional image (PET scan – positron emission tomography). The images generated by the gamma camera depend on how the radiopharmacon is absorbed, distributed, metabolized, or excreted in the body.

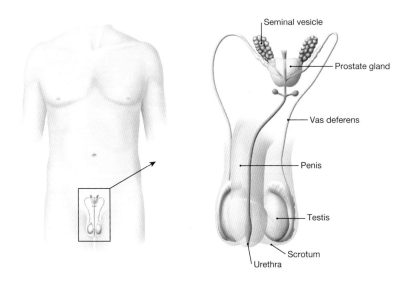

Fig. 1.65 Male reproductive system. [L275]
The male reproductive system includes the scrotum, testes, spermatic ducts, sex glands, and penis. These organs work together to produce, maintain, and transport sperm (the male reproductive cells) and protective fluid (semen) to discharge sperm within the female reproductive tract during sex and to produce and secrete male sex hormones responsible for maintaining the male reproductive system. Unlike the female reproductive system, a majority of the male reproductive system is located outside the body (penis, scrotum and testicles).

Fig. 1.66 Female reproductive system. [L275]
The female reproductive system includes the ovaries, uterine tubes (FALLOPIAN tubes), uterus, vagina, and vulva. The ovaries produce the female egg cells, called the ova or oocytes. The oocytes are then transported to the FALLOPIAN tube where fertilization by a sperm may occur. The fertilized egg then moves to the uterus, where the uterine lining has thickened in response to the normal hormones of the reproductive cycle. Once in the uterus the fertilized egg can implant into the thickened uterine lining and continue to develop. If fertilization does not take place, the uterine lining is shed as menstrual flow. In addition, the female reproductive system produces female sex hormones that maintain the reproductive cycle.

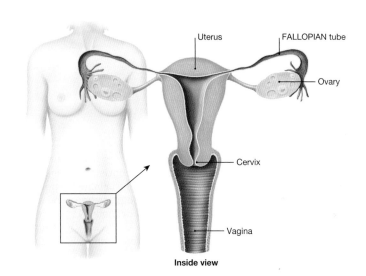

Inside view

Fig. 1.67 Sonography, an ultrasound image of a fetus at week 28 of pregnancy; lateral view.
Physical examinations employing ultrasound are common in all medical specialties. Ultrasound uses a series of high-frequency sound waves (not an electromagnetic beam) generated by electric impulses in piezo-electric crystals to visualize soft tissue structures of the body in real time. These sound waves are reflected from inner organs and their content (fetus in the uterus), analyzed by a computer and presented on a screen. This way, the movements of the extremities and opening of the mouth can be viewed as a live image. Because ultrasound imaging techniques do not employ ionizing radiation to generate images (unlike radiography, and CT scans), they are generally considered safer and are therefore more common in obstetrical imaging. But the quality of images obtained using ultrasound is highly dependent on the skills of the examiner (ultrasonographer) and the patient's body size.

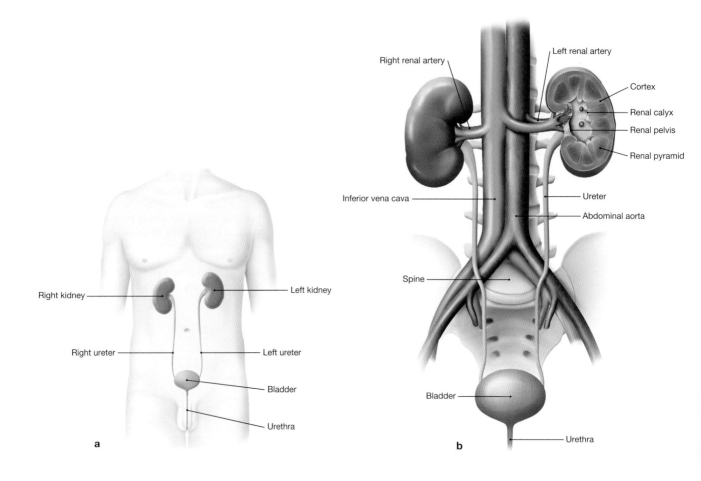

a

Right kidney — **Left kidney**

Right ureter — **Left ureter**

Bladder

Urethra

a

Fig. 1.68a and b Urinary system; anterior view. [L275]
a The **urinary system** (also known as the **renal system**) consists of the **kidneys, ureters, bladder and urethra.** It functions to eliminate waste from the body, regulate blood volume and blood pressure, control the level of electrolytes and metabolites, and determines blood pH.
b The renal arteries transport blood to the kidneys for filtration. Waste from the blood is removed by the kidneys and becomes

urine, which is transported via the ureters (tubes made of smooth muscle fibers) to the urinary bladder. Here the urine collects and is stored before it is subsequently transported through the urethra to be expelled from the body by urination (voiding). The male and female urinary systems are very similar, differing only in the length of the urethra.

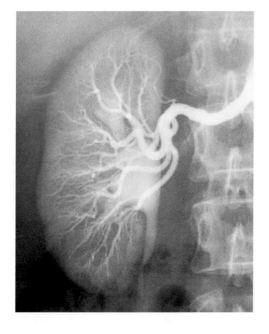

Fig. 1.69 Angiography of the kidney. [G570]
Angiography is a special application of X-ray imaging. Arteries and veins are poor in contrast, and in order to be visualized radiographically, they need to be filled with a substance that absorbs X-rays to increase contrast. For vessels, iodine-containing molecules are usually employed. These substances are safe and well-tolerated by most patients and can also be used to image the kidneys, ureters, and bladder as they are excreted by the kidneys.

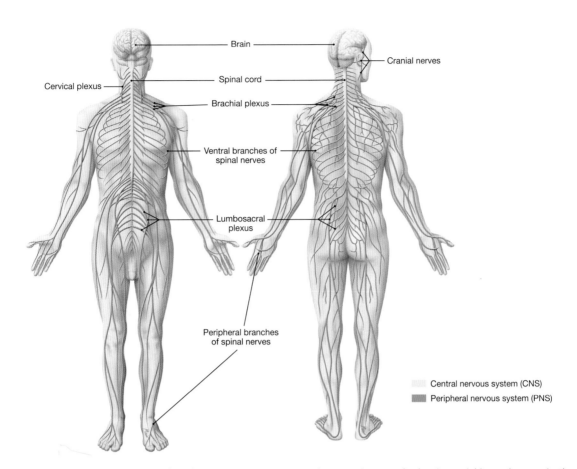

Fig. 1.70 Organization of the nervous system. [L127]
Structurally, the nervous system is comprised of the **central** (brain and spinal cord) **and peripheral nervous system** (spinal and cranial nerves). The nervous system is involved in complex functions including the regulation of the activities of the muscles and the intestines, the communication with the environment and the inner self, and memorizing past experiences (memory). The nervous system is also essential for conceptualizing imaginations (thinking), generating emotions, and adapting quickly to changes in the surrounding world and the body interior. Functionally, the nervous system can be organized into the **autonomic** (visceral, regulating the activities of the intestines, predominantly involuntary) and the **somatic** (innervation of skeletal muscles, cognitive perception of sensory input) **nervous system**. Both systems interact and affect each other. Apart from the nervous system, overall body functions are also regulated by the endocrine system.

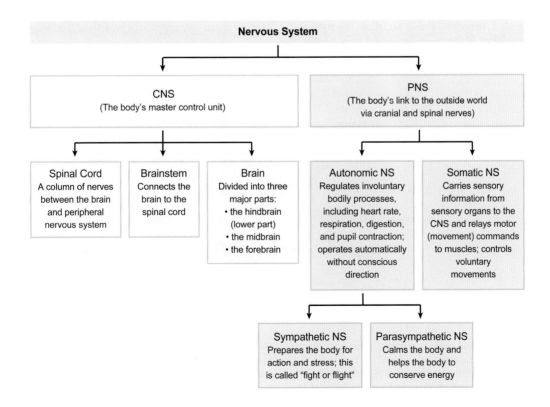

Fig. 1.71 Organization of the nervous system. [L126]

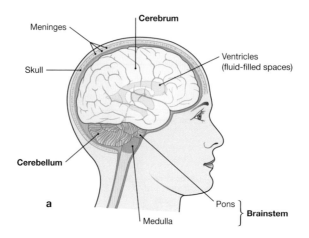

a

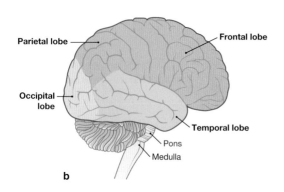

b

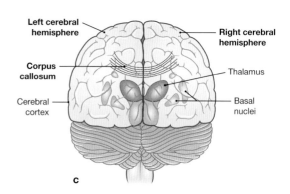

c

Fig. 1.72 a to c Schematic representation of the brain; sagittal and frontal view. [L126]
The brain is composed of three main parts: the **brainstem, cerebellum,** and **cerebrum.** The cerebrum is divided into four lobes: **1. frontal, 2. parietal, 3. temporal,** and **4. occipital.** The **right and left cerebral hemispheres** of the brain are joined by a bundle of fibers called the **corpus callosum** that delivers messages from one side to the other. Each hemisphere controls the opposite side of the body, but not all functions of the hemispheres are shared (left controls speech, comprehension, arithmetic, and writing; right controls creativity, spatial ability, artistic, and musical skills.

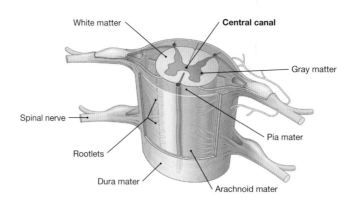

Fig. 1.73 Anatomy of the spinal cord; schematic representation of the spinal cord, in cross-section. [E402]
The spinal cord is the part of the central nervous system (CNS) located within the vertebral canal. It extends from the base of the skull down to the level of the first and second lumbar vertebrae (in the adult), and is covered by the three membranes of the CNS, i.e., the dura mater, arachnoid and the innermost pia mater. Unlike the brain, in the spinal cord the grey matter is surrounded by the white matter at its circumference. Rootlets which carry motor and sensory information to and from the spinal cord extend outward along its length to form spinal nerves.

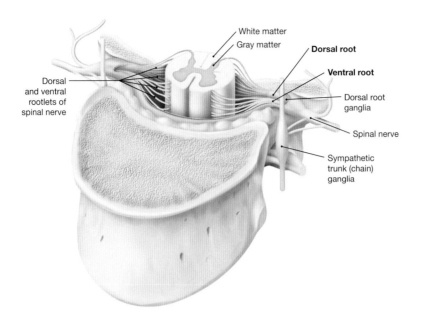

Fig. 1.74 Schematic representation of a spinal nerve (spinal cord segment) exemplified by two thoracic nerves; viewed from above in an oblique lateral angle. [L275]
The ventral and dorsal roots of the spinal cord come together at each vertebral level to form the 31 pairs of spinal nerves of the peripheral nervous system (eight cervical, twelve thoracic, five lumbar, five sacral pairs, one coccygeal pair). Each spinal nerve is composed of a ventral root and a dorsal root. The cell bodies of motor nerves are located in the gray matter within the spinal cord. Their axons leave the spinal cord forming the **ventral root.** The cell bodies of sensory nerves are located in the dorsal root ganglia. Their processes enter the spinal cord via the **dorsal roots.** Communicating branches connect the spinal cord with the chain of sympathetic ganglia of the sympathetic trunk.

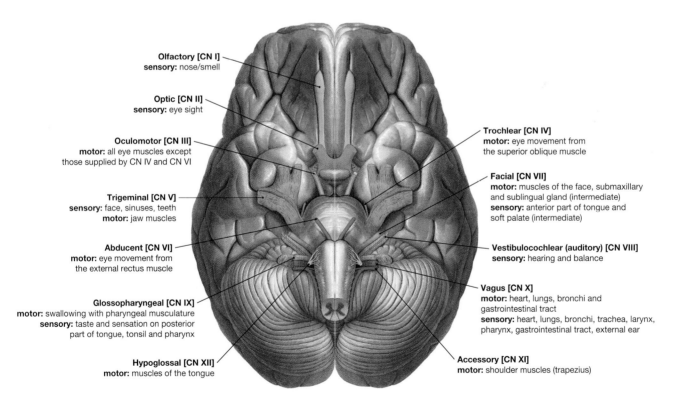

Fig. 1.75 Schematic representation and organization of the twelve cranial nerves arising from the brainstem region of the brain.
There are twelve pairs of cranial nerves that can be seen on the inferior aspect of the brain. Cranial nerves are a component of the peripheral nervous system (PNS) that emerge directly from the brain (not the spinal cord) and relay information from the sense organs (such as the eyes, ears, nose, mouth and tongue) to the brain, control motor function (e.g. contraction of trapezius muscle), or are connected to glands or internal organs such as the heart and lungs. Unlike spinal nerves (which contain both a motor and sensory component), some cranial nerves relay only motor or sensory information, while others may relay both types of information (like a spinal nerve).

Back and Spine

Surface Anatomy of the Back 41

Organization of the Spine 42

Curvatures of the Spine 43

Vertebrae – Basic Features 44

Vertebrae – Foramina 45

Vertebral Column –
Segmental Motion 47

Intervertebral Discs 48

Facet Joints 49

Vertebral Ligaments 50

Cervical Spine 53

Cervical Vertebrae –
Distinguishing Features 55

Occiput (C0) and Atlas (C1) 56

Axis (C2) 57

Atlanto-occipital and
Atlantoaxial Joints 58

Cervical Spine – Ligaments 59

Cervical Spine – Movements 60

Anterior Muscles of
the Cervical Region – Superficial ... 61

Anterior Muscles of
the Cervical Region – Deep 62

Posterior Muscles of
the Cervical Region – Superficial ... 63

Posterior Muscles of
the Cervical Region – Deep 64

Thoracic Spine 65

Thoracic Vertebrae –
Distinguishing Features 66

Lumbar Spine 67

Lumbar Vertebrae –
Distinguishing Features 69

Thoracolumbar Movements 70

Muscles of the Back –
Superficial and Intermediate 71

Muscles of the Back –
Intermediate 72

Muscles of the Back – Deep 73

Sacrum 74

Coccyx 76

Abdominal Muscles 77

Anterior Abdominal Wall 78

Posterior Abdominal Wall 80

Vessels of the Vertebral Column 81

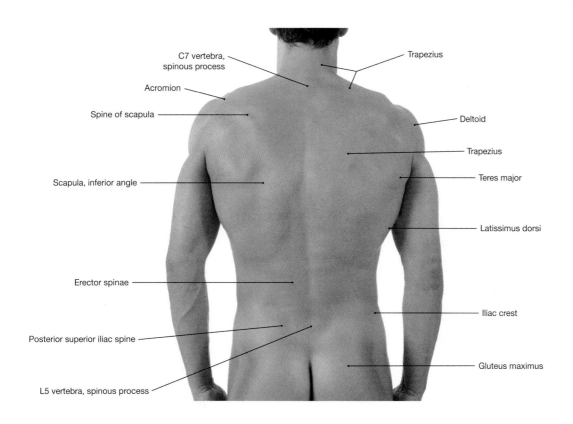

C7 vertebra, spinous process
Acromion
Spine of scapula
Scapula, inferior angle
Erector spinae
Posterior superior iliac spine
L5 vertebra, spinous process

Trapezius
Deltoid
Trapezius
Teres major
Latissimus dorsi
Iliac crest
Gluteus maximus

Fig. 2.1 Surface anatomy of the back; posterior view.

The contours of the back provide useful landmarks to determine different regions of the vertebral column, pelvis, muscles, and the approximate position for the end of the spinal cord.

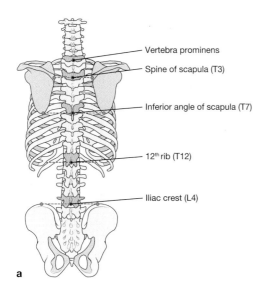

Vertebra prominens
Spine of scapula (T3)
Inferior angle of scapula (T7)
12th rib (T12)
Iliac crest (L4)

a

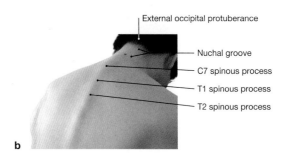

External occipital protuberance
Nuchal groove
C7 spinous process
T1 spinous process
T2 spinous process

b

Fig. 2.2a and b Skeleton and back with bony landmarks. a [L126], b [L271]

a Bony landmarks such as the **vertebra prominens** (the spinous process of the C7 vertebra) are easily palpated. Other vertebrae can be located via their relationship to other easily palpated structures, including the spine of scapula (T3 vertebra), the inferior angle of scapula (T7 vertebra), the 12th rib (T12 vertebra), and the iliac crests (L4 vertebra).

b Forward flexion of the cervical spine allows many of the bony features of the cervical and upper thoracic spine to be more easily identified on palpation.

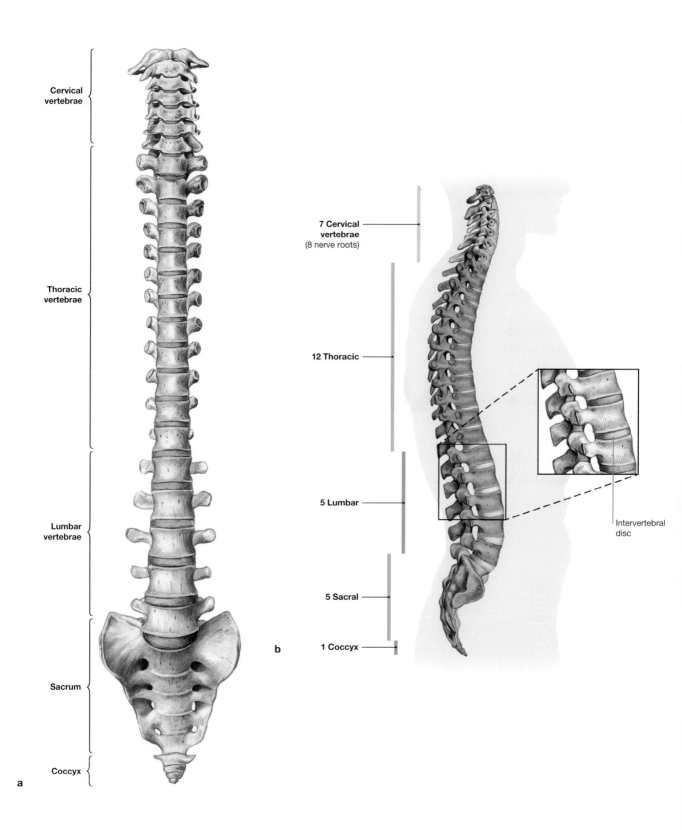

Cervical
vertebrae

Thoracic
vertebrae

Lumbar
vertebrae

Sacrum

Coccyx

a

7 Cervical
vertebrae
(8 nerve roots)

12 Thoracic

5 Lumbar

5 Sacral

1 Coccyx

b

Intervertebral
disc

Fig. 2.3a and b Vertebral column; anterior **(a)** and lateral **(b)** views. b [L127]
The vertebral column accounts for approximately 40 % of the overall height of a healthy human, with ¼ of its length due to the intervertebral discs. The vertebral column is typically described as consisting of **30 vertebrae (7 cervical, 12 thoracic, 5 lumbar, 5 sacral, and 1 coccyx).** The vertebrae of the sacral and coccygeal regions are each fused together to form one distinct segment (sacrum and coccyx). The thoracic vertebrae connect with the twelve paired ribs, the sacrum articulates with the innominate (or hip) bones of the pelvis. In the upright standing position, the physical forces to which the spine is exposed increase as one moves from head to toe. This is reflected by the increase in vertebral size as one progresses inferiorly down the spine (➤ Fig. 12.72).

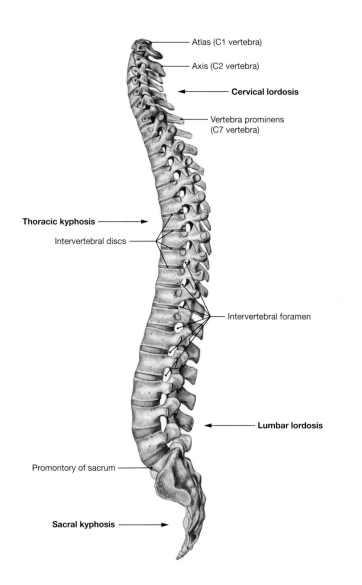

Atlas (C1 vertebra)

Axis (C2 vertebra)

Cervical lordosis

Vertebra prominens (C7 vertebra)

Thoracic kyphosis

Intervertebral discs

Intervertebral foramen

Lumbar lordosis

Promontory of sacrum

Sacral kyphosis

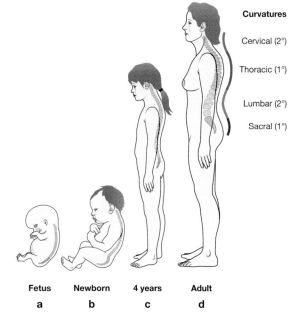

Curvatures

Cervical (2°)

Thoracic (1°)

Lumbar (2°)

Sacral (1°)

Fetus	Newborn	4 years	Adult
a	b	c	d

Fig. 2.4 Vertebral column; view from the left side.
When viewed in the sagittal plane the vertebral column has several normal curvatures:
1. Cervical lordosis
2. Thoracic kyphosis
3. Lumbar lordosis
4. Sacral kyphosis

Lordosis and kyphosis are medical terms used to describe the concave **(lordosis)** or convex **(kyphosis)** curves of the vertebral column (viewed from the side).

Fig. 2.5a to d Vertebral column, curvatures. [L126]
At birth, all sections of the vertebral column show a convex bend – these are referred to as primary curves of the spine. During the first year of life, secondary or concave curvatures of both the cervical and lumbar regions begin to form. These changes in spinal alignment facilitate the child's ability to lift and control head posture and movements, sitting upright (unassisted), standing upright, and learning to walk. The secondary curves of the vertebral column continue to develop as the child grows, and are accentuated by the forward tilt of the pelvis which is necessitated for effective bipedal gait.

Structure/Function

Excessive curvature of the spine can occur as a result of postural changes associated with habitual activities of work or play, or can be secondary to abnormal spinal development. **Scoliosis** is a growth deformity of the spine that results in a fixed lateral curvature, torsion, and rotation of the vertebral column. **(Hyper-)Kyphosis** describes an abnormal increase in the primary convex curvature of the thoracic spine. **(Hyper-)Lordosis** is an exaggeration of the secondary concave curvature in the lumbar spine. [L126]

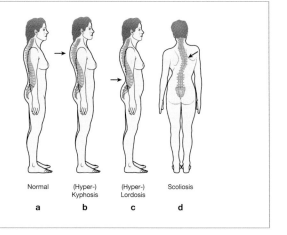

Normal	(Hyper-)Kyphosis	(Hyper-)Lordosis	Scoliosis
a	b	c	d

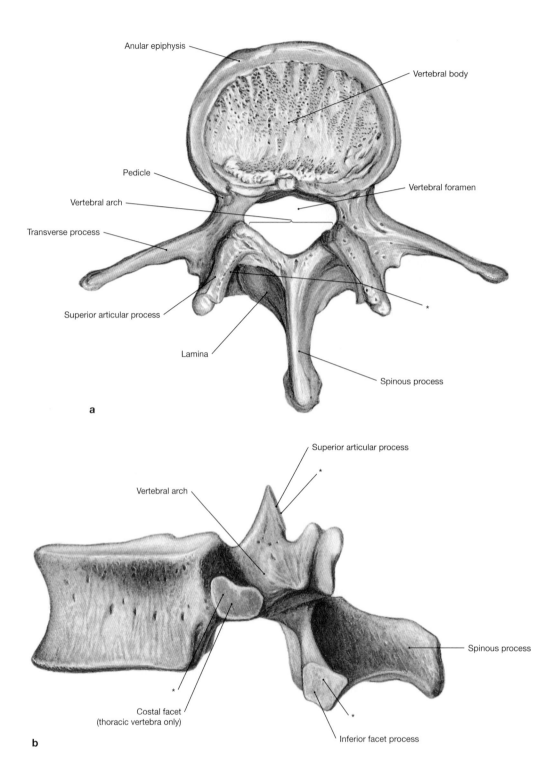

Anular epiphysis

Vertebral body

Pedicle

Vertebral foramen

Vertebral arch

Transverse process

Superior articular process

*

Lamina

Spinous process

a

Superior articular process

*

Vertebral arch

Spinous process

*

Costal facet
(thoracic vertebra only)

*

Inferior facet process

b

Fig. 2.6a and b Lumbar vertebra (L4), superior view **(a); thoracic vertebra (T12),** view from the left side **(b).**
Like the basic construct of the human body (one head/two arms/ one torso/two legs), the vertebrae of the cervical, thoracic and lumbar region each are comprised of similar bony features. These include eight basic components:

1. Vertebral body: the anterior component of the vertebrae. It serves to bear the weight of the body.
2. Vertebral arch: the posterior portion of the vertebrae, forms a closed circle or arch which surrounds and protects the spinal cord.
3. Pedicle: extends posteriorly from both sides of the vertebral body to form the anterior portion of the vertebral arch.

4. Lamina: forms the posterior portion of the vertebral arch.
5. Transverse processes: 'bony arms' which extend laterally from the junction between the pedicle and lamina.
6. Spinous process: 'bony tail' which extends posteriorly from the junction of the two laminae; represents the most posterior aspect of a vertebra.
7. Superior and inferior articular processes: serve as the primary points of articulation between adjacent vertebrae.
8. Vertebral foramen: the opening between vertebral body and vertebral arch. Opening through which the spinal cord travels.

* denotes articular surface

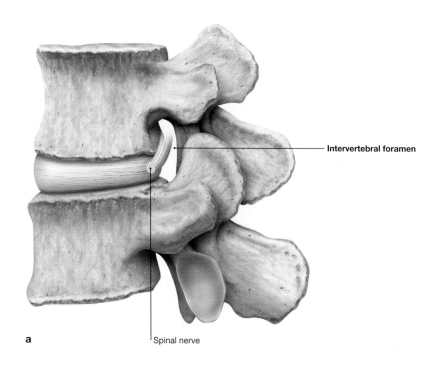

Intervertebral foramen

Spinal nerve

a

Facet joint

Vertebral canal
(with spinal cord)

Vertebral arch

Vertebral body

Intervertebral disc

b

Nucleus pulposus
(core of intervertebral disc)

Vertebral foramen
(with spinal cord)

Spinous process

Anulus fibrosus
(connective tissue ring of intervertebral disc)

c

**Fig. 2.7a to c Intervertebral and vertebral foramina, lateral (a, b)
and superior views (c). [L127]**
The **intervertebral foramen** (also called neural foramen) is a laterally directed tunnel (present on both the left and right sides) which is formed by the articulation of two adjacent vertebrae in the cervical, thoracic and lumbar regions. It facilitates the passage of several structures between the inside/outside of the **vertebral canal,** including:
1. Spinal nerves
2. Dorsal root ganglia
3. Spinal arteries

4. Communicating veins
5. Recurrent meningeal nerves
The **vertebral foramen** is an opening formed by the vertebral arch of the individual vertebrae that creates an opening for passage of the spinal cord. The linkage of multiple **vertebral foramina** of adjacent vertebrae creates the **vertebral canal.** It runs the length of the vertebral column and serves to form a 'bony cage' which protects the spinal cord. The size of the vertebral foramina (and canal) is variable, and can be influenced by spinal location, pathology, spinal loading, and posture.

Clinical Remarks

Posterolateral disc herniations, spondylophytes, or tumors can lead to a **narrowing of an intervertebral foramen** and compression of the spinal nerve roots causing deficits in nerve function. [L126]

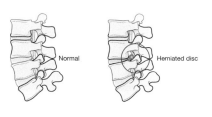

Normal

Herniated disc

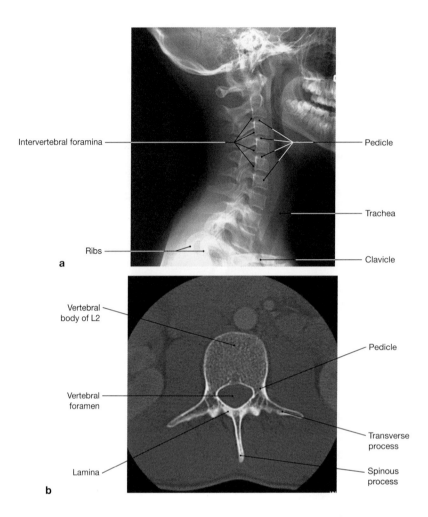

Intervertebral foramina

Pedicle

Trachea

Ribs

Clavicle

a

Vertebral body of L2

Pedicle

Vertebral foramen

Lamina

Transverse process

Spinous process

b

Fig. 2.8a and b Lateral radiograph of the cervical spine (a); CT image of the lumbar spine (L2 vertebra), axial reconstruction (b).
a [E404], b [E458]

Clinical Remarks

Spinal stenosis refers to an abnormal narrowing of a (vertebral or intervertebral) foramen within the vertebral column that can lead to pressure on or compression of the spinal cord and spinal nerve roots. It is most commonly caused by wear-and-tear degenerative changes in the spine (e.g. osteoarthritis). Stenosis can lead to symptoms such as pain, numbness, paresthesia, and loss of motor control. The location of the stenosis will deter-mine which area of the body is affected. Approximately 75% of all spinal stenoses occur in the lumbar spine – leading to symptoms of **sciatica** (tingling, weakness, or numbness that radiates from the low back into the buttocks and legs). In severe cases, physicians may recommend surgery to create additional space for the spinal cord or nerves within the narrowed foramen. [E684]

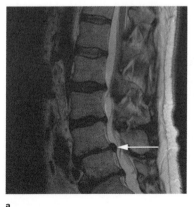

a

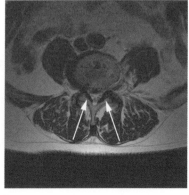

b

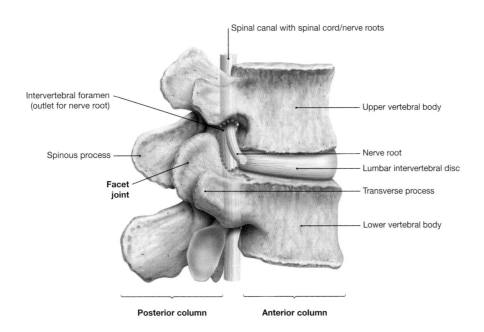

Spinal canal with spinal cord/nerve roots

Intervertebral foramen
(outlet for nerve root)

Upper vertebral body

Spinous process

Nerve root

Lumbar intervertebral disc

Facet joint

Transverse process

Lower vertebral body

Posterior column   **Anterior column**

Fig. 2.9 Lateral view of the spine; right side. [L127]
All movements of the spine are facilitated by segmental motion that occurs between two adjacent vertebrae (called a motion segment). Each **motion segment** of the spine consists of:
- two vertebral bodies;
- an intervertebral disc;
- left and right facet joints; and
- their associated ligamentous structures.

A motion segment can be divided into two columns or regions:
1. **The anterior column is built for stability.** It is formed by the vertebral bodies and the intervertebral disc that sits between them, and is stabilized by a tremendous number of ligamen-

tous structures. It is a fibrocartilaginous joint (symphysis) that is capable of subtle motion and is designed to support the majority of body weight.

2. **The posterior column is built for mobility.** It consists of the vertebral arches and the superior and inferior articular processes of the two adjacent vertebrae. Movements of the posterior column are facilitated by the **left and right facet joints** which are formed by articulation between the superior and inferior articular processes of two adjacent vertebrae. These small synovial joints allow flexion, extension, lateral flexion, and rotation movements to occur between adjacent vertebrae.

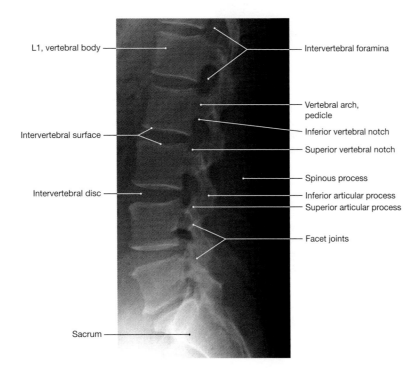

L1, vertebral body

Intervertebral foramina

Vertebral arch, pedicle

Inferior vertebral notch

Superior vertebral notch

Intervertebral surface

Spinous process

Intervertebral disc

Inferior articular process

Superior articular process

Facet joints

Sacrum

Fig. 2.10 Lumbar vertebrae; lateral radiograph of the lumbar part of the vertebral column; upright position; central beam is directed onto the 2nd lumbar vertebra.

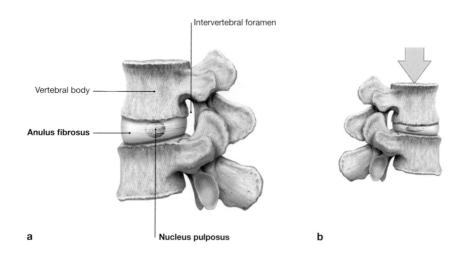

Fig. 2.11a and b Intervertebral discs. Normal (a) and compressed intervertebral disc (b) in a weight-bearing situation. [L127]
One **intervertebral disc** (or **intervertebral fibrocartilage**) is located between the bodies of two adjacent cervical (except at C1/C2 junction), thoracic, and lumbar vertebrae along the length of the verte-

bral column. Each disc helps to form a fibrocartilaginous joint (or symphysis) between two articulating vertebrae, and functions to:
1. add height to the vertebral column;
2. allow subtle movements between vertebrae;
3. serve as a shock absorber within the spine.

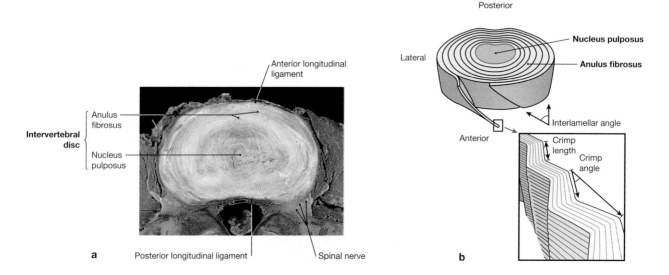

Fig. 2.12a and b Lumbar intervertebral disc; superior view. b [L126]
Each intervertebral disc is comprised of a central jelly-like **nucleus pulposus,** and a fibrous ring – **anulus fibrosus** – which surrounds the nucleus pulposus. The nucleus pulposus helps to distribute

pressure evenly across the disc, while the anulus fibrosus consists of several layers (lamellae) of fibrocartilage made up of type I and type II collagen. The type I is concentrated towards the edge of the ring where it provides greater strength.

Clinical Remarks

Approximately 25 % of individuals under 40 years of age, and 60 % of people older than 40 years show some evidence of disc degeneration. Degenerative changes of an intervertebral disc are most frequently observed in the lumbar and cervical regions of the spine. It can result in disc protrusion or disc prolapse, with the disc tissue most commonly shifting to the posterior and lateral sides. This can lead to compression of the spinal nerves (radiculopathy) as they exit through the intervertebral foramen. The discs located between L4/L5 and L5/S1 are the most common areas of injury.
[L127]

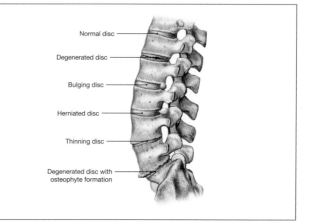

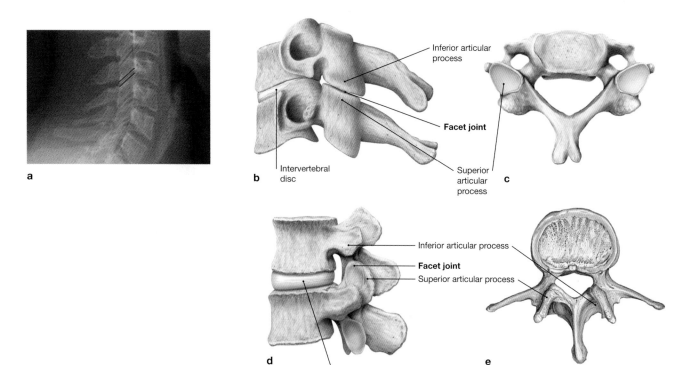

a

b Intervertebral disc

c

Inferior articular process

Facet joint

Superior articular process

Inferior articular process

Facet joint

Superior articular process

d

e

Intervertebral disc

Fig. 2.13a to e Lateral radiograph of the cervical region (a) and lateral and superior views of spinal motion segments (b and c, cervical region; d and e, lumbar region). a [G723], b,d [L127], c [L266]

Facet joints (also referred to as zygapophysial, apophysial, or Z-joints) are a set of synovial joints which occupy the posterior column of a motion segment of the spine. They are formed between the articular processes of two adjacent vertebrae and function to guide and limit movements of each motion segment. The orientation of the facet joint is different in each region of the spine (see Structure/Function below), and thus influences the range of motion possible in each region. Cavitation of the synovial fluid within the facet joints is responsible for the popping sound (crepitus) associated with spinal manipulation, commonly referred to as 'cracking the back'.

Structure/Function

Plane of orientation of facet joints **(a)**; spinal range of motion **(b)**. The facet joints in the lower **cervical region** are oriented 45° to the transverse plane and lie parallel to the frontal plane, with the superior articular processes facing posterior and up and the inferior articular processes facing anterior and down. This facilitates a large range of motion during flexion, extension, lateral flexion, and rotation. The facet joints between adjacent **thoracic vertebrae** are angled at 60° to the transverse plane and 20° to the frontal plane, with the superior facets facing posterolaterally (and a little upwards) and the inferior facets facing anteromedially (and slightly downwards). This facilitates the movements of lateral flexion and rotation, but allows only limited flexion and extension movements. The facet joints in the **lumbar region** are oriented at right angles (90°) to the transverse plane and 45° to the frontal plane. The superior facets face medially, and the inferior facets face laterally (this changes at the lumbosacral junction in order to keep the vertebral column stable on the sacrum). The orientation of the lumbar facets facilitates flexion and extension movements of the lumbar spine, but limits the ability of the region to rotate. [L126]

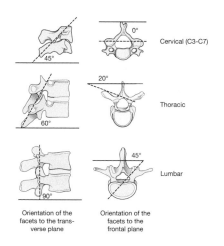

a Orientation of the facets to the transverse plane

Orientation of the facets to the frontal plane

Cervical (C3–C7)

Thoracic

Lumbar

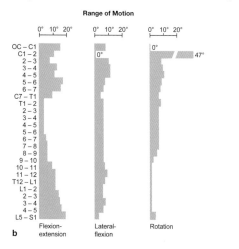

Range of Motion

b Flexion-extension   Lateral-flexion   Rotation

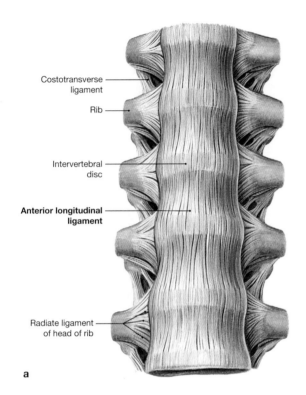

Costotransverse ligament

Rib

Intervertebral disc

Anterior longitudinal ligament

Radiate ligament of head of rib

a

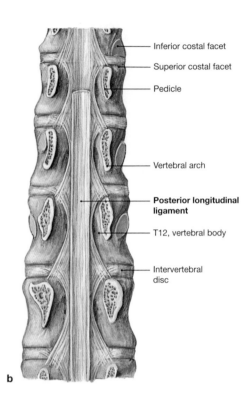

Inferior costal facet

Superior costal facet

Pedicle

Vertebral arch

Posterior longitudinal ligament

T12, vertebral body

Intervertebral disc

b

Fig. 2.14a and b Ligaments of the vertebral column; anterior **(a)** and posterior **(b)** views.

The **anterior longitudinal ligament** ranges from the anterior tubercle of atlas to the sacrum. It is fixed to the anterior surface of the vertebral bodies and to the intervertebral discs. This ligament increases the stability of the vertebral column during extension.

The **posterior longitudinal ligament** is a continuation of the tectorial membrane and extends to the sacral canal. It is fixed to the intervertebral discs and the rims of the intervertebral surfaces and secures the intervertebral discs. It increases the stability of the vertebral column during flexion.

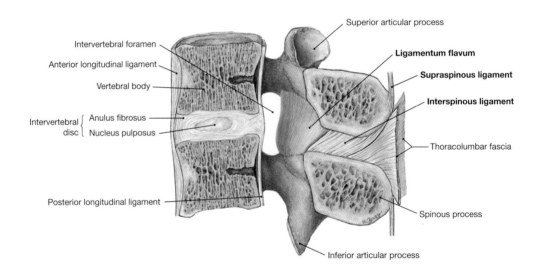

Intervertebral foramen

Anterior longitudinal ligament

Vertebral body

Intervertebral disc { Anulus fibrosus / Nucleus pulposus

Posterior longitudinal ligament

Superior articular process

Ligamentum flavum

Supraspinous ligament

Interspinous ligament

Thoracolumbar fascia

Spinous process

Inferior articular process

Fig. 2.15 Lumbar region; median section; view from the left side.

The **supraspinous ligament** connects the tips of the spinous processes from the C7 vertebrae to the sacrum and functions to limit hyperflexion of the spine. Above the level of C7 it is continuous with the nuchal ligament. The **interspinous ligament** fills in and connects adjoining spinous processes of the vertebral column and functions to limit flexion of the spine. In the thoracolumbar region, the interspinous ligament projects into the thoracolumbar fascia. The **Ligamentum flava** connects the laminae of adjacent vertebrae. They are highly elastic structures which help maintain an upright posture, and assist the vertebral column to resume its normal posture following trunk flexion.

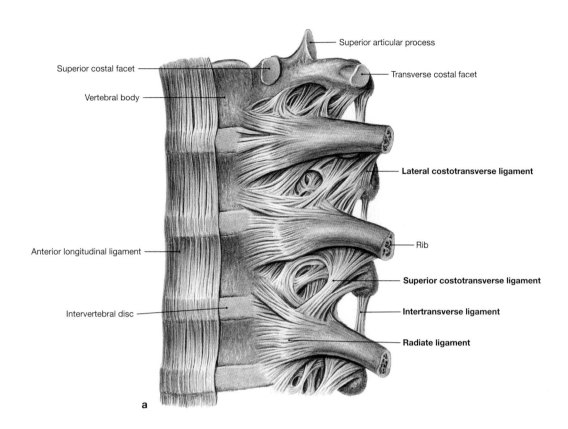

Superior costal facet

Vertebral body

Anterior longitudinal ligament

Intervertebral disc

Superior articular process

Transverse costal facet

Lateral costotransverse ligament

Rib

Superior costotransverse ligament

Intertransverse ligament

Radiate ligament

a

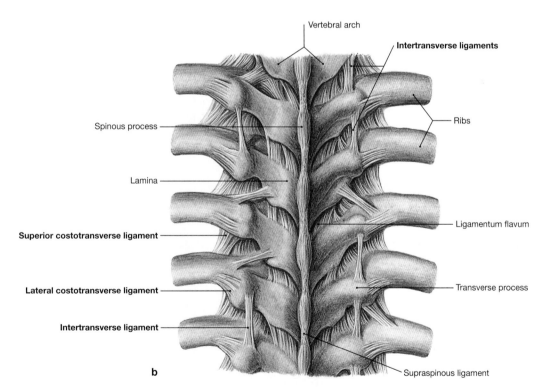

Vertebral arch

Intertransverse ligaments

Spinous process

Lamina

Superior costotransverse ligament

Lateral costotransverse ligament

Intertransverse ligament

Ribs

Ligamentum flavum

Transverse process

Supraspinous ligament

b

Fig. 2.16a and b Ligaments of the vertebral column and the costovertebral joints; view from the left side – lateral parts of the anterior longitudinal ligament removed **(a)**; posterior view **(b)**.
The **radiate ligaments** connect the anterior part of the head of each rib with the sides of two adjacent vertebral bodies, and the intervertebral fibrocartilage between them. The costotransverse joints are supported by the **lateral and superior costotransverse ligaments** which function to prevent dislocation of the ribs from the vertebrae. The **intertransverse ligaments** are located between adjacent transverse processes along the length of the spine, and function to limit lateral flexion of the spine.

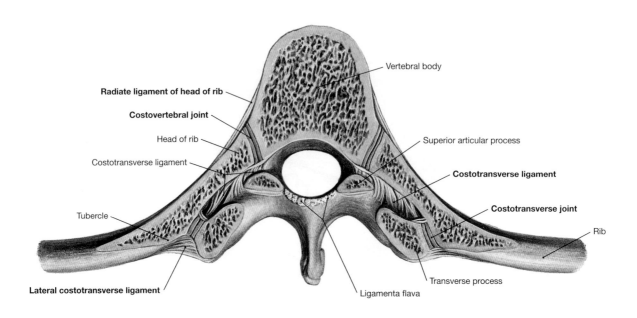

Fig. 2.17 Costovertebral joints; transverse section through the lower part of the costovertebral joint; superior view.
With the exception of the ribs I, XI and XII, two regions of each rib articulate with each thoracic vertebrae. The first point of articulation **(costovertebral joint)** is an articulation between the convex facets of each rib (head), and the bodies of the two adjacent verte-

brae (➤ Fig. 5.21). The second point of articulation **(costotransverse joint)** occurs between the tubercle of each rib and the transverse process of each vertebrae. These two joints are stabilized by the **radiate ligament of the head of the rib,** the **costotransverse ligament,** and the **lateral costotransverse ligament.**

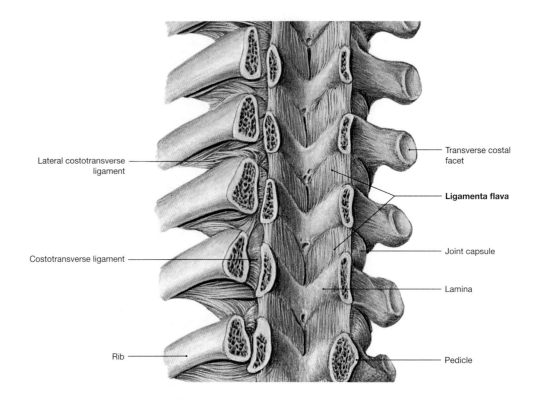

Fig. 2.18 Connections of the vertebral arches; anterior view.
The **ligamenta flava** (yellow color results from the high content of elastic fibers oriented perpendicular to each other) are located between the vertebral arches and extend from the C2 vertebra to the

S1 segment. They line the posterior aspect of the intervertebral foramina and help to support the muscles of the back when extending the vertebral column from all flexed positions.

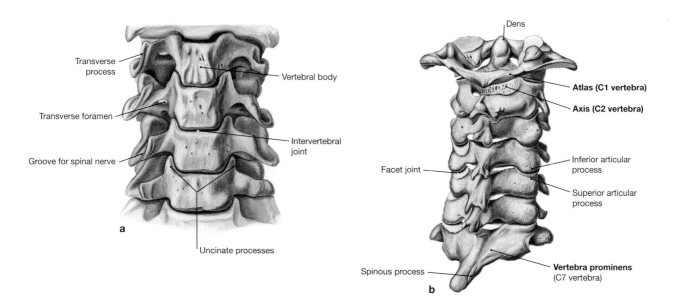

Fig. 2.19a and b **Cervical vertebrae;** anterior view **(a)**; postero-lateral view **(b)**.
The **cervical spine** consists of seven vertebrae, which become progressively larger as you extend down the spine from the C1 to C7 level. The first cervical vertebra (C1) articulates with the base of the skull, and is known as the **atlas.** The C2 vertebra sits directly below it, and is referred to as the **axis.** The C7 vertebra, the **vertebra prominens,** represents the most identifiable and easily palpated vertebra of the cervical region because of its distinctively long and prominent spinous process.

Fig. 2.20a and b **Normal cervical spine;** schematic drawing **(a)** and lateral radiograph **(b)**.
a [L126], b [G724]
A lateral cervical spine X-ray is useful for detecting ominous injuries of the neck. The **anterior vertebral line** (drawn along the anterior margin of the vertebral bodies) should form a smooth curve anteriorly. The **posterior vertebral line** (drawn along the posterior margin of the vertebral bodies) should depict vertebral bodies that are well aligned and positioned with even and consistent **intervertebral disc spaces** – a narrowed space can be a clue that extrusion of a disc has occurred into the spinal canal. Disruption of the **spinolaminar line** (a line drawn along the posterior margin of the vertebral canal) is an important indicator that a vertebral subluxation may have occurred. Loss of continuity of the **posterior spinous line** (a line connecting the tips of the spinous processes) may be indicative of ligamentous injury or bone fracture.

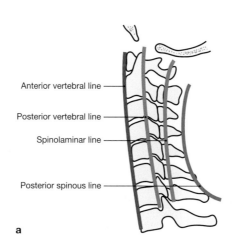
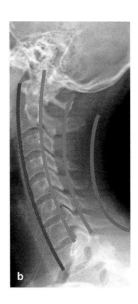

Structure/Function

The normal architecture of a healthy C-spine allows the neck to assume a naturally lordotic posture. This lordosis allows for controlled motion and transmission of forces to the supporting muscles and soft tissues. **a** When the neck is in flexion, the normal lordotic position of the neck is lost, making it highly susceptible to injuries such as a cervical fracture and/or dislocation. **b** As the neck moves into an extended position, the size of the lordotic curve increases.
[G724]

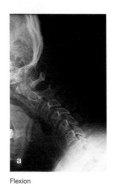
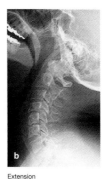

Flexion   Extension

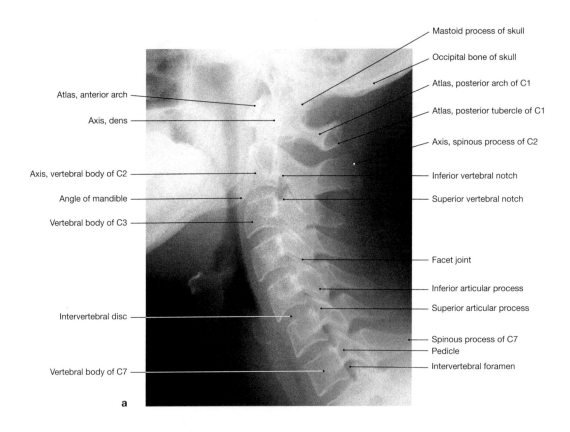

Atlas, anterior arch

Axis, dens

Axis, vertebral body of C2

Angle of mandible

Vertebral body of C3

Intervertebral disc

Vertebral body of C7

Mastoid process of skull

Occipital bone of skull

Atlas, posterior arch of C1

Atlas, posterior tubercle of C1

Axis, spinous process of C2

Inferior vertebral notch

Superior vertebral notch

Facet joint

Inferior articular process

Superior articular process

Spinous process of C7

Pedicle

Intervertebral foramen

a

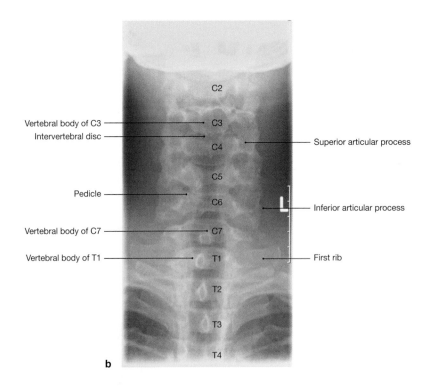

Vertebral body of C3

Intervertebral disc

Pedicle

Vertebral body of C7

Vertebral body of T1

C2
C3
C4
C5
C6
C7
T1
T2
T3
T4

Superior articular process

Inferior articular process

First rib

b

Fig. 2.21a and b Cervical vertebrae, lateral **(a)** and anteroposterior **(b)** radiograph of the cervical spine; upright position; the central beam is directed onto the third cervical vertebra (C3); shoulders are pulled downwards **(a)**. b [R382]

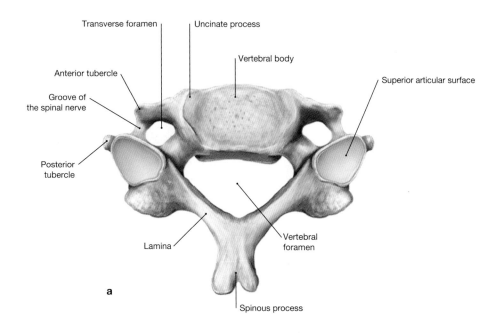

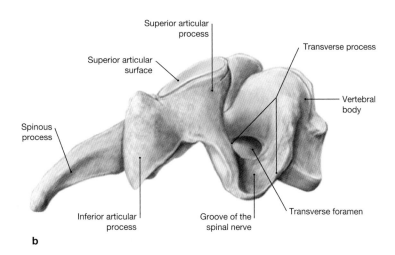

Fig. 2.22a and b Cervical vertebrae; superior **(a)** and lateral **(b)** views. [L266]

The 5th cervical vertebra exemplifies the normal structure of the 3rd to 6th cervical vertebrae – which are considered to be 'typical' cervical vertebrae. The C1 and C2 vertebrae are considered unique or specialized vertebrae. The C7 vertebra (vertebra prominens) is so named for its prominent spinous process.

Cervical vertebrae – distinguishing features
1. Small bodies with uncinate processes
2. Bifid spinous process (except C7)
3. Large, triangular vertebral foramina

4. Small gutter-shaped transverse processes for passage of the spinal nerves
5. Transverse foramina for the passage of the vertebral artery (the vertebral artery passes through the transverse foramen of C1–C6, not C7; ➤ Fig. 11.17)
6. Short articular processes which are oriented 45° to the transverse plane and lie parallel to the frontal plane, with the superior articular processes facing posterior and up and the inferior articular processes facing anterior and down. This facilitates a large range of motion during flexion, extension, lateral flexion, and rotation movements.

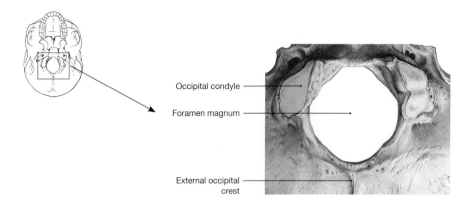

Occipital condyle

Foramen magnum

External occipital crest

Fig. 2.23 Base of occipital bone, region of the foramen magnum and the occipital condyles of the atlanto-occipital joint; inferior view.

The occipital condyles are located lateral to the foramen magnum.

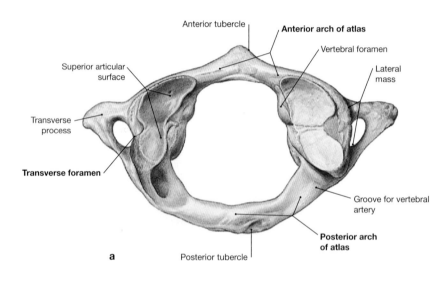

Anterior tubercle

Anterior arch of atlas

Vertebral foramen

Superior articular surface

Lateral mass

Transverse process

Transverse foramen

Groove for vertebral artery

Posterior arch of atlas

a Posterior tubercle

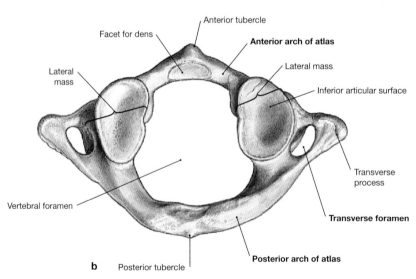

Anterior tubercle

Facet for dens

Anterior arch of atlas

Lateral mass

Lateral mass

Inferior articular surface

Transverse process

Vertebral foramen

Transverse foramen

Posterior arch of atlas

b Posterior tubercle

Fig. 2.24a and b First cervical vertebra (C1), atlas; superior **(a)** and inferior **(b)** views.
The C1 vertebra (or 'atlas') does not possess a vertebral body. The **anterior arch** of the atlas is positioned anterior to and articulates with the dens of the C2 vertebrae. At the **posterior arch,** the spinous process is replaced by a small posterior tubercle. Compared to other cervical vertebrae, the atlas has slightly longer **transverse processes,** with a transverse foramen on both sides, that facilitate passage of the vertebral arteries. Its inferior articular surface is shallow, concave, and tilted at a 30° angle to the transverse plane.

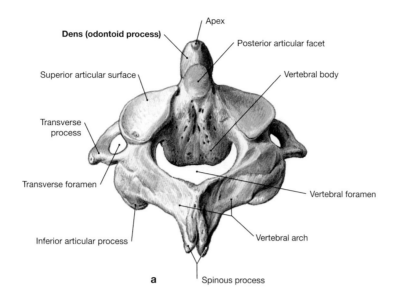

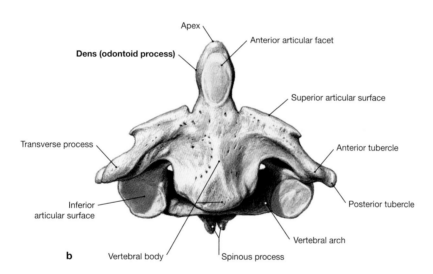

Fig. 2.25a and b Second cervical vertebra (C2), axis; posterior superior **(a)** and anterior **(b)** views.
A distinct feature that sets the axis apart from the other cervical vertebrae is the **dens (odontoid process).** The anterior and posterior surfaces of the dens are covered by articular facets. The articular facets of the superior articular processes are sloped to the outside and the inferior articular processes are positioned in an oblique angle to the frontal plane. The transverse processes of the axis are short and the spinous process is frequently split in two.

Fig. 2.26 First and second cervical vertebrae (C1 and C2), atlas and axis; median section – view from the left side.
A median section permits the inspection of the vertebral canal. The atlas and axis articulate via the **facet for dens** and the **anterior articular facet** forming the median atlantoaxial joint. The posterior arch of the atlas is considerably smaller in relation to the vertebral arch of the axis.

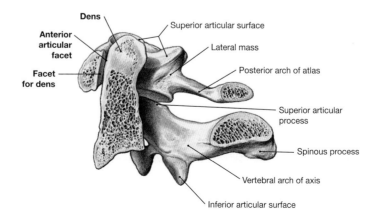

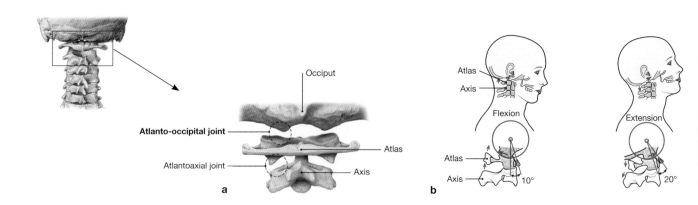

Fig. 2.27a and b Atlanto-occipital joint and atlantoaxial joints, posterior view **(a)**, and range of motion **(b)**. a [L127], b [L126]
a The **atlanto-occipital articulation** is comprised of a pair of condylar synovial joints that connect the **occiput** (C0) to the **atlas** (C1). The joints are comprised of two concave articular surfaces on the superior aspect of the lateral mass of the atlas which articulate with a convex surface on the occipital condyle.

b The primary motions which occur at this joint are flexion and extension (total ROM = 30°, approximately 10° flexion and 20° extension) and slight lateral flexion (total ROM = 15°, approximately 8–10° in each direction).

Movements of C0/C1 Joint	Muscles Active During Movement(s)
Flexion	Longus capitis, rectus capitis anterior
Extension	Rectus capitis posterior, semispinalis capitis, splenius capitis, obliquus capitis superior, sternocleidomastoid, trapezius (upper fibers)
Lateral flexion	Rectus capitis lateralis, splenius capitis, semispinalis capitis, sternocleidomastoid (same side), trapezius (same side)

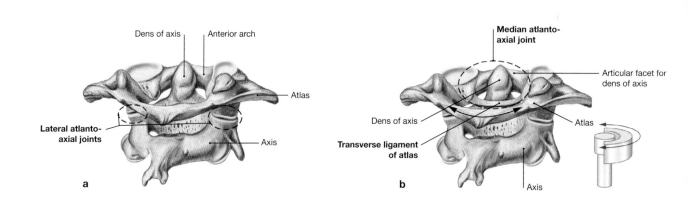

Fig. 2.28a and b Atlantoaxial joints; posterior views, planar type of joint **(a)** and pivot type **(b)**. [L127]
Primary joint motion at the atlantoaxial articulation is maintained by three synovial joints which connect the C1 and C2 vertebrae. The **paired lateral atlantoaxial joints** are classified as planar type synovial joints and are located between the superior and inferior articular processes of the C1 and C2 vertebrae. The midline or **median atlantoaxial joint** is a pivot type of synovial joint formed between the anterior and posterior articular surfaces of the dens (odontoid process) of C2 and the anterior arch and transverse ligament of C1. The primary movement at this joint is rotation – approximately 50°.

Movements of C1/C2 Joint	Muscles Active During Movement(s)
Rotation – ipsilateral contraction	Obliquus capitis superior and inferior, rectus capitis posterior, splenius capitis, longissimus capitis
Rotation – contralateral contraction	Sternocleidomastoid, semispinalis capitis

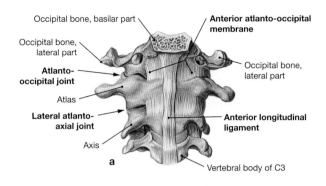

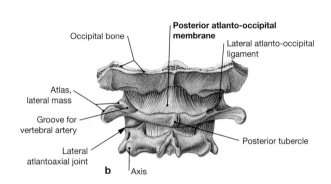

Fig. 2.29a and b Superficial ligaments; anterior **(a)** and posterior **(b)** views.
The **atlanto-occipital joint** is located between the occiput (C0) of the skull and the first cervical vertebra (atlas/C1). It is supported by an **anterior atlanto-occipital membrane** – which is a dense, broad fibrous structure which connects the anterior arch of atlas to the skull, and is a continuation of the **anterior longitudinal ligament** which prevents excessive extension of the neck. The **posterior atlanto-occipital membrane** forms a broad but thin fibrous membrane which connects the foramen magnum to the superior aspect of the posterior arch of the atlas and blends with the joint capsule laterally.

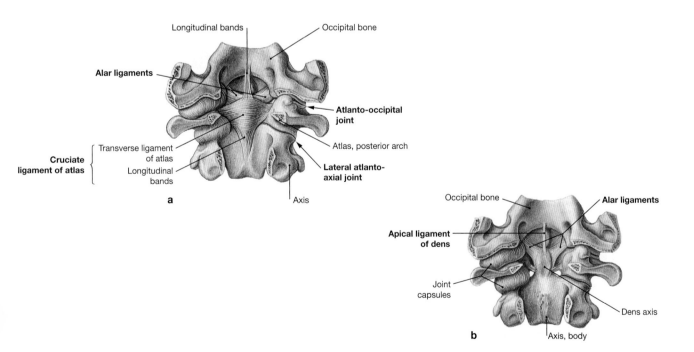

Fig. 2.30a and b Deep ligaments; posterior views – after removal of the tectorial membrane **(a)** and after removal of the cruciate ligament of atlas **(b)**.
Centrally located is the **cruciate ligament of atlas** composed of the transverse ligament of the atlas and the two longitudinal bands. Behind this ligament the **alar (winged) ligaments** are located which originate from the tip and the lateral surface of the dens; they project upwards at an oblique angle. On the left side **(a)**, the joint capsules of the **atlanto-occipital joint** and the lateral **atlantoaxial joint** are shown. On the right side **(b)**, the joint capsules have been removed and the joint cavity is visible. This facilitates visualization of the alar ligaments which frequently insert on the lateral mass of the atlas and the thin **apical ligament of dens.**

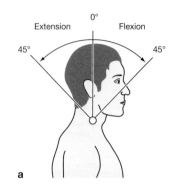

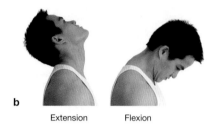

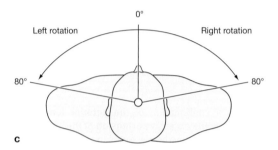

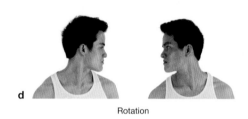

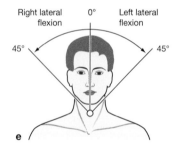

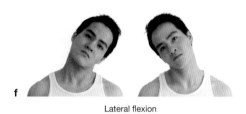

Fig. 2.31a to f Range of motion of the cervical region. a, c, e [L126], b, d, f [L271]

The cervical region can be divided into an upper cervical region – consisting of the atlanto-occipital (C0–C1) and atlantoaxial (C1–C2) joints; and a lower cervical region – consisting of connections between the cervical vertebrae C2–C3 through C6–C7, which all have a similar type of anatomy including intervertebral discs and facet joints. There are six movements possible in the normal range of motion of the cervical spine (**b** flexion/extension, **d** rotation right/left, **f** lateral flexion right/left). The range of motion at each motion segment (i.e. between two adjacent vertebrae) is significantly influenced by the orientation of the facet joints at each level.

Movements of Cervical Spine (C2–C7)	Muscles Active During Movement(s)
Flexion	Sternocleidomastoid; scalenes, longus coli, longus capitis, rectus capitis anterior
Extension	Splenius capitis, semispinalis capitis, semispinalis cervicis, splenius cervicis, semispinalis thoracis, rectus capitis posterior, obliquus capitis
Lateral flexion	Scalenes, longus capitis, rectus capitis lateralis, longus colli, semispinalis capitis, semispinalis cervicis, semispinalis thoracis
Rotation	Sternocleidomastoid, splenius capitis, longus capitis, longus colli, rectus capitis posterior, obliquus capitis, semispinalis thoracis, semispinalis capitis, semispinalis cervicis, splenius cervicis

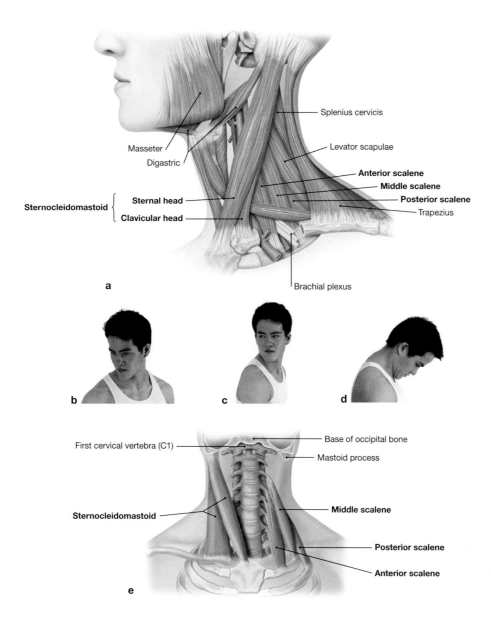

Fig. 2.32a to e **Muscles of the neck;** anterolateral **(a)** and anterior **(e)** views; superficial layer. a [L127], b–d [L271], e [L238]
Superficial muscles of the neck (➤ Fig. 11.11) can function both in a unilateral and bilateral manner to power everyday movements of the head and neck region:

b neck flexion and rotation to contralateral side – i.e. tilting your head and neck forward and looking over opposite shoulder;
c neck rotation – i.e. looking over your shoulder;
d neck flexion – i.e. bringing your chin to your chest.

Muscle	Attachments (P = proximal, D = distal)	Action/Function	Innervation
Sternocleidomastoid	**P:** mastoid process of temporal bone, lateral ½ of superior nuchal line **D:** anterior surface of manubrium of sternum (sternal head); medial ⅓ of clavicle (clavicular head)	Bilateral contraction: neck flexion; Unilateral contraction: tilts head to contralateral side – i.e. flexes and rotates neck so that face is turned superiorly to the opposite side	Spinal root of accessory nerve (motor), C2 and C3 nerves (pain and proprioception)
Scalenes	**Anterior** **P:** anterior surface of transverse processes of C3–C7 **D:** 1st rib **Middle** **P:** posterior surface of transverse processes of C3–C7 **D:** 1st rib **Posterior** **P:** posterior surface of transverse processes of C4–C6 **D:** 2nd rib	Bilateral contraction: neck flexion; rib elevation during deep inspiration Unilateral contraction: lateral flexion of the neck to the ipsilateral side.	**Anterior:** anterior rami of cervical spinal nerves C4–C6 **Middle:** anterior rami of cervical spinal nerves C3–C7 **Posterior:** anterior rami of cervical spinal nerves C7 and C8

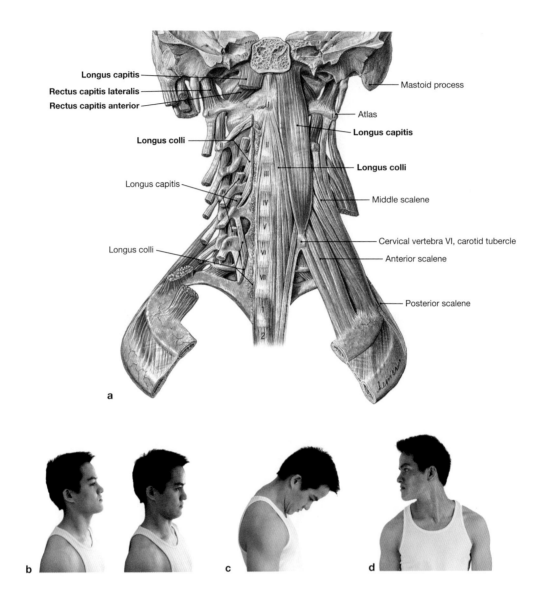

Fig. 2.33a to d Muscles of the neck; anterior view; deep layer.
b–d [L271]
a Deep muscles of the neck help to control precise movements of both the head and the cervical spine such as:

b stabilizing the head and cervical spine – i.e. tucking your chin;
c neck flexion – i.e. bringing your chin to your chest;
d neck rotation – i.e. looking over your shoulder.

Muscle	Attachments (P = proximal, D = distal)	Action/Function	Innervation
Longus capitis	**P:** basilar part of occipital bone **D:** anterior surface of transverse processes C3–C6	Bilateral contraction: cervical flexion Unilateral contraction: rotation and lateral flexion to the ipsilateral side	Anterior rami of cervical nerves C1–C4.
Rectus capitis	**Anterior** **P:** base of skull: anterior to occipital condyle **D:** anterior surface of lateral mass of atlas (C1) **Lateralis** **P:** jugular process of occipital bone **D:** transverse process of C1 vertebra	Anterior: aids in neck flexion Lateralis: head stabilization, lateral flexion	C1 and C2 cervical nerves
Longus colli	**P:** anterior surface of C1 vertebra, bodies of C1–C3 vertebrae, transverse processes of C3–C6 vertebrae **D:** bodies of C5–T3 vertebrae, transverse processes of C3–C6	Bilateral contraction: flexion of head and neck Unilateral contraction: rotation to the ipsilateral side	Anterior rami of cervical nerves C2–C6

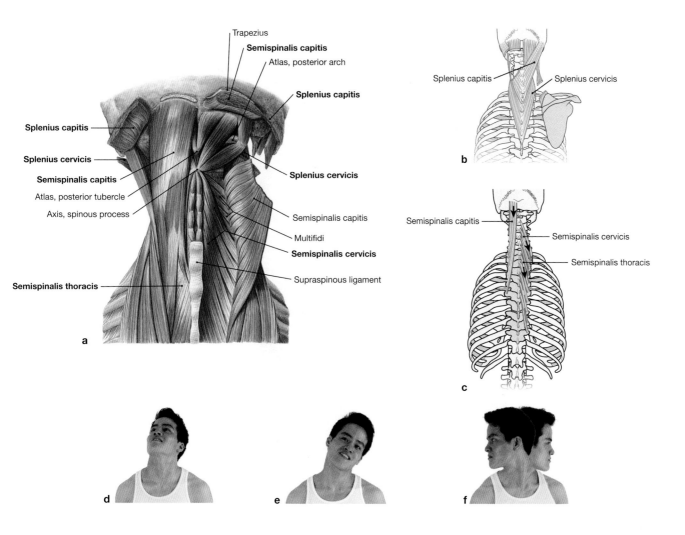

Fig. 2.34a to f Muscles of the neck; posterior view; superficial layer; overview **(a)**, splenius **(b)** and semispinalis muscles **(c).** b, c [L126], d–f [L271]
Superficial muscles of the posterior aspect of the neck contract bilaterally to primarily power extension movements of the head and neck; they also contract unilaterally and work in concert with muscles located on the anterior side of the neck to power lateral flexion and rotation of the neck.
d Extension of the head and neck – i.e. looking up to the sky;
e lateral flexion of the neck – i.e. moving your ear towards your shoulder;
f rotation of neck – i.e. looking over your shoulder.

Muscle	Attachments (P = proximal, D = distal)	Action/Function	Innervation
Splenius	**Capitis** **P:** mastoid process **D:** nuchal ligament and spinous processes of C7–T3 **Cervicis** **P:** transverse processes of C1–C3 **D:** spinous processes of T3–T6	**Capitis and Cervicis:** Bilateral contraction: extension of head and neck Unilateral contraction: lateral flexion and rotation to the ipsilateral side	**Capitis:** posterior rami of spinal nerves C3 and C4 **Cervicis:** posterior rami of lower cervical nerves
Semispinalis	**Capitis** **P:** between superior and inferior nuchal lines of occipital bones **D:** transverse processes of C7, T1–T6 **Cervicis** **P:** spinous processes of C1–C5 **D:** transverse processes of T1–T6 **Thoracis** **P:** spinous processes of C6 and C7, T1–T4 **D:** transverse processes of T6–T10	**Capitis and Cervicis:** Bilateral contraction: extension of head and neck Unilateral contraction: lateral flexion of neck to same side; rotation of head to the contralateral side **Thoracis:** Bilateral contraction: extension of the cervical and thoracic region Unilateral contraction: lateral flexion of the cervical and thoracic region to same side; rotation to the contralateral side	**Capitis:** posterior rami of lower cervical nerves **Cervicis:** posterior rami of lower cervical nerves **Thoracis:** posterior rami of upper thoracic nerves

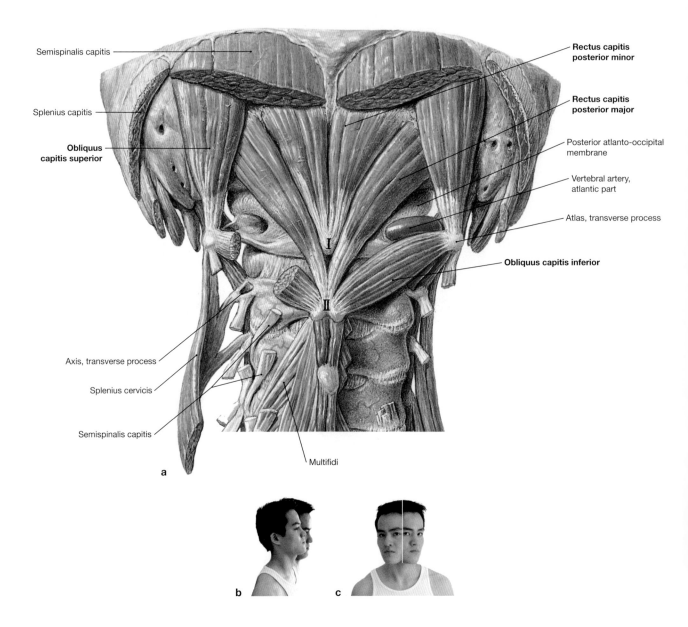

Fig. 2.35a to c Suboccipital muscles; posterior view; deep layer.
b, c [L271]
a The **rectus capitis posterior** and **obliquus capitis muscles** create
the margins of the **suboccipital triangle**.

They are responsible for statically stabilizing the head on the cervical spine and powering subtle movements of the head, such as
b nodding your head – i.e. saying yes; or
c shaking your head – i.e. saying no.

Muscle	Attachments (P = proximal, D = distal)	Action/Function	Innervation
Rectus capitis posterior	**Major** **P:** lateral aspect of inferior nuchal line of the occipital bone **D:** spinous process of C2 **Minor** **P:** medial ⅓ of inferior nuchal line **D:** posterior arch of C1 vertebra	Extension of head on C1 vertebra, rotation of the head and C1 on C2 vertebra	Suboccipital nerve (posterior ramus of C1)
Obliquus capitis	**Superior** **P:** between superior and inferior nuchal lines of the occipital bone **D:** transverse process of C1 vertebra **Inferior*** **P:** transverse process of C1 vertebra **D:** spinous process of C2 vertebra * Only capitis muscle does not attach directly to cranium	Extension of head on C1 vertebra, rotation of the head and C1 on C2 vertebra	Suboccipital nerve (posterior ramus of C1)

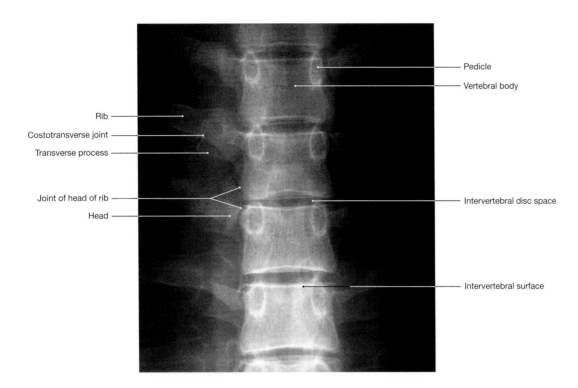

Rib
Costotransverse joint
Transverse process

Joint of head of rib
Head

Pedicle
Vertebral body

Intervertebral disc space

Intervertebral surface

Fig. 2.36 Thoracic vertebrae; anteroposterior (A/P) radiograph of the thoracic region of the vertebral column; upright position with thorax in inspiration; central beam is directed onto the thoracic vertebra T6.

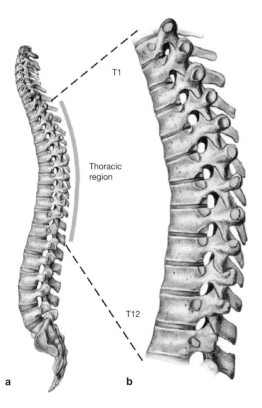

T1

Thoracic region

T12

a   b

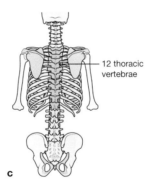

12 thoracic vertebrae

c

Fig. 2.37a to c Thoracic vertebrae (T1–T12); lateral **(a, b)** and posterior **(c)** views. a, b [L127], c [L126]
The thoracic spine is located in the upper-to-middle back – extending down about five inches past the bottom of the shoulder blades, where it connects with the lumbar spine. It is built for stability and plays an important role in holding the body upright and providing protection for the vital organs in the chest. It assists in the formation of the rib cage, as each of the 12 pairs of ribs connect with a thoracic vertebra at the corresponding level.

Clinical Remarks

(Hyper-)Kyphosis refers to an exaggeration in the primary or normal anterior convex curvature of the vertebral column. With extreme anterior curvature of the thoracic region, a pronounced kyphotic curve can lead to a hump formation (gibbus deformity), which can present in various forms, depending on the age of the affected individual – in early childhood as **humpback;** in adolescence as juvenile or **adolescent kyphosis** (SCHEUERMANN's disease); in adults as **senile kyphosis** due to loss of elasticity and disc degeneration. Congenital kyphosis usually results from hemi- or fused vertebrae.   [G725]

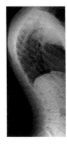

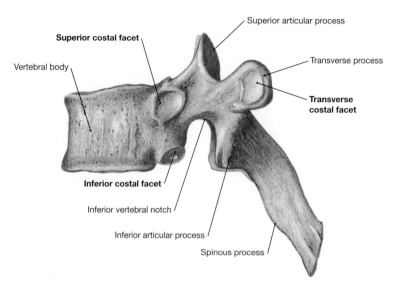

Fig. 2.38 Thoracic vertebra (T6); view from the left side.
Illustration of the **superior and inferior costal facets** for the head(s) of rib(s), the superior and inferior articular processes of the facet joints positioned almost in the frontal plane, the **transverse costal facets** for the articulation with the tubercle of the ribs, the inferior vertebral notch, and the spinous process pointing sharply downwards.

Thoracic vertebrae – distinguishing features
1. Heart-shaped vertebral bodies.
2. Small, circular vertebral foramina.

3. Long spinous processes that slope posteroinferiorly and extend to the level of the next vertebral body below.
4. Costal facets (superior, inferior and transverse) are found on the vertebral bodies and transverse processes for articulation with the heads of the rib(s).
5. The facet joints are angled at 60° to the transverse plane and 20° to the frontal plane, with the superior facets facing posterolaterally (and a little upwards) and the inferior facets facing anteromedially (and slightly downwards). This facilitates lateral flexion and rotation, but allows only limited flexion and extension movements.

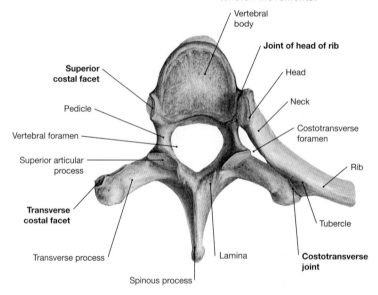

Fig. 2.39 Thoracic vertebra; detailing the typical structure of a thoracic vertebra; superior view.
In the thoracic region, each vertebral body possesses laterally located **superior and inferior facets** for articulation with the head of each rib. The **costotransverse joint** is formed by articulation of each transverse process with the tubercle of each corresponding rib (➤ Fig. 5.17).

Clinical Remarks

Osteoporosis is a metabolic bone disease which is characterized by localized or universal reduction of bone tissue without changing the external shape of the bone. This condition mostly affects women over 55 and men over 70 years of age. Genetic predisposition, low physical activity, malnutrition, and unfavorable estrogen levels contribute to the development of osteoporosis. As a result of the weakened bone structure, fractures of the vertebral column, distal radius, and of the head of femur can occur.
[L126]

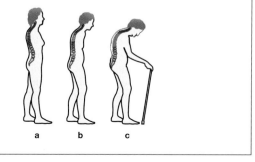

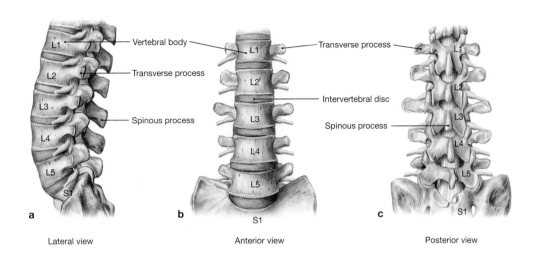

a — Lateral view

b — Anterior view

c — Posterior view

Fig. 2.40a to c Lumbar vertebrae; lateral **(a)**, anterior **(b)**, and posterior **(c)** views. [L127]
The lumbar spine refers to the lower back region. It begins approximately 5 to 6 inches below the shoulder blades, and extends into the pelvis, where it connects with the sacral region of the spine. The word 'lumbar' is derived from the Latin word 'lumbus' meaning loin. It is built for both power and stability – enabling common activities of daily living such as lifting and bending.

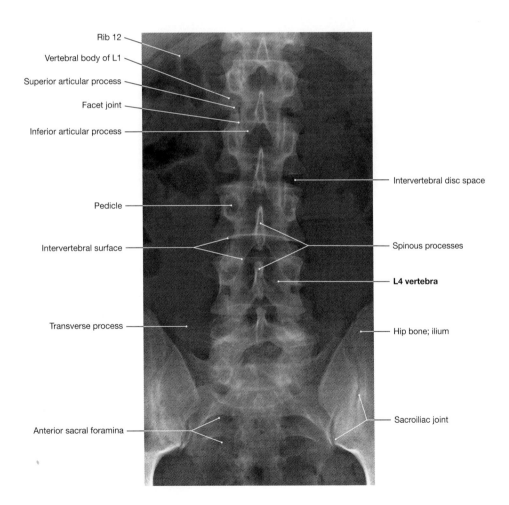

Fig. 2.41 Lumbar vertebrae and sacrum; A/P-radiograph of the lumbar part of the vertebral column and sacrum; upright position; central beam is directed onto the L2 vertebra. The **L4 vertebra** can be found at the level of the iliac crests of the innominate bone.

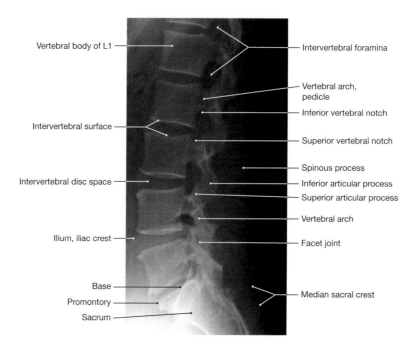

Vertebral body of L1 — Intervertebral foramina

Vertebral arch, pedicle

Inferior vertebral notch

Intervertebral surface — Superior vertebral notch

Spinous process

Intervertebral disc space — Inferior articular process

Superior articular process

Vertebral arch

Ilium, iliac crest — Facet joint

Base —

Promontory — Median sacral crest

Sacrum —

Fig. 2.42 Lumbar vertebrae; lateral radiograph of the lumbar part of the vertebral column; upright position; central beam is directed onto the L2 vertebra. The anterior edges of the lower lumbar vertebrae are oblique and an initial sign of degenerative changes.

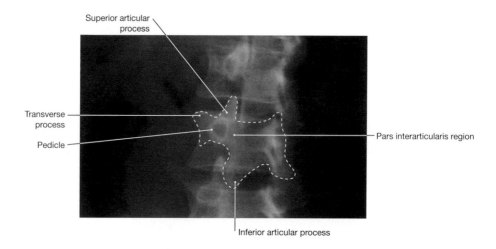

Superior articular process

Transverse process

Pedicle — Pars interarticularis region

Inferior articular process

Fig. 2.43 Lumbar vertebrae; radiograph with beam in an oblique angle; upright position. [E402]

The experienced radiologist can recognize a dog-like figure in this oblique radiograph image. The posterior elements of the vertebrae form the figure of a **'scotty dog'**.

Clinical Remarks

Scotty dog sign with a collar

If a **spondylolysis** deformity is present (a fracture of the pars interarticularis region of the vertebrae) in the lumbar spine, the neck of the scotty dog will have a defect or break (arrow on X-ray), and often looks as though the scotty dog is wearing a collar around its neck.

[E329-002]

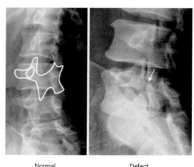

Normal   Defect

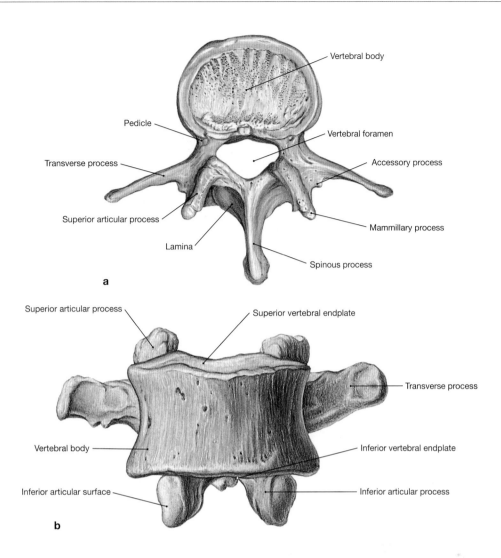

a

b

Fig. 2.44a and b Typical lumbar vertebra (L4); superior (a) and anterior (b) views.
The lumbar vertebrae are larger and structurally more compact in order to withstand the large compression forces imposed by body weight. The first lumbar vertebra is positioned at the same level as the anterior end of rib IX. This level is also referred to as the transpyloric plane – as the pylorus of the stomach is at this level. The fifth lumbar vertebra (L5) is characterized by its body being much deeper in front than behind (due to its articulation with the base of the sacrum).

Lumbar vertebrae – distinguishing features
1. Large kidney-shaped vertebral bodies.
2. Triangular vertebral foramina.
3. Large, short, thick spinous processes.
4. Long, slender, transverse processes.
5. Articular processes are orientated in the sagittal plane; the articular facets are at right angles to the transverse plane and 45° to the frontal plane. The superior facets face medially, and the inferior facets face laterally (this changes at the lumbosacral junction in order to keep the vertebral column from sliding forward on the sacrum). The orientation of the lumbar facets allows flexion and extension movements, but limits the ability of the region to rotate or laterally flex.

Clinical Remarks

Spondylolysis (spon-dee-low-lye-sis) and **spondylolisthesis** (spon-dee-low-lis-thee-sis) are two separate, yet related conditions that cause pain within the lumbar spine. Spondylolysis comes from the term 'spondylo', which means 'spine', and 'lysis', which means to divide. It refers to a fracturing of the pars interarticularis region of a vertebra (most commonly occurring at the level of L4 or L5 vertebrae). The fracture can occur on one side (unilateral) or both sides (bilateral) of the vertebra. If a spondylolysis is present, then there is potential to develop a spondylolisthesis. It refers to an actual slippage of one vertebra forward upon another (the term 'listhesis' means 'to slip forward'). This occurs when the pars interarticularis separates and allows the vertebral body to move forward and out of position.

Slippage is measured on a scale from grade 1 slippage (25 %) to grade 4 (100 %), and significantly influences the size of a patient's lordotic curve (the steeper the grade, the larger the lordotic curve). [L126]

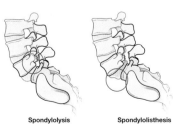

Spondylolysis   Spondylolisthesis

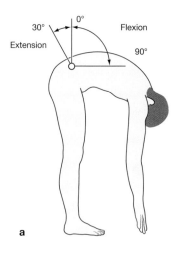

a

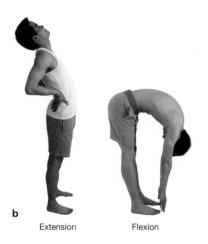

b

Extension   Flexion

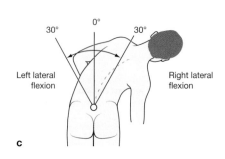

c

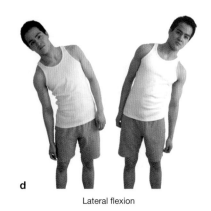

d

Lateral flexion

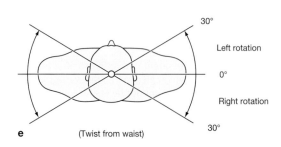

e   (Twist from waist)

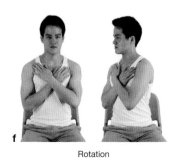

f

Rotation

Fig. 2.45a to f Range of motion of the thoracolumbar region.
a, c, e [L126], b, d, f [L271]
It is very difficult to isolate movements of back and spine to either
the thoracic or lumbar regions. Instead, the movements of
b flexion/extension,
d lateral flexion, and

f rotation of the trunk are described as **thoracolumbar movements,**
in recognition of the fact that both the thoracic and lumbar regions
of the spine work in concert to facilitate normal trunk motion.

Thoracolumbar Movements	Muscles Active During this Movement(s)
Flexion	Rectus abdominis, psoas major, internal oblique, external oblique, psoas major, ilipsoas
Extension	Erector spinae, multifidus, semispinalis thoracis, quadratus lumborum, serratus posterior inferior
Lateral flexion	Multifidus, external and internal oblique muscles, quadratus lumborum, erector spinae, psoas major
Rotation	Rotatores, multifidus, external oblique (acting together with opposite internal oblique), semispinalis thoracis

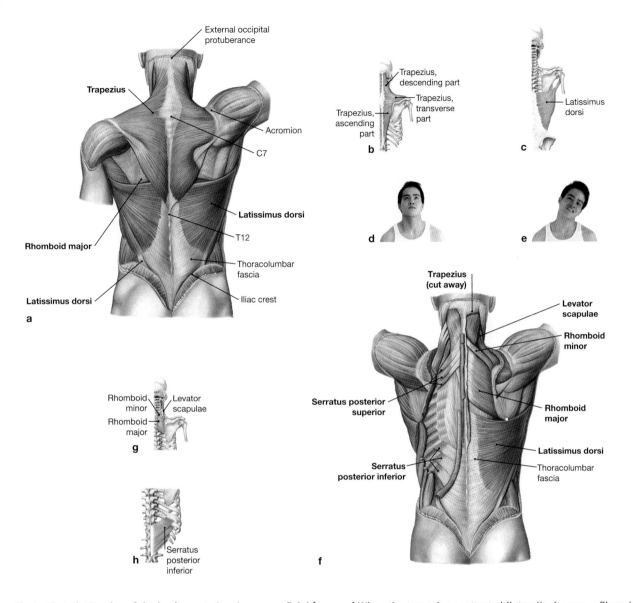

Fig. 2.46a to i Muscles of the back; posterior view; superficial **(a to c)** and intermediate layers **(g to h)**. b, c, g [L266], d, e [L271], h [L284]

The **trapezius** (b) and **latissimus dorsi** (c) are the most superficial muscles of the back and can be easily palpated (➤ Fig. 3.25a). Immediately beneath the superficial back muscles are the **rhomboids (h), levator scapulae (h),** and **serratus posterior (i)** muscles.

d When the trapezius contracts bilaterally, its upper fibers help to **power forceful extension** of the neck – i.e. extending your neck against a resistance.

e When upper muscle fibers of the trapezius contract unilaterally they **power ipsilateral lateral flexion** – i.e. bringing your ear closer to the shoulder.

Muscle	Attachments (P = proximal, D = distal)	Action/Function	Innervation
Trapezius	**P:** Medial $^1/_3$ of superior nuchal line of occiput; external occipital protuberance; spinous processes of C7–T12 vertebrae **D:** Lateral $^1/_3$ of clavicle, acromion and spine of scapula	Bilateral contraction: when shoulder is stabilized – neck extension. Unilateral contraction: neck lateral flexion	Spinal root of accessory nerve (CN XI), and cervical plexus (C3 and C4)
Latissimus dorsi	**P:** Spinous processes of lower 6 thoracic vertebrae; thoracolumbar fascia; iliac crest **D:** Floor of bicipital groove of humerus	Bilateral contraction: functions synergistically to stabilize lumbar spine, and assists with lateral flexion to the ipsilateral side	Thoracodorsal nerve (C6, C7, C8)
Rhomboid major and minor	**P:** Nuchal ligament and C7–T1 spinous processes (minor); T2–T5 spinous processes (major) **D:** Medial border of the scapula	Scapular retraction; holds scapula flat against thoracic wall	Dorsal scapular nerve (C4 and C5)
Levator scapulae	**P:** Transverse processes of C1–C4 vertebrae **D:** Superior aspect of medial border of scapula	When shoulder is stabilized – rotation and lateral flexion to the ipsilateral side. Bilateral contraction produces cervical extension	Dorsal scapular nerve (C5) and cervical plexus (C3 and C4)
Serratus posterior inferior	**P:** Spinous processes of T11–L2 **D:** Inferior borders of ribs IX–XII	Thoracolumbar extension (bilateral contraction) and rotation to the ipsilateral side	Segmental innervation – intercostal nerves T9–T12

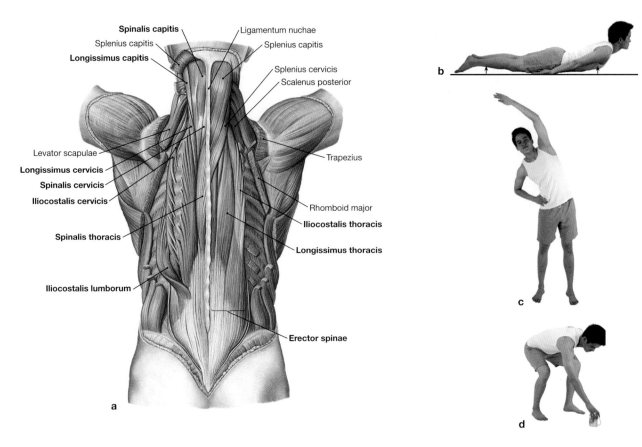

Fig. 2.47a to d Erector spinae muscles of the back; posterior view (a). b–d [L271]

The **erector spinae** muscles are a set of vertically positioned muscles that run parallel to the spine along its entire length from the sacral region to the upper cervical vertebrae. Anatomically, they are classically described as being comprised of three distinct columns of muscles – **iliocostalis** (lateral column), **longissimus** (intermediate column) and **spinalis** (medial column).

b From a functional standpoint, the three sections work together to **power extension movements of the spine** during bilateral contraction;

c lateral flexion movements of the spine when contracting unilaterally; and

d function primarily in an 'anti-gravity' capacity during forward flexion movements of the spine – eccentric contraction of the erector spine muscles allows the spine to be slowly flexed and lowered in a controlled and coordinated manner against gravity (i.e. slowly lowering or forward bending your trunk to pick up an object on the floor).

Sections of Erector spinae	Attachments (P = proximal, D = distal)	Action and Innervation
Iliocostalis (lateral column)	**Cervicis** **P:** C4–C6 transverse processes **D:** angles of ribs I–VI **Thoracis** **P:** angles of ribs I–VI, C7 transverse process **D:** angles of ribs VI–XII **Lumborum** **P:** angles of ribs VI–XII **D:** posterior sacrum, iliac crest, sacrotuberous ligament, posterior sacroiliac ligament, transverse processes of T11–L5 vertebrae	Actions: spine extension (bilateral contraction) and side flexion to ipsilateral side Innervation: segmental innervation by posterior rami of spinal nerves
Longissimus (intermediate column)	**Capitis** **P:** T1–T3 transverse processes, C3–C7 articular processes **D:** mastoid process of temporal bone **Cervicis** **P:** T1–T6 transverse processes **D:** C2–C7 transverse processes **Thoracis** **P:** L1–L5 transverse processes **D:** T1–T12 transverse processes, ribs III to XII	Actions: spine extension (bilateral contraction) and side flexion to ipsilateral side Innervation: segmental innervation by posterior rami of spinal nerves
Spinalis (medial column)	**Capitis** **P:** C7–T6 transverse processes, and articular processes of C4–C6 vertebrae **D:** superior and inferior nuchal lines of the occiput bone **Cervicis** **P:** C6–T2 spinous processes **D:** C2–C4 spinous processes **Thoracis** **P:** T10–L3 spinous processes **D:** T2–T8 spinous processes	Actions: spine extension (bilateral contraction) and side flexion to ipsilateral side Innervation: segmental innervation by posterior rami of spinal nerves

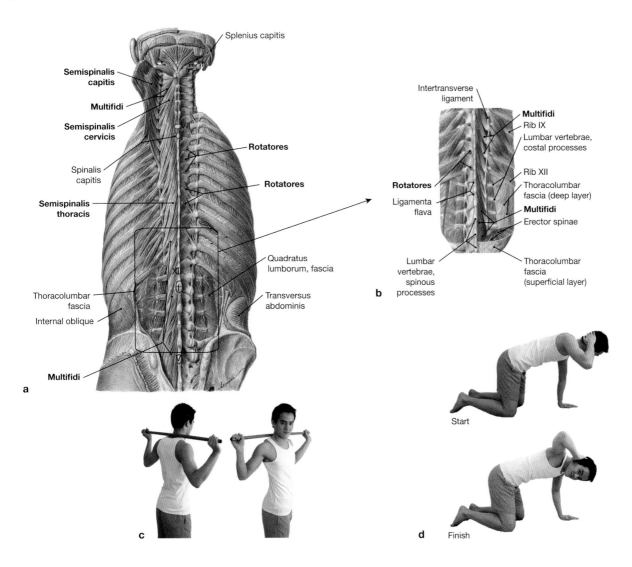

Fig. 2.48a to d Deep muscles of the back; posterior view of the whole vertebral column **(a)**; magnified posterior view of lower thoracic and lumbar regions **(b)**. c, d [L271]

The **transversospinalis muscle** of the back is comprised of three smaller muscles (**semispinalis, multifidus, and rotatores**) that span the length of the vertebral column and course from the transverse process of one vertebra to the spinous process of the superiorly positioned vertebra.

c Together these small muscles function as one **muscle,** and **contribute to rotational and extension movements of the vertebral column** (in general),

d as well **as control rotational and extension movements of specific regions** of the spine (i.e. thoracic) at a segmental level **(d)**.

Muscle	Attachments (P = proximal, D = distal)	Action/Function	Innervation
Semispinalis	**Capitis** **P:** between superior and inferior nuchal lines of occipital bones **D:** transverse processes of C7, T1–T6 **Cervicis** **P:** spinous processes of C1–C5 **D:** transverse processes of T1–T6 **Thoracis** **P:** spinous processes of C6 and C7, T1–T4 **D:** transverse processes of T6–T10	**Capitis and Cervicis:** Bilateral contraction: extension of head and neck Unilateral contraction: lateral flexion of neck to same side; rotation of head to the contralateral side **Thoracis:** Bilateral contraction: extension of the cervical and thoracic region Unilateral contraction: lateral flexion of the cervical and thoracic region to same side; rotation to the contralateral side	**Capitis:** posterior rami of lower cervical nerves **Cervicis:** posterior rami of lower cervical nerves **Thoracis:** posterior rami of upper thoracic nerves
Multifidi	**P:** Muscle fibers pass superomedially to the spinous processes of vertebrae 2–4 segments above **D:** arise from sacrum, posterior ilium, mammillary processes of lumbar vertebrae, transverse processes of thoracic vertebrae, articular processes of C4–C7	Stabilize vertebral segments during localized movements of the spine	* Same as above
Rotatores	**P:** Each muscle spans 1–2 vertebral segments in a superomedial orientation to attach to the lamina and transverse process of above vertebra **D:** arise from transverse processes of each vertebra	Stabilize vertebral segments and assist with segmental extension and rotational movements	* Same as above

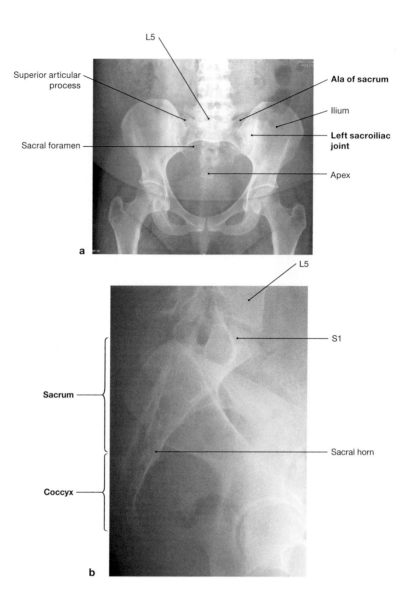

Fig. 2.49a and b **Radiograph of the sacrum;** A/P radiograph **(a)** and lateral radiograph **(b)**. a [M500], b [F274-002]

The sacral region **(sacrum)** is at the bottom of the spine and sits between the **5th segment of the lumbar spine** (L5) and the **coccyx** (tailbone). It consists of five segments (S1–S5) that are fused together into 1 triangular bone. The first three sacral vertebrae have transverse processes that come together to form wide lateral wings

called **alae** – which articulate with the iliac region of the innominate (hip) bones to form the pelvic girdle via the **sacroiliac joints** (➤ Fig. 4.4). The sacrum contains a bilateral series of four openings on each side of the median sacral crest (through which the sacral nerves and blood vessels run), and a centrally located sacral canal that runs down the middle of the sacrum (it represents the end of the vertebral canal).

Structure/Function

Congenital anomalies in the structure of the sacrum and base of the spine are quite common and can influence the function of the lumbar region of the spine. **Lumbarization** refers to a condition in which the S1 vertebra is not fused to the sacrum, but instead functions like a lumbar vertebra (L6). **Sacralization** refers to a condition in which the lowest lumbar vertebra (L5, mainly its transverse process) gets fused or semi-fused to the base of the sacrum, the ilium, or both. Both conditions can change the kinematic function of the lower back region.
a [F903-004], b [G533]

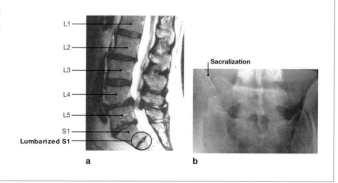

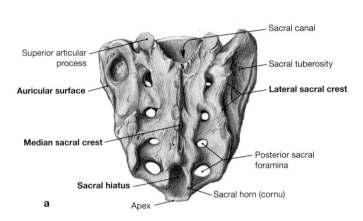

a

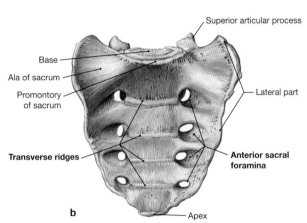

b

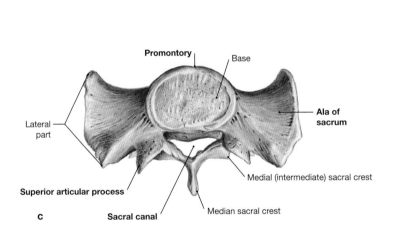

c

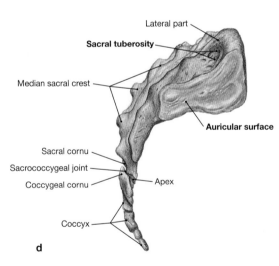

d

Fig. 2.50a to d Sacrum; posterior **(a)**, anterior **(b)**, superior **(c)** and lateral **(d)** views.

The **posterior surface (a)** displays five longitudinal crests formed by the fusion of the corresponding vertebral processes. The **median sacral crest** results from the fusion of the spinous processes; and the **lateral sacral crest** represents the fusion of the rudimentary transverse processes. The median sacral crest terminates above the **sacral hiatus** which represents the inferior opening of the vertebral canal. The **anterior or pelvic surface (b)** displays the fused margins of the sacral vertebrae **(transverse ridges)** and the paired **anterior sacral foramina,** where the branches of the spinal nerves exit. The lateral part of sacrum is located lateral to the anterior sacral foramina. Visible from the top **(c)**, the **base of sacrum** is the contact surface for the intervertebral disc of the L5 vertebra. The anterior rim of the base, is named the **promontory.** Lateral to the base, the **alae** extend as cranial portion of the lateral parts of the sacrum. Located posterior to the base is the triangular **sacral canal,** and the **superior articular processes** for articulation with the L5 vertebra are located laterally. The lateral view **(d)** shows the **auricular surface** that helps form the sacroiliac joint. The **sacral tuberosity** is located at the dorsal aspect and serves as an insertion region for ligaments.

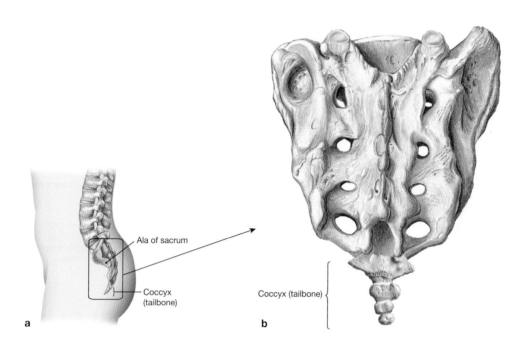

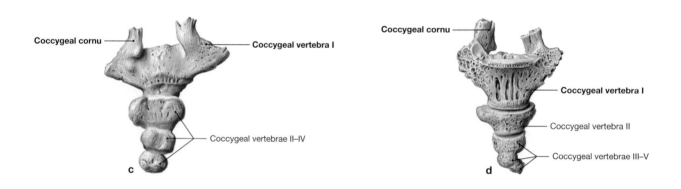

Fig. 2.51a to d   Coccyx; lateral **(a)**, posterior **(b)**, anterior **(c)** and posterior **(d)** views. a [L127]

The **coccyx** represents the most distal end of the vertebral column (i.e. the 'tailbone') and is formed by the **fusion of 3–5 coccygeal vertebrae,** which decrease in size towards the distal end of the ver-

tebral column. Of all coccygeal vertebrae, only the coccygeal verte-bra I resembles a typical vertebral structure. The coccyx is connect-ed to the sacrum via the **coccygeal cornua** and the rudimentary vertebral body of **coccygeal vertebrae I.**

Clinical Remarks

Most tailbone injuries (bruise, dislocation, or fracture) are caused by a trauma to the coccyx area – a fall onto the coccyx in the seated position; a direct blow to the tailbone (such as those that occur during contact sports); or due to repetitive straining or friction against the coccyx (activities such as bicycling or row-ing). Injuries result in significant pain and discomfort in the coc-cygeal region, and while they may be slow to heal, the majority of injuries respond well to rest and conservative treatment. [J787]

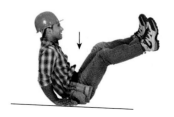

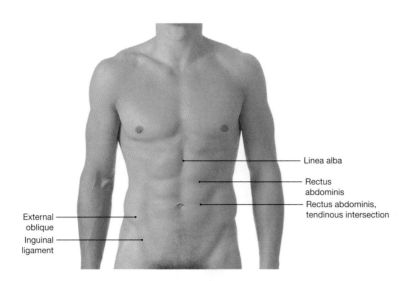

Fig. 2.52 Surface anatomy of the abdominal wall of the male.

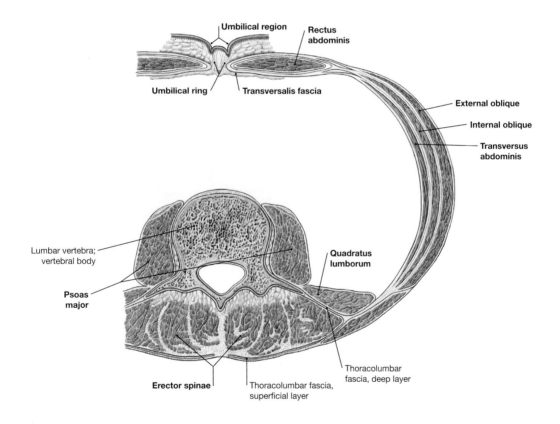

Fig. 2.53 Muscles of the anterior and posterior abdominal wall; cross-section; superior view.
The anterior abdominal wall is comprised of three flat muscles (**external oblique, internal oblique, and transversus abdominis**), that are supplemented in front on each side of the midline by the **rectus abdominis muscle** (➤ Fig. 6.10). The posterior abdominal wall is supported by the lumbar vertebrae and comprised of the **quadratus lumborum, psoas major, iliacus** (not depicted), **and erector spinae muscles.** Together the anterior and posterior abdominal walls function to:
1. **stabilize the spine** when upright and influence body posture (via isometric contraction);

2. **power trunk movements** such as flexion (anterior abdominal wall), extension (posterior abdominal wall), lateral flexion and rotation;
3. **cause changes in size and pressure of the abdominal cavity.**
The anterior layer of the rectus sheath is formed by the aponeurosis of the external oblique and the anterior part of the aponeurosis of the internal oblique; the posterior layer is comprised of the posterior part of the aponeurosis of the internal oblique, the aponeurosis of the transversus abdominis as well as the transversalis fascia and the parietal peritoneum.

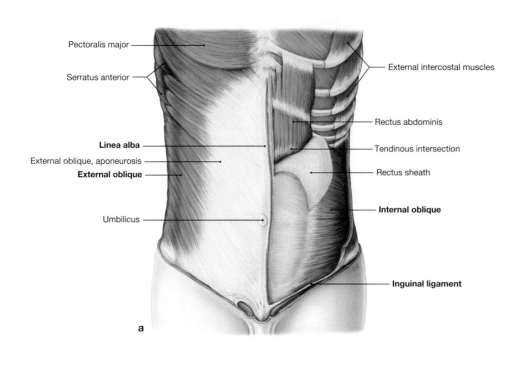

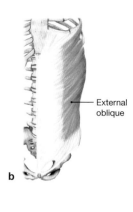

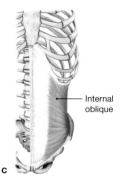

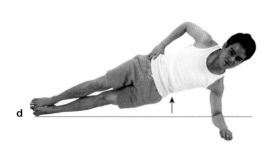

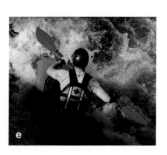

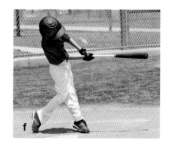

Fig. 2.54a to f Muscles of the anterior abdominal wall; anterior **(a)** and anterolateral **(b and c)** views; superficial layer. a [L285], b, c [L284], d [L271], e, f [J787]

The **internal and external oblique muscles** help to form the anterolateral aspect of the anterior abdominal wall (➤ Fig. 6.11). The external oblique is most superficial and its fiber direction and line of pull is best described as a 'hands in pocket' orientation. The internal oblique is positioned deep to the external oblique and its fiber direction is described by a 'hands on hips' orientation.

Bilateral contraction of these abdominal muscles will result in stabilization and compression of the abdominal viscera, while unilateral contraction **(d)** will result in **lateral flexion of the trunk to the ipsilateral side** – (e.g. raising your trunk off the floor while side lying); and

e, f trunk rotation to the contralateral side – (e.g. while paddling or swinging a golf club or baseball bat).

Muscle	Attachments (P = proximal, D = distal)	Action/Function	Innervation
External oblique	**P:** ribs V–XII **D:** anterior ½ of iliac crest, pubic tubercle, linea alba	Bilateral contraction: compress and support abdominal viscera Unilateral contraction: sidebending/lateral flexion of trunk to the same side (when in the lying position); rotation of trunk to the opposite side (when in the upright position).	Segmental innervation via thoracic nerves T7–T12, and subcostal nerve
Internal oblique	**P:** linea alba, pecten pubis, ribs X–XII **D:** inguinal ligament, anterior ⅔ of iliac crest, and thoracolumbar fascia	Bilateral contraction: compress and support abdominal viscera Unilateral contraction: lateral flexion of trunk to the same side (when in the lying position); rotation of trunk to the same side (when in the upright position)	Segmental innervation via thoracic nerves T7–T12, and subcostal nerve

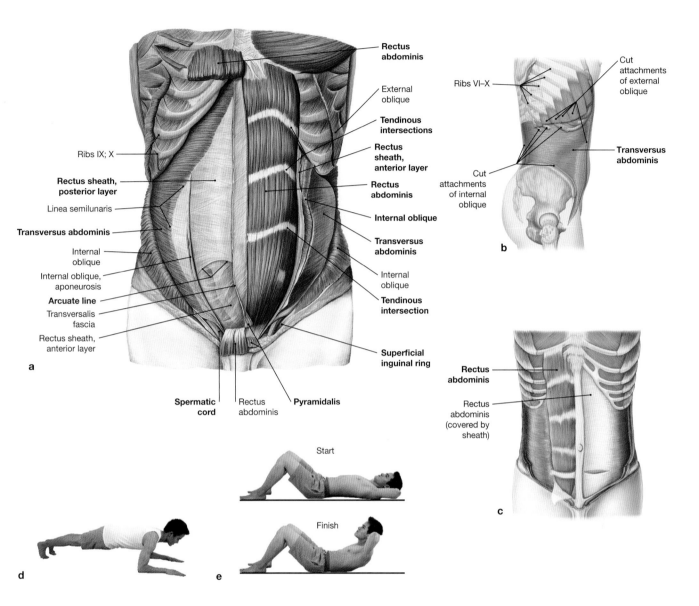

a

b

c

Start

Finish

d   e

Fig. 2.55a to e Muscles of the anterior abdominal wall; anterior **(a and c)** and lateral **(b)** views; deep layer. b [L127], c [L285], d, e [L271]
The **transversus abdominis** is the innermost abdominal muscle, sitting deep to the internal oblique. Its fibers run horizontally, and traverse across the abdomen from its most lateral aspect to its midline (➤ Fig. 6.11).
d It functions to compress the ribs and viscera and provides thoracic and pelvic stability (i.e. when performing a 'plank' exercise), thus enabling a person to compress their belly button in towards their spine. The **rectus abdominis** is a long and flat muscle that

runs vertically on each side of the belly button, extending from the pubic region of the pelvis to the base of sternum. This paired muscle is separated by a midline band of connective tissue called the **linea alba,** as well as by **tendinous intersections** (from the rectus sheath) that divide the muscle horizontally into eight distinct muscle bellies (i.e. 'six pack' abdominal configuration in extremely fit or lean people).
e The rectus abdominis **functions to flex the trunk** (i.e. when performing an abdominal crunch exercise).

Muscle	Attachments (P = proximal, D = distal)	Action/Function	Innervation
Transversus abdominis	**P:** xiphoid process, linea alba, pubic crest, and pecten pubis **D:** iliac crest, inguinal ligament, thoracolumbar fascia, and costal cartilage of ribs VII–XII	Compress abdominal contents (i.e. brings belly button to spine)	Thoracoabdominal nerve (T6–T11); subcostal nerve (T12); iliohypogastric nerve (L1); ilioinguinal nerve (L1)
Rectus abdominis	**P:** costal cartilage of ribs V–VII, xiphoid process of sternum **D:** crest of pubis, pubic symphysis	Flexion of lumbar spine, compress and support abdominal contents	Segmental innervation via thoraco-abdominal nerves T7–T12

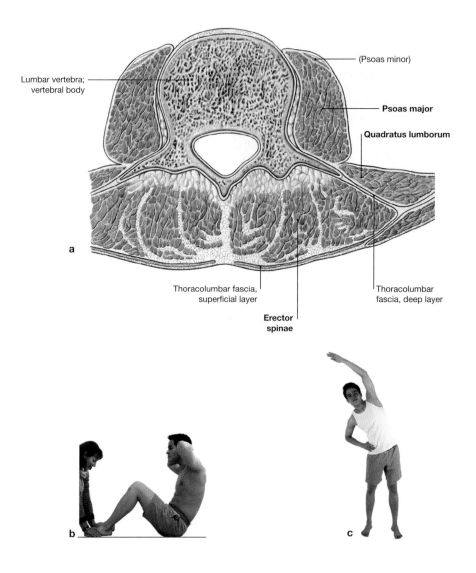

Fig. 2.56a to c Muscles of the posterior abdominal wall, cross-section; superior view **(a)**. b, c [L271]

The posterior abdominal wall is comprised of the lumbar vertebrae and the **psoas major, iliacus, quadratus lumborum, and erector spinae** muscles. They function to **stabilize the lumbar spine** when in an upright standing position, influence body posture, and serve as a scaffold for the retroperitoneal viscera and neurovascular structures that travel through the region. The deep layer of the thoracolumbar fascia is a diamond-shaped area of connective tissue that separates the erector spinae muscles from the other muscles of the posterior abdominal wall.

b Bilateral contraction of the psoas major and iliacus when the feet are fixed in place **helps to power trunk flexion** – i.e. performing a sit up. **c** Unilateral contraction of the erector spinae and quadratus lumborum muscles **assists with lateral flexion movements of the trunk.**

Muscle	Attachments (P = proximal, D = distal)	Action/Function	Innervation
Psoas major	**P:** transverse processes of T12–L5 vertebrae **D:** lesser trochanter of femur	Unilateral contraction: lateral flexion of trunk Bilateral contraction: flexion of trunk from a supine position, works in conjunction with iliacus to flex hip	Segmental innervation: anterior rami of lumbar nerves (L1, L2, L3)
Iliacus (not illustrated)	**P:** iliac crest, iliac fossa, ala of sacrum **D:** lesser trochanter of femur via tendon of psoas major	Functions as part of iliopsoas muscle to flex trunk from a supine position (bilateral contraction)	Femoral nerve (L2, L3)
Quadratus lumborum	**P:** iliac crest, iliolumbar ligament **D:** transverse processes of L1–L4, rib XII (inferior border)	Bilateral contraction: thoracolumbar extension Unilateral contraction: lateral flexion	Segmental innervation: anterior rami of T12–L4 nerves
Erector spinae (in general)	**P:** iliac crest, sacrum, iliolumbar ligament, transverse and spinous processes of lumbar vertebrae **D:** angles of lower ribs, transverse and spinous processes of lumbar and thoracic vertebrae	Bilateral contraction: spine extension Unilateral contraction: lateral flexion to ipsilateral side	Segmental innervation by posterior rami of spinal nerves

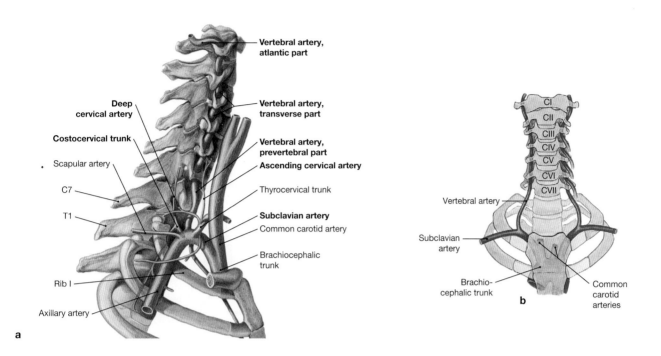

a

b

Fig. 2.57a and b Arteries of the cervical region.
Two vertebral arteries, one on each side of the cervical vertebrae, arise from the right and left **subclavian arteries.** They ascend through the transverse foramina of C6 through C1, and enter the skull via the foramen magnum where they join together to form the basilar artery.

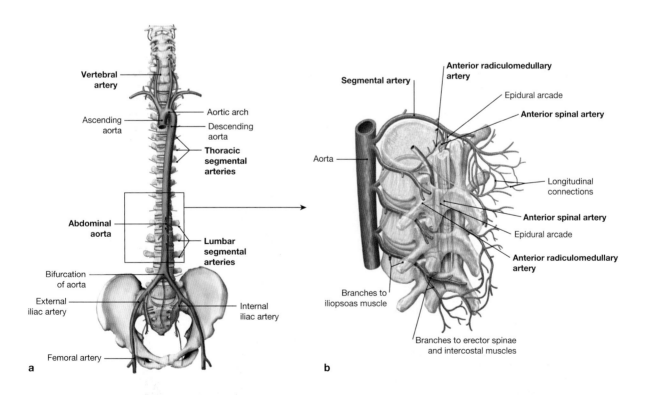

a

b

Fig. 2.58a and b Arteries of the thoracic and lumbosacral regions;
a anterior view, **b** cross-section. a [L284], b [L127]

Segmental arteries arise from the posterior region of the aorta and run in a posterolateral direction, behind the sympathetic trunk, to intervals between adjacent transverse processes of each vertebra.

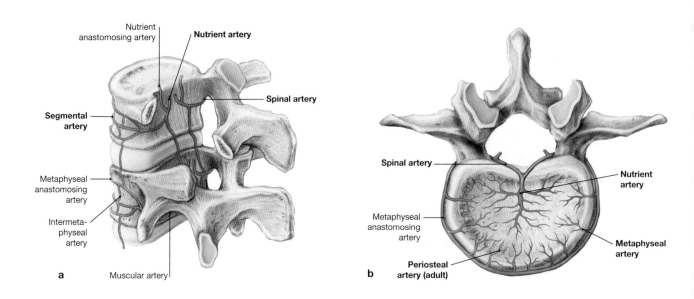

a

Nutrient anastomosing artery

Nutrient artery

Spinal artery

Segmental artery

Metaphyseal anastomosing artery

Intermetaphyseal artery

Muscular artery

b

Spinal artery

Metaphyseal anastomosing artery

Periosteal artery (adult)

Nutrient artery

Metaphyseal artery

Fig. 2.59a and b Arterial supply of the vertebral body and intervertebral anastomoses; posterior oblique **(a)**, and superior **(b)** views. [L285]

These images demonstrate the arterial anatomy of an individual vertebral segment or vertebrae. The major supply to the vertebral body is from the **nutrient artery,** which is formed from **paired spinal arteries** (which arise from **segmental arteries**). Each nutrient artery courses along the dorsal surface of the vertebral body and then enters the body at its mid-portion. At each vertebral level, there are multiple small, **peripheral periosteal branches** along the surface of the vertebral body, which supply the peripheral ⅓ of the lateral and anterior aspects of the vertebral bodies. In addition, there are smaller, **metaphyseal arterial branches** supplying the metaphyseal regions of the vertebral bodies.

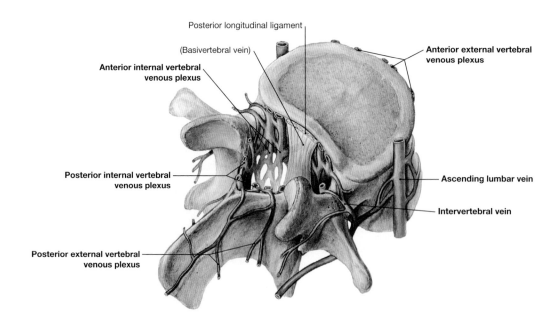

Posterior longitudinal ligament

(Basivertebral vein)

Anterior internal vertebral venous plexus

Anterior external vertebral venous plexus

Posterior internal vertebral venous plexus

Ascending lumbar vein

Intervertebral vein

Posterior external vertebral venous plexus

Fig. 2.60 Veins of the vertebral canal; view from the right side in an oblique posterior angle.

The vertebral canal is filled with a dense network of veins which form the **anterior and posterior internal vertebral venous plexus. Intervertebral veins** (which accompany the spinal nerves as they exit through the intervertebral foramina) drain blood from the spinal cord and vertebral venous plexus. They connect with the **anterior external vertebral venous plexus** (draining the anterior side of the vertebral bodies and the intervertebral discs) and **posterior external vertebral venous plexus** and drain into the paravertebral ascending lumbar veins (lumbar region), the azygos, hemiazygos, and accessory hemiazygos veins (thoracic region), and the internal jugular vein (cervical region).

Upper Extremity

Surface Anatomy of the Shoulder
Region and Upper Trunk 86

Surface Anatomy of the Arm,
Forearm, Wrist and Hand 87

Overview of Bones 88

Shoulder Girdle 89

Clavicle 90

Scapula 91

Proximal Humerus 92

Sternoclavicular Joint 94

Acromioclavicular Joint 95

Glenohumeral Joint 96

Shoulder Movements 99

Scapulohumeral Movement 100

Muscles of the Anterior Shoulder ... 101

Muscles of the Posterior Shoulder –
Superficial and Deep 102

Muscles of the Shoulder –
Rotator Cuff 104

Axilla 105

Innervation of the Shoulder –
Brachial Plexus.................... 106

Arteries of the Shoulder 107

Neurovascular Structures of the Arm . 108

Surface Anatomy of
the Arm and Elbow 109

Bones of the Elbow Joint 110

Elbow Joint and Ligaments 111

Elbow Joint Alignment 112

Elbow Joint Movements 113

Muscles of the Anterior Arm –
Biceps Region 114

Muscles of the Posterior Arm –
Triceps Region 115

Cubital Fossa 116

Neurovascular Structures
of the Elbow Region 117

Surface Anatomy of the Forearm,
Wrist and Hand 118

Bones of the Forearm,
Wrist and Hand 119

Ulna 120

Radius 121

Bones of Wrist and Hand 122

Wrist Joints 123

Wrist Ligaments 124

Wrist Movements 125

Joints and Ligaments of the Fingers .. 126

Finger and Thumb Movements 127

Muscles of the Forearm –
An Overview 128

Muscles of the Anterior Forearm –
Superficial and Deep 129

Muscles of the Posterior Forearm –
Superficial and Deep 131

Neurovascular Structures
of Forearm 133

Flexor Retinaculum
and Carpal Tunnel 134

Extensor Retinaculum 135

Muscles of the Hand –
Thenar Region 136

Muscles of the Hand –
Hypothenar Region 137

Muscles of the Hand –
Central Compartment 138

Neurovascular Structures
of the Wrist and Hand 139

Arterial Arches of the Hand 140

Brachial Plexus of Nerves 141

Brachial Plexus –
Supraclavicular Branches 142

Brachial Plexus – Infraclavicular
Branches of the Posterior Cord 143

Brachial Plexus –
Infraclavicular Branches
of the Lateral and Medial Cord 145

Sensory Innervation – Cutaneous
Nerves and Dermatomes 147

Arteries 149

Veins and Lymphatic
Nodes/Vessels 150

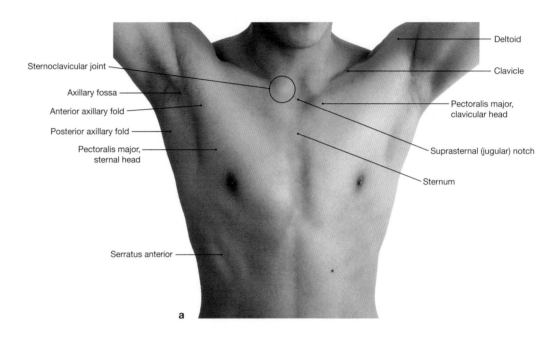

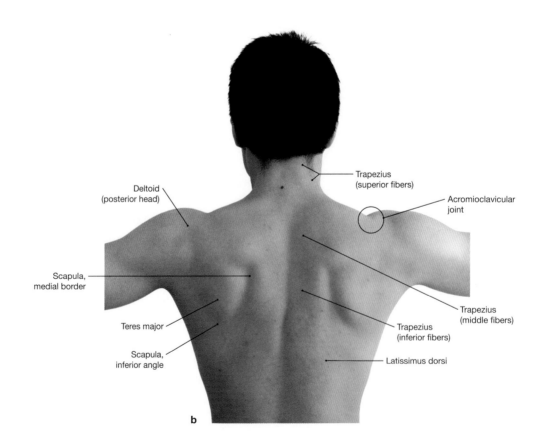

Fig. 3.1a and b Surface anatomy of the shoulder and upper trunk; anterior view **(a);** posterior view **(b).** [L271]
The shape and contour of the shoulder and upper trunk are influenced by muscles that are structurally related to the function of the

upper extremity. It is important to include palpation of many of these surface landmarks when performing a physical examination of the upper extremity.

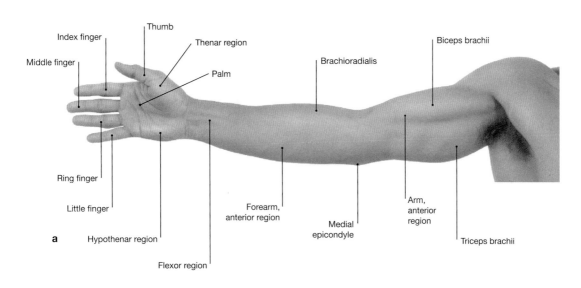

Thumb
Index finger
Middle finger
Thenar region
Palm
Brachioradialis
Biceps brachii
Ring finger
Little finger
Forearm, anterior region
Medial epicondyle
Arm, anterior region
Triceps brachii
a Hypothenar region
Flexor region

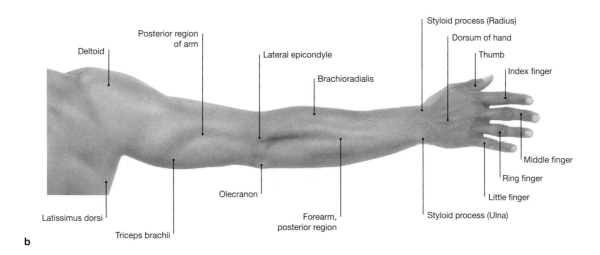

Deltoid
Posterior region of arm
Lateral epicondyle
Brachioradialis
Styloid process (Radius)
Dorsum of hand
Thumb
Index finger
Middle finger
Ring finger
Little finger
Styloid process (Ulna)
Olecranon
Forearm, posterior region
Latissimus dorsi
Triceps brachii
b

Fig. 3.2a and b Surface anatomy of the arm, forearm, wrist and hand, right side; anterior view **(a)**; posterior view **(b)**.
The shape and contour of the upper extremity are determined by superficial muscles and bony alignment. The surface landmarks which are palpable through the skin are important for physical examination.

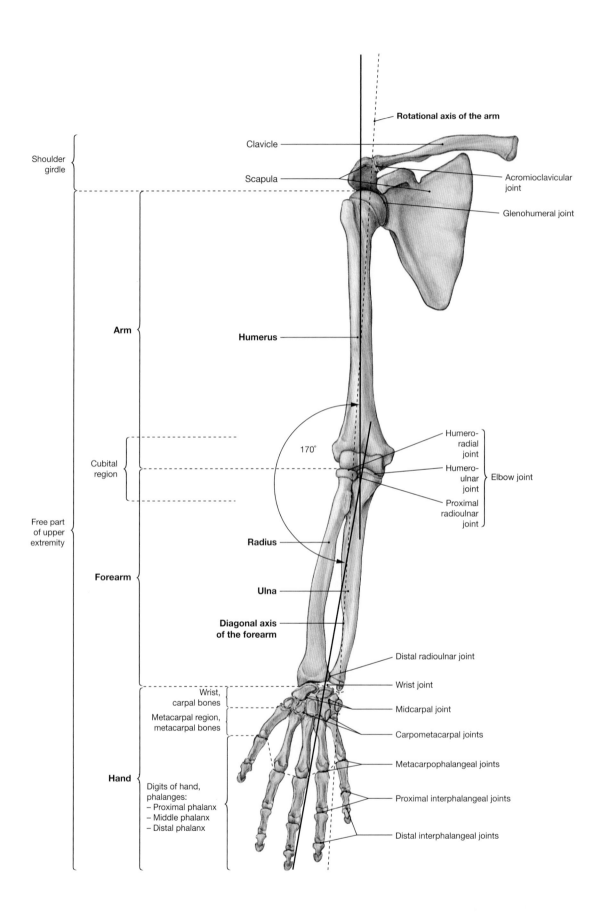

Fig. 3.3 Bones and joints of the upper extremity, right side; ante-rior view.
Similar to the lower extremity, the **arm (brachium)** and **forearm (an-tebrachium)** form a lateral open angle of 170° which is divided in half by the transverse axis of the elbow joint. The connecting line between the head of **humerus** and the head of **ulna** depicts the **ro-tational axis of the upper arm.** The **diagonal axis of the forearm** is the rotational axis for movements of the **radius** around the **ulna** (pronation/supination).

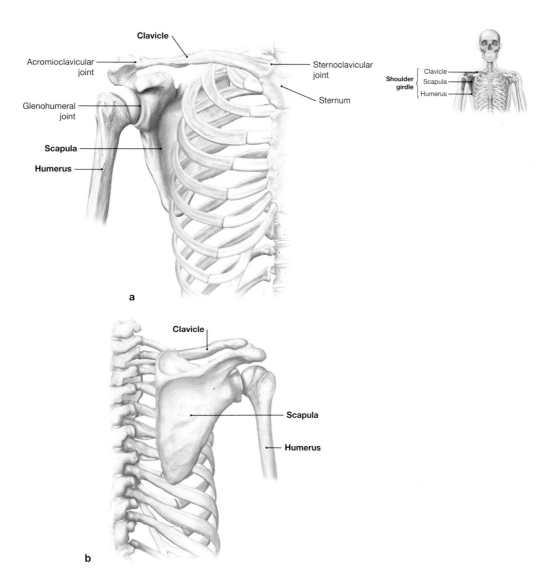

Fig. 3.4a and b Shoulder girdle, right side; anterior view (a); posterior view (b); trunk. [L127]
The shoulder (pectoral) girdle is formed by the **clavicle** (collarbone), **scapula** (shoulder blade) and upper portion of the **humerus** (long bone of upper arm). The clavicle represents the only bony connection of the upper extremity to the sternum and trunk.

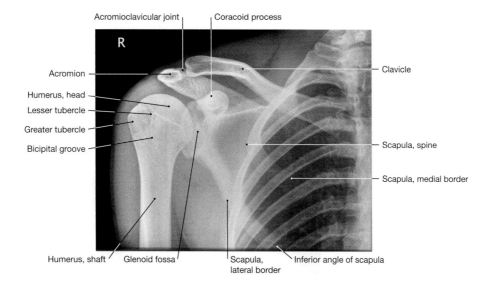

Fig. 3.5 A/P radiograph of the shoulder girdle, right side; anterior view. [G305]

Many of the main articulations (joints) and key bony features of the clavicle, scapula and upper humerus are visible on a radiograph.

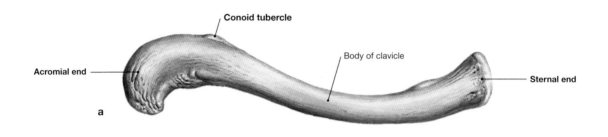

Conoid tubercle

Body of clavicle

Acromial end

Sternal end

a

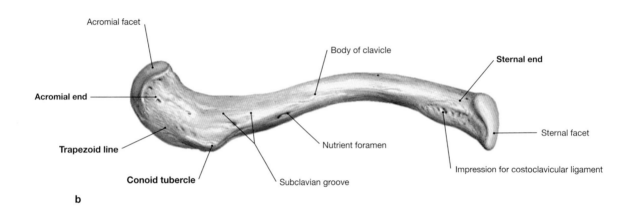

Acromial facet

Body of clavicle

Sternal end

Acromial end

Trapezoid line

Nutrient foramen

Sternal facet

Conoid tubercle

Impression for costoclavicular ligament

Subclavian groove

b

Fig. 3.6a and b Clavicle, right side; superior view **(a)**; inferior view **(b)**.
Matching an isolated clavicle to either side of the body is often difficult. It helps to know that the **sternal end is larger and rounded, while the acromial end is more pointed.** When positioned on the skeleton, the sternal convexity is oriented towards the front. The inferior aspect of the clavicle also shows two characteristic apophyses for the attachment of both parts of the coracoclavicular ligament. The **conoid tubercle** is positioned medially, while the **trapezoid line** is located laterally.

Clinical Remarks

The clavicle is a bone of the upper extremity which is commonly fractured – often by a fall on an outstretched arm and hand, a fall on the point of the shoulder, or a direct blow to the clavicle.
a The fracture site is most commonly observed in the middle ⅓ of the bone – a region of transition between the concave and convex orientation of the bone.
b On clinical examination, the region demonstrates marked deformity and swelling, and the patient is often unable to support the weight of the affected limb. Beyond this, physical examination of the region should be used to help rule out lesions of underlying structures such as the subclavian artery, brachial plexus, and superior lobe of the lung.
c A/P radiograph of the shoulder girdle (➤ Fig. 5.19) allows the location and extent of the fracture to be easily visualized.
a [L231], b [G721], c [G305]

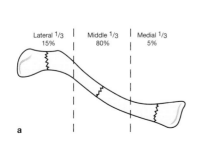

Lateral ⅓
15%

Middle ⅓
80%

Medial ⅓
5%

a

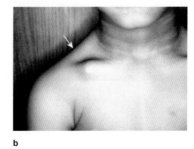

b

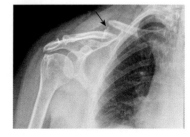

c

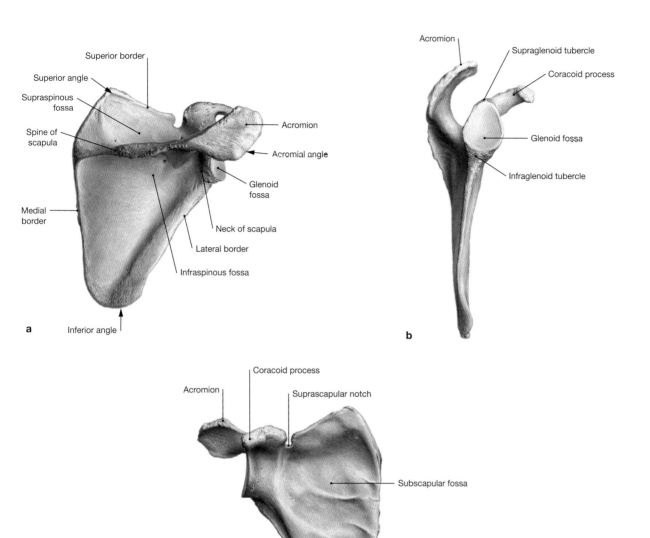

Fig. 3.7a to c Scapula, right side; posterior view **(a)**; lateral view **(b)**; anterior view **(c)**.
The scapula (or shoulder blade) is a flat bone with four important borders (medial, lateral, vertebral, and superior) and angles (inferi-or, superior, acromial). The T-shaped protrusion on the posterior aspect of the scapula (spine of scapula), is an important apophysis for the attachment of muscles, and serves to separate the supraspinous fossa from the infraspinous fossa.

Clinical Remarks

The position of the scapulae on the posterior thorax allows one to quickly approximate the level of the thoracic vertebrae during clinical examination. The **T3 vertebra** is intersected by a line that connects the root of the spines of the left and right scapulae. A line that connects the inferior angles of the left and right scapulae also intersects the vertebral column at the **T7 level.** [L126]

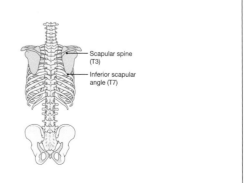

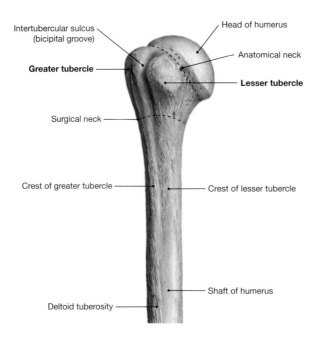

Fig. 3.8 Humerus, bony features of the upper one-third of the arm, right side; anterior view.

The head of the humerus is positioned at an angle of 150–180° relative to the long axis of the shaft of humerus. The **greater tubercle** and the **lesser tubercle** are located laterally and medially on the proximal shaft (respectively), and provide important attachment for muscles of the shoulder that arise from both the thorax (e.g. – pectoralis major, latissimus dorsi) and the scapula (e.g. – supraspinatus, infraspinatus, teres minor, teres major, subscapularis).

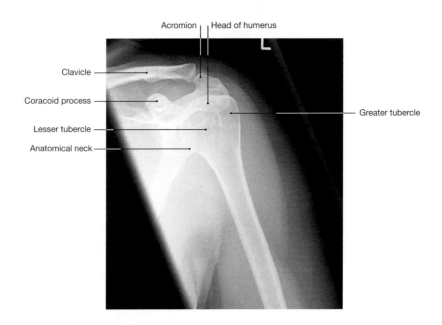

Fig. 3.9 A/P radiograph of the upper arm, left side; anterior view.
[G305]

Many of the key bony features and the position of the humerus in relation to the scapula are visible on radiograph.

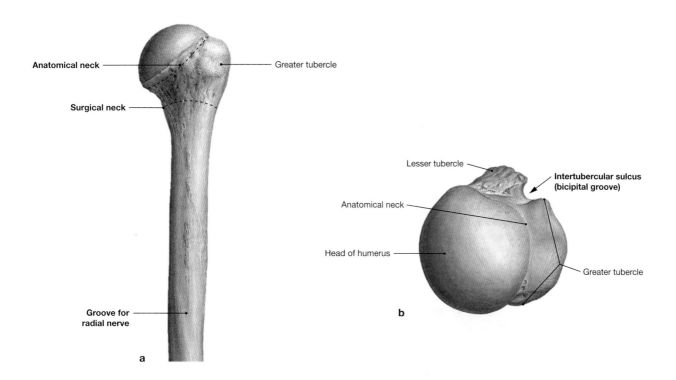

Anatomical neck
Greater tubercle
Surgical neck

Lesser tubercle
**Intertubercular sulcus
(bicipital groove)**
Anatomical neck
Head of humerus
Greater tubercle
b

**Groove for
radial nerve**

a

Fig. 3.10a and b Humerus, proximal one-third of arm, right side;
posterior view **(a)**; superior view **(b)**.
The **surgical neck** of the humerus represents the transition zone
between the head and the shaft of humerus. The **anatomical neck**
refers to an area that is used to distinguish between the articular
(covered by hyaline cartilage) and non-articular portion of the head

of humerus. It provides attachment for the articular capsule of the
glenohumeral joint and serves to separate the head of humerus
from the two tubercles (greater and lesser). The **groove for radial
nerve** spirals around the posterior shaft of humerus guiding the
radial nerve. The greater and the lesser tubercles are separated
from one another by the **intertubercular sulcus (bicipital groove).**

Clinical Remarks

Humeral fractures are classified by their location (proximal end/
mid-shaft/distal end).
a Proximal fractures commonly occur in the region of the surgical neck, and can result in lesions of the axillary nerve. The
'NEER classification' system is often used to describe proximal
humeral fractures according to:
1. number of fractured pieces,
2. degree of displacement of the fractured bone.
b A midshaft fracture can be associated with damage to the radial nerve as it courses distally within its groove on the posterior
aspect of the shaft of humerus. Radial nerve injury will impair
function of muscles on the posterior forearm which power wrist
extension, and will result in a **'wrist drop'** deformity. In addition,
a sensory deficit may occur on the posterior aspect of the forearm, in the first interdigital space (autonomic region) of the
hand, and on the posterior surfaces of fingers 2 through 4.
a [R234], b [E402]

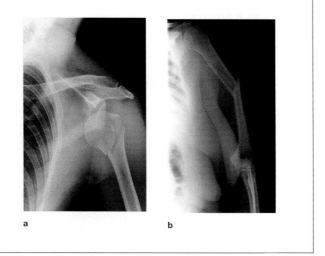

a b

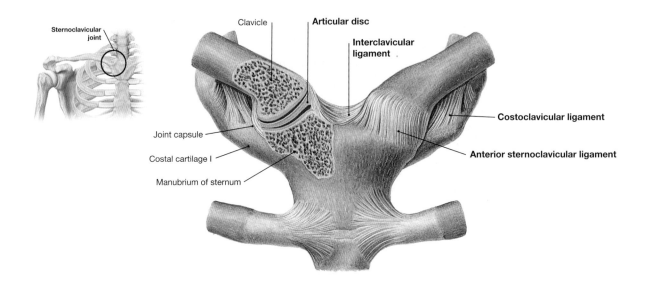

Fig. 3.11 Sternoclavicular joints; anterior view. [L127]
Articular surfaces of the sternoclavicular joint with key ligaments and articular disc which support the joint.

The sternoclavicular (S/C) joint is a saddle type of synovial joint, and represents the only articular connection between the upper extremity and the skeleton of the trunk (➤ Fig. 5.37). The articular surfaces of the sternum and clavicle are separated by a fibrocartilaginous **articular disc** which functions to absorb joint forces and enhance articulation. The joint is stabilized by strong ligaments – the **anterior and posterior** (not depicted) **sternoclavicular ligaments** span the joint on both the anterior and posterior surfaces and function to resist anterior/posterior movements of the clavicle on the sternum, while an **interclavicular ligament** connects and stabilizes both clavicles superiorly. A **costoclavicular ligament** also extends from the cartilage of rib I to the sternal end of the clavicle, functioning to anchor the proximal end of the clavicle.

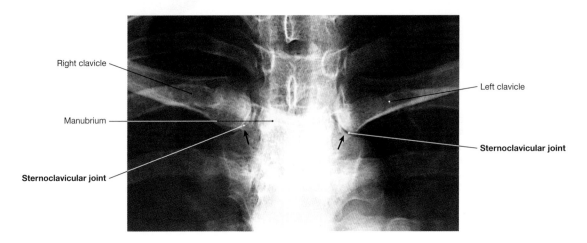

Fig. 3.12 A/P radiograph of the sternoclavicular joints, right and left side; anterior view. [E530]

The orientation of the **left and right sternoclavicular joints** relative to the sternum and ribs are **clearly** visible on this radiograph.

Clinical Remarks

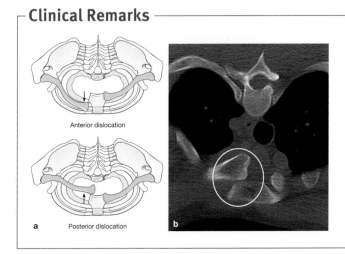

a While the strong ligamentous support of the S/C joint make it very stable, dislocations can occur as a result of significant direct or indirect force to the shoulder.
b A posterior dislocation has the potential to result in life threatening complications due to the proximity of the joint to the lung, trachea, key neurovascular structures, and the esophagus.
a [L126], b [H064-001]

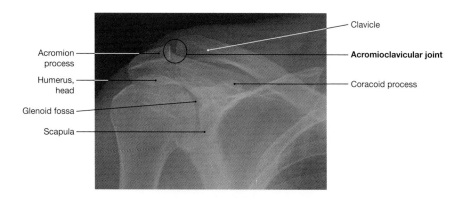

Fig. 3.13 Acromioclavicular joint, right side; A/P radiograph in anteroposterior beam projection. [G568]

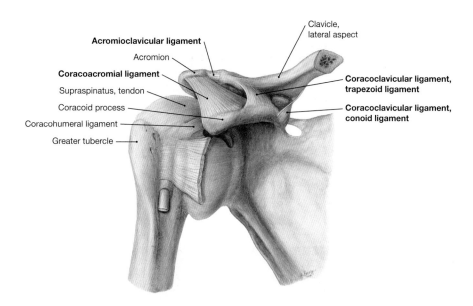

Fig. 3.14 Acromioclavicular joint, right side; anterior view.
The acromioclavicular (A/C) joint connects the lateral clavicle to the acromion of the scapula. This plane synovial joint is directly stabilized by the **acromioclavicular ligament** and the **coracoclavicular ligament** (which consists of two parts – **conoid ligament and trapezoid ligament**) inserting laterally on the inferior and acromial aspects of the clavicle along the trapezoid line. The anterior aspect of the shoulder joint is also reinforced by the **coracoacrominal ligament**.

Clinical Remarks

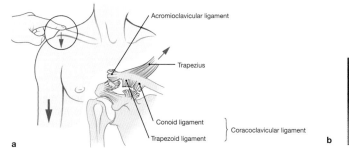
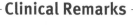

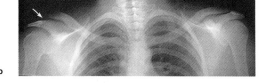

a Injury or displacement of the A/C joint is referred to as a **'shoulder separation'**. The extent of clavicular displacement is used to classify the injury as mild/moderate/severe. In a mild injury, the acromioclavicular ligament is injured. In a moderate injury, the acromioclavicular ligament is completely disrupted, and the coracoclavicular ligament is damaged. With a severe injury, the acromioclavicular and coracoclavicular ligaments are both severly damaged.
b A/C joint separations can be easily identified because of the high riding clavicle which is visible on A/P radiograph. In general, the more severe the A/C joint injury, the further the lateral end of the clavicle is displaced.   a [L126], b [G718]

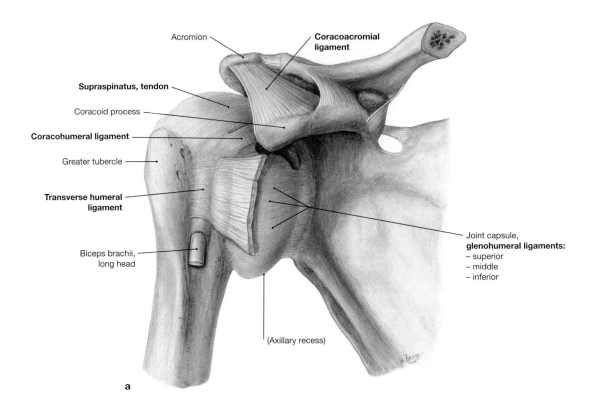

Acromion

Coracoacromial ligament

Supraspinatus, tendon

Coracoid process

Coracohumeral ligament

Greater tubercle

Transverse humeral ligament

Biceps brachii, long head

(Axillary recess)

Joint capsule, **glenohumeral ligaments:**
– superior
– middle
– inferior

a

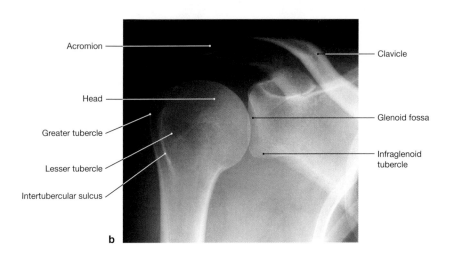

Acromion

Head

Greater tubercle

Lesser tubercle

Intertubercular sulcus

Clavicle

Glenoid fossa

Infraglenoid tubercle

b

Fig. 3.15a and b Glenohumeral joint, right side; anterior view **(a)** and radiograph in anteroposterior (A/P) beam projection **(b).**

a The glenohumeral (G/H) joint is supported by various ligaments, as well as the tendons of the rotator cuff muscles. The **glenohumeral ligaments** (superior, middle and inferior) reinforce the anterior and inferior aspects of the capsule and function to stabilize the anterior part of the joint. The **coracohumeral ligament** is positioned superiorly, and functions to resist inferior displacement of the head of humerus on the glenoid fossa. The **tendons of the rotator cuff muscles** (only the **supraspinatus** tendon is depicted) also radiate into the G/H joint capsule from anterior, superior, and posterior directions, functioning to limit excessive movements in

these directions. The **coracoacromial ligament,** together with the coracoid process and the acromion, form the roof of the shoulder outside of the joint capsule. The roof of the shoulder functions as an additional support for the glenoid fossa by stabilizing the head of humerus, and resisting a superior migration. The **transverse humeral ligament** also functions to stabilize the long head of biceps as it enters the G/H joint from below.

b The glenoid fossa of the shoulder joint is relatively small. Only about one-third of the head of humerus is in direct contact with the glenoid fossa during movements, making it prone to injury. Dislocations (luxations) of the shoulder joint are among the most common injuries of the shoulder girdle.

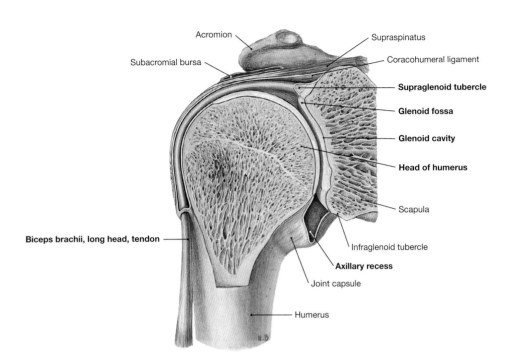

Acromion

Subacromial bursa

Supraspinatus

Coracohumeral ligament

Supraglenoid tubercle

Glenoid fossa

Glenoid cavity

Head of humerus

Scapula

Infraglenoid tubercle

Axillary recess

Joint capsule

Biceps brachii, long head, tendon

Humerus

Fig. 3.16 Shoulder joint, right side; anterior cross-section of the joint socket.

The glenohumeral (G/H) joint is a classical ball-and-socket type synovial joint in which the **head of humerus articulates with the glenoid fossa of the scapula.** The glenoid fossa anchors a ring of fibrocartilage called the **glenoid labrum.** The labrum functions to deepen the socket by as much as 50%, serving to enhance joint stability, functioning as a shock absorber, and helping to promote the circulation of synovial fluid throughout the joint. The joint capsule originates from the glenoid labrum and envelopes the **tendon of the long head of biceps brachii** (at the superior aspect of the glenoid labrum). Originating from the **supraglenoid tubercle,** the **long head tendon of biceps brachii** projects through the shoulder joint while the long head of triceps brachii has its origin at the infraglenoid tubercle outside of the shoulder joint capsule (not depicted). The capsule inserts at the anatomical neck of humerus, leaving the greater and lesser tubercles extraarticular. Inferiorly, the joint capsule extends to form a fold called the **axillary recess.**

Clinical Remarks

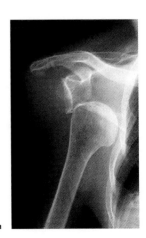

a

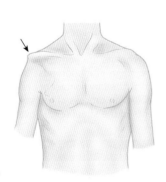

b

a Dislocation of the G/H joint is a frequent injury of the shoulder girdle. The joint is prone to injury because of the weak bony and ligamentous support which guides movements of the head of humerus on the smaller glenoid fossa. G/H joint dislocations most frequently occur in an anterior and inferior direction and result in the head of humerus being positioned inferior to the coracoid process in the subcoracoid region.

b On examination, the contour (or dome appearance) of the shoulder is reduced and the arm appears longer.

a [R234], b [E748]

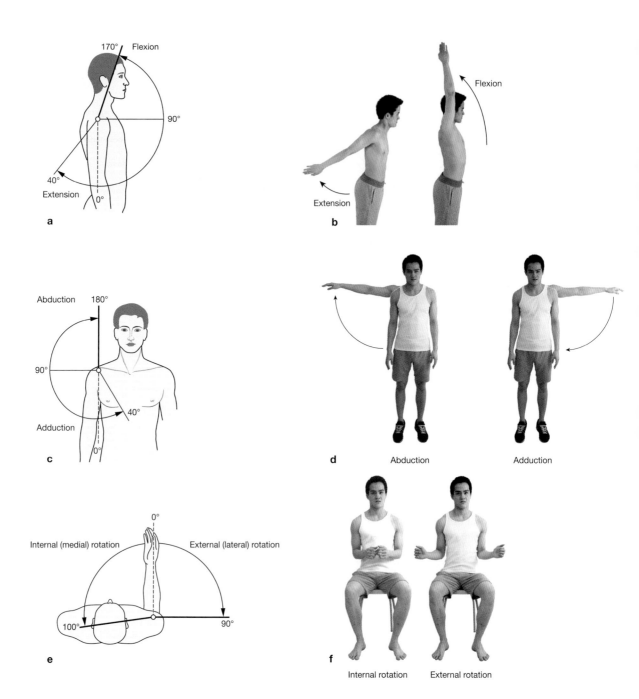

Fig. 3.17a to f Range of motion of the shoulder – glenohumeral joint. a, c, e [L126], b, d, f [L271]

The glenohumeral joint is the joint primarily responsible for shoulder motion. It is a tri-axial, **ball-and-socket type of synovial joint** that provides the greatest degree of mobility of all joints in the human body. When movements are performed by the glenohumeral joint in isolation, the range of motion possible during abduction and forward flexion is limited by contact or opposition of the head of humerus on the acromion process of the scapula (roof of shoulder). Some movements of the shoulder (ie. overhead movements)

require the orientation of the glenoid fossa to be changed (example – tilted upward). This tilting is facilitated by movements of the scapula on the thoracic wall and influences the range of motion that the glenohumeral joint can move through during forward flexion and abduction.

a and b Shoulder extension – flexion: 40° – 0° – 170°
c and d Shoulder abduction – adduction: 180 – 0° – 40°
e and f Shoulder external (lateral) rotation – internal (medial) rotation: 90° – 0° – 100°

Glenohumeral Joint Movements	Muscles Active During Movements
Flexion	Pectoralis major, deltoid – anterior head, biceps brachii, coracobrachilis
Extension	Latissimus dorsi, deltoid – posterior head, triceps – long head, teres major
Abduction	Deltoid – middle head, supraspinatus
Adduction	Latissimus dorsi, pectoralis major, teres major
Internal rotation	Subscapularis, pectoralis major, latissimus dorsi, teres major
External rotation	Infraspinatus, teres minor

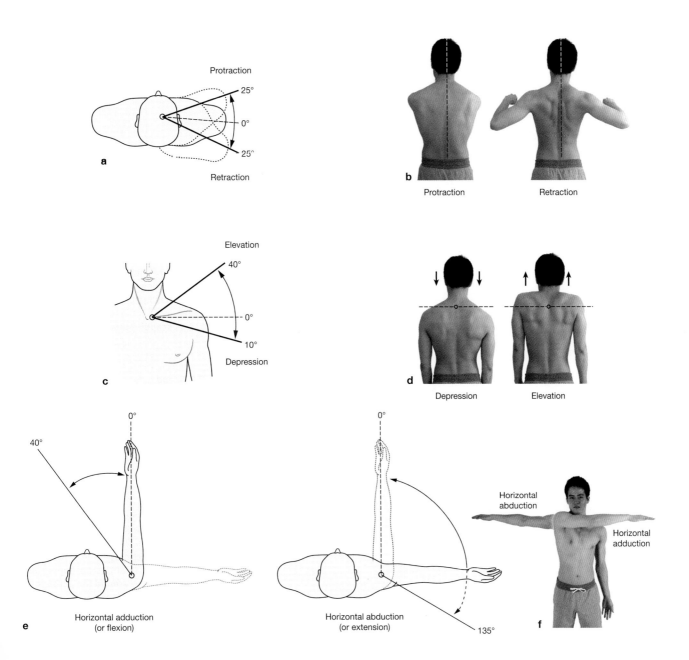

Fig. 3.18a to f Range of motion of the shoulder – shoulder girdle.
a, c, e [L126], b, d, f [L271]
Many of the movements of the shoulder girdle do not occur exclusively at one joint. Instead they require simultaneous motion and interaction (in varying degrees) at the sternoclavicular, acromioclavicular, and glenohumeral joints, as well as between the scapula and thoracic wall (i.e. scapulothoracic region).

a and b Shoulder protraction – retraction: 25° – 0° – 25°
c and d Shoulder elevation – depression: 40° – 0° – 10°
e and f Shoulder horizontal adduction (flexion) – horizontal abduction (extension): 40° – 0° – 135°

Movements of Shoulder Girdle	Muscles Active During Movements
Protraction	Serratus anterior, pectoralis minor
Retraction	Rhomboids (major and minor), trapezius – middle fibers
Elevation	Trapezius – superior fibers, levator scapulae
Depression	Trapezius – inferior fibers
Horizontal adduction/flexion	Deltoid – anterior and middle head, pectoralis major, coracobrachialis
Horizontal abduction/extension	Deltoid – posterior and middle head, latissimus dorsi, teres major

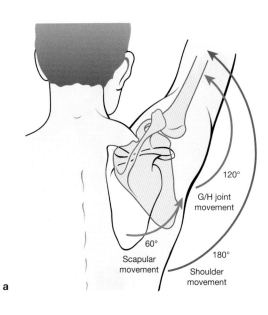
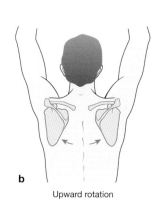
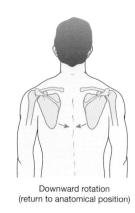

a

b
Upward rotation

c
Downward rotation
(return to anatomical position)

120°
G/H joint movement

60°
Scapular movement

180°
Shoulder movement

Fig. 3.19a to c Scapulohumeral movement. [L126]
a During overhead movements of the shoulder, the scapula and humerus move in a 1 : 2 ratio (i.e. when the arm is abducted overhead to 180°, 60° of the motion occurs as a result of movement of the scapula on the thoracic wall, and 120° of the movement occurs at the glenohumeral joint).
b and c Movement of the scapula on the thorax facilitates **upward and downward rotation** of the glenoid fossa of the scapula in association with movements of the humerus, and is described as **scapulohumeral motion.**

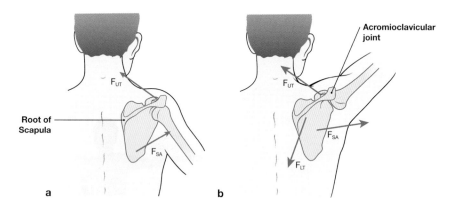

Root of Scapula

F_{UT}

F_{SA}

a

Acromioclavicular joint

F_{UT}

F_{SA}

F_{LT}

b

Fig. 3.20a and b Scapulohumeral force couples. [L126]
Upwards rotation of the glenoid fossa of scapula during shoulder abduction is controlled by **'force couples'** which are created by muscles about the shoulder.
a At less than 100° of abduction, upward **rotation occurs around the root of the scapula** – the force of the upper fibers of the trapezius muscle (F_{UT}) counteract the lateral pull of the deltoid muscle, while the force of the serratus anterior (F_{SA}) protracts the scapula and pulls the inferior angle in an anterolateral direction.
b When the arm is abducted above 100°, **the scapula rotates around the acromioclavicular joint** – the force of the lower trapezius (F_{LT}) becomes more active in order to counteract the force of the serratus anterior (F_{SA}). This functions to hold the scapula against the thoracic wall, while the upper fibers of trapezius (F_{UT}) contract and rotate the scapula upwards.

Clinical Remarks

Impairment of normal **scapulohumeral motion** can lead to alterations in the subacromial space and degenerative changes in structures such as the supraspinatus tendon which passes through the subacromial space (identified by the white arrow in the A/P radiograph). As a result, patients experience pain when lifting the arm overhead because this movement results in compression of the supraspinatus tendon underneath the acromion of the scapula (i.e. the roof of the shoulder). This phenomenon is commonly referred to as **shoulder impingement syndrome.**
a [G217], b [L126]

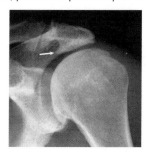

a

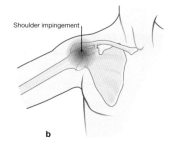

Shoulder impingement

b

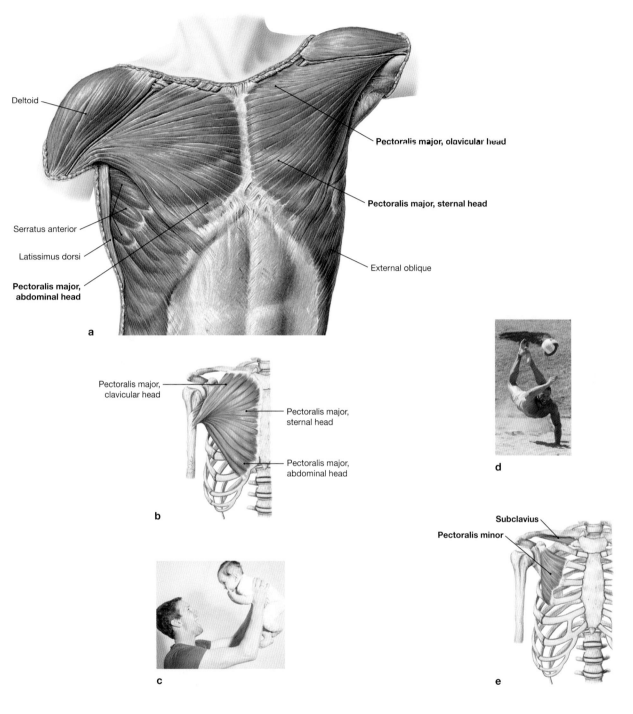

Deltoid

Serratus anterior

Latissimus dorsi

Pectoralis major, abdominal head

Pectoralis major, olavicular head

Pectoralis major, sternal head

External oblique

a

Pectoralis major, clavicular head

Pectoralis major, sternal head

Pectoralis major, abdominal head

b

c

d

Subclavius

Pectoralis minor

e

Fig. 3.21a to e Muscles of the shoulder; anterior view; superficial **(a and b)** to deep layers **(e).** b, e [L266, L127], c [K383], d [J787]
a and b The **pectoralis major** is the largest and most superficial muscle in the anterior shoulder region. It has three distinct attachment points or 'heads' at the midline – clavicular, sternal and abdominal.

c It functions to power activities such as lifting an object out in front of you or overhead.
d It also functions to brace or catch yourself during a fall.
e The **pectoralis minor** and **subclavius** muscles both lie deep to the pectoralis major, and function to stabilize and guide motion of the scapula and clavicle.

Muscle	Attachments (P = proximal, D = distal)	Action/Function	Innervation
Pectoralis major	**P:** Anterior surface of medial half of clavicle (clavicular head); anterior surface of sternum, upper six costal cartilages (sternal head); aponeurosis of external oblique muscle (abdominal part) **D:** Lateral lip of bicipital groove of humerus	Shoulder adduction and medial rotation; clavicular head acts alone to power shoulder flexion; sternal head acts alone to extend shoulder from a flexed position.	Medial and lateral pectoral nerves: clavicular head (C5 and C6); sternal head (C7, C8 and T1).
Pectoralis minor	**P:** Ribs III to V, near costal cartilage **D:** Coracoid process of scapula	Scapular protraction; powers reach-beyond-reach motion at shoulder	Medial pectoral nerve (C8, T1)
Subclavius	**P:** Medial boundary of 1st rib and costal cartilage **D:** Middle one-third of clavicle (inferior surface)	Clavicular depression; anchors clavicle	Nerve to subclavius (C5, C6)

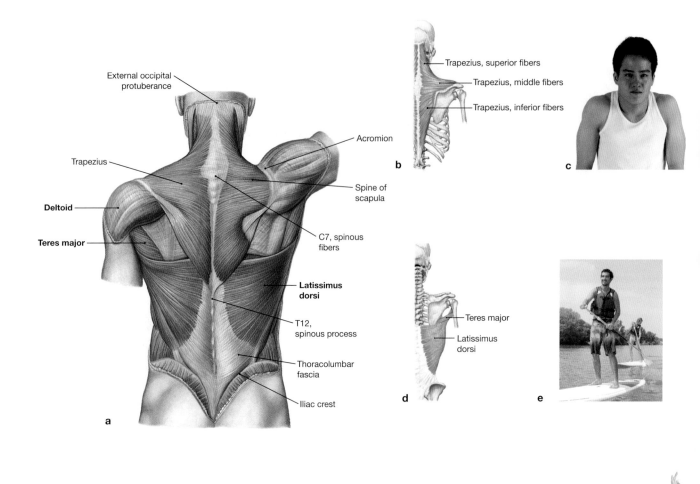

Fig. 3.22a to g Superficial muscles of the shoulder; posterior **(a, b, d)** and lateral **(f)** views. b, d, f [L266, L127], c [L271], e, g [J787]

a The **trapezius**, **latissimus dorsi**, **teres major** and **deltoid** are all superficial muscles which occupy the posterior regions of the shoulder and back (➤ Fig. 2.46).

b and c The trapezius (superior fibers) function to **elevate the shoulders** during an activity such as shrugging your shoulders.

d and e The latissimus dorsi and teres major muscles power movements such as **shoulder adduction, extension, and internal rotation** during sporting activities like paddling.

f and g The deltoid is comprised of three heads – the **anterior head powers forward flexion** of the shoulder during an activity such as raising your hand to ask a question.

Muscle	Attachments (P = proximal, D = distal)	Action/Function	Innervation
Trapezius	**P:** Medial one-third of superior nuchal line; external occipital protuberance; spinous processes of C7–T12 vertebrae **D:** Lateral one-third of clavicle, acromion and spine of scapula	Superior fibers – scapular elevation Middle fibers – scapular retraction Inferior fibers – scapular depression see ➤ chapter 2 for details regarding trapezius function and the spine	Root of accessory nerve (CN XI; ➤ Fig. 12.63), and cervical plexus (C3 and C4)
Latissimus dorsi	**P:** Spinous processes of lower six thoracic vertebrae; thoracolumbar fascia; iliac crest **D:** Floor of bicipital groove of humerus	Shoulder extension, adduction and medial rotation	Thoracodorsal nerve (C6, C7, C8)
Deltoid	**P:** Lateral one-third of clavicle, acromion and spine of scapula **D:** Deltoid tuberosity of proximal humerus	Anterior head – shoulder flexion, middle head – shoulder abduction, posterior head – shoulder extension	Axillary nerve (C5, C6)
Teres major	**P:** Inferior angle of scapula – posterior surface **D:** Medial lip of bicipital groove	Shoulder adduction and medial rotation	Lower subscapular nerve (C6, C7), and thoracodorsal nerve (C6, C7, C8)

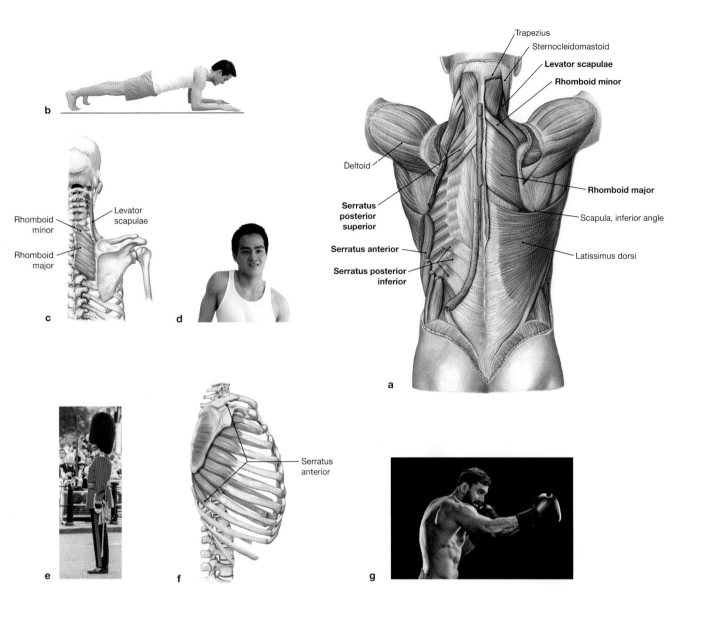

Fig. 3.23a to g Deep muscles of the shoulder; posterior **(a, c)** and lateral **(f)** views. b, d [L271], c, f [L266, L127], e, g [J787]
a The **levator scapulae, rhomboid muscles** and **serratus muscles** (➤ Fig. 2.46) are each located deep to trapezius and latissimus dorsi.
b With assistance from trapezius, they each function to 'fix' or stabilize the scapula against the thoracic wall during activities such as a push-up or when performing a plank exercise.

c to e The levator scapulae functions to **elevate the scapula unilaterally.** The rhomboids (major and minor) function to power **scapular retraction;** for example: squeezing shoulder blades together when standing at attention).
f and g The serratus anterior functions to **protract the scapula** during activities such as punching an object.

Muscle	Attachments (P = proximal, D = distal)	Action/Function	Innervation
Rhomboid major and minor	**P:** Nuchal ligament and C7–T1 spinous processes (minor); T2–T5 spinous processes (major) **D:** Medial border of the scapula below the spine of scapula	Scapular retraction; holds scapula flat against thoracic wall	Dorsal scapular nerve (C4 and C5)
Levator scapulae	**P:** Transverse processes of C1–C4 vertebrae **D:** Medial border of scapula above spine of scapula	Scapular elevation; tilts glenoid fossa inferiorly by rotating vertebral border of scapula upward	Dorsal scapular nerve (C5) and cervical plexus (C3 and C4)
Serratus anterior	**P:** Lateral surfaces of ribs I–VIII. **D:** Anterior surface of the medial border of scapula	Scapular protraction; holds scapula flat against thoracic wall	Long thoracic nerve (C5, C6 and C7)
Serratus posterior superior and inferior	**P:** Nuchal ligament and C7–T3 spinous processes (superior); T11–L2 spinous processes (inferior) **D:** upper border of ribs II–V (superior); lower border of ribs IX–XII (inferior)	Elevate upper rib cage during deep-inspiration (superior); depress lower rib cage during forced expiration (inferior)	Intercostal nerves 2–5 (superior); intercostal nerves T9–T12 (inferior)

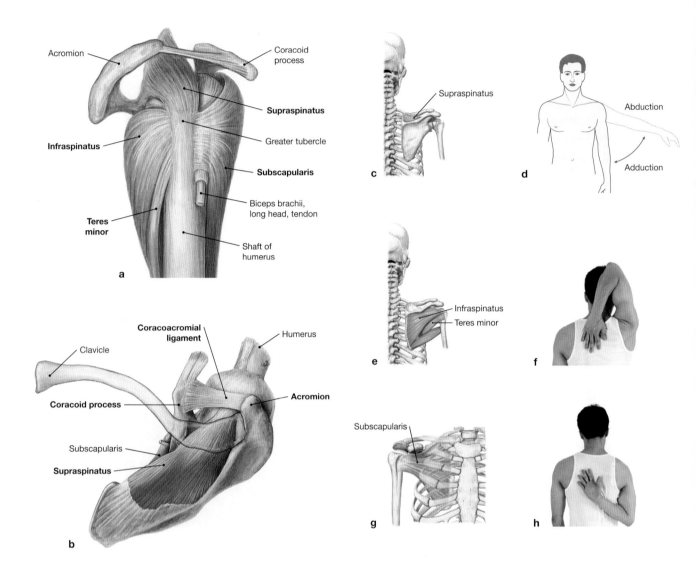

Fig. 3.24a to h Rotator cuff muscles of the shoulder; lateral view (a), superior view (b), posterior view (c, e), anterior view (g). c, e, g [L266, L127], d [L126], f, h [L271]

a and b The **rotator cuff** is comprised of four distinct muscles which are often referred to as the **'SITS' muscle group** (**s**upraspinatus, **i**nfraspinatus, **t**eres minor, **s**ubscapularis). They are responsible for powering internal and external rotation movements of the shoulder, e.g. when throwing a ball from an overhead position.

c and d The **supraspinatus** passes through the subacromial space (under the acromioclavicular joint) and functions as a primary stabilizer of the head of humerus within the glenoid labrum; **it initiates and powers shoulder abduction (f).**

e and f The **infraspinatus and teres minor** wrap around the lateral aspect of the shoulder and are active when performing functional movements of the shoulder such as reaching overhead to scratch the back.

g and h The **subscapularis** arises from the anterior surface of the scapula and is active when performing functional movements of the shoulder such as reaching behind the back to scratch between your shoulder blades.

Muscle	Attachments (P = proximal, D = distal)	Action/Function	Innervation
Supraspinatus	**P:** Supraspinous fossa of scapula **D:** Greater tubercle of humerus – superior facet	Initiates shoulder abduction; assists deltoid with shoulder abduction; intrinsic stabilization of G/H joint	Suprascapular nerve (C4, C5, C6)
Infraspinatus	**P:** Infraspinous fossa of scapula **D:** Greater tubercle of humerus – middle facet	External (lateral) rotation of shoulder	Suprascapular nerve (C5, C6)
Teres minor	**P:** Superior portion of lateral border of scapula **D:** Greater tubercle of humerus – inferior facet	External (lateral) rotation of shoulder	Axillary nerve (C5, C6)
Subscapularis	**P:** Subscapular fossa **D:** Lesser tubercle of humerus	Internal (medial) rotation of shoulder	Upper and lower subscapular nerves (C5, C6, C7)

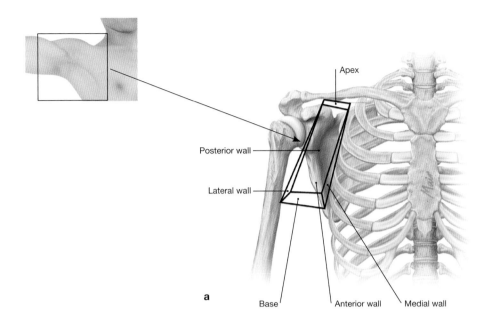

a

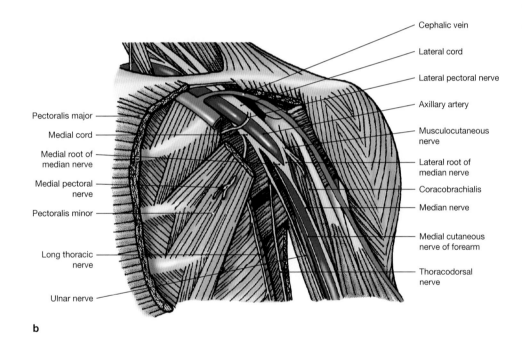

b

Fig. 3.25a and b Axillary region of the right shoulder; anterior view. [L271], a [L127], b [E877]

The **axilla** (armpit) is the area of the shoulder (➤ Fig. 11.14) directly under the glenohumeral joint, where the arm connects to the thorax.

a The size and shape of the axilla are defined by six features: **apex** – formed by the cervicoaxillary canal, bordered by the clavicle, first rib, and the top of the scapula; **base** – formed by the skin that stretches from the arm to the thorax; forms an indentation known as the axillary fossa; **anterior wall** – formed by the pectoralis major and minor muscles (anterior axillary fold); **posterior wall** – formed by the subscapularis, latissimus dorsi, and teres major muscles (posterior axillary fold); **medial wall** – comprised of the thorax and the serratus anterior muscle; **lateral wall** – formed by the humerus.

b Major blood vessels, lymphatic vessels, and nerves going to and from the upper extremity pass through the axillary region.

Contents of the axilla:
- Cords and branches of the brachial plexus
- Axillary artery and its branches
- Axillary vein and its tributaries
- Axillary lymph nodes
- Axillary lymphatic vessels
- Axillary fat
- Loose connective tissue

The neurovascular bundle is enclosed in connective tissue, called the 'axillary sheath'.

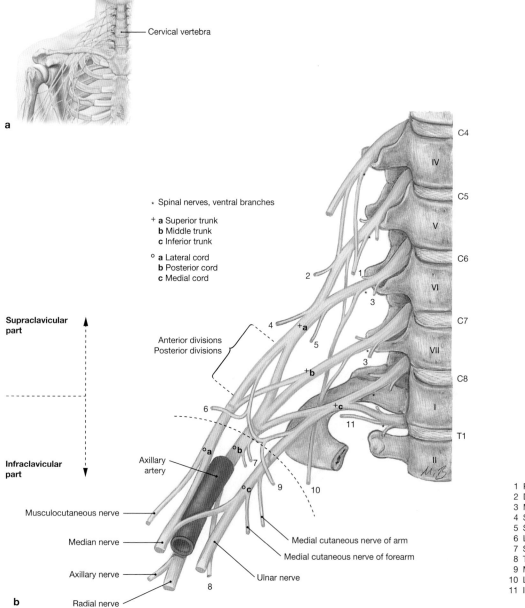

— Cervical vertebra

a

∗ Spinal nerves, ventral branches

+ **a** Superior trunk
  b Middle trunk
  c Inferior trunk

° **a** Lateral cord
  b Posterior cord
  c Medial cord

Supraclavicular part

Anterior divisions
Posterior divisions

Infraclavicular part

Axillary artery

Musculocutaneous nerve

Median nerve

Axillary nerve

Radial nerve

b

Medial cutaneous nerve of arm

Medial cutaneous nerve of forearm

Ulnar nerve

C4
IV
C5
V
C6
VI
C7
VII
C8
I
T1
II

1 Phrenic nerve (cervical plexus)
2 Dorsal scapular nerve
3 Muscular branches
4 Suprascapular nerve
5 Subclavian nerve
6 Lateral pectoral nerve
7 Subscapular nerve
8 Thoracodorsal nerve
9 Medial pectoral nerve
10 Long thoracic nerve
11 Intercostal nerve

Fig. 3.26a and b Brachial plexus (C5–T1): segmental arrangement and nerves of the shoulder and arm, right side; anterior view.
a [L127]
Innervation of the shoulder and arm is derived from the brachial plexus (C5–T1 spinal nerves), which is organized into two distinct parts:
1. a supraclavicular part – which supplies nerves that innervate a majority of the muscles that power movements of the shoulder;
2. an infraclavicular part – which supplies nerves that innervate muscles of the shoulder, as well as terminal nerves that innervate muscles of the arm, forearm and hand.

Supraclavicular branches include:
- Dorsal scapular nerve (C3–C5)
- Long thoracic nerve (C5–C7)
- Suprascapular nerve (C4–C6)
- Subclavian nerve (C5–C6)

Infraclavicular branches of the brachial plexus are organized according to the cord from which they arise (see table below).

Posterior Cord (C5–T1)	Lateral Cord (C5–C7)	Medial Cord (C8–T1)
Thoracodorsal nerve (C6–C8)	Lateral pectoral nerve (C5–C7)	Medial pectoral nerve (C8–T1)
Subscapular nerves (C5–C7)	Musculocutaneous nerve (C5–C7)*	Ulnar nerve (C8–T1)*
Axillary nerve (C5–C6)*	Median nerve, lateral root (C6–C7)*	Median nerve, medial root (C8–T1)*
Radial nerve (C5–T1)*		Medial cutaneous nerve of arm (C8–T1)

* Denotes the five terminal branches of the brachial plexus.

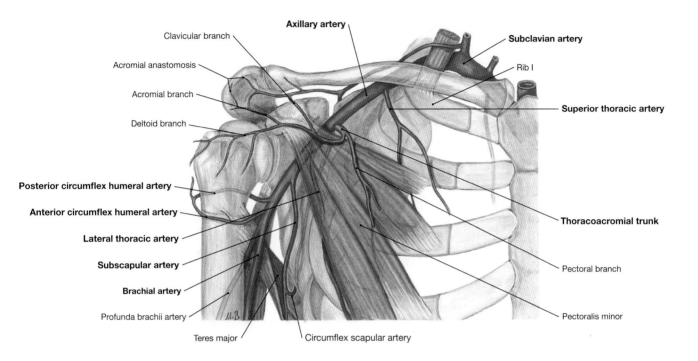

Fig. 3.27 Arteries of the shoulder region, right side; anterior view. The **axillary artery** is a continuation of the **subclavian artery** and stretches from the lateral border of the first rib to the inferior border of the pectoralis major (➤ Fig. 2.57 and ➤ Fig. 5.96). It is positioned between the three cords of the brachial plexus and the two roots of the median nerve. The inferior border of the teres major (tm) marks the end of the axillary artery and the beginning of the **brachial artery.** Anatomically, the axillary artery can be divided into three sections according to its position in relation to the pectoralis minor (pm) muscle:

- **Section 1:** located above or superior to the pectoralis minor and gives rise to one small branch – the **superior thoracic artery** which supplies the first intercostal space
- **Section 2:** located behind or posterior to the pectoralis minor and gives rise to two main branches – the **thoracoacromial**

trunk which has four branches (supplying the clavicular, pectoral, deltoid and acromial regions of the shoulder); and the **lateral thoracic artery** which supplies the muscles of the lateral thoracic wall

- **Section 3:** located below or inferior to the pectoralis minor and gives rise to three main branches – the **subscapular artery** which supplies the subscapular region and the latissimus dorsi muscle; the **anterior circumflex humeral artery** which provides blood supply to head of humerus and anterior aspect of G/H joint; and the **posterior circumflex humeral artery** which is the larger of the two circumflex arteries, and accompanies the axillary nerve to the posterior humerus where it provides blood supply to head of humerus and posterior aspect of the joint.

Clinical Remarks

An angiogram of the axillary region of the shoulder can be used to visualize the different branches of the axillary artery. The coracoid process serves as a key visual landmark for orienting oneself to the three sections of the axillary artery, as it represents the superior attachment for the pectoralis minor. [H063-001]

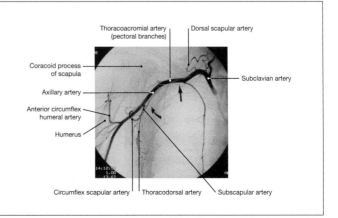

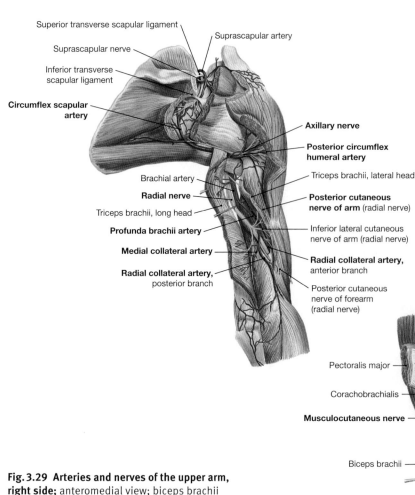

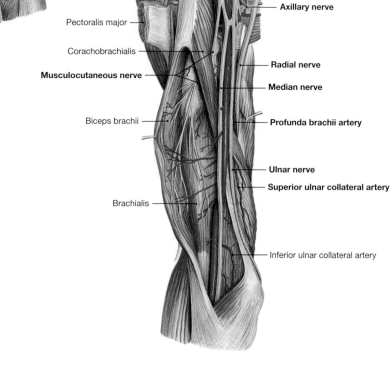

Fig. 3.28 Arteries and nerves of the upper arm, right side; posterolateral view.
This illustration depicts the branches of the **radial nerve**. The **profunda brachii artery** runs together with the radial nerve and splits into the **medial collateral artery** (to the medial epicondyle) and the **radial collateral artery** (concomitant with the nerve). The **axillary nerve** and **posterior circumflex humeral artery** pass through the quadrangular axillary space (QAS). The **circumflex scapular artery** passes through the triangular axillary space to the posterior side.

Fig. 3.29 Arteries and nerves of the upper arm, right side; anteromedial view; biceps brachii held apart.
The biceps brachii is lifted off laterally to show the course of the **musculocutaneous nerve.** The **median nerve** descends together with the brachial artery in the medial bicipital groove to reach the cubital fossa. The **ulnar nerve** continues together with the **superior ulnar collateral artery** to the posterior side of the medial epicondyle. The **axillary nerve** branches off the posterior cord proximally and passes through the quadrangular axillary space. The **radial nerve** courses together with the **profunda brachii artery through the triceps slit.**

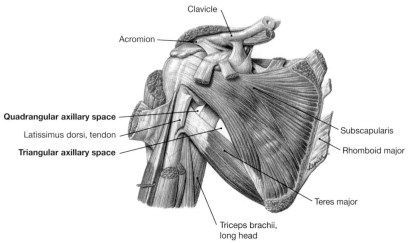

Fig. 3.30 Triangular and quadrangular axillary spaces, right side; anterior view.
The axillary spaces are located between the teres major and teres minor muscles (with the humerus as their lateral border). Both muscles diverge from one another as they move away from the scapula, leaving a gap which is divided by the long head of triceps brachii into a medially positioned **triangular axillary space (TAS)** and the laterally positioned **quadrangular axillary space (QAS).** The TAS allows passage of the circumflex scapular artery and vein to the posterior side of the scapula. The QAS provides passage for the axillary nerve and the posterior circumflex humeral artery and vein.

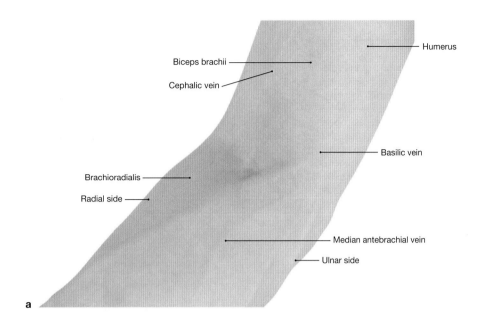

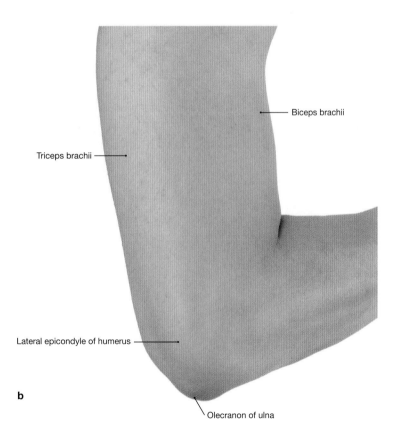

Fig. 3.31a and b Surface anatomy of the arm and elbow, right side; anteriomedial view **(a),** posterolateral view **(b).** [L271]
The shape and contour of the upper extremity is determined by superficial muscles and bony alignment. The surface landmarks which are palpable through the skin are important for physical examination.

Fig. 3.32 Bones of the elbow joint; anterior view.

The elbow is where the two bones of the forearm – the **radius** (thumb side) and **ulna** (little finger side) – meet with the **humerus.** At its distal end, the humerus flares out into two rounded protrusions called **epicondyles.** The upper end of the ulna also has two protrusions – the **olecranon and coronoid process.** These protrusions fit around the distal end of the humerus (**trochlea**) to form the **humeroulnar joint.** Beyond this, the **head of radius** also articulates with the **capitulum** portion of the distal humerus to form the **humeroradial joint.** Finally the proximal aspects of both the radius and ulna also articulate with each other – **proximal radioulnar joint.** The articular surfaces of each of the bones (depicted in blue color) are covered with a layer of thick, shiny articular cartilage that absorbs shock and allows the bones to glide smoothly against one another.

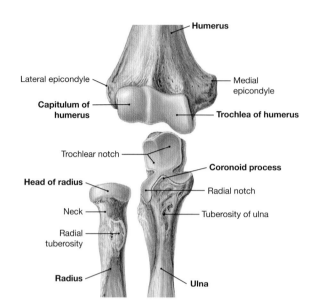

Fig. 3.33a and b Elbow joint, right side.

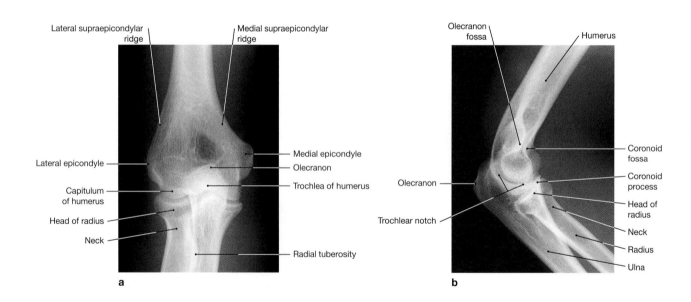

Radiographs in anteroposterior (A/P; **a**) and lateral **(b)** beam projections.

Clinical Remarks

The anterior fat pad of the elbow is located within the confines of the coronoid fossa of the humerus – it is considered intraarticular, but extrasynovial. When there is effusion within the elbow joint, the fat pad becomes elevated. On radiograph, the elevation of the anterior fat pad creates a silhouette similar to a billowing spinnaker sail from a boat. This **'sail sign'** is indicative of joint effusion within the elbow, and may suggest the presence of an intraarticular fracture of the elbow (i.e. head of radius or supracondylar fracture of humerus).   [E373]

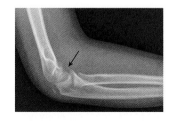

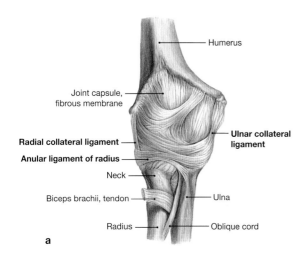

Humerus

Joint capsule, fibrous membrane

Radial collateral ligament

Anular ligament of radius

Neck

Biceps brachii, tendon

Radius

Ulnar collateral ligament

Ulna

Oblique cord

a

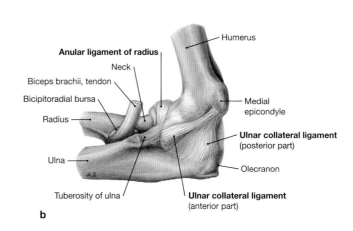

Humerus

Anular ligament of radius

Neck

Biceps brachii, tendon

Bicipitoradial bursa

Radius

Ulna

Tuberosity of ulna

Medial epicondyle

Ulnar collateral ligament (posterior part)

Olecranon

Ulnar collateral ligament (anterior part)

b

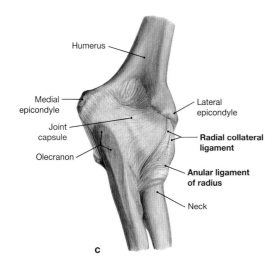

Humerus

Medial epicondyle

Joint capsule

Olecranon

Lateral epicondyle

Radial collateral ligament

Anular ligament of radius

Neck

c

Fig. 3.34a to c Elbow joint, right side; anterior view **(a)**, medial view **(b)**, and posterior view **(c)**.

The elbow joint is a hinge type synovial joint that is composed of three partial joints.

1. **Humeroulnar joint:** a hinge type of synovial joint formed by articulation between the trochlea of humerus and the trochlear notch of ulna. It allows movement around a single axis – flexion and extension.

2. **Humeroradial joint:** a hinge type of synovial joint involving articulation of the capitulum of humerus and the head of radius.

3. **Proximal radioulnar joint:** an uni-axial pivot joint involving articulation of the head of radius (ball) and the radial notch of ulna (socket). It allows pronation and supination movements of the forearm region.

The joint capsule encloses the cartilaginous articular surfaces of all three bones. The capsule is reinforced by strong accessory ligaments. Medially, the **ulnar collateral ligament** connects the medial epicondyle of the humerus with the coronoid process (anterior part) and the olecranon (posterior part) of the ulna – it resists valgus loads at the elbow. The **radial collateral ligament** (which resists varus loads at the elbow) originates from the lateral epicondyle and radiates out to join the **anular ligament of radius** which is attached to the anterior and posterior sides of the ulna, and loops around the head of radius. The **anular ligament** allows for guided rotational movements (pronation/supination) at the proximal radioulnar joint.

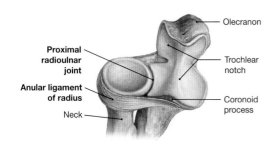

Olecranon

Proximal radioulnar joint

Trochlear notch

Anular ligament of radius

Neck

Coronoid process

Fig. 3.35 Articulating bones of the elbow joint; anterior-superior view.

Articular surfaces covered by hyaline cartilage are illustrated in blue.

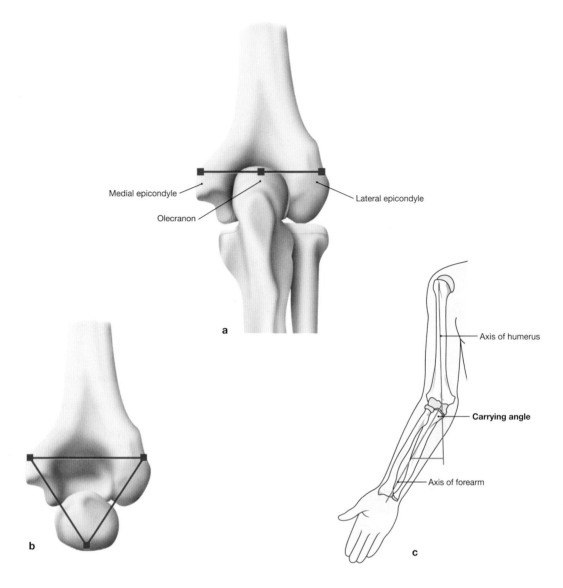

a

b

c

Medial epicondyle

Olecranon

Lateral epicondyle

Axis of humerus

Carrying angle

Axis of forearm

Fig. 3.36a to c Elbow alignment. a, b [L127], c [L231]
a In the extended position of the elbow joint, the epicondyles of the humerus are in line with the olecranon.
b In a flexed position, however, the epicondyles form an equilateral triangle – HUETER's triangle. The HUETER's triangle has radiological relevance since fractures and dislocations may result in deviations from this triangular orientation of the epicondyles.

c Carrying angle refers to the degree of cubital valgus present at the elbow. When the arms are held out beside the thorax and the palms are facing forwards, the forearms and hands should normally be 5 to 15 degrees away from the body. This angle allows the forearm to clear the hips when the arms swing during activities such as walking. Fractures of the elbow can increase or decrease the carrying angle.

Clinical Remarks

The elbow is a very stable joint, but dislocations can occur as a result of high impulse traumas such as falls from heights or motor vehicle accidents – they account for 10–25 % of all elbow injuries in the adult population. A posterior dislocation is most common and can be associated with fractures of various parts of the elbow (i.e. fracture of the humerus, radius, ulna or a combination of all three bones). Patients with a dislocated elbow will experience considerable pain, obvious deformity (loss of HUETER's triangle) and swelling. They may also have numbness or tingling in their hand after injury. Complex fracture-dislocations require surgical management that involves reduction of the dislocation, management of the fracture and repair of surrounding damaged soft tissues. These complex injuries are far more likely to have a poor outcome, including secondary osteoarthritis, limited range of motion, instability and recurrent dislocation.   [E813]

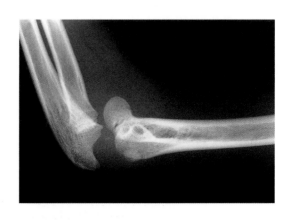

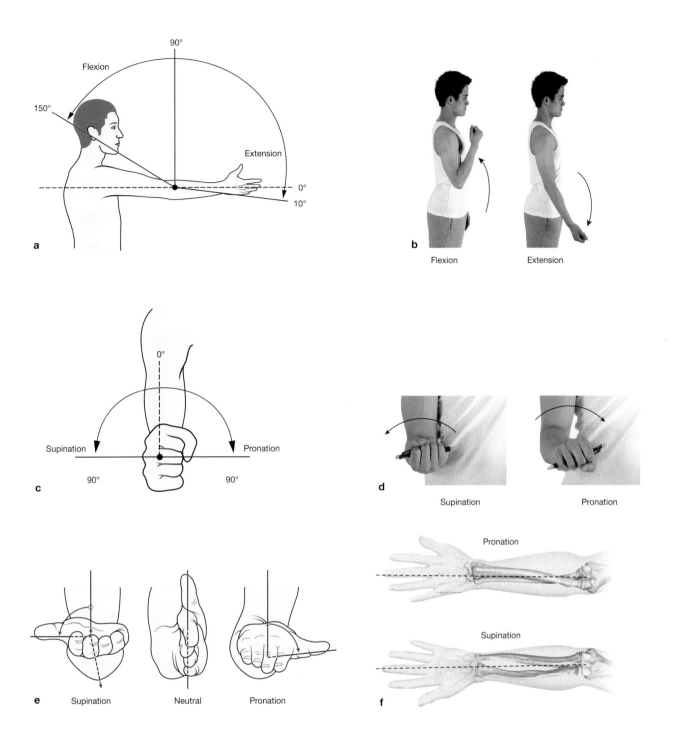

Fig. 3.37a to f Range of motion at the elbow joint. a, c, e [L126], b, d [L271], f [L127]

The elbow joint enables two distinct movements:

a and b Hinge movements (flexion and extension) between humerus and ulna, and between humerus and radius. Extension – flexion: 10° – 0° – 150°

c to f Rotational movements of pronation (palm facing downwards) and supination (palm facing upwards) between the radius and ulna. Elbow supination – pronation: 90° – 0° – 90°

The possible range of motion during elbow flexion is limited by soft tissue approximation (i.e. soft tissue contact between the muscles of the forearm and biceps region), while the range of motion of elbow extension is limited by the bony structure of the olecranon. Pronation and supination movements of the radius around the ulna are guided by the anular ligament and occur at both the proximal and distal radioulnar joints.

Elbow Movement	Muscles Active During Movements
Flexion	Brachialis, biceps brachii, brachioradialis (semi-pronated forearm)
Extension	Triceps – long, medial and lateral heads, anconeus
Supination	Biceps brachii, supinator
Pronation	Pronator teres, pronator quadratus

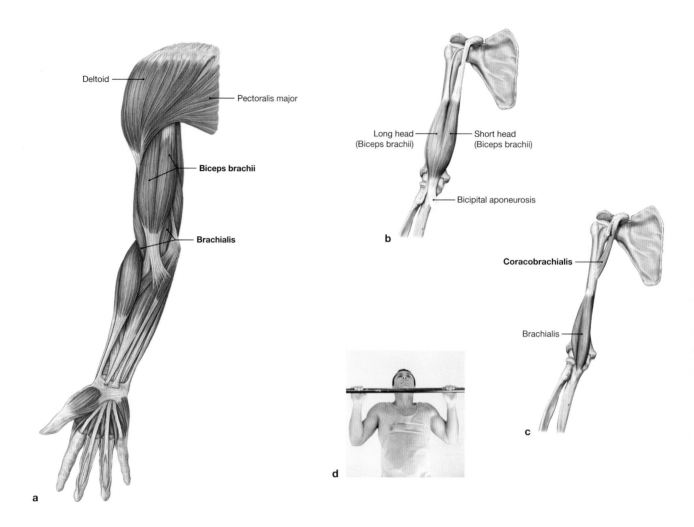

Fig. 3.38a to d **Muscles of the arm, right side;** anterior view.
b, c [L266, L127], d [J787]

The biceps region **(a)** is comprised of three separate and distinct muscles – **biceps brachii (b), coracobrachialis (c), and brachialis (c).** The biceps brachii is the most superficial muscle of the group, and is the only muscle that crosses both the shoulder and elbow joints – thus it powers motion at both joints. Together, the three anterior arm muscles power shoulder and elbow flexion movements such as would be required when **performing a chin-up maneuver (d).** Beyond this, the biceps brachii also serves as the strongest supinator of the forearm.

Muscle	Attachments (P = proximal, D = distal)	Action/Function	Innervation
Biceps brachii	**P:** Coracoid process of scapula (short head); supraglenoid tubercle of scapula (long head) **D:** Radial tuberosity, bicipital aponeurosis of forearm	Forearm supination, elbow flexion, assists with shoulder flexion	Musculocutaneous nerve (C5 and C6)
Brachialis	**P:** Anterior surface of humerus (distal half) **D:** Coronoid process and tuberosity of ulna	Elbow flexion	Musculocutaneous nerve (C5 and C6)
Coracobrachialis	**P:** Coracoid process of scapula **D:** Middle one-third of humerus (medial surface)	Assists with shoulder flexion	Musculocutaneous nerve (C5, C6, C7)

Clinical Remarks

Rupture of the proximal tendon of the biceps brachii can occur secondary to wear and tear conditions (tendinitis/tendopathy) of the shoulder.

a It is characterized by detachment of the long head from the supraglenoid tubercle of scapula.

b It is a common injury observed in older individuals, with the detached muscle belly falling inferiorly to form a 'ball' of muscle ('Popeye deformity') near the center of the distal portion of the humerus. This injury is frequently treated via conservative management, as it results in limited alteration of strength or function at the elbow.   a [L126], b [F276-005]

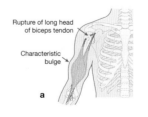

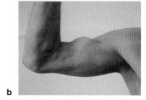

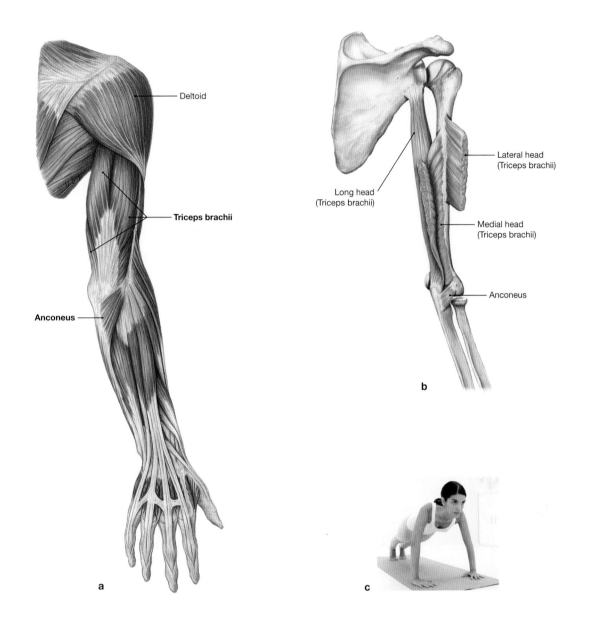

a

b

c

Fig. 3.39a to c Posterior muscles of the arm, triceps brachii and anconeus, right side; posterior view. b [L266, L127], c [J787]
The **triceps brachii (a)** is positioned on the posterior side of the humerus and is comprised of three separate heads **(long, medial, lateral; b)** which all are involved in powering elbow extension during activities such as **performing a push-up** or when catching/bracing yourself when falling forward (c). Because the long head crosses the G/H joint, it is also active during activities which involve shoulder extension. The functions of the triceps muscle group are also supported by the **anconeus,** which reinforces and helps to stabilize the posterolateral aspect of the elbow as it reaches full extension.

Muscle	Attachments (P = proximal, D = distal)	Action/Function	Innervation
Triceps brachii	**P:** Infraglenoid tubercle of scapula (long head), posterior surface of humerus – superior to radial groove (lateral head), posterior surface of humerus – inferior to radial groove (medial head) **D:** Olecranon of ulna	Elbow extension, assists with shoulder extension (long head)	Radial nerve (C6, C7 and C8)
Anconeus	**P:** Lateral epicondyle of humerus **D:** Lateral surface of olecranon, posterior surface of proximal ulna	Stabilizes elbow posteriorly, assists with elbow extension	Radial nerve (C7, C8 and T1)

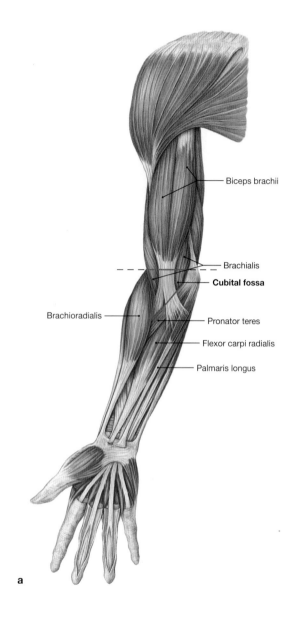

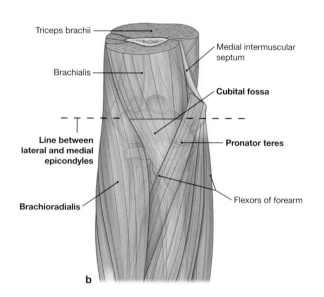

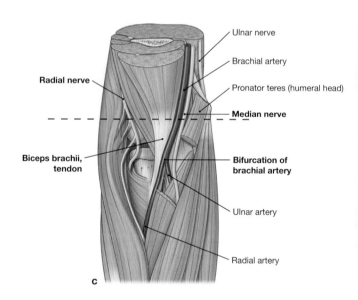

Fig. 3.40a to c Cubital fossa of the arm, right side; anterior view. b, c [E402]

a The **cubital fossa** is a region of the upper extremity located on the anterior surface of the elbow. It contains key neurovascular structures of the forearm, wrist and hand.

b It is a triangular area that is bordered by: laterally – **brachioradialis;** medially – **pronator teres;** superiorly – an **imaginary line that**

connects the medial and lateral epicondyles of the humerus; floor – **brachialis** and **supinator** muscles.

c From medial to lateral its contents include:
1. Median nerve
2. Bifurcation of the brachial artery
3. Biceps brachii tendon
4. Radial nerve

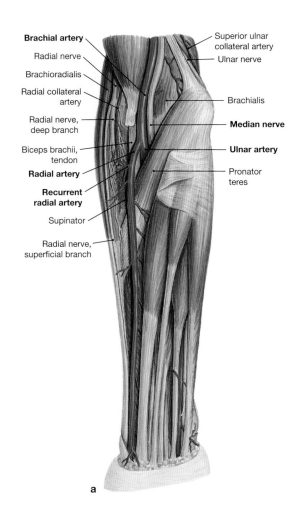

Brachial artery
Radial nerve
Brachioradialis
Radial collateral artery
Radial nerve, deep branch
Biceps brachii, tendon
Radial artery
Recurrent radial artery
Supinator
Radial nerve, superficial branch

Superior ulnar collateral artery
Ulnar nerve
Brachialis
Median nerve
Ulnar artery
Pronator teres

a

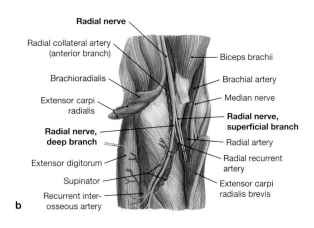

Radial nerve
Radial collateral artery (anterior branch)
Brachioradialis
Extensor carpi radialis
Radial nerve, deep branch
Extensor digitorum
Supinator
Recurrent interosseous artery

Biceps brachii
Brachial artery
Median nerve
Radial nerve, superficial branch
Radial artery
Radial recurrent artery
Extensor carpi radialis brevis

b

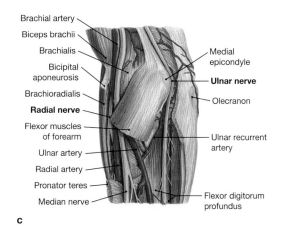

Brachial artery
Biceps brachii
Brachialis
Bicipital aponeurosis
Brachioradialis
Radial nerve
Flexor muscles of forearm
Ulnar artery
Radial artery
Pronator teres
Median nerve

Medial epicondyle
Ulnar nerve
Olecranon
Ulnar recurrent artery
Flexor digitorum profundus

c

Fig. 3.41a to c Arteries and nerves of the elbow region, right side; anterior view **(a)**; lateral (radial) view **(b)**; medial (ulnar) view **(c)**.
a The brachioradialis and distal biceps brachii have been removed to visualize branching of the **brachial artery into radial and ulnar arteries** in the forearm. The **radial artery** continues its course beneath the brachioradialis and reaches the radial side of the wrist. The **ulnar artery** branches off below the pronator teres and descends next to the ulnar nerve beneath the flexor carpi ulnaris to the ulnar side of the wrist. Together with the brachial artery, the **median nerve** enters the cubital fossa on the medial side.

b and c The **radial nerve** enters the cubital fossa on the lateral side between the brachioradialis and brachialis together with the radial collateral artery. Here it divides into two terminal branches – the **superficial branch** continues beneath the brachioradialis, while the **deep branch** reaches the posterior side of the forearm through the supinator muscle (supinator canal). The **ulnar nerve** is directly adjacent to the bone in the groove for ulnar nerve. It courses beneath the flexor carpi ulnaris to the flexor side of the forearm.

Clinical Remarks

a **Compression or entrapment of the ulnar nerve** can occur where it passes through the ulnar groove behind the medial epicondyle of the humerus (i.e. 'funny bone region').
b Symptoms (such as muscle weakness, numbness or tingling) may affect the fourth and fifth digits – the ring and little fingers – of the hand, with severity being dependent upon the duration and extent of nerve entrapment.
a, b [L126]

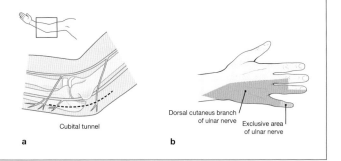

Cubital tunnel

Dorsal cutaneus branch of ulnar nerve
Exclusive area of ulnar nerve

a   b

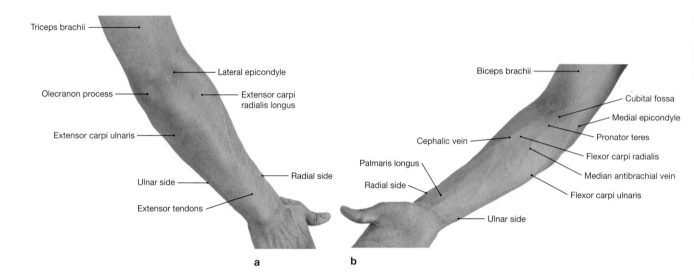

a

b

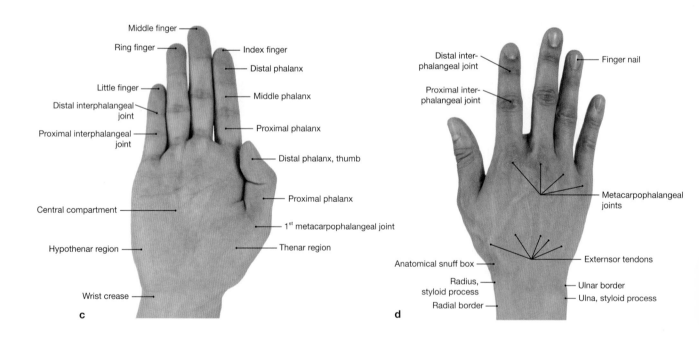

c

d

Fig. 3.42a to d Surface anatomy of the forearm, wrist and hand, right side; posterior **(a)**, anterior **(b)**, palmar **(c)** and dorsal **(d)** views. [L271]

The shape and contour of the forearm, wrist and hand regions are determined by superficial muscles and the alignment of underlying bones. The surface landmarks which are palpable through the skin are important for the physical examination.

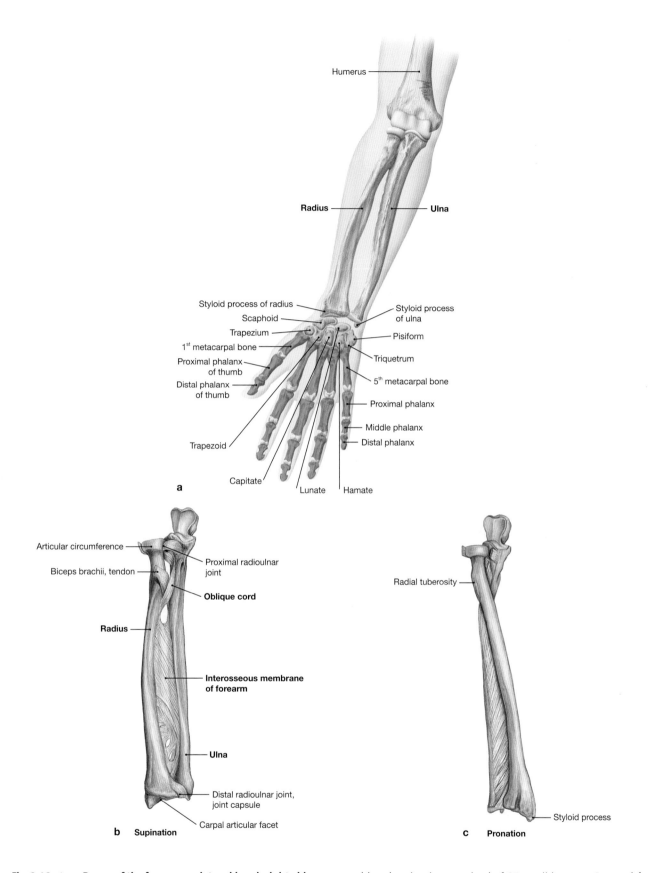

Fig. 3.43a to c Bones of the forearm, wrist and hand, right side; anterior view. a [L127]

a The forearm region is comprised of two long bones arranged in parallel: the ulna and the radius. The **ulna** is the longer and larger of the two bones, residing on the medial (little finger) side of the forearm. It is widest at its proximal end and narrows considerably at its distal end. The **radius** is slightly shorter, thinner, and located on the lateral (thumb) side of the forearm. The radius is narrowest at the elbow and widens as it descends towards the wrist. The wrist and hand region is comprised of 27 small bones – **8 carpal (yellow), 5 metacarpal (orange) bones, and 14 phalanges (green).**

The bones of the forearm are connected by the tough **interosseous membrane** of forearm with collagen fibers which are predominantly oriented from the radius proximally to the ulna distally.

These figures demonstrate the rotation of the radius around the ulna. The radius and ulna are positioned parallel during **supination** of the forearm **(b)** but they cross during **pronation** of the forearm **(c)**.

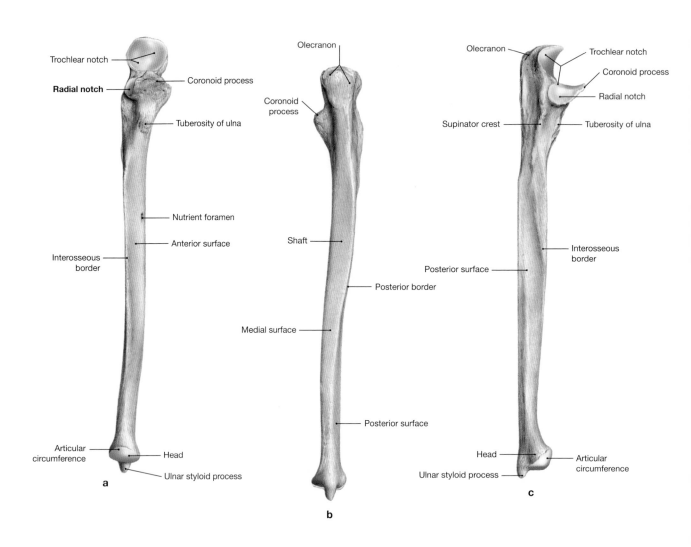

Fig. 3.44a to c Ulna, right side; anterior **(a)**, posterior **(b)** and lateral **(c)** views.

Matching an isolated ulna to one side of the body is aided by the position of the **radial notch** which points laterally.

Clinical Remarks

a There are several bursae which are located in the olecranon region of the proximal ulna (at the elbow).
b Olecranon bursitis can occur secondary to trauma, inflammation or infection. It results in a large mass of swelling that appears at the point of elbow, making the region very painful to touch (it can be painful to even wear a long sleeve shirt), and often makes elbow flexion movements difficult.
a [L126], b [G463]

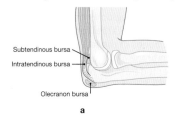

a

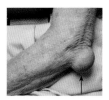

b

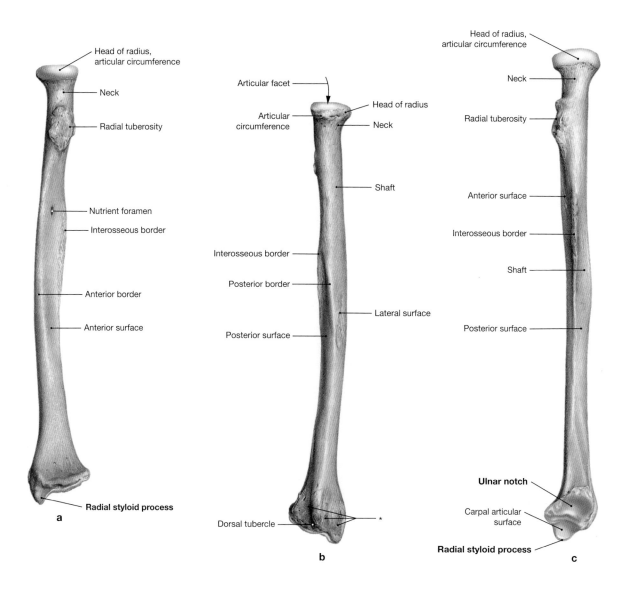

Fig. 3.45a to c Radius, right side; anterior **(a)**, posterior **(b)** and medial **(c)** views.

Matching an isolated radius to one side of the body is aided by the position of the **radial styloid process** which points laterally. The **ulnar notch,** however, points in the direction of the ulna.

* Grooves and bony crests for the extensor tendons

Clinical Remarks

A COLLES fracture refers to a fracture of the distal radius, usually about an inch or two proximal to the radiocarpal joint (but without involvement of the articular surface). It frequently occurs as a result of a fall onto an outstretched hand (i.e. trying to catch yourself when falling onto a hard surface) and is visualized on lateral radiographs as a 'dinner fork'- or 'bayonet'-like deformity because of the posterior and lateral displacement of the distal fragment. It is the most common type of distal radius fracture, and can occur across all age groups and demographics – with patients diagnosed with osteoporosis being particularly at risk. [G645]

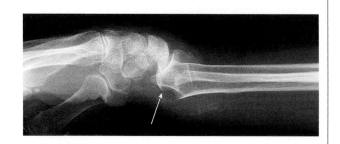

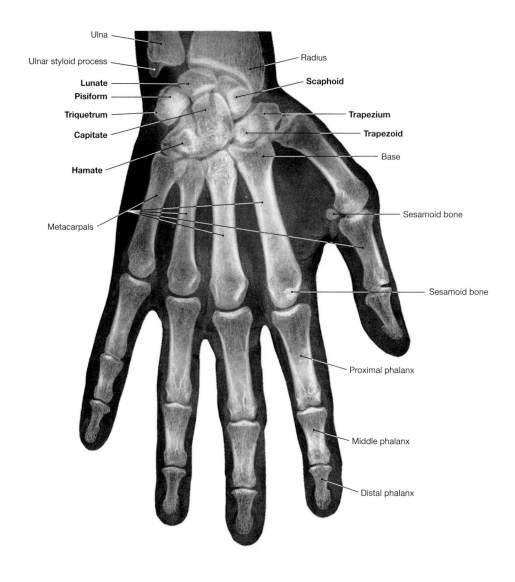

Fig. 3.46 Hand, right side; radiograph in anteroposterior (A/P) beam projection.
This radiograph depicts the wrist (with carpal bones), the palm (with metacarpal bones) and the digits of the hand (with phalanges). The wrist is comprised of a proximal and a distal row of carpal bones. Arranged from the radial to ulnar side, the proximal row contains the **scaphoid, lunate and triquetrum.** The **pisiform** (a sesamoid bone within the tendon of the flexor carpi ulnaris) is adjacent to the triquetrum on the palmar surface of the wrist. The distal row (again organized from the radial to ulnar side) is comprised of the **trapezium, trapezoid, capitate and hamate.** Students use the mnemonic 'She Likes To Play, Try To Catch Her' to help remember the sequence of the carpal bones. The bones of the wrist also help to form the carpal groove which builds the base of the carpal tunnel – it is bordered by the scaphoid and the trapezium on the radial side and by the pisiform and the hamate on the ulnar side. The five metacarpal bones serve to form the palm of the hand. The five digits each consist of several phalanges.

Clinical Remarks

Fractures of the wrist and hand are very common.
a A fracture of the 5th metacarpal bone immediately proximal to the head is referred to as a **'boxer's' fracture.** It can occur as a result of striking an object with a glancing blow in which only the medial aspect of the hand – 4th and 5th digits – make contact.
b The scaphoid bone is the most commonly fractured carpal bone. Concomitant injuries of the supplying blood vessels may result in necrosis of the scaphoid bone and show a reduced bone density on radiographic imaging. In addition, injuries may cause degenerative alterations (e.g. osteoarthritis) within the joints of the hand and fingers.   a [G719], b [E513-002]

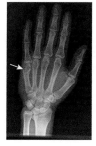

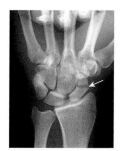

a   **b**

Fig. 3.47 Distal radioulnar joint; inferior view. The **distal radioulnar** joint is a pivot joint (pronation/supination) that is located superior to the proximal row of carpal bones at the wrist. The joint is comprised of the head of ulna and the ulnar notch of the radius. At the wrist, the **carpal articular facet** of the distal radius and the **articular disc** of the distal radioulnar joint articulate with the proximal carpal bones.

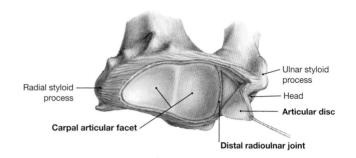

Radial styloid process

Carpal articular facet

Ulnar styloid process

Head

Articular disc

Distal radioulnar joint

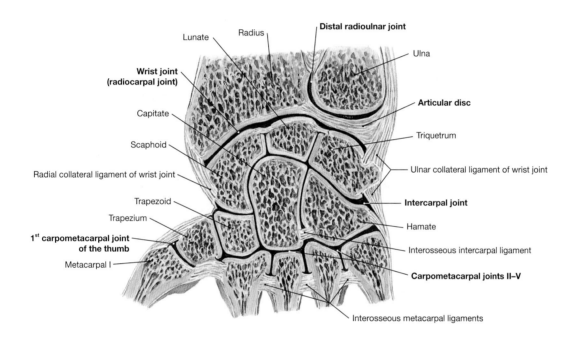

Lunate

Radius

Distal radioulnar joint

Ulna

Wrist joint (radiocarpal joint)

Articular disc

Capitate

Triquetrum

Scaphoid

Ulnar collateral ligament of wrist joint

Radial collateral ligament of wrist joint

Intercarpal joint

Trapezoid

Hamate

Trapezium

1ˢᵗ carpometacarpal joint of the thumb

Interosseous intercarpal ligament

Metacarpal I

Carpometacarpal joints II–V

Interosseous metacarpal ligaments

Fig. 3.48 Joints of the wrist and metacarpus, right side; palmar view, section parallel to the dorsum of hand.
The proximal wrist joint – **radiocarpal joint** – is a condyloid synovial joint which connects the forearm bones (radius and ulna) with the proximal row of carpal bones. An **articular disc** is positioned between the distal ulna and triquetrum bone. **Intercarpal joints** – plane synovial joints – connect the proximal and distal rows of carpal bones and only allow a small range of motion between two adjacent bones. The **carpometacarpal joints II–V** and the **intermetacarpal joints** are also plane synovial joints which allow only limited movement. In contrast, **the 1ˢᵗ carpometacarpal joint of the thumb** is a saddle type of synovial joint that is highly mobile and facilitates flexion/extension, abduction/adduction, and finger opposition movements of the thumb.

Structure/Function

a A/P radiograph illustrating the normal alignment of the carpal bones at the wrist. Normally, the orientation of the bones should form three smooth curves – GILULA arcs – which outline the proximal and distal surfaces of the proximal carpal row, as well as the proximal cortical margins of the capitate and hamate bones.
b A lateral radiograph depicts the normal orientation of the radius, lunate and capitate bones – the apple (capitate) should sit in the cup (lunate), which is positioned in the saucer (radius). The articular surfaces of each bone should be arranged in a straight line and be congruent (parallel).
a [G425], b [E372]

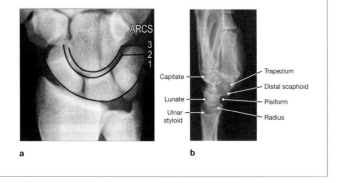

ARCS
3
2
1

Capitate

Lunate

Ulnar styloid

Trapezium

Distal scaphoid

Pisiform

Radius

a

b

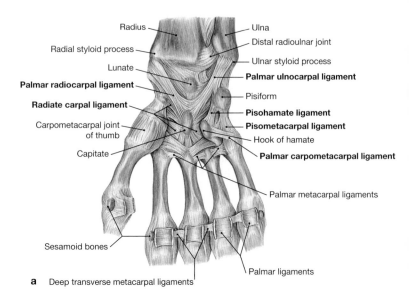

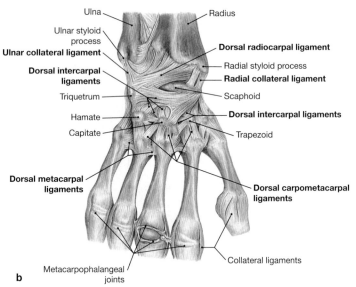

Fig. 3.49a and b Joints and ligaments of the hand, right side; palmar view **(a)** and dorsal view **(b)**.

Ligaments of Wrist and Metacarpus	
• Palmar and dorsal radiocarpal ligaments, and palmar ulnocarpal ligament	• Pisohamate ligament: continuation of the flexor carpi ulnaris tendon to the hamate
• Radial and ulnar collateral ligaments of wrist joint: from the styloid processes	• Pisometacarpal ligament: continuation of the flexor carpi ulnaris tendon to the metacarpals IV and V
• Palmar, dorsal, and interosseous intercarpal ligaments	• Palmar and dorsal carpometacarpal ligaments
• Radiate carpal ligament: ligament radiating from the capitate	• Palmar, dorsal, and interosseous metacarpal ligaments

Clinical Remarks

a A/P radiograph depicting injury of the scapholunate ligamentous complex which results in an internal derangement of bones (loss of GILULA arcs) which form the radiocarpal and intercarpal joints.
b A lateral view radiograph depicting abnormal orientation of the radius, lunate and capitate bones – a line drawn along the long axis of the radius crosses the lunate, but not the capitate which is dislocated posteriorly. This is indicative of a perilunate dislocation.
a [G493], b [E380]

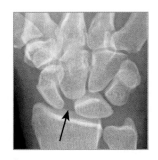

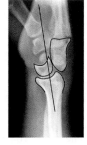

a

b

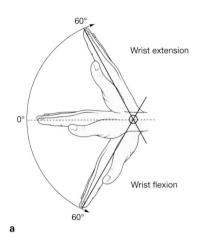

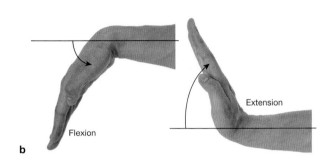

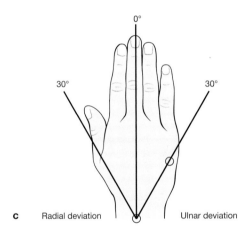

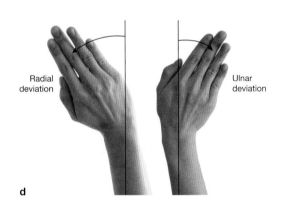

Fig. 3.50a to d Wrist movements. a, c [L126], b, d [L271]
a and b Flexion – extension: 60° – 0° – 60°
c and d Radial deviation – ulnar deviation: 30° – 0° – 30°

Wrist Movement	Muscles Active During Movements
Flexion	Palmaris longus, flexor carpi radialis, flexor carpi ulnaris, flexor digitorum superficialis, flexor digitorum profundus
Extension	Extensor digitorum, extensor carpi radialis longus, extensor carpi radialis brevis, extensor carpi ulnaris, extensor digiti minimi, extensor indicis
Ulnar deviation	Flexor carpi ulnaris, extensor carpi ulnaris
Radial deviation	Flexor carpi radialis, extensor carpi radialis longus, extensor carpi radialis brevis

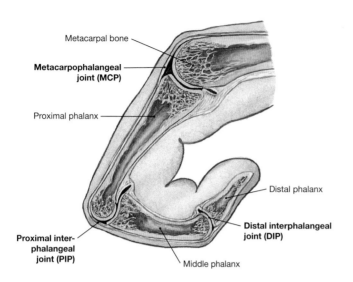

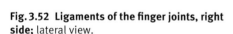

Fig. 3.51 Finger joints, right side; lateral view, sagittal section.

The finger joints are comprised of the metacarpophalangeal and interphalangeal joints. The **metacarpophalangeal joints** are condyloid synovial joints in which the distal parts (or head region) of the metacarpal bones articulate with the bases of the proximal phalanges. The **proximal and distal interphalangeal joints** are all hinge type synovial joints which are located between the heads and the bases of the respective phalanges of each of the fingers.

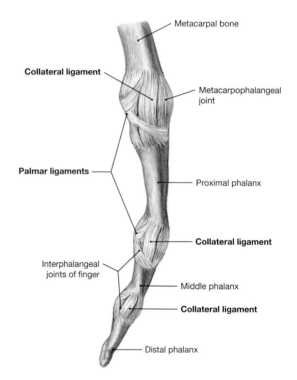

Fig. 3.52 Ligaments of the finger joints, right side; lateral view.

The metacarpophalangeal and interphalangeal joints are each supported by several ligaments:

1. **Deep transverse metacarpal ligament** (not depicted): connects palmar ligaments at adjacent metacarpophalangeal joints
2. **Collateral ligaments:** lateral and medial collateral ligaments resist varus/valgus stresses
3. **Palmar ligaments:** anterior surface of joints – resist A/P directed forces

Clinical Remarks

The small joints of hands and fingers are easily injured during sports, work, or even everyday activities. Injuries are characterized by pain, significant swelling, an inability to move the affected joint, and sometimes deformity immediately following the traumatic event.

a Lateral radiograph which illustrates a dislocated proximal interphalangeal joint.

b Severe articular and ligamentous injury frequently results in small fractures around the affected joint, such as when a ligament 'pulls' a piece of bone away from the main bone mass – an avulsion fracture.

a [E339], b [E380]

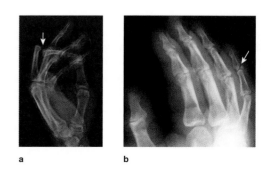

a　　　　　b

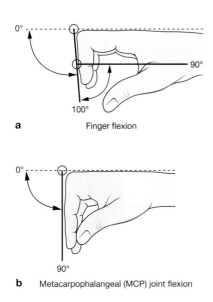

a Finger flexion

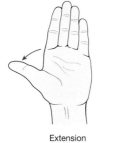

b Metacarpophalangeal (MCP) joint flexion

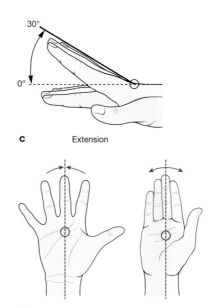

c Extension

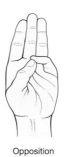
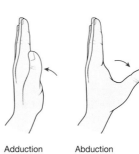

d MCP adduction MCP abduction

Fig. 3.53a to d Range of motion of the finger joints. [L126]
Movements of the fingers (digits II–V) are powered by both extrinsic muscles (originating outside of the hand) and intrinsic muscles (originating within the hand).
a to c The **proximal interphalangeal joints (PIP)** and **distal interphalangeal joints (DIP)** of digits II–V allow only flexion and extension movements to occur.

The **metacarpophalangeal (MCP)** joints allow flexion and extension movements, as well as adduction and abduction movements away from the midline axis of the hand which runs through the middle finger (digit II). **Flexion – extension movements:** MCP joints 90° – 0° – 30°; PIP joints 90° – 0° – 0°; DIP joints 90° – 0° – 0°
d Adduction – abduction movements: MCP joints of fingers II–V (20–40)° – 0° – (20–40)°

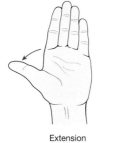

Extension Flexion Opposition Adduction Abduction

Fig. 3.54 Thumb motion. [L126]
The **carpometacarpal (CMC) joint of the thumb** (saddle joint) facilitates a large range of motion not only in thumb flexion/extension, but also during adduction/abduction. These movements can be combined for circumduction and finger opposition movements of the thumb, both of which are important when grasping objects.

The **MCP joint of the thumb** enables only hinge (flexion/extension) movements, as does the PIP joint of the thumb.
- **1st CMC (saddle) joint:** Extension – flexion 30° – 0° – 40°, abduction – adduction 10° – 0° – 40°
- **1st MCP joint:** Extension – flexion 0° – 0° – 50°
- **1st PIP joint:** Extension – flexion 0° – 0° – 80°

Finger Movement	Extrinsic Muscles of Hand	Intrinsic Muscles of Hand
Flexion	Flexor digitorum superficialis, flexor digitorum profundus, flexor pollicis longus	Flexor pollicis brevis, flexor digiti minimi, lumbricals
Extension	Extensor digitorum, extensor pollicis longus, extensor pollicis brevis	
Abduction	Abductor pollicis longus	Dorsal interossei, abductor pollicis brevis
Adduction		Palmar interossei, adductor pollicis
Opposition		Opponens pollicis, opponens digiti minimi

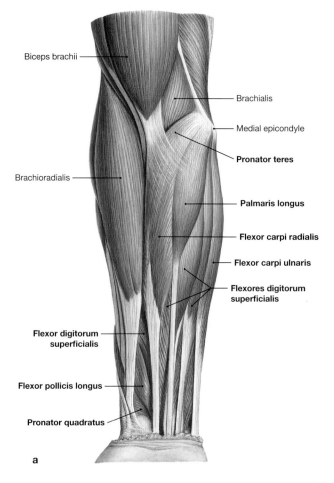

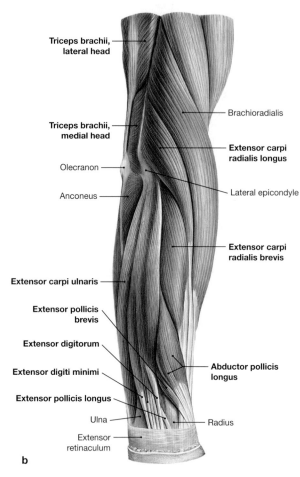

Fig. 3.55a and b Muscles of the forearm, right side; anterior view **(a)**, posterior view **(b)**.

The forearm can be organized into two **compartments – anterior and posterior**. Each compartment contains **a superficial and a deep layer of muscles.**

The superficial layer of muscles in both compartments arises from the epicondylar region of the humerus **(anterior arises from the medial epicondyle/posterior arises from the lateral epicondyle)**, while the deep layer of muscles in each compartment arises from the ulna, radius or interosseous membrane (distal to the elbow).

The muscles which occupy the **posterior compartment are all innervated by the radial nerve,** and function to power extension and supination movements. The muscles which occupy the **anterior compartment are primarily innervated by the median nerve** (the ulnar nerve innervates one and a half muscles), and powers flexion and pronation movements. Muscles of both compartments equally assist with powering radial and ulnar deviation of the wrist.

Note: The supinator and extensor indicis muscles are not visualized on the above images.

Anterior Compartment	Posterior Compartment
• Comprised of eight muscles in total	• Comprised of ten muscles in total
• Organized into superficial and deep layers	• Organized into superficial and deep layers
• Five superficial muscles/three deep muscles	• Six superficial muscles/four deep muscles
• All superficial muscles arise from the medial epicondyle	• All superficial muscles arise from the lateral epicondyle
• Muscles function to either flex (wrist/thumb/fingers) or pronate wrist	• Muscles function to either extend (wrist/thumb/fingers) or supinate wrist
• Assist with ulnar and radial deviations at the wrist	• Assist with ulnar and radial deviation at the wrist

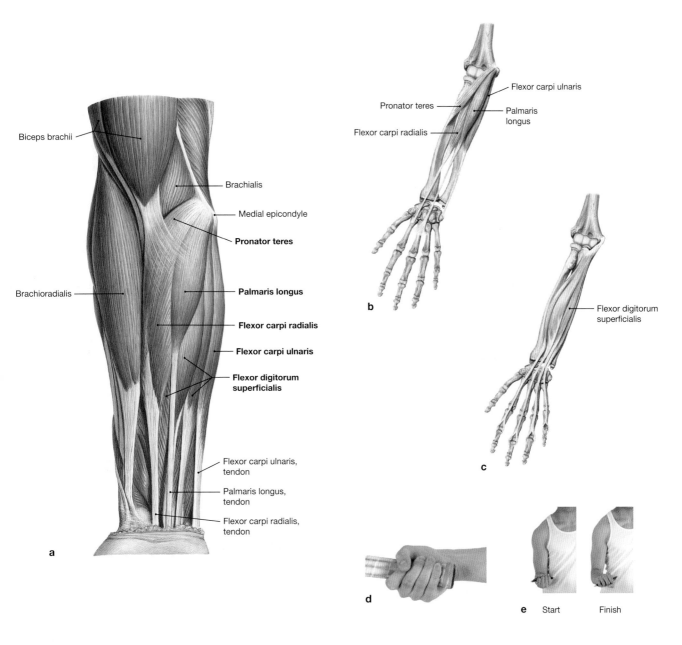

Fig. 3.56a to e Superficial layer of muscles located in the anterior compartment of the forearm, right side; anterior view. b, c [L266, L127], d, e [L271]

A total of **five muscles are located in the superficial layer of the anterior forearm.** All arise from the common flexor tendon which attaches proximally to the medial epicondyle of the distal humer-us. These muscles are primarily **innervated by the median nerve** (the ulnar nerve only innervates the flexor carpi ulnaris) and func-tion to power everyday gripping activities such as **flexing the wrist and fingers** to grasp a handle **(d)**, and **pronation** or rotation of the palm to face downwards **(e)**. They also assist with radial and ulnar deviation of the wrist.

Muscle	Attachments (P = proximal, D = distal)	Action/Function	Innervation (spinal root)
Pronator teres	**P:** Medial epicondyle of humerus; coronoid process of ulna **D:** Lateral edge of middle one-third of radius	Wrist pronation; assists with elbow flexion	Median nerve (C6, C7)
Flexor carpi radialis	**P:** Medial epicondyle of humerus **D:** Base of metacarpal II	Radial deviation of wrist; wrist flexion	Median nerve (C7, C8)
Palmaris longus	**P:** Medial epicondyle of humerus **D:** Flexor retinaculum; palmar aponeurosis	Tightening of palmar aponeurosis; wrist flexion	Median nerve (C7, C8)
Flexor carpi ulnaris	**P:** Medial epicondyle of humerus, olecranon and anterior border of ulna **D:** Pisiform, hook of hamate, base of metacarpal V	Ulnar deviation of wrist; wrist flexion	Ulnar nerve (C7, C8)
Flexor digitorum superficialis	**P:** Medial epicondyle of humerus, ulnar collateral ligament, coronoid process of ulna, superior half of anterior border of radius **D:** Middle phalanges of the medial four digits	Flexes proximal interphalan-geal joint of medial four digits; assists with flexion of metacar-palphalengal and wrist joints	Median nerve (C7, C8, T1)

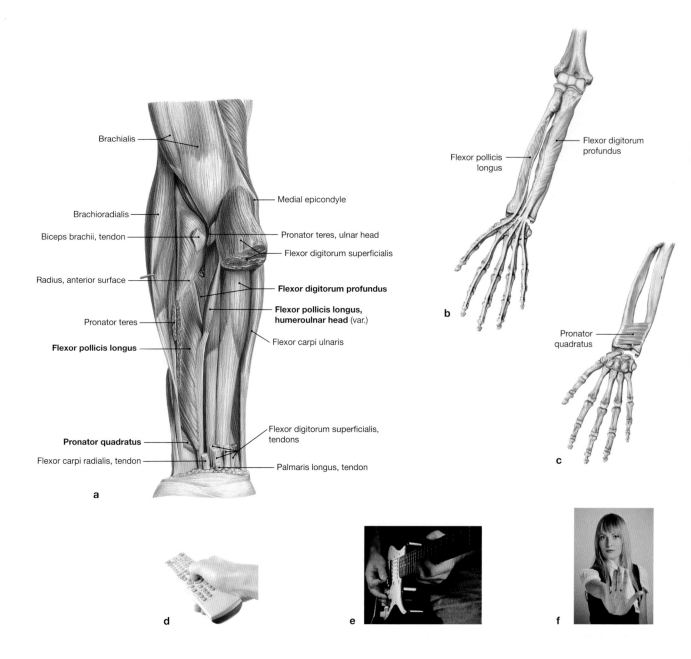

Fig. 3.57a to f Deep layer of muscles located in the anterior compartment of the forearm, right side; anterior view. b, c [L266, L127], d [L271], e, f [J787]
Following removal of the superficial layer of muscles within the anterior compartment, the **three deep muscles** become visible. These muscles all arise from the anterior surface of the ulna, radius, or interosseous membrane (distal to the elbow), and are primarily **innervated by the median nerve** (the ulnar nerve only innervates a

portion of the flexor digitorum profundus). They are important for performing activities such:
d Flexion of the MCP and PIP joints of the thumb (e.g. pressing a button) with your thumb;
e Flexion of the DIP joints of digits I–IV (e.g. playing a musical instrument);
f Pronation of the forearm (e.g. signalling someone to stop).

Muscle	Attachments (P = proximal, D = distal)	Action/Function	Innervation
Flexor digitorum profundus	**P:** Medial and anterior aspects of proximal ulna; interosseous membrane **D:** Distal phalanges of medial four digits	Flexes distal interphalangeal joint of medial four digits; assist with flexion of the hand	Median nerve (C8, T1) – tendons to 3rd and 4th digits, ulnar nerve (C8, T1) – tendons to 1st and 2nd digits
Flexor pollicis longus	**P:** Anterior surface of radius; interosseous membrane **D:** Base of distal phalanx of thumb	Radial deviation of wrist; wrist flexion	Median nerve via anterior interosseous nerve (C8, T1)
Pronator quadratus	**P:** Anterior aspect of distal ulna **D:** Anterior aspect of distal radius	Wrist pronation; stabilization of distal radioulnar joint	Median nerve via anterior interosseous nerve (C8, T1)

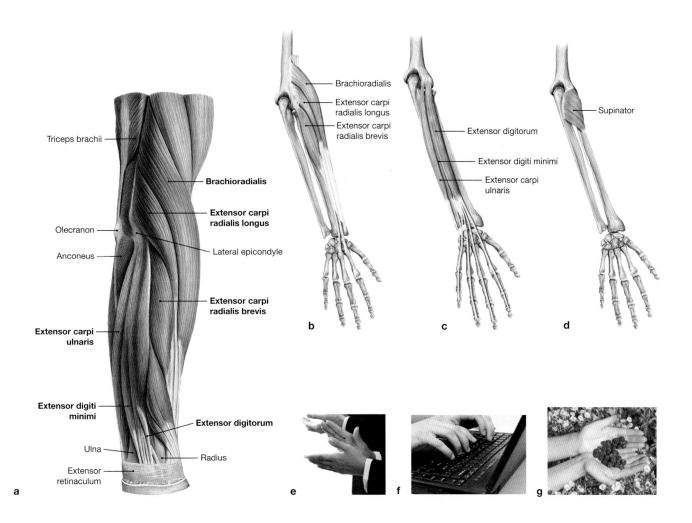

Fig. 3.58a to g Superficial layer of muscles located in the posterior compartment of the forearm, right side; posterolateral views. b–d [L266, L127], e–g [J787]

The anterior and posterior compartments of the forearm are separated on the lateral side by the **brachioradialis muscle.** It powers elbow flexion of a semi-pronated forearm i.e. lifting a cup/glass up to your mouth to drink. The superficial layer of the posterior forearm is comprised of six muscles which all arise from the lateral epicondyle of the humerus (proximal to the elbow) via the common extensor tendon, and are all innervated by the radial nerve. Each of these muscles functions to power **extension and supination movements** of the wrist and hand during everyday activities such as clapping your hands **(e)** or typing on a computer **(f).** Muscles in the superficial layer also assist with radial and ulnar deviation of the wrist; turning your palms upwards (supination) when gesturing or asking for something **(g).**

Muscle	Attachments (P = proximal, D = distal)	Action/Function	Innervation (spinal root)
Brachioradialis	**P:** Lateral supracondylar ridge – proximal two-third **D:** Lateral surface of distal radius	Flexes semipronated elbow	Radial nerve (C5, C6, C7)
Extensor carpi radialis longus	**P:** Lateral epicondyle of humerus **D:** Base of metacarpal II	Radial deviation of wrist; wrist extension	Radial nerve (C6, C7)
Extensor carpi radialis brevis	**P:** Lateral epicondyle of humerus **D:** Base of metacarpal III	Radial deviation of wrist; wrist extension	Radial nerve (C7, C8)
Extensor digitorum	**P:** Lateral epicondyle of humerus **D:** Extensor expansion of the four medial digits	Extends the proximal and distal interphalangeal and metacarpophalangeal joints of medial four digits; assists with wrist extension	Posterior interosseous branch of radial nerve (C7, C8)
Extensor digiti minimi	**P:** Lateral epicondyle of humerus **D:** Extensor expansion of digit V	Extends the proximal and distal interphalangeal and metacarpophalangeal joints of digit V	Posterior interosseous branch of radial nerve (C7, C8)
Extensor carpi ulnaris	**P:** Lateral epicondyle of humerus, posterior border of ulna **D:** Base of metacarpal V	Ulnar deviation of wrist; wrist extension	Posterior interosseous branch of radial nerve (C7, C8)
Supinator	**P:** Lateral epicondyle; radial collateral ligament; anular ligament, supinator fossa, crest of ulna **D:** Proximal one-third of radius (posterior, lateral and anterior surfaces)	Supination of wrist	Radial nerve (C5, C6)

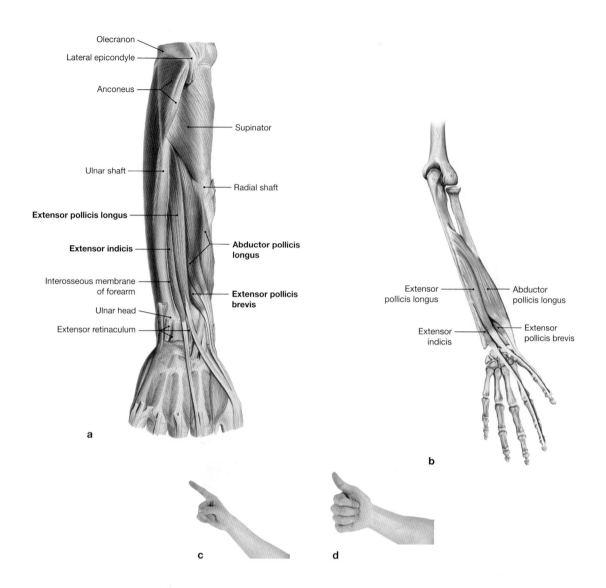

a

b

c

d

Fig. 3.59a to d Deep layer of muscles located in the posterior compartment of the forearm, right side; posterior view. b [L266, L127], c, d [L271]

Removal of the superficial extensor muscles of the forearm enables visualization of the four muscles which comprise the deep lay-er of the extensor compartment. These muscles all arise from the posterior surface of the ulna, radius, or interosseous membrane and are all innervated by the radial nerve. They are important for performing everyday manual activities such as pointing with your index finger **(c)** or giving the thumbs-up sign **(d)**.

Muscle	Attachments (P = proximal, D = distal)	Action/Function	Innervation (spinal root)
Abductor pollicis longus	**P:** Posterior surface of ulna, radius, and interosseous membrane **D:** Base of metacarpal I	Abduction of 1st carpometacarpal joint	Posterior interosseous branch of radial nerve (C7, C8)
Extensor pollicis brevis	**P:** Posterior surface of radius and inter-osseous membrane **D:** Base of proximal phalanx of thumb	Extension of proximal phalanx of thumb at carpometacarpal joint	Posterior interosseous branch of radial nerve (C7, C8)
Extensor pollicis longus	**P:** Posterior surface of middle one-third of ulna and interosseous membrane **D:** Base of distal phalanx of thumb	Extension of distal phalanx of thumb in the interphalangeal and carpome-tacarpal joints	Posterior interosseous branch of radial nerve (C7, C8)
Extensor indicis	**P:** Posterior surface of middle one-third of ulna and interosseous membrane **D:** Extensor expansion of digit II	Extension of digit II (index finger)	Posterior interosseous branch of radial nerve (C7, C8)

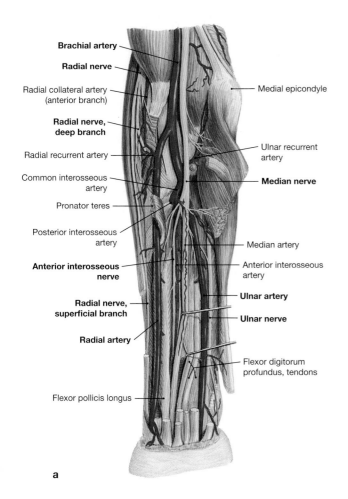

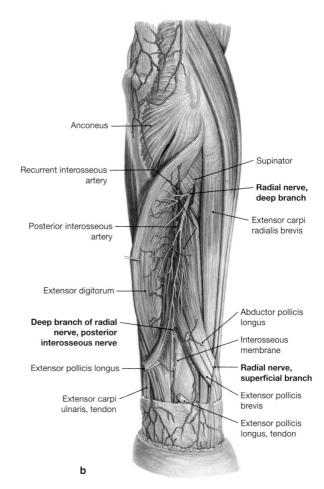

Fig. 3.60a and b Arteries and nerves of the forearm, right side; anterior view – all superficial flexor muscles have been removed **(a)**, lateral view **(b)**.

Below the elbow, the **brachial artery** splits into radial and ulnar arteries. The **radial artery** descends beneath the brachioradialis on the radial side of the forearm to the level of the wrist. Palpation of arterial pulses is predominantly performed on the radial artery just above the proximal wrist joint. The **ulnar artery** branches off below the pronator teres and descends next to the ulnar nerve beneath the flexor carpi ulnaris to the ulnar side of the wrist. Between the brachioradialis and brachialis muscles, the **radial nerve** enters the cubital fossa from lateral and splits into superficial and deep branches. The **superficial branch** runs adjacent to the radial artery and to the posterior side in the distal third of the forearm. The **deep branch** innervates and pierces the supinator. The **median nerve** descends distally along the midline of the forearm between the deep and superficial flexor muscles and is commonly accompanied by a thin artery (median artery). In the proximal forearm, the **anterior interosseous nerve** branches off the median nerve to provide motor innervation to the deep flexor muscles and provide sensory function to the wrist joint. The **ulnar nerve** courses beneath the flexor carpi ulnaris to the flexor side of the forearm.

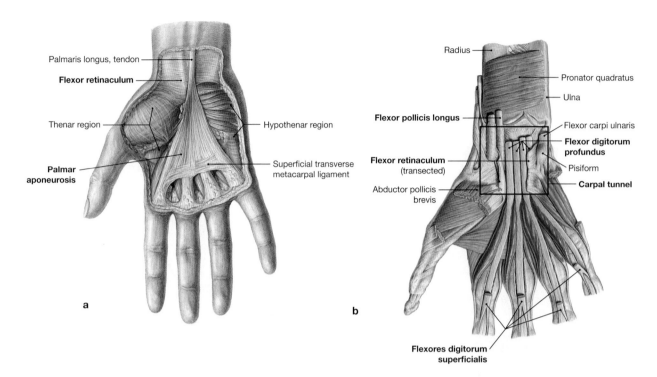

Fig. 3.61a and b Superficial and deep tendons of the wrist and hand, right side; palmar view **(a)**, after removal of the palmar aponeurosis, flexor retinaculum, and the superficial muscles **(b)**. The **palmar aponeurosis** is located in the superficial hand and consists of longitudinal and transverse fibers. It is fixed proximally to the **flexor retinaculum,** and distally to the tendinous sheaths of the finger flexors and to the ligaments of the metacarpophalangeal

joints **(a)**. Transecting the flexor retinaculum reveals the **contents of the carpal tunnel** which include **(b)**:
1. **Flexor digitorum superficialis** (four transected tendons)
2. **Flexor digitorum profundus** (four tendons)
3. **Flexor pollicis longus** (one tendon)
4. Median nerve (not displayed)

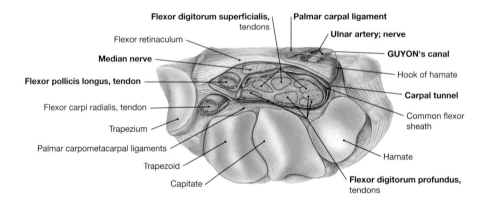

Fig. 3.62 Carpal tunnel and GUYON's canal, right side; distal view; transverse section at the level of the carpometacarpal joints. Together with the carpal bones the flexor retinaculum forms the **carpal tunnel** (outlined in red) which is traversed by the median

nerve and the tendons of the long flexor muscles. **GUYON's canal** (outlined in green) is formed by the flexor retinaculum and its superficial separation, the **'palmar carpal ligament'**. The ulnar nerve, together with the ulnar artery and vein, traverses GUYON's canal.

Clinical Remarks

Inflammatory reactions of the tendinous sheaths or swelling in the area of the carpal tunnel may result in compression of the median nerve. Functional deficits associated with compression of the median nerve in the carpal tunnel are referred to as **carpal tunnel syndrome.**
[L284]

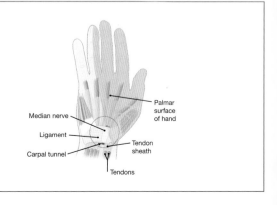

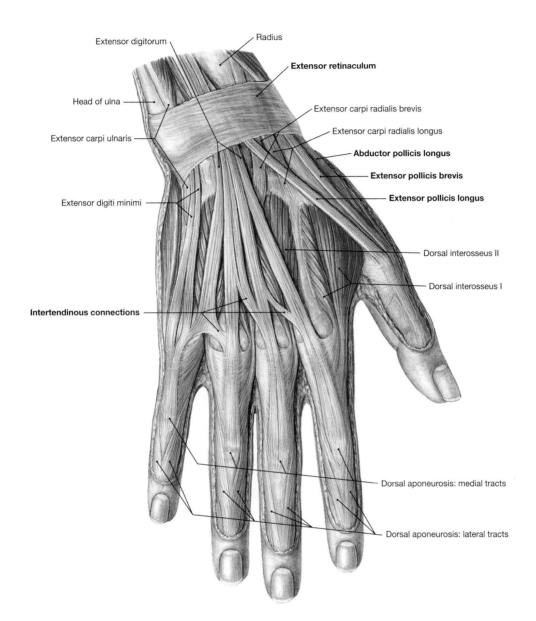

Extensor digitorum

Radius

Extensor retinaculum

Head of ulna

Extensor carpi ulnaris

Extensor carpi radialis brevis

Extensor carpi radialis longus

Abductor pollicis longus

Extensor pollicis brevis

Extensor pollicis longus

Extensor digiti minimi

Dorsal interosseus II

Dorsal interosseus I

Intertendinous connections

Dorsal aponeurosis: medial tracts

Dorsal aponeurosis: lateral tracts

Fig. 3.63 Retinacula and superficial tendons of the wrist and hand, right side; posterior view.

The tendons of the extensor muscles run beneath the **extensor retinaculum** to reach the dorsal surface of the thumb and the dorsal aponeuroses of the fingers. The distinct tendons of the extensor digitorum are linked by **intertendinous connections** which limit the separate mobility of each finger. There are no intrinsic muscles on the dorsal surface of the hand. According to their developmental origin and innervation, the dorsal interossei belong to the palmar muscles.

Structure/Function

The **anatomical snuff box** is a surface anatomy feature. It appears as a triangular depression on the posterolateral surface of the wrist, when the thumb is extended. **Tendons of extensor pollicis longus (medial) and extensor pollicis brevis and abductor pollicis longus (lateral) form the borders** of the indented space, while the scaphoid and trapezium bones of the wrist can be palpated on the floor of this space. Contents of the space include:

1. radial artery
2. superficial branch of radial nerve
3. cephalic vein

Clinically, localized tenderness on palpation within the anatomical snuff box is frequently associated with a fracture of the scaphoid bone.
[L271]

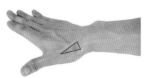

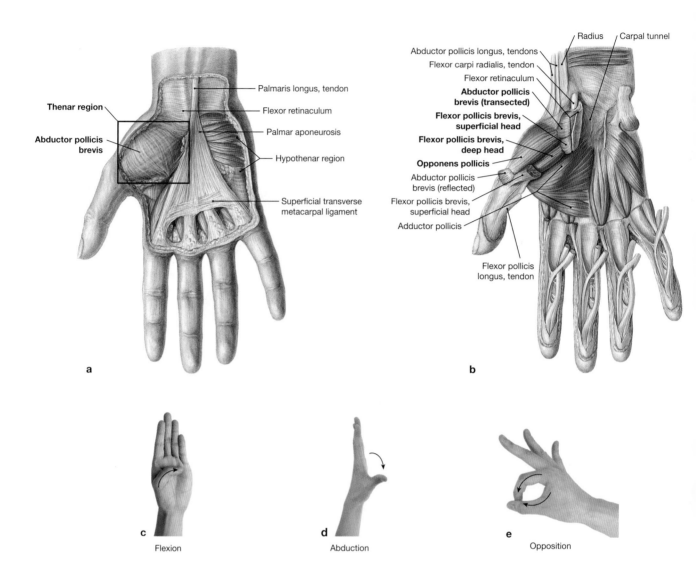

Thenar region			Radius Carpal tunnel
Abductor pollicis brevis	Palmaris longus, tendon		Abductor pollicis longus, tendons
	Flexor retinaculum		Flexor carpi radialis, tendon
	Palmar aponeurosis		Flexor retinaculum
	Hypothenar region		**Abductor pollicis brevis (transected)**
	Superficial transverse metacarpal ligament		**Flexor pollicis brevis, superficial head**

a

b

c
Flexion

d
Abduction

e
Opposition

Fig. 3.64a to e Thenar muscles in the palm of hand, right side; palmar view. c–e [L271]
The **thenar region** of the hand is located on the thumb side of the palmar surface. It is comprised of **three small intrinsic muscles** (both the proximal and distal attachments of each muscle are located within the hand) which are all innervated by the median nerve. These muscles function together to help guide precise movements of the thumb when performing typical activities of daily living such as manipulating a pen while writing; texting on a smartphone; or threading a needle for sewing. Individually each of the muscles is responsible for a specific thumb movement: **thumb flexion (c); thumb abduction (d), thumb opposition (e).**

Muscle	Attachments (P = proximal, D = distal)	Action/Function	Innervation
Abductor pollicis brevis	**P:** Flexor retinaculum and tubercles of scaphoid and trapezium **D:** Proximal phalanx of thumb – lateral side	Abducts thumb	Median nerve – recurrent branch (C8, T1)
Flexor pollicis brevis	**P:** Flexor retinaculum and tubercles of scaphoid and trapezium **D:** Proximal phalanx of thumb	Flexes thumb	Median nerve – recurrent branch (C8, T1)
Opponens pollicis	**P:** Flexor retinaculum and tubercles of scaphoid and trapezium **D:** Metacarpal I – lateral side	Thumb opposition to the four medial digits	Median nerve – recurrent branch (C8, T1)

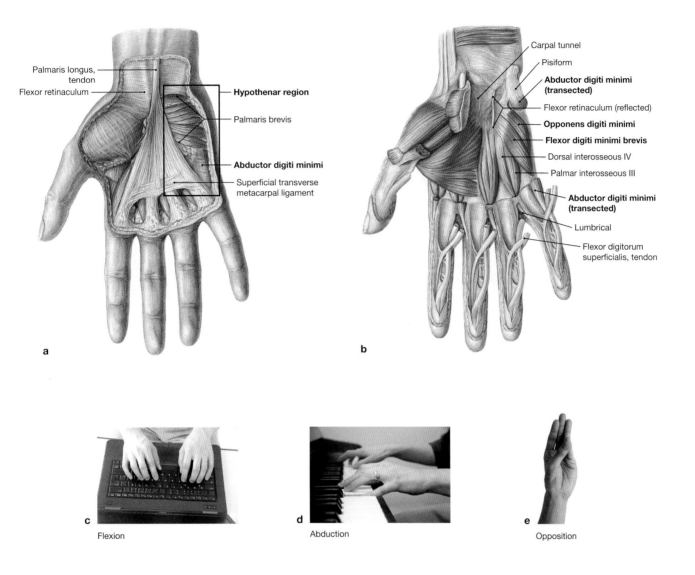

Fig. 3.65a to e Hypothenar muscles in the palm of hand, right side; palmar view. c, e [L271], d [J787]

The **hypothenar region** of the hand is located on the lateral side of the palmar surface and helps to control precise movements of the fifth digit (little finger). It is comprised of **three small intrinsic muscles** (both the proximal and distal attachments of each muscle are located within the hand) that are all innervated by the ulnar nerve. These muscles function together to help guide everyday movements of the fifth digit such as typing on a computer keyboard **(fifth digit flexion, c)**; playing piano **(fifth digit abduction, d)** or pinching your fifth digit and thumb together **(finger opposition, e).**

Muscle	Attachments (P = proximal, D = distal)	Action/Function	Innervation
Abductor digiti minimi	**P:** Pisiform and flexor retinaculum **D:** Base of proximal phalanx of digit V	Abducts digit V (pinky finger)	Ulnar nerve – deep branch (C8, T1)
Flexor digiti minimi brevis	**P:** Hamate and flexor retinaculum **D:** Base of proximal phalanx of digit V (ulnar side).	Flexes proximal phalanx of digit V	Ulnar nerve – deep branch (C8, T1)
Opponens digiti minimi	**P:** Hamate and flexor retinaculum **D:** Medial border of metacarpal V	Digit V opposition to thumb	Ulnar nerve – deep branch (C8, T1)

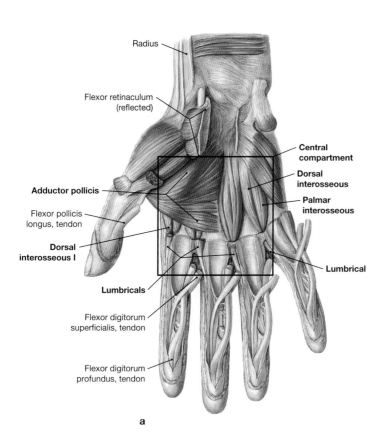

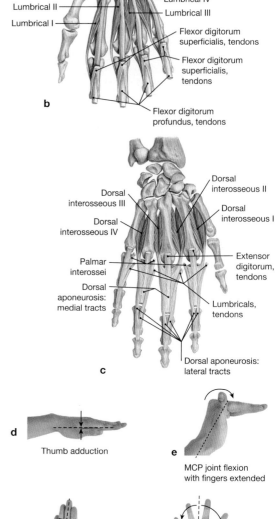

Fig. 3.66a to g Central compartment of muscles in the palm of hand, right side; palmar view **(a, b);** dorsal view **(c).** d–g [L271]
The **central compartment** of the hand is located deep to the palmar aponeurosis, between the hypothenar and thenar regions. It is comprised of **twelve small intrinsic muscles,** that can be organized into three major groups:

1. **Adductor pollicis** (one)
2. **Lumbricals** (four)
3. **Interossei** (three palmar and four dorsal)

These muscles function together to help guide everyday movements of the thumb and fingers such as squeezing your thumb to the side of your index finger **(adductor pollicis, d);** waving with your fingers to gesture good-bye **(lumbricals, e);** squeezing your fingers together **(palmar interossei, f)** and splaying your fingers apart **(dorsal interossei, g).**

Muscle	Attachments (P = proximal, D = distal)	Action/Function	Innervation (spinal roots)
Adductor pollicis	**P:** Body of metacarpal III (transverse head); base of metacarpals II and III, trapezoid and capitate (oblique head) **D:** Proximal phalanx of thumb (medial side)	Adducts thumb towards midline of hand	Ulnar nerve – deep branch (C8, T1)
Lumbricals (four muscles)	**P:** Lumbricals I and II arise from lateral two tendons of flexor digitorum profundus (FDP); lumbricals III and IV arise from medial three tendons of FDP **D:** Lateral side of extensor expansions of digits II–V	Flexes the four medial metacarpophalangeal joints while extending the interphalangeal joints of fingers	Lumbricals I and II – median nerve (C8, T1); Lumbricals III and IV – ulnar nerve – deep branch (C8, T1)
Palmar interossei (three muscles)	**P:** Palmar surface of metacarpals II, IV and V **D:** Extensor expansions and base of proximal phalanges of digits II, IV and V	Adducts digits II, IV and V towards midline of hand (middle finger)	Ulnar nerve – deep branch (C8, T1)
Dorsal interossei (four muscles)	**P:** Adjacent sides of metacarpals I–IV **D:** Extensor expansions and base of proximal phalanges of digits II–IV	Abducts digits towards the midline of hand (middle finger)	Ulnar nerve – deep branch (C8, T1)

Fig. 3.67 Arteries and nerves of the wrist and hand, right side; palmar view; after removal of the palmar aponeurosis.

The **superficial palmar arch** is primarily formed by the ulnar artery and frequently anastomoses with a branch from the radial artery (superficial palmar branch). The **palmar digital arteries** supplying the ulnar 3½ digits branch off the superficial palmar arch while it crosses the tendons of the long flexor muscles of the fingers. The **ulnar nerve** accompanies the **ulnar artery** through the GUYON's canal. Distal to the pisiform, the **ulnar nerve splits into its deep and superficial branches.** The **superficial branch** divides into palmar digital nerves for sensory innervation of the ulnar 1½ digits. The radial 3½ digits are supplied by the branches of the **median nerve** which enter the palm of hand through the **carpal tunnel** beneath the flexor retinaculum.

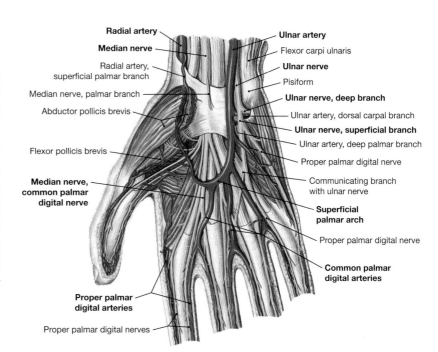

Radial artery
Median nerve
Radial artery, superficial palmar branch
Median nerve, palmar branch
Abductor pollicis brevis
Flexor pollicis brevis
Median nerve, common palmar digital nerve
Proper palmar digital arteries
Proper palmar digital nerves

Ulnar artery
Flexor carpi ulnaris
Ulnar nerve
Pisiform
Ulnar nerve, deep branch
Ulnar artery, dorsal carpal branch
Ulnar nerve, superficial branch
Ulnar artery, deep palmar branch
Proper palmar digital nerve
Communicating branch with ulnar nerve
Superficial palmar arch
Proper palmar digital nerve
Common palmar digital arteries

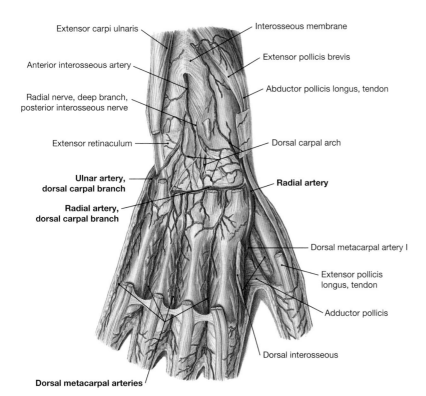

Extensor carpi ulnaris
Anterior interosseous artery
Radial nerve, deep branch, posterior interosseous nerve
Extensor retinaculum
Ulnar artery, dorsal carpal branch
Radial artery, dorsal carpal branch
Dorsal metacarpal arteries

Interosseous membrane
Extensor pollicis brevis
Abductor pollicis longus, tendon
Dorsal carpal arch
Radial artery
Dorsal metacarpal artery I
Extensor pollicis longus, tendon
Adductor pollicis
Dorsal interosseous

Fig. 3.68 Arteries and nerves of the wrist and hand, right side; posterior view; after removal of the long tendons of the extensor muscles.
Both, the **radial artery** and **ulnar artery** send a **dorsal carpal branch** to the dorsum of hand where they communicate. The radial branch is usually stronger and predominantly supplies the **dorsal metacarpal** and the dorsal digital (not depicted) arteries of hand for the fingers up to the proximal interphalangeal joints. The intermediate and distal phalanges are supplied by the palmar digital arteries.

┌─ **Clinical Remarks** ─────────────────────────

Injuries or entrapment of the terminal branches of the brachial plexus within the wrist can lead to muscle weakness or wasting of intrinsic muscles of the hand.
a Entrapment of the median nerve within the carpal tunnel can result in atrophy of the thenar muscles.
b Injury or **compression of the ulnar nerve** within the GUYON's canal can result in wasting of the hypothenar and interosseous muscles of the hand.
a [G056], b [G720]

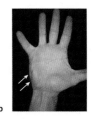

Thenar wasting

a   b

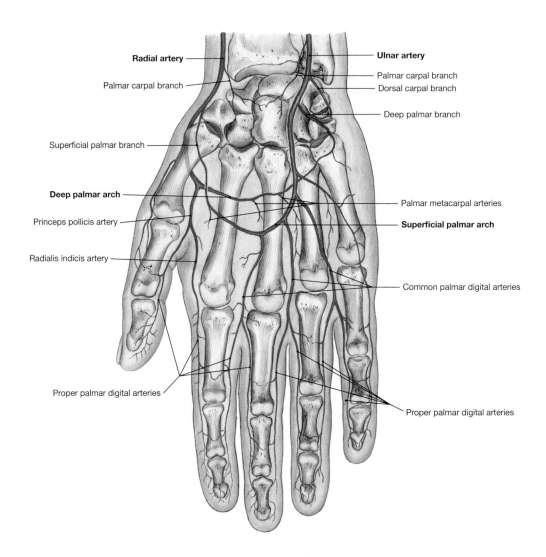

Fig. 3.69 Arteries of the hand, right side; palmar view.
The palm of hand is supplied by the radial and ulnar arteries which usually both contribute to the two arterial palmar arches. The **radial artery** terminates in the **deep palmar arch** and contributes with a communicating branch to the superficial palmar arch, whereas the **ulnar artery** terminates in the **superficial palmar arch** and provides a branch to the deep palmar arch.

Clinical Remarks

ALLEN's test can be used to test function of either the radial or ulnar arteries. It is routinely used to evaluate the risk of ischemia within the hand, and is often performed prior to radial cannulation or catheterization (because placement of such a catheter can result in thrombosis). The test involves the patient first making a fist with his/her hand and elevating it for approximately 30 seconds. Pressure is then applied by the clinician over both the radial and ulnar arteries as they cross the wrist. The hand is then opened – and should remain pale (as both arteries are being occluded). Ulnar pressure is now released and the normal color of the hand should return within five to ten seconds. If color fails to return to the hand, the test would be considered 'positive', and indicative of an inefficient blood supply of the hand by the ulnar artery – the radial artery should therefore not be cannulated or catheterized.
[L126]

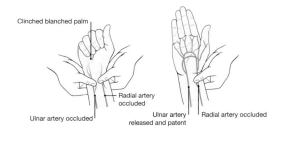

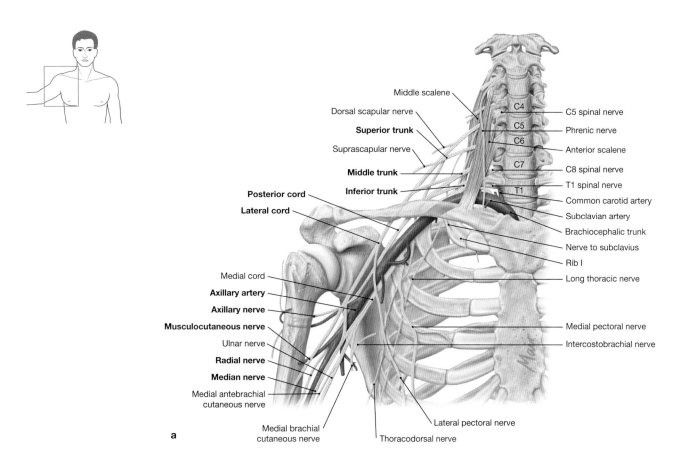

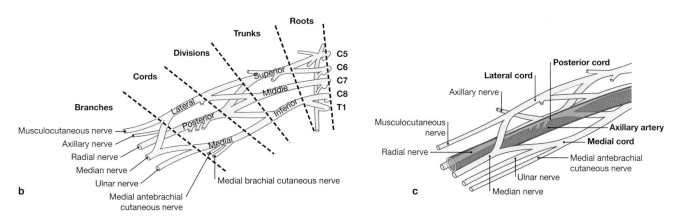

Fig. 3.70a to c Brachial plexus of nerves; anterior view. [L126], a [L127], b, c [L126]

The brachial plexus arises from the spinal cord (➤ Fig. 12.73) and passes under the clavicle and through the axillary region to provide sensory and motor innervation to the entire upper extremity **(a)**. It has a specific pattern of organization: **R**oots, **T**runks, **D**ivisions, **C**ords, **B**ranches (terminal). The mnemonic 'Robert Thompson Drinks Cold Beer' is often used to remember its structural organization. The **R**oots of the brachial plexus are formed by the anterior rami from the spinal segments **C5–T1,** which combine to form three **T**runks. Nerve fibers from C5 and C6 assemble into a **superior trunk;** fibers from C7 into a **middle trunk;** and fibers from C8 to T1 into an **inferior trunk.** Each trunk then divides into **two divisions**

(anterior and posterior), which then rearrange at the level of the clavicle to form **three cords (b).** The posterior divisions of all three trunks form the **posterior cord** (fibers from C5–T1). The anterior divisions of the superior and middle trunk continue as **lateral cord** (fibers from C5–C7), the anterior divisions of the inferior trunk continue as **medial cord** (fibers from C8–T1). The three cords are named according to their position in relation to the **axillary artery (c).** Finally, the **infraclavicular portion** of the brachial plexus terminates as five **branches** which arise from the three cords:

1. Lateral cord – **musculoculaneous nerve,** lateral root of **median nerve**
2. Posterior cord – **axillary nerve, radial nerve**
3. Medial cord – **ulnar nerve,** medial root of **median nerve**

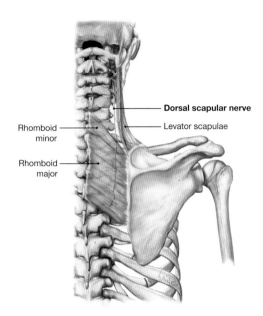

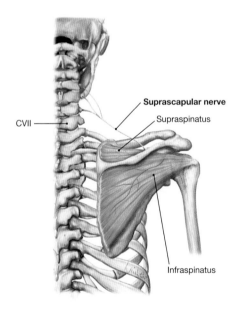

Fig. 3.71 Dorsal scapular nerve (C3–C5), right side; posterior view. [L127]

The **dorsal scapular nerve** innervates the rhomboids and the levator scapulae. It is the first supraclavicular nerve to branch off the brachial plexus, and pierces through the medial scalene muscle to run posteriorly along the inferior border of the levator scapulae.

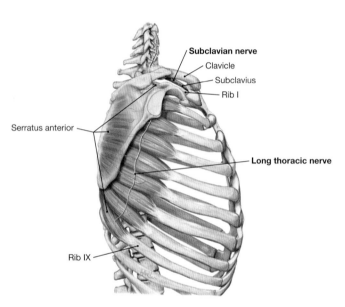

Fig. 3.72 Long thoracic (C5–C7) and subclavian nerves (C5–C6), right side; lateral view. [L127]

The **long thoracic nerve** innervates the serratus anterior. It pierces the medial scalene muscle and travels underneath the brachial plexus and clavicle to the lateral side of the thorax to descend along the outer surface of the serratus anterior. The **subclavian nerve** innervates its corresponding muscle. It runs adjacent to the subclavius muscle and often sends a branch to the phrenic nerve ('accessory phrenic nerve').

Fig. 3.73 Suprascapular nerve (C4–C6), right side; posterior view. [L127]

The **suprascapular nerve** innervates the supraspinatus and infraspinatus muscles of the rotator cuff. It is derived from the superior trunk, runs dorsally along the clavicle, and reaches the dorsal aspect of the shoulder blade by traversing the suprascapular notch.

Structure/Function

The appearance of a winging scapula – the medial border of the scapula protrudes in a wing-like fashion away from the body – during activities in which the scapula must be stabilized against the wall of the thorax (e.g. performing a push-up extensively) – may be indicative of injury to the **long thoracic nerve** which innervates the serratus anterior. This lesion can result from carrying heavy loads on the back (e. g. backpacker's palsy) because the nerve can be easily compressed by the shoulder straps of a backpack.
[G042]

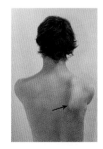

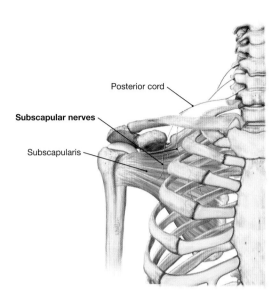

Fig. 3.74 Subscapular nerve (C5–C7), right side; anterior view. [L127]

The **subscapular nerve** innervates the subscapularis. It branches off the posterior cord and immediately descends to the anterior side of the scapula (where it is well protected from injury).

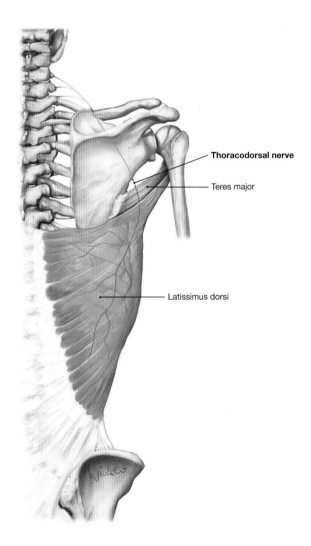

Fig. 3.75 Thoracodorsal nerve (C6–C8), right side; posterior view. [L127]

Together with its corresponding artery, the **thoracodorsal nerve** courses to the medial side of the latissimus dorsi, to innervate this muscle and the teres major.

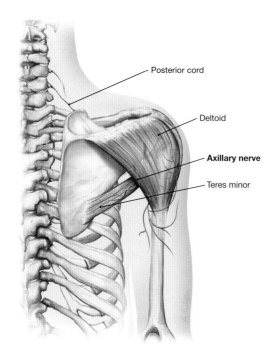

Posterior cord

Deltoid

Axillary nerve

Teres minor

Fig. 3.76 Axillary nerve (C5–C6), right side; posterior view. Sensory cutaneous branches are shown in purple. [L266]

The **axillary nerve** originates from the posterior cord and traverses the quadrangular axillary **space** in the axillary region together with the posterior circumflex humeral artery to reach the posterior side of the arm. The axillary nerve innervates the deltoid and teres minor muscles.

Fig. 3.77 Radial nerve (C5–T1), right side; anterior view (posterior side not visible because of pronation of the forearm). Sensory cutaneous branches are shown in purple. [L266]

The **radial nerve** is derived from the posterior cord and reaches the dorsal side of humerus through the **'triceps slit'** between the long and lateral heads of the triceps brachii muscle. It sends motor branches to the triceps brachii and a sensory branch to the posterior side of the arm. The radial nerve then enters the cubital fossa from lateral between the brachioradialis and brachialis muscles, and divides into a superficial branch and deep branch. The **superficial branch** courses to the dorsum of the hand for the sensory innervation of the skin between the thumb and the index finger and the radial 2½ fingers. The **deep branch** pierces the supinator and reaches the posterior side of the forearm to provide motor innervation to all extensor muscles of the forearm.

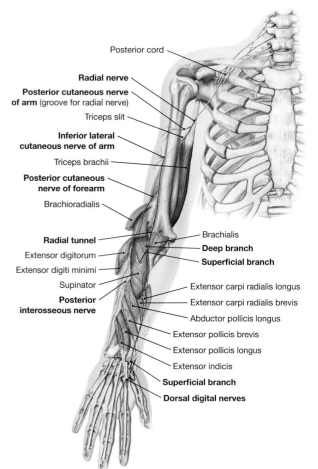

Posterior cord

Radial nerve
Posterior cutaneous nerve of arm (groove for radial nerve)
Triceps slit
Inferior lateral cutaneous nerve of arm
Triceps brachii
Posterior cutaneous nerve of forearm
Brachioradialis

Radial tunnel
Extensor digitorum
Extensor digiti minimi
Supinator
Posterior interosseous nerve

Brachialis
Deep branch
Superficial branch

Extensor carpi radialis longus
Extensor carpi radialis brevis
Abductor pollicis longus
Extensor pollicis brevis
Extensor pollicis longus
Extensor indicis
Superficial branch
Dorsal digital nerves

Clinical Remarks

The **axillary nerve** may be injured in association with proximal humeral fractures or shoulder dislocations. Following injury, abduction of the arm is severely impaired, and sensory input from the lateral side of the shoulder is lost. Long-lasting injury causes muscle atrophy, such that the dome shaped appearance of the shoulder is lost.

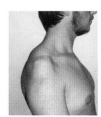

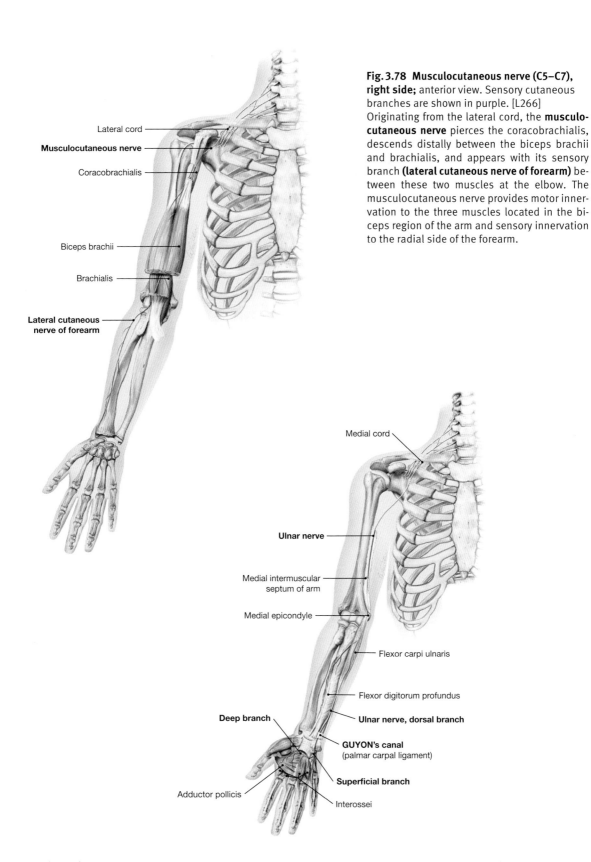

Fig. 3.78 Musculocutaneous nerve (C5–C7), right side; anterior view. Sensory cutaneous branches are shown in purple. [L266]
Originating from the lateral cord, the **musculocutaneous nerve** pierces the coracobrachialis, descends distally between the biceps brachii and brachialis, and appears with its sensory branch **(lateral cutaneous nerve of forearm)** between these two muscles at the elbow. The musculocutaneous nerve provides motor innervation to the three muscles located in the biceps region of the arm and sensory innervation to the radial side of the forearm.

Lateral cord
Musculocutaneous nerve
Coracobrachialis
Biceps brachii
Brachialis
Lateral cutaneous nerve of forearm

Medial cord
Ulnar nerve
Medial intermuscular septum of arm
Medial epicondyle
Flexor carpi ulnaris
Flexor digitorum profundus
Ulnar nerve, dorsal branch
Deep branch
GUYON's canal (palmar carpal ligament)
Superficial branch
Adductor pollicis
Interossei

Fig. 3.79 Ulnar nerve (C8–T1), right side; anterior view. Sensory cutaneous branches are shown in purple. [L266]
The **ulnar nerve** originates from the medial cord and courses along the medial arm. After piercing the medial intermuscular septum of arm, the ulnar nerve appears on the posterior side of the medial epicondyle and runs directly adjacent to the bone in the ulnar groove ('funny bone'). The ulnar nerve has no branches in the upper arm. In the forearm, it courses together with the ulnar artery beneath the flexor carpi ulnaris muscle to the wrist and enters the palm of hand through the **GUYON's canal** (a semi-rigid longitudinal canal on the ulnar side of the wrist that provides passage for the ulnar nerve and artery into the hand). In the forearm, the ulnar nerve provides motor innervation to the flexor carpi ulnaris and the ulnar head of the flexor digitorum profundus. In the palm of hand, its **deep branch** provides motor innervation to the muscles of the hypothenar region, all interossei muscles, the 3rd and 4th lumbricals and adductor pollicis. The **superficial branch** continues as the sensory common palmar digital branch, which divides into the terminal branches innervating the palmar side of the ulnar 1½ fingers (and the dorsal sides of their distal phalanges).

145

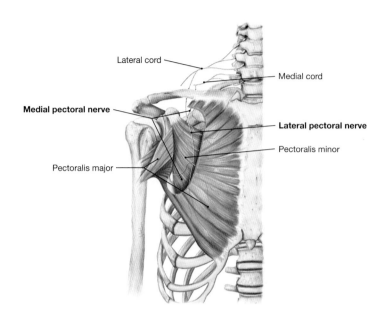

Lateral cord

Medial cord

Medial pectoral nerve

Lateral pectoral nerve

Pectoralis minor

Pectoralis major

Fig. 3.80 Lateral (C5–C7) and medial (C8–T1) pectoral nerves, right side; anterior view. [L127] The terms 'lateral' and 'medial' are related to the origins of each nerve from the lateral or medial cord, respectively (not to the topographical position of each nerve). Both nerves innervate the pectoralis major and pectoralis minor muscles.

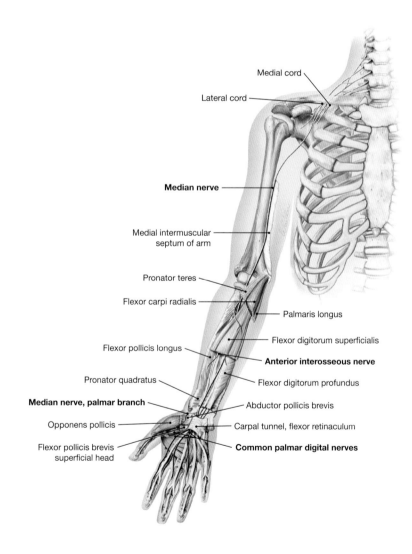

Medial cord

Lateral cord

Median nerve

Medial intermuscular septum of arm

Pronator teres

Flexor carpi radialis

Palmaris longus

Flexor digitorum superficialis

Flexor pollicis longus

Anterior interosseous nerve

Pronator quadratus

Flexor digitorum profundus

Median nerve, palmar branch

Abductor pollicis brevis

Opponens pollicis

Carpal tunnel, flexor retinaculum

Flexor pollicis brevis superficial head

Common palmar digital nerves

Fig. 3.81 Median nerve (C6–T1), right side; anterior view. Sensory cutaneous branches are shown in purple. [L266]

The **median nerve** receives contributions from both the lateral and medial cords, and initially descends along the medial side of the arm in the medial bicipital groove without providing any branches. The nerve then enters the cubital fossa from the medial side and traverses between both heads of the pronator teres into the intermuscular layer between the superficial and deep flexor muscles of the forearm.

The **median nerve** innervates all flexor muscles of the anterior forearm – with the exception of the flexor carpi ulnaris and the medial aspect (which flexes the 4th and 5th digits) of the flexor digitorum profundus. The deep flexors are innervated by the **anterior interosseous nerve** which also provides sensory innervation to the palmar side of the wrist joints. The median nerve enters the palm of hand via the **carpal tunnel** between the tendons of the flexor muscles. In the palm of hand, the median nerve divides into three **common palmar digital nerves,** which provide motor innervation to the muscles of the thumb (except for the adductor pollicis) and the 1st and 2nd lumbricals. Their terminal branches provide sensory innervation on the palmar aspect of the lateral 3½ fingers and the dorsal side of the distal phalanges.

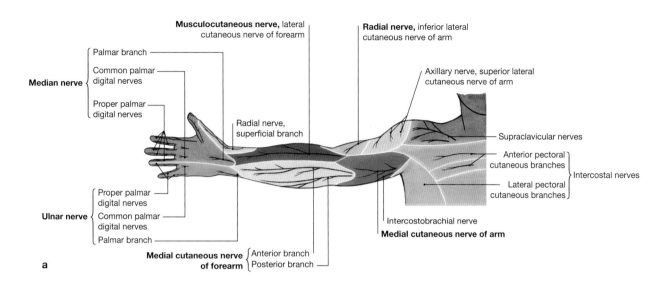

Musculocutaneous nerve, lateral cutaneous nerve of forearm

Radial nerve, inferior lateral cutaneous nerve of arm

Median nerve
- Palmar branch
- Common palmar digital nerves
- Proper palmar digital nerves

Radial nerve, superficial branch

Axillary nerve, superior lateral cutaneous nerve of arm

Supraclavicular nerves

Anterior pectoral cutaneous branches

Intercostal nerves

Lateral pectoral cutaneous branches

Ulnar nerve
- Proper palmar digital nerves
- Common palmar digital nerves
- Palmar branch

Intercostobrachial nerve
Medial cutaneous nerve of arm

Medial cutaneous nerve of forearm { Anterior branch, Posterior branch }

a

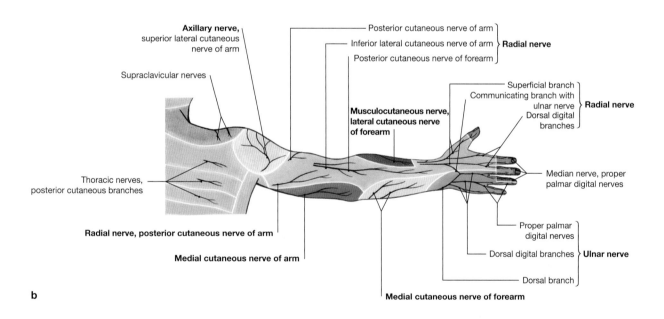

Axillary nerve, superior lateral cutaneous nerve of arm

Posterior cutaneous nerve of arm
Inferior lateral cutaneous nerve of arm } **Radial nerve**
Posterior cutaneous nerve of forearm

Supraclavicular nerves

Superficial branch
Communicating branch with ulnar nerve } **Radial nerve**
Dorsal digital branches

Musculocutaneous nerve, lateral cutaneous nerve of forearm

Median nerve, proper palmar digital nerves

Thoracic nerves, posterior cutaneous branches

Proper palmar digital nerves

Radial nerve, posterior cutaneous nerve of arm

Dorsal digital branches } **Ulnar nerve**

Medial cutaneous nerve of arm

Dorsal branch

b

Medial cutaneous nerve of forearm

Fig. 3.82a and b Cutaneous nerves of the upper extremity, right side; anterior view **(a)** and posterior view **(b).**
All terminal branches of the **brachial plexus** contribute to the sensory innervation of **shoulder, arm, forearm, wrist and hand.** The lateral aspect of the shoulder is innervated by the **axillary nerve.** The lateral and posterior sides of the arm, the posterior aspect of the forearm, and the dorsal surface of the radial 2½ fingers are innervated by the **radial nerve.** The **musculocutaneous nerve** (via the lateral cutaneous nerve) conveys sensory innervation to the lateral aspect of the forearm. The **medial cutaneous nerves of arm and forearm** innervate the medial aspect of the arm. The **median nerve** (palmar surface of the radial 3½ fingers) and **ulnar nerve** (palmar surface of the ulnar 2½ fingers) innervate the hand.

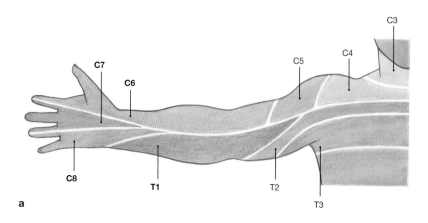

a

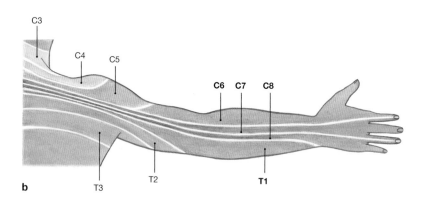

b

Fig. 3.83a and b Dermatome map of the upper extremity, right side; anterior view **(a)** and posterior view **(b).**
Specific areas of the skin are innervated by one single spinal root. These areas of the skin are termed **dermatomes** (➤ Fig. 12.75). As peripheral cutaneous nerves of the arm contain sensory fibers from several spinal roots, dermatomes are not exactly congruent with the cutaneous area supplied by the peripheral nerves. In contrast to the belt-like orientation of the dermatomes of the trunk, dermatomes of the upper extremity are **oriented along the longitudinal axis.**

Clinical Remarks

MR image depicting compression of the spinal cord at the C3/C4 and C5/C6 vertebral levels. Demarcation of dermatomes is of significance in the clinical diagnosis of herniated discs and narrowing (stenosis) of the vertebral canal and intervertebral foramina. Impairment of the C4 spinal root would result in altered sensory function on the top of the shoulder. Impairment of the C6 spinal root would result in altered sensory function along the radial side of the forearm and thumb.
[F371-003]

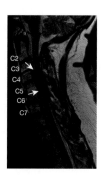

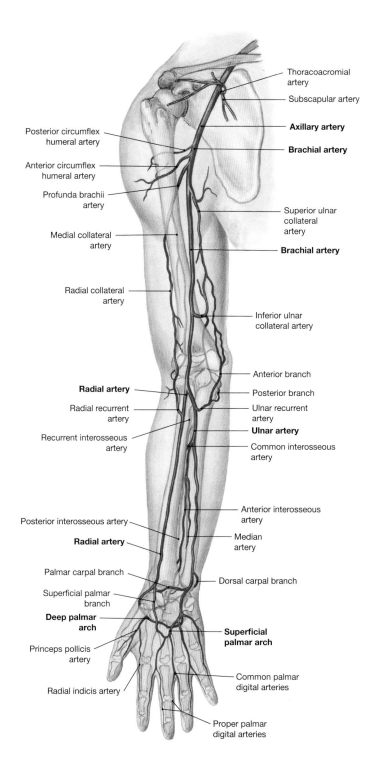

Thoracoacromial artery

Subscapular artery

Axillary artery

Brachial artery

Posterior circumflex humeral artery

Anterior circumflex humeral artery

Profunda brachii artery

Medial collateral artery

Superior ulnar collateral artery

Brachial artery

Radial collateral artery

Inferior ulnar collateral artery

Anterior branch

Radial artery

Posterior branch

Radial recurrent artery

Ulnar recurrent artery

Recurrent interosseous artery

Ulnar artery

Common interosseous artery

Anterior interosseous artery

Posterior interosseous artery

Median artery

Radial artery

Palmar carpal branch

Dorsal carpal branch

Superficial palmar branch

Deep palmar arch

Superficial palmar arch

Princeps pollicis artery

Common palmar digital arteries

Radial indicis artery

Proper palmar digital arteries

Branches of the Axillary Artery

1. Superior thoracic artery
2. Thoracoacromial artery
   - Clavicular branch
   - Pectoral branch
   - Deltoid branch
   - Acromial branch
3. Lateral thoracic artery
4. Subscapular artery
   - Circumflex scapular artery
   - Thoracodorsal artery
5. Posterior circumflex humeral artery
6. Anterior circumflex humeral artery

Branches of the Brachial Artery

1. Profunda brachii artery
   - Medial collateral artery
   - Radial collateral artery
2. Superior ulnar collateral artery
3. Inferior ulnar collateral artery

Branches of the Radial Artery

1. Radial recurrent artery
2. Palmar carpal branch
3. Dorsal carpal branch ⟶ dorsal carpal arch ⟶ dorsal metacarpal arteries ⟶ dorsal digital arteries
4. Superficial palmar branch ⟶ superficial palmar arch
5. Princeps pollicis artery
6. Radialis indicis artery
7. Deep palmar arch ⟶ palmar metacarpal arteries

Branches of the Ulnar Artery

1. Ulnar recurrent artery
2. Common interosseous artery
3. Dorsal carpal branch
4. Palmar carpal branch
5. Deep palmar branch ⟶ deep palmar arch
6. Superficial palmar arch ⟶ palmar digital arteries

Fig. 3.84 Arteries of the upper extremity, right side; anterior view.

The **axillary artery** is a continuation of the subclavian artery and stretches from the first rib to the inferior margin of the pectoralis major. It is positioned between the three cords of the brachial plexus and the two roots of the median nerve. At the inferior border of the teres major, the axillary artery becomes the **brachial artery** and courses together with the median nerve to enter the cubital fossa, where it divides into the radial artery and ulnar artery. The **radial artery** descends between the superficial and deep flexor muscles of the forearm to the wrist. Traversing the anatomical snuff box, the radial artery enters the palm of hand to provide the major input for the **deep palmar arch**. Below the elbow, the **ulnar artery** gives off the common interosseous artery and then runs together with the ulnar nerve through the GUYON's canal (at the wrist) to enter the palm of hand. Here, it provides the major input to the **superficial palmar arch.**

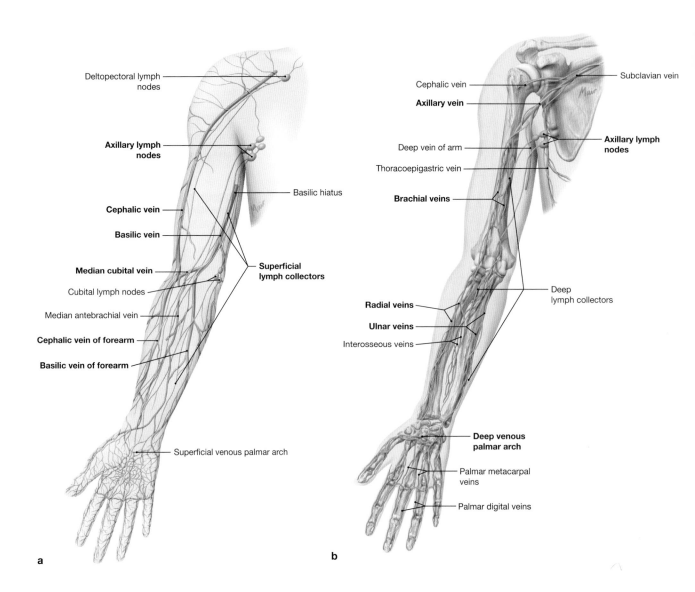

Fig. 3.85a and b Superficial (a) and deep (b) veins and lymphatic vessels, right side; anterior view. [L127]

a The **superficial venous system** of the arm consists of two major vessels which collect venous blood from the hand:

The **cephalic vein of forearm** collects blood from the posterior venous network of the hand and runs on the radial side of the forearm to the cubital fossa to join the **basilic vein** via the **median cubital vein.** In the arm, the cephalic vein courses in the lateral bicipital groove and merges in the clavipectoral triangle with the **axillary vein.** The **basilic vein of forearm** begins on the ulnar side of the hand, continues up the ulnar side of the forearm and enters the **brachial veins** at the basilic hiatus of the distal portion of the arm.

The **superficial lymph collectors** form a radial, ulnar and medial bundle in the forearm. In the arm, the medial bundle follows the basilic vein and drains into the **axillary lymph nodes.** The posterolateral bundle courses along with the cephalic vein and additionally drains into the supraclavicular lymph nodes. The regional lymph node stations for both systems are positioned in the axilla **(axillary lymph nodes).** There are only a few lymph nodes in the cubital fossa (cubital lymph nodes).

b The **deep venous systems** and the deep lymph collectors accompany the respective arteries.

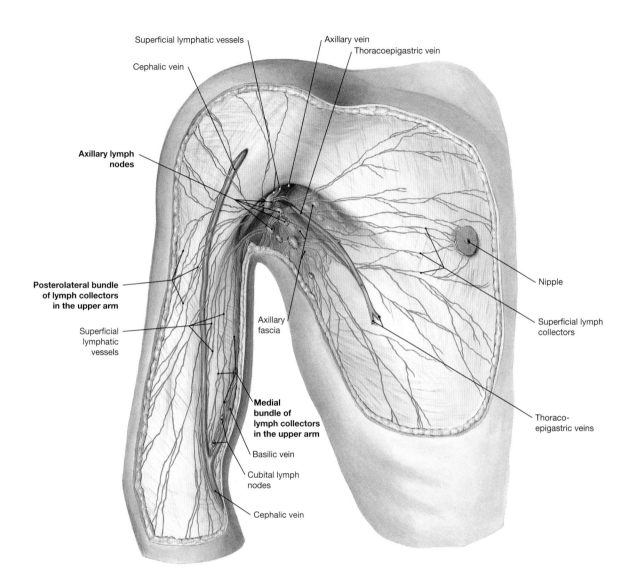

Superficial lymphatic vessels

Cephalic vein

Axillary vein

Thoracoepigastric vein

Axillary lymph nodes

Posterolateral bundle of lymph collectors in the upper arm

Superficial lymphatic vessels

Axillary fascia

Medial bundle of lymph collectors in the upper arm

Basilic vein

Cubital lymph nodes

Cephalic vein

Nipple

Superficial lymph collectors

Thoraco-epigastric veins

Fig. 3.86 Superficial lymphatic vessels and lymph nodes in the axilla and the lateral wall of the thorax, right side; anterior view. In the upper arm, the superficial lymph collectors constitute a **medial bundle** along the basilic vein and a **posterolateral bundle** along the cephalic vein, both of which connect to the axillary lymph nodes. The **axillary lymph nodes** not only serve as regional lymph nodes of the arm but also for the wall of the upper thorax and back (> Fig. 5.14).

Lower Extremity

Surface Anatomy – Overview 156

Surface Anatomy
of the Pelvis and Thigh 157

Pelvic Girdle 158

Hip Bone – Os coxae 159

Joints and Ligaments of the Pelvis .. 160

Pelvic Foramina 161

Femur 162

Hip Joint 163

Hip Joint – Functional Anatomy 165

Hip Joint Movements 166

Muscles of the Posterior Hip 167

Muscles of the Posterior Hip – Deep .. 168

Muscles of the Anterior Hip 169

Muscles of the Anterior Hip – Deep .. 170

Muscles of the Anterior Thigh –
Quadriceps 171

Muscles of the Medial Thigh –
Groin 172

Muscles of the Posterior Thigh –
Hamstrings 173

Neurovascular Structures – Gluteal
Region and Posterior Thigh 174

Neurovascular Structures –
Anterior and Medial Thigh 175

Surface Anatomy of the Knee 176

Knee Joint 177

Bones of the Knee 178

Knee Joint Movements 180

Knee – Functional Anatomy 181

Collateral Ligaments of the Knee ... 182

Cruciate Ligaments of the Knee 183

Menisci of the Knee 184

Patella 185

Patellofemoral Joint 186

Knee Bursae 187

Popliteal Region of the Knee 188

Neurovascular Structures
of the Knee 189

Surface Anatomy of the
Lower Leg, Ankle and Foot 190

Bones of the Lower Leg 191

Tibia 192

Fibula 193

Bones of the Foot 194

Ankle Movements 196

Ankle – Talocrural Joint 197

Ankle – Subtalar Joint 198

Ankle Ligaments 199

Joints of the Foot 200

Muscular Compartments
of the Lower Leg 201

Muscles of the
Anterior Compartment 202

Muscles of the
Lateral Compartment 203

Muscles of the Posterior Compartment –
Superficial and Deep 204

Retinacula and Tendinous Sheaths . . 206

Muscles of the Foot – Dorsum 207

Muscles of the Foot –
1st and 2nd Plantar Layers 208

Muscles of the Foot –
3rd and 4th Plantar Layers 209

Arches of the Foot 210

Gait 211

Neurovascular Structures
of the Lower Leg, Ankle and Foot . . . 212

Lumbosacral Plexus of Nerves 214

Lumbar Plexus – Motor Innervation . . 215

Sacral Plexus – Motor Innervation . . 216

Sensory Innervation –
Cutaneous Nerves 217

Sensory Innervation – Dermatomes . . 218

Arteries 219

Veins 221

Lymphatic Vessels 222

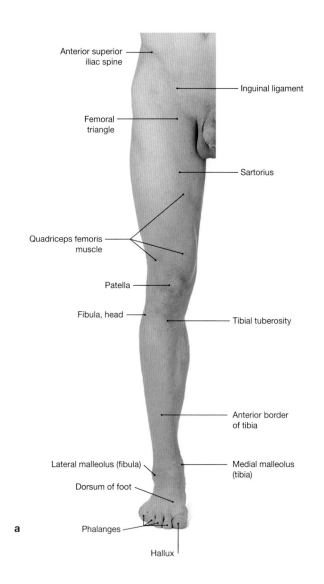

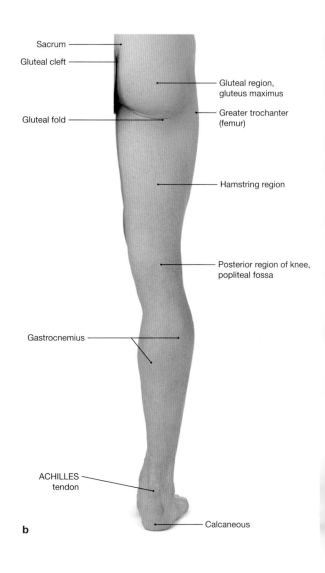

Fig. 4.1a and b Surface anatomy of the lower extremity, right side; anterior **(a)** and posterior **(b)** views. [K340]
The shape and contours of the lower extremity are determined by superficial muscles and bony alignment. The surface landmarks which are palpable through the skin are important for physical examination.

Structure/Function

Surface anatomy (or living anatomy as it is sometimes called) is important for understanding the human body and its function. When examining a patient, structures are often more difficult to locate than on an anatomical specimen. Much of what we are looking for is not necessarily visible to the naked eye. To further complicate matters, people are different! While most humans fall within a 'normal' range of size and proportion, there is a great deal of variability between individuals. The structures that you find displayed clearly and concretely in an anatomy text-book may not always appear that way on a living person. As an example, leg alignment of the lower extremity can vary among patients. As a clinician, it is important to appreciate this variability and develop skill in locating the same structure on different people. The best way to learn how to do this is to practice palpation on as many people as you can, paying close attention to variations in such things as size, shape and gender. [L126]

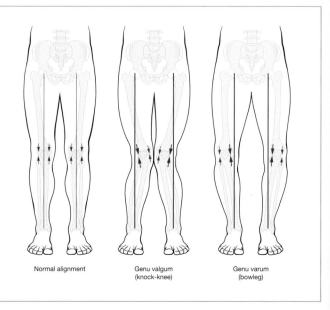

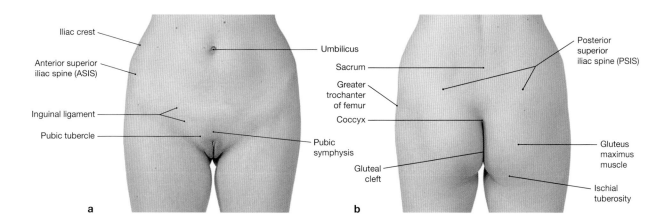

Fig. 4.2a and b Surface anatomy of the pelvis and gluteal region; anterior (**a**) and posterior (**b**) views. [K340]
Many of the bony and muscular landmarks of the pelvis and gluteal region can be palpated on the surface of the body. Their position, alignment, and symmetry from side-to-side can often provide valuable information to the clinician during the observation component of a musculoskeletal examination.

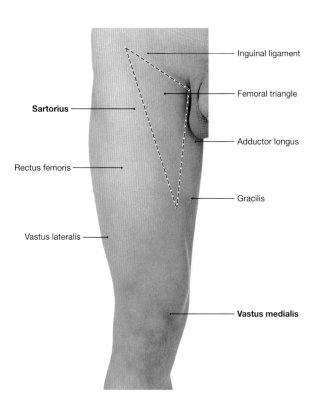

Fig. 4.3 Anterior thigh, right side; anterior view. [K340]
The anterior thigh extends from the inguinal ligament superiorly, to the knee joint inferiorly. The **sartorius** muscle serves as a key superficial landmark that can be used to anatomically separate the anterior 'quads' compartment from the medial 'groin' compartment. Hypertrophy and atrophy of the **vastus medialis** component of the quadriceps femoris muscle can be easily visualized because of its distinct position in the anterior inferior thigh.

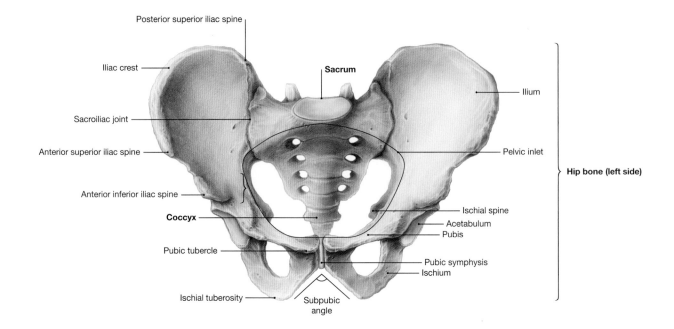

Fig. 4.4 Pelvis; anterior view. [L285]
The pelvis forms a stable ring that encompasses the viscera with its iliac bones, and transfers the weight of the upper body to the lower extremities (➤ Fig. 7.5). It is made up of four bones: **one sacrum, one coccyx and two hip bones (left and right).**

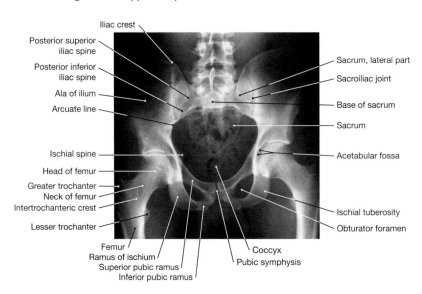

Fig. 4.5 Pelvic girdle; anteroposterior (AP) radiograph; upright standing position.
Plain radiographies of the pelvis are frequently used in the diagnosis of fractures and malpositions of the skeletal elements of the pelvic girdle (➤ Fig. 7.6). They also enable the detection of degenerative changes (osteoarthritis) or local alterations of the bones, such as metastases.

Clinical Remarks

Anteroposterior radiographs allow key aspects of the hip bone and pelvis to be visualized.
a Fractures can occur as a result of high-energy trauma that leads to a disturbance in the shape and orientation of the pelvic inlet or outlet.
b Violent muscle contraction can also result in an 'avulsion type' fracture to areas of the pelvis that provide attachment for large muscles.
a [G198], b [E513-002]

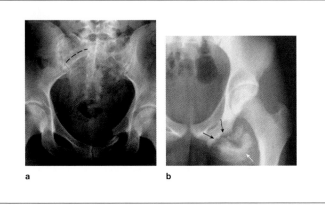

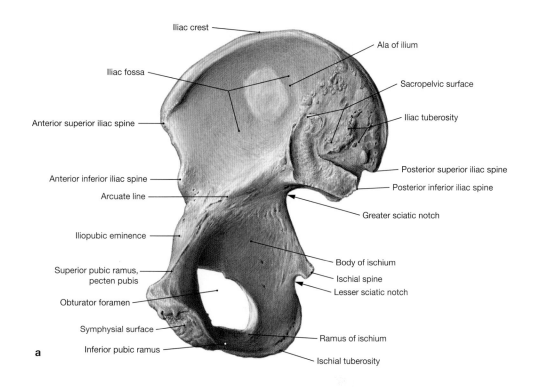

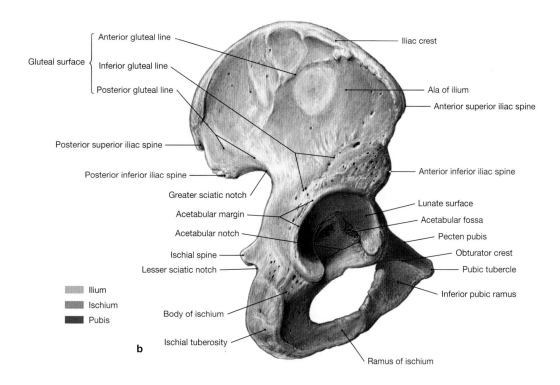

Fig. 4.6a and b Right hip bone; medial **(a)** and lateral **(b)** views.
Each os coxae **(hip bone)** is comprised of three distinct regions:
1. **Ilium:** superior aspect of the hip bone
2. **Pubis:** anterior inferior aspect of the hip bone

3. **Ischium:** posterior inferior aspect of the hip bone
All three regions of the hip bone (➤ Fig. 7.5) contribute to the formation of the acetabular fossa (acetabulum) of the hip joint.

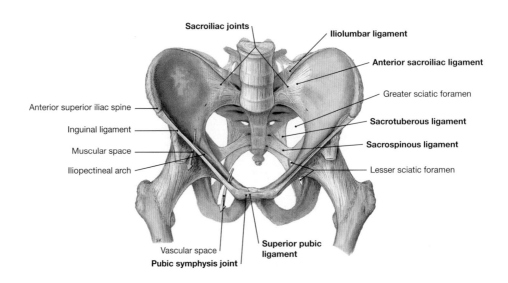

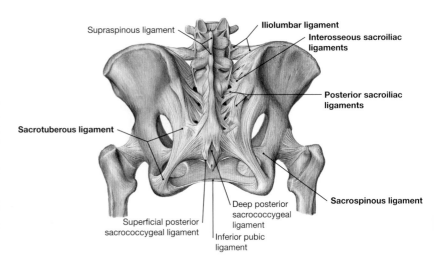

Fig. 4.7 Joints and supporting ligaments of the pelvis; anterior view.
The pelvis is formed by the sacral region of the distal vertebral spine connecting to the two hip bones. Posteriorly, this articulation

forms the left and right **sacroiliac joints.** In the anterior region, the paired hip bones connect at the midline to form the **pubic symphysis.**

Fig. 4.8 Sacroiliac joints; posterior view.
Each sacroiliac (SI) joint – a plane type of synovial joint – is stabilized **by anterior and posterior SI ligaments, an interosseous sacroiliac ligament,** and superiorly by an **iliolumbar ligament** that connects the costal processes of the lumbar vertebrae L4/L5 with the iliac crest (➤ Fig. 2.49). The posterior inferior aspect of each sacroiliac joint is also reinforced by the **sacrospinous** and **sacrotuberous ligaments.** Unlike other synovial joints, the SI joints allow only a limited range of motion (subtle gliding and rotational movements).

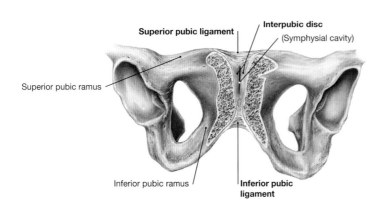

Fig. 4.9 Pubic symphysis joint; anterior view.
The pubic symphysis – fibrocartilage type joint, is stabilized by the **superior and inferior pubic ligaments,** as well as an **interpubic disc** comprised of fibrocartilage.

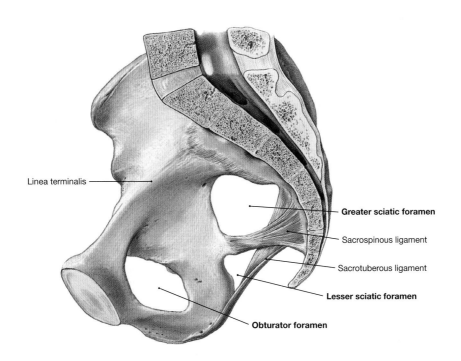

Linea terminalis

Greater sciatic foramen

Sacrospinous ligament

Sacrotuberous ligament

Lesser sciatic foramen

Obturator foramen

Fig. 4.10 Pelvic foramina; lateral view.
The sacrospinous and sacrotuberous ligaments are strong thick ligaments which reinforce the posterior-inferior aspect of the pelvis, and function to stabilize the bony articulations. Beyond this, they assist in the formation of the **greater sciatic foramen,** and the **lesser sciatic foramen. The obturator foramen** is also most easily visualized using a hemisectioned, lateral view of the pelvis. Each of these foramina allow important neurovascular structures to exit the pelvis (➤ Fig. 7.108, ➤ Fig. 7.109, ➤ Fig. 7.115, ➤ Fig. 7.116).

Foramen	Nerves	Vessels	Muscle
Greater Sciatic	Sciatic, superior gluteal, inferior gluteal, pudendal, posterior femoral cutaneous, nerve to quadratus femoris, nerve to obturator internus	Superior gluteal artery and vein, inferior gluteal artery and vein, internal pudendal artery and vein	Piriformis
Lesser Sciatic	Pudendal nerve, nerve to obturator internus	Internal pudendal artery and vein	Tendon of obturator internus
Obturator	Obturator	Obturator artery and vein	Covered by obturator membrane which serves as the pelvic attachment for both obturator internus and externus muscles

Structure/Function

A total of 14 structures (seven nerves, six vessels, one muscle) passes through the **greater sciatic foramen,** while four structures (two nerves, one vessel, one muscle) pass through the **lesser sciatic foramen.** The piriformis muscle serves as a key anatomical landmark for locating the greater and lesser sciatic foramina. It arises from the anterior (pelvic) surface of the sacrum, courses through the greater sciatic foramen, and attaches to the greater trochanter of femur. Only the superior gluteal nerve and vessels are located superior to the piriformis muscle, as they exit the pelvis.

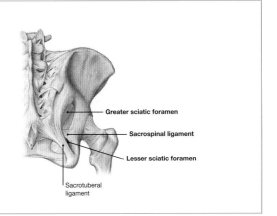

Greater sciatic foramen

Sacrospinal ligament

Lesser sciatic foramen

Sacrotuberal ligament

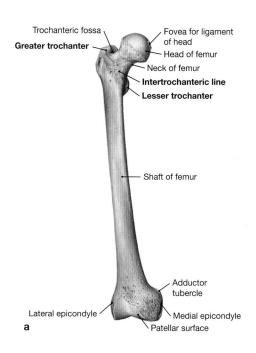

Trochanteric fossa
Fovea for ligament of head
Greater trochanter
Head of femur
Neck of femur
Intertrochanteric line
Lesser trochanter

Shaft of femur

Adductor tubercle
Lateral epicondyle
Medial epicondyle
a
Patellar surface

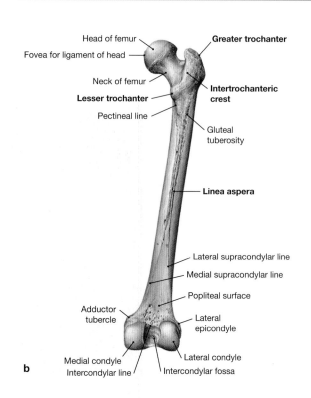

Head of femur
Greater trochanter
Fovea for ligament of head
Neck of femur
Intertrochanteric crest
Lesser trochanter
Pectineal line
Gluteal tuberosity

Linea aspera

Lateral supracondylar line
Medial supracondylar line
Popliteal surface
Adductor tubercle
Lateral epicondyle
Medial condyle
Lateral condyle
b
Intercondylar line
Intercondylar fossa

Fig. 4.11a and b Key features of the proximal third of femur; anterior **(a)** and posterior **(b)** views.
On the proximal femur, the **greater trochanter** is positioned laterally and the **lesser trochanter** posteromedially.

The **linea aspera** serves as the proximal attachment for the quadriceps femoris muscle, as well as the distal attachment for several muscles of the adductor muscle group. Note the prominence of the **intertrochanteric crest** on the posterior surface of the femur, as compared to the thin **intertrochanteric line** on the anterior surface.

Clinical Remarks

a A **'hip fracture'** refers to a fracture of the proximal $1/3$ of the femur. It is commonly observed as a result of a low-energy impact (e.g. a fall to the side while walking) in an elderly patient population, with the incidence of injury doubling for each decade past 50 years of age.
b Hip fractures typically occur in either the neck of femur or intertrochanteric regions.
c In adults, the medial circumflex femoral artery is the primary blood vessel for the head of femur. The lateral circumflex femoral artery mainly supplies the neck of femur. The acetabulum is supplied by the obturator artery and superior gluteal artery. Intracapsular fractures of the neck of femur can lead to disruption of the blood supply to the head of femur and result in complications such as non-union and avascular necrosis (AVN). While intertrochanteric fractures typically have lower rates of avualar necrosis (AVN) and non-union (because it is a fracture in the extracapsular region), they often require more robust stabilization.   a [M614], b [L126], c [L266, L127]

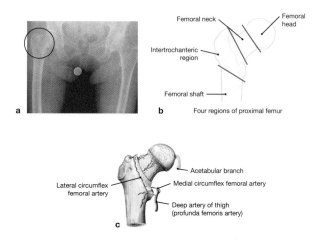

Femoral neck
Femoral head
Intertrochanteric region
Femoral shaft
a
b Four regions of proximal femur

Lateral circumflex femoral artery
Acetabular branch
Medial circumflex femoral artery
Deep artery of thigh (profunda femoris artery)
c

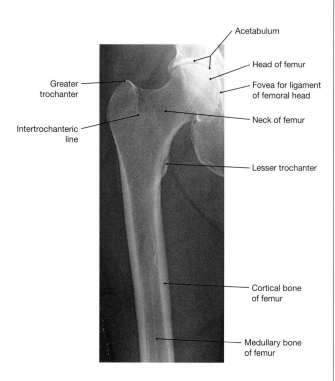

Acetabulum
Head of femur
Greater trochanter
Fovea for ligament of femoral head
Neck of femur
Intertrochanteric line
Lesser trochanter
Cortical bone of femur
Medullary bone of femur

Fig. 4.12 Right proximal femur and hip joint; anteroposterior (A/P) radiograph. [F264-004]

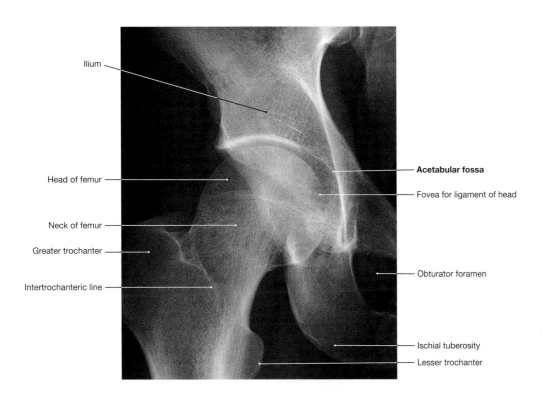

Ilium

Head of femur

Neck of femur

Greater trochanter

Intertrochanteric line

Acetabular fossa

Fovea for ligament of head

Obturator foramen

Ischial tuberosity

Lesser trochanter

Fig. 4.13 Hip joint, right side; anteroposterior (A/P) radiograph, upright standing position.

The hip joint is a very stable ball-and-socket type of synovial joint in which the socket is formed by the **acetabular fossa** of the hip bone.

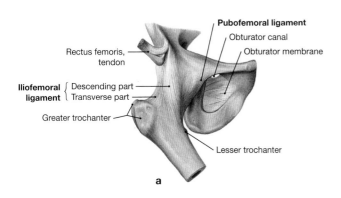

Rectus femoris, tendon

Iliofemoral ligament { Descending part / Transverse part }

Greater trochanter

Pubofemoral ligament

Obturator canal

Obturator membrane

Lesser trochanter

a

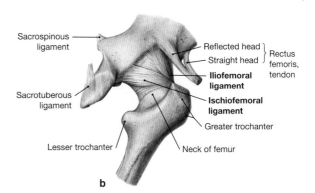

Sacrospinous ligament

Sacrotuberous ligament

Lesser trochanter

Reflected head / Straight head } Rectus femoris, tendon

Iliofemoral ligament

Ischiofemoral ligament

Greater trochanter

Neck of femur

b

Fig. 4.14a and b Hip joint, right side; anterior **(a)** and posterior **(b)** views.
There are three major ligaments of the hip joint which surround the femoral head in a spiral manner. Their principal function is to limit the range of hip extension and to prevent the backward tilting of the pelvis:

1. **Iliofemoral ligament:** inhibits extension and adduction
2. **Pubofemoral ligament:** inhibits extension, abduction, and lateral rotation
3. **Ischiofemoral ligament:** inhibits extension, medial rotation, and adduction.

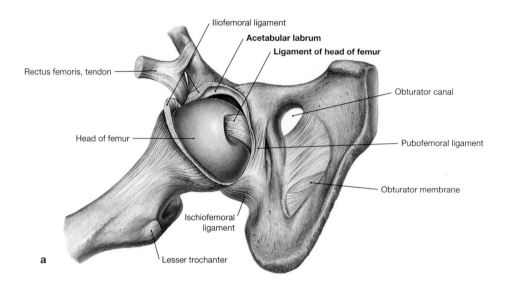

Iliofemoral ligament

Acetabular labrum

Ligament of head of femur

Rectus femoris, tendon

Obturator canal

Head of femur

Pubofemoral ligament

Obturator membrane

Ischiofemoral
ligament

a

Lesser trochanter

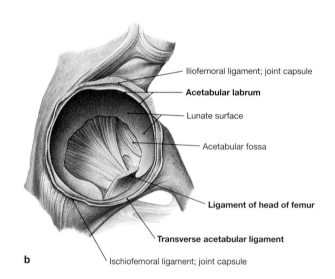

Iliofemoral ligament; joint capsule

Acetabular labrum

Lunate surface

Acetabular fossa

Ligament of head of femur

Transverse acetabular ligament

b

Ischiofemoral ligament; joint capsule

Fig. 4.15a and b Hip joint, right side; anterior view; after opening of the capsule and partial **(a)** or complete **(b)** disarticulation of the femoral head.
Hip joint: the **transverse acetabular ligament** inferiorly closes the acetabulum, and together with the **acetabular labrum,** it serves to guide the head of femur. While the **ligament of head of femur** lacks a mechanical function, it serves to protect an important blood supply to the hip joint – the acetabular branch of the obturator artery.

Clinical Remarks

a Orthopedic research suggests that the position and shape of the acetabulum and the head of femur are important factors that may be associated with the onset and progression of degenerative conditions of the hip joint such as **osteoarthritis.**
b Degenerative changes may result in the hip joint needing to be replaced with an 'artifical ball-and-socket style joint' via hip arthroplasty.
[M614]

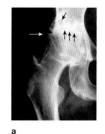

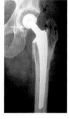

a   b

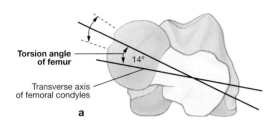

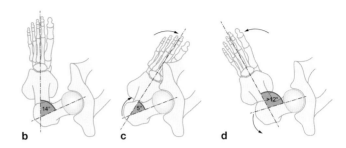

Fig. 4.16 a to d Proximal femur; the proximal and distal ends of the femur are projected on top of each other. b–d [L231]
a The neck of femur is normally rotated anteriorly by 12–14° against the axis connecting both femoral condyles (transverse axis of the femoral condyles). This is referred to as the **torsion angle of the femur.**
b Normal hip.

c In the case of **femoral anteversion** the torsion angle of the femur is smaller than 14°, resulting in the head of femur being rotated anteriorly and the patient walking with a 'toed in' gait pattern.
d In the case of **femoral retroversion** the torsion angle of the femur is greater than 12°, resulting in the head of femur being rotated posteriorly and the patient walking with a 'toed out' gait pattern.

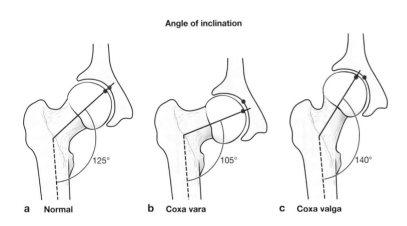

Angle of inclination

a Normal   **b Coxa vara**   **c Coxa valga**

Fig. 4.17 a to c Proximal end of the femur; frontal plane; illustration of variances to the normal femoral neck-shaft angle. [L126]
The **angle of inclination** refers to an angle formed by the long axis of the neck of femur and the long axis of the shaft. This angle can vary with age, sex, and development.
a The neck of femur normally forms an angle of approximately 125° with the shaft of femur.
b When the angle between the neck and shaft of femur is significantly diminished, it leads to a condition referred to as **coxa vara.**
c When the angle of inclination is significantly larger than normal, the alignment is referred to as **coxa valga.**

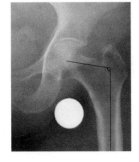

Fig. 4.18 Coxa vara; anteroposterior (A/P) radiograph of left hip joint. [R333]

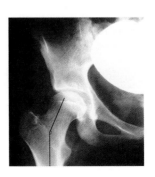

Fig. 4.19 Coxa valga; anteroposterior (A/P) radiograph of right hip joint. [R333]

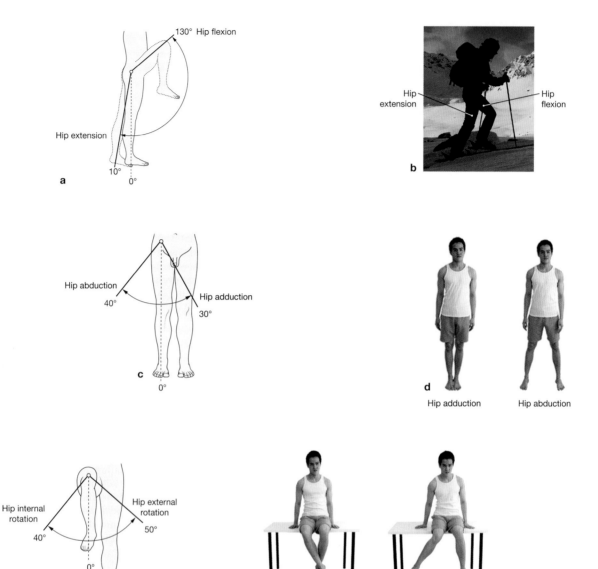

Fig. 4.20a to f Range of motion of the hip joint. a, c, e [L126], b [J787], d, f [L271]

The hip joint is one of the most important joints in the human body. It allows humans to walk, run and jump, and serves as the primary connection of the lower extremity to the axial skeleton. It is a tri-axial, ball-and-socket type of synovial joint that is stabilized by large ligaments and muscle from the pelvic girdle.

a and b Hip extension – flexion: 10°–0°–130°.
c and d Hip abduction – adduction: 40°–0°–30°.
e and f Hip external (lateral) rotation – internal (medial) rotation: 50°–0°–40°.

Hip Movement	Muscles Active During Movements
Flexion	Iliopsoas, sartorius, rectus femoris, pectineus
Extension	Gluteus maximus, biceps femoris, semitendinosus, semimembranosus, adductor magnus
Abduction	Gluteus medius, gluteus minimus, tensor fasciae latae/iliotibial band
Adduction	Pectineus, adductor longus, adductor brevis, adductor magnus, gracilis
Internal rotation	Gluteus medius, gluteus minimus
External rotation	Piriformis, gluteus maximus, quadratus femoris, gemellus superior and inferior, obturator internus and externus

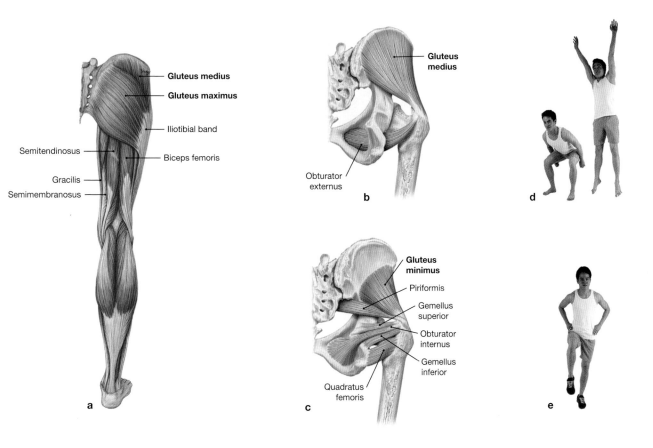

Fig. 4.21a to e Muscles of the posterior hip and gluteal region, right side; posterior view. b, c [L127], d, e [L271]

The posterior hip or buttocks region is occupied by three gluteal muscles: gluteus maximus **(a)**, gluteus medius **(b)**, and gluteus minimus **(c)**. The **gluteus maximus** is the most superficial muscle of the region, and functions to power **hip extension movements** during activities such as running, jumping and ice skating **(d)**. The smaller and deeper **gluteus medius and minimus** muscles function to keep the pelvis level when the opposite leg is raised such as during the **single leg stance** phase of walking or running, or when standing on one leg **(e)**.

Muscle	Attachments (P = proximal, D = distal)	Action/Function	Innervation
Gluteus maximus	**P:** Ilium, posterior to gluteal line, posterior sacrum and coccyx, sacrotuberous ligament **D:** Iliotibial band, gluteal tuberosity of femur	Hip extension, hip external rotation	Inferior gluteal nerve (L5, S1, S2)
Gluteus medius	**P:** Ilium, between anterior and posterior gluteal lines **D:** Greater trochanter of femur	Hip adduction, hip internal rotation keep pelvis level when opposite leg is raised	Superior gluteal nerve (L5, S1)
Gluteus minimus	**P:** Ilium between anterior and inferior gluteal lines **D:** Greater trochanter of femur	Hip adduction, hip internal rotation keep pelvis level when opposite leg is raised	Superior gluteal nerve (L5, S1)

Clinical Remarks

The muscles of the gluteal region play a key role in stabilizing the hip joint during change of direction movements in sport, as well as when landing from a jump. Weakness of the gluteus medius and minimus muscles or injury to the superior gluteal nerve (which innervates these muscles) can result in ineffective stabilization of the hip joint, and lead to the knee joint experiencing a **large valgus force (or knee adduction moment) during movement.** This abnormal knee movement may be associated with the occurrence of traumatic knee injuries such as a torn anterior cruciate ligament.
a [G728], b [L231]

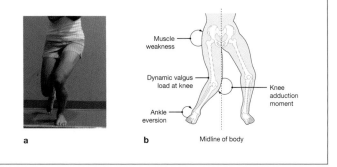

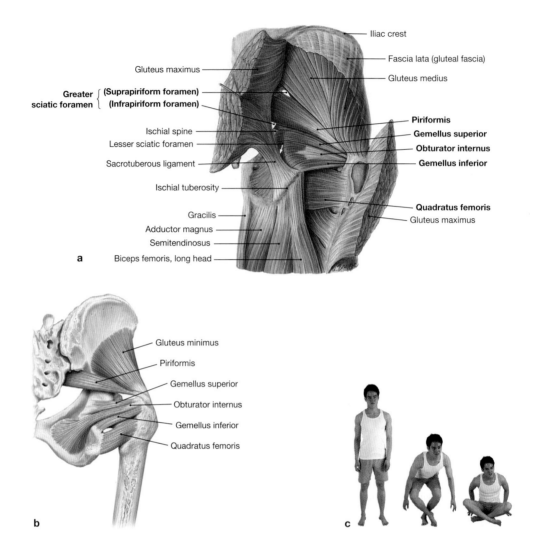

Fig. 4.22a to c Deep muscles of the posterior hip and gluteal region, right side; posterior view. b [L127], c [L271]
The **pelvitrochanteric muscle group (piriformis, obturator internus, obturator externus, gemellus superior, gemellus inferior, quadratus femoris)** function exclusively as lateral (external) rotators of the hip **(a)**. The **piriformis** is the largest and most identifiable muscle of this group, and can be used to divide the **greater sciatic foramen** into the **suprapiriform** and **infrapiriform foramina**

(b). It also serves as important anatomical landmark for the identification of key neurovascular structures that enter the gluteal region via the **greater sciatic foramen.** Piriformis, together with the smaller muscles of the deep gluteal region – obturator internus, obturator externus, gemellus superior, gemellus inferior, quadratus femoris control **hip external rotation** – such as when lowering from a standing to cross-legged sitting position **(c)**.

Muscle	Attachments (P = proximal, D = distal)	Action/Function	Innervation
Piriformis	**P:** Anterior surface of sacrum, superior margin of greater sciatic notch, sacrotuberous ligament **D:** Greater trochanter of femur	Hip external rotation	Anterior rami of S1 and S2
Obturator internus	**P:** Pelvic surface of ilium and ischium, obturator membrane **D:** Greater trochanter of femur	Hip external rotation	Nerve to obturator internus (L5, S1)
Obturator externus (not displayed)	**P:** Margins of obturator foramen and obturator membrane **D:** Trochanteric fossa of femur	Hip external rotation	Obturator nerve (L3, L4)
Gemellus superior	**P:** Ischial spine **D:** Greater trochanter of femur	Hip external rotation	Nerve to obturator internus (L5, S1)
Gemellus inferior	**P:** Ischial tuberosity **D:** Greater trochanter of femur	Hip external rotation	Nerve to quadratus femoris (L5, S1)
Quadratus femoris	**P:** Ischial tuberosity – lateral border **D:** Intertrochanteric crest of femur	Hip external rotation	Nerve to quadratus femoris (L5, S1)

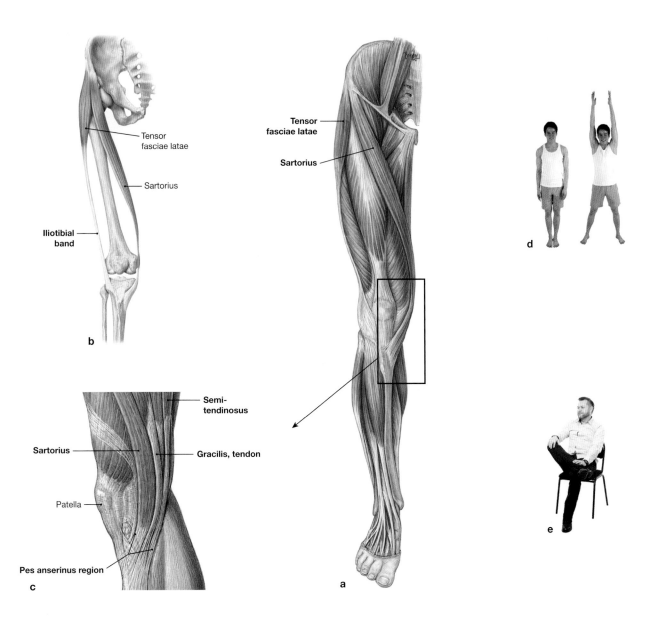

Fig. 4.23a to e Superficial muscles of the anterior hip, right side; anterior view. b [L127], d [L271], e [J787]

Fig. 4.23a to e Superficial muscles of the anterior hip, right side;
anterior view. b [L127], d [L271], e [J787]
The **tensor fasciae latae (TFL)** muscle is located at the superior lateral aspect of the thigh, and acts as a tension band of the lateral thigh via its insertion into the **iliotibial band (ITB).** The **sartorius** shares its distal attachment on the medial condyle of the tibia (region called the **pes anserinus)** with the **gracilis** (adductor muscle group), and **semitendinosus** (hamstring muscle group) muscles.

The **TFL/ITB** complex functions together to power **hip abduction with a straight knee** – i.e. when performing a jumping jack movement pattern **(d)**. The **sartorius** crosses both the hip and knee joints, and thus actively assists with flexion of these joints. It is often described as the **FABER muscle** of the hip (because it simultaneously powers hip **f**lexion, **ab**duction and **e**xternal **r**otation), assisting a person to move their leg into a cross-legged sitting position **(e)**.

Muscle	Attachments (P = proximal, D = distal)	Action/Function	Innervation
Tensor fasciae latae (TFL)	**P:** Anterior superior iliac spine (ASIS), iliac crest **D:** Iliotibial band (ITB) which attaches on the lateral condyle of tibia (region called GERDY's tubercle)	TFL – abducts and flexes hip joint. ITB – helps to maintain the knee in an extended position when the hip is performing a straight-legged abduction movement.	Superior gluteal nerve (L4, L5)
Sartorius	**P:** ASIS **D:** Pes anserinus region located on superior portion of medial tibia	Flexes, abducts and external rotates hip joint (FABER), flexes knee joint	Femoral nerve (L2, L3)

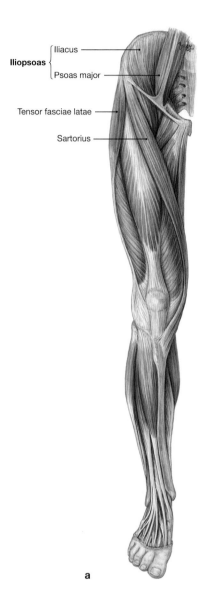

Iliopsoas { Iliacus
Psoas major

Tensor fasciae latae

Sartorius

a

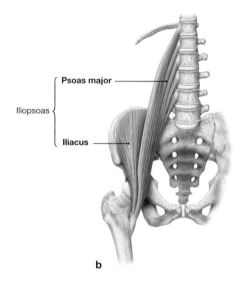

Psoas major

Iliopsoas {

Iliacus

b

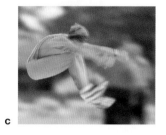

c

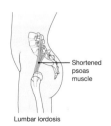

d

Fig. 4.24a to d Deep muscles of the anterior hip, right side; anterior view. b [L127], c, d [J787]
The **iliopsoas** is comprised of two different muscles: 1. Psoas major, 2. Iliacus. The iliopsoas muscle functions as a **powerful hip flexor,** and undergoes significant hypertrophy (enlargement) in individuals who participate in activities such as cycling or track and field **(c and d).**

Muscle	Attachments (P = proximal, D = distal)	Action/Function	Innervation
Iliopsoas – psoas major	**P:** T12 to L5 vertebrae – sides, discs between, and transverse processes **D:** Lesser trochanter of femur	Flexes hip joint	Anterior rami of lumbar nerves (L1, L2, L3)
Iliopsoas – iliacus	**P:** Iliac crest, iliac fossa, ala of sacrum **D:** Lesser trochanter of femur via tendon of psoas major	Flexes hip joint	Femoral nerve (L2, L3)

Structure/Function

As a result of its attachment to the vertebrae of the lumbar spine, **tightness of the psoas major** component of the iliopsoas muscle complex can lead to an increased lordotic curve of the lumbar spine. This muscle tightness/inflexibility can result in low back pain which occurs following vigorous activities that involve hip extension movements during which the 'tight' psoas muscle repeatedly lengthens. Prolonged sitting (i.e. working at a desk or driving a vehicle) with the hips in a flexed position (which places the iliopsoas muscle in a shortened position) is believed to be one possible cause of psoas major muscle tightness.   [L231]

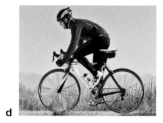

Normal psoas muscle

Shortened psoas muscle

Normal psoas posture   Lumbar lordosis

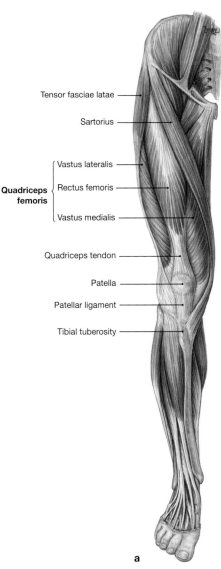

Tensor fasciae latae

Sartorius

Quadriceps femoris
- Vastus lateralis
- Rectus femoris
- Vastus medialis

Quadriceps tendon

Patella

Patellar ligament

Tibial tuberosity

a

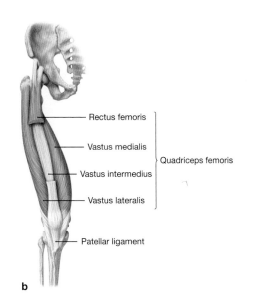

Rectus femoris

Vastus medialis

Vastus intermedius

Vastus lateralis

Patellar ligament

Quadriceps femoris

b

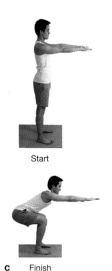

Start

c   Finish

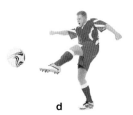

d

Fig. 4.25a to d Muscles of the anterior thigh, right side; anterior view; superficial to deep.
b [L127], c [L271], d [J787]

The muscles of the anterior thigh are collectively referred to as the **'quadriceps femoris'** muscle group **(a).** It is comprised of four distinct sections, each of which shares a common distal attachment to the tibial tuberosity via the patella ligament and quadriceps tendons **(b).** All four sections of the quadriceps femoris muscle are active when performing a squat; **moving from a sit-to-stand/stand-to-sit position (c).** Because the rectus femoris muscle also crosses the hip, it helps to power both **hip flexion and knee extension** when performing a powerful kicking movement **(d).**

Quadriceps femoris Muscle	Attachments (P = proximal, D = distal)	Action/Function	Innervation
Rectus femoris	**P:** Anterior inferior iliac spine, ilium superior to acetabulum **D:** Tibial tuberosity via patella ligament	Hip flexion; knee extension	Femoral nerve (L2, L3, L4)
Vastus lateralis	**P:** Greater trochanter, lateral lip of linea aspera **D:** Tibial tuberosity via patella ligament	Knee extension	Femoral nerve (L2, L3, L4)
Vastus medialis	**P:** Intertrochanteric line, medial lip of linea aspera **D:** Tibial tuberosity via patella ligament	Knee extension	Femoral nerve (L2, L3, L4)
Vastus intermedius	**P:** Femoral shaft **D:** Tibial tuberosity via patella ligament	Knee extension	Femoral nerve (L2, L3, L4)

Clinical Remarks

The anterior thigh or 'quads' region can be severely contused as a result of a blunt force trauma. As the magnitude of the force increases, so does the damage to the region. Severe contusions can result in a dramatic loss of muscle strength, restricted range of motion, and cause a significant amount of pain and skin discoloration **(ecchymosis)** in the region. A complication that can be associated with severe bruising in the quadriceps region is a condition known as **myositis ossificans**. It occurs as a result of ectopic calcification that is associated with trauma to both the quadriceps muscle and the underlying bone.
a [J787], b [E969], c [J787-046]

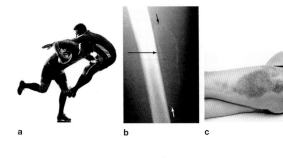

a   b   c

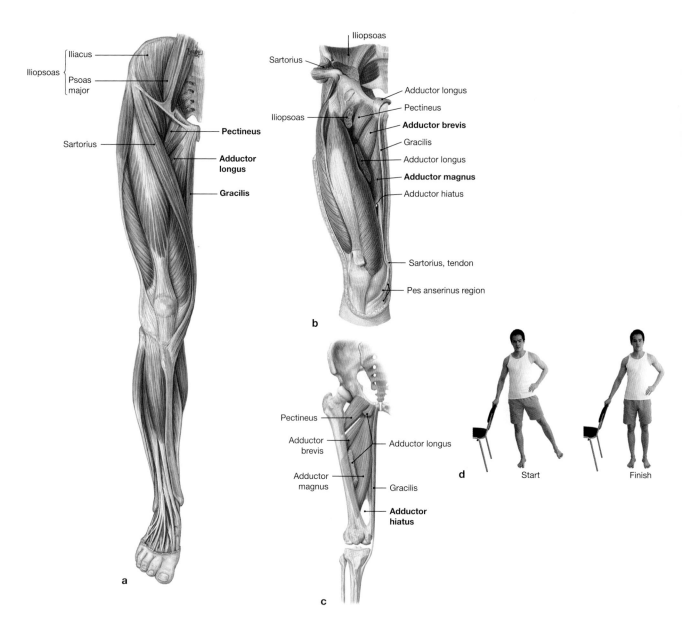

Fig. 4.26a to d Muscles of the medial thigh, right side; anterior view; superficial to deep. c [L127], d [L271]

The muscles of the medial thigh are separated from the quadriceps femoris muscle group by the sartorius muscle. There are a total of five **'groin muscles'** that are organized into two layers, of which only the **pectineus, adductor longus,** and **gracilis** are visible **(a)**. Removal of the sartorius and adductor longus muscles reveals the two deep adductor muscles **(adductor brevis** and **adductor magnus; b)**. The adductor magnus and its tendon form an **adductor hiatus (canal)** through which the blood vessels of the anterior thigh (femoral artery/vein) pass to reach the popliteal region in the back of the knee **(c)**. The groin muscles function to **bring the leg towards the midline,** hip adduction **(d)**.

Groin Muscles	Attachments (P = proximal, D = distal)	Action/Function	Innervation
Pectineus	**P:** Superior ramus of pubis **D:** Pectineal line of femur, inferior to lesser trochanter	Hip adduction, assists with hip flexion	Femoral nerve (L2, L3)
Adductor brevis	**P:** Body and inferior ramus of pubis **D:** Pectineal line of femur, linea aspera of femur	Hip adduction	Obturator nerve (L2, L3, L4)
Adductor longus	**P:** Body of pubis inferior to pubic crest **D:** Middle ⅓ of linea aspera of femur	Hip adduction	Obturator nerve (L2, L3, L4)
Adductor magnus	**Adductor part:** **P:** Inferior ramus of pubis, ramus of ischium; **D:** Gluteal tuberosity, linea aspera, medial supracondylar line	Hip adduction	Adductor part: obturator nerve (L2, L3, L4)
	Hamstring part: **P:** Ischial tuberosity **D:** Adductor tubercle of femur	Assists with hip extension	Hamstring part: tibial division of sciatic nerve (L4)
Gracilis	**P:** Body and inferior ramus of pubis **D:** Pes anserinus region on superior portion of medial tibia	Hip adduction	Obturator nerve (L2, L3)

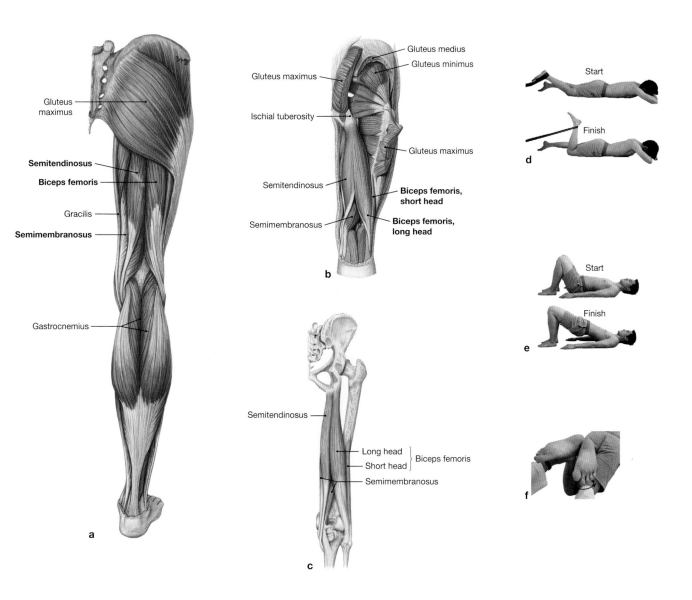

Fig. 4.27a to f Muscles of the posterior thigh, right side; posterior view; superficial to deep. c [L127], d–f [271]

The three **hamstring muscles** all share a common proximal attachment, the ischial tuberosity of the hip bone. The **biceps femoris** courses in an inferolateral direction to attach distally on the head of fibula. The **semimembranosus** and **semitendinosus** both course in an inferomedial direction to attach to the proximal tibia. Together the hamstring muscles function to power: **knee flexion (d)**; **hip extension** about a stable knee – i. e. performing a bridge activity at the trunk **(e)**; and to power **internal** (semimembranosus and semitendinosus) and **external** (biceps femoris) **rotation** when knee is flexed **(f)**.

Hamstring Muscles	Attachments (P = proximal, D = distal)	Action/Function	Innervation
Biceps femoris	**P:** Long head: ischial tuberosity; short head: linea aspera and lateral supracondylar region of femur **D:** Head of fibula	Hip extension Knee flexion External rotation of a flexed knee	Long head: sciatic nerve – tibial division (L5, S1, S2) Short head: sciatic nerve – common fibular division (L5, S1, S2)
Semimembranosus	**P:** Ischial tuberosity **D:** Posterior aspect of medial condyle of tibia	Hip extension Knee flexion Internal rotation of a flexed knee	Sciatic nerve – tibial division (L5, S1, S2)
Semitendinosus	**P:** Ischial tuberosity **D:** Pes anserinus region on superior portion of medial tibia	Hip extension Knee flexion Internal rotation of a flexed knee	Sciatic nerve – tibial division (L5, S1, S2)

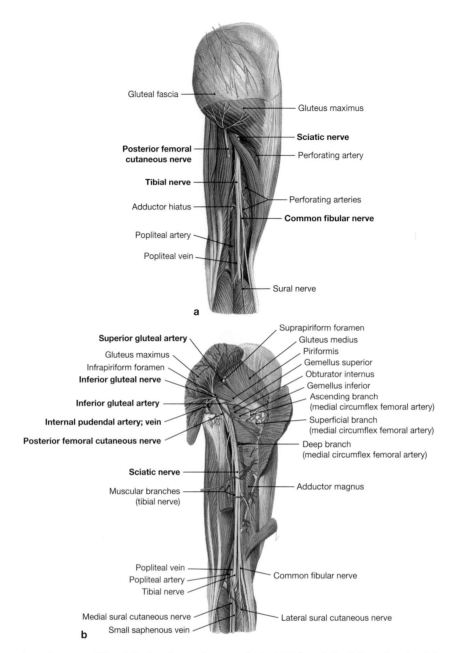

Gluteal fascia

Gluteus maximus

Sciatic nerve

Perforating artery

Posterior femoral cutaneous nerve

Tibial nerve

Perforating arteries

Adductor hiatus

Common fibular nerve

Popliteal artery

Popliteal vein

Sural nerve

a

Superior gluteal artery

Suprapiriform foramen

Gluteus medius

Piriformis

Gluteus maximus

Gemellus superior

Infrapiriform foramen

Obturator internus

Inferior gluteal nerve

Gemellus inferior

Ascending branch
(medial circumflex femoral artery)

Inferior gluteal artery

Superficial branch
(medial circumflex femoral artery)

Internal pudendal artery; vein

Deep branch
(medial circumflex femoral artery)

Posterior femoral cutaneous nerve

Sciatic nerve

Adductor magnus

Muscular branches
(tibial nerve)

Popliteal vein

Common fibular nerve

Popliteal artery

Tibial nerve

Medial sural cutaneous nerve

Lateral sural cutaneous nerve

Small saphenous vein

b

Fig. 4.28a and b Vessels and nerves of the gluteal region and posterior thigh, right side.
The **superior gluteal nerve** (not visible), **artery and vein** exit the pelvis through the suprapiriform foramen but remain deep to the gluteus medius. The **sciatic nerve** exits the pelvis via the infrapiriform foramen together with the **posterior femoral cutaneous nerve**, and the **inferior gluteal nerve, artery and vein.** The pudendal nerve

(not visible) and the **internal pudendal artery and vein** also exit here, but immediately wind around the sacrospinous ligament and re-enter the pelvis via the lesser sciatic foramen. The **sciatic nerve** descends through the posterior thigh (under the biceps femoris muscle) and divides into its terminal branches: the **tibial and common fibular nerves.**

Clinical Remarks

a The topography of the gluteal region explains why **intramuscular injections** must be applied into the **gluteus medius,** not into the gluteus maximus. Incorrectly placed injections may cause bleeding and injuries to the nerves which innervate the muscles that power movements of the hip (superior and inferior gluteal nerves) and the knee (sciatic nerve). **Lesions of the superior gluteal nerve** can lead to paralysis of the gluteus medius and minimus muscles or the tensor fasciae latae.
b This type of injury may manifest itself as a positive **TRENDELENBURG's sign** – an inability to keep the pelvis level when performing single leg balance on the affected side.
a [L126], b [L127]

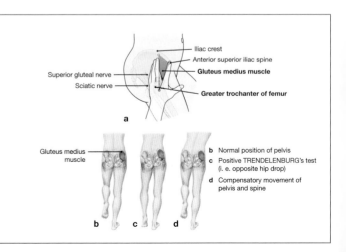

Iliac crest

Anterior superior iliac spine

Gluteus medius muscle

Superior gluteal nerve

Sciatic nerve

Greater trochanter of femur

a

Gluteus medius muscle

b Normal position of pelvis

c Positive TRENDELENBURG's test
(i. e. opposite hip drop)

d Compensatory movement of
pelvis and spine

b   c   d

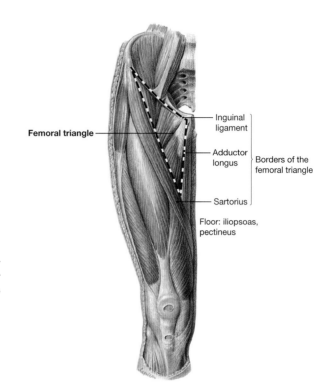

Femoral triangle

Inguinal ligament

Adductor longus

Sartorius

Borders of the femoral triangle

Floor: iliopsoas, pectineus

Fig. 4.29 Femoral triangle, right side; anterior view.
The **femoral triangle** is a triangular space located in the superomedial ⅓ of the anterior thigh. Its boundaries include the inguinal ligament (superior/base), adductor longus (medial), sartorius (lateral), and iliapsoas, pectineus (floor).

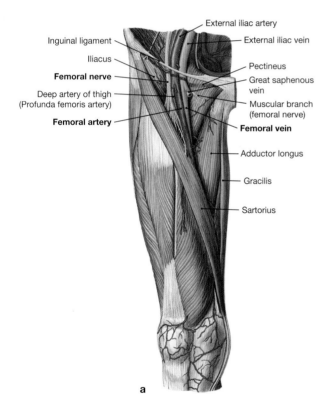

External iliac artery

Inguinal ligament

Iliacus

Femoral nerve

Deep artery of thigh (Profunda femoris artery)

Femoral artery

External iliac vein

Pectineus

Great saphenous vein

Muscular branch (femoral nerve)

Femoral vein

Adductor longus

Gracilis

Sartorius

a

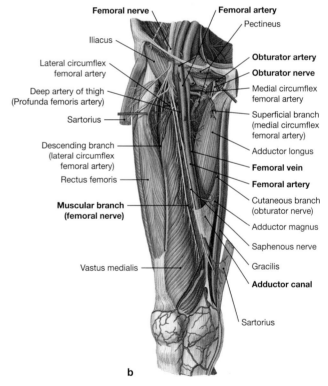

Femoral nerve

Iliacus

Lateral circumflex femoral artery

Deep artery of thigh (Profunda femoris artery)

Sartorius

Descending branch (lateral circumflex femoral artery)

Rectus femoris

Muscular branch (femoral nerve)

Vastus medialis

Femoral artery

Pectineus

Obturator artery

Obturator nerve

Medial circumflex femoral artery

Superficial branch (medial circumflex femoral artery)

Adductor longus

Femoral vein

Femoral artery

Cutaneous branch (obturator nerve)

Adductor magnus

Saphenous nerve

Gracilis

Adductor canal

Sartorius

b

Fig. 4.30a and b Vessels and nerves of the thigh, right side; anterior view. The **femoral triangle** contains (organized medial to lateral): **femoral vein, femoral artery** (➤ Fig. 6.133), **and femoral nerve** (both the vein and artery are enclosed in a fascial envelope called the femoral sheath, **a**). The femoral nerve creates a fan-shaped branching and divides into:
1. the saphenous nerve;
2. several motor branches (which innervate the quadriceps femoris, sartorius, pectineus, and iliacus muscles);
3. the anterior cutaneous branches which provide sensory innervation to the skin of the anterior thigh.

The femoral artery and vein and the saphenous nerve course together beneath the sartorius muscle to their entrance into the **adductor canal (b).** Following passage through the adductor canal the femoral artery is then referred to as popliteal artery (arterial supply of the knee joint). In the superior thigh, the obturator canal allows the **obturator nerve, artery and vein** to exit the pelvis and course into the medial thigh or 'groin' region.

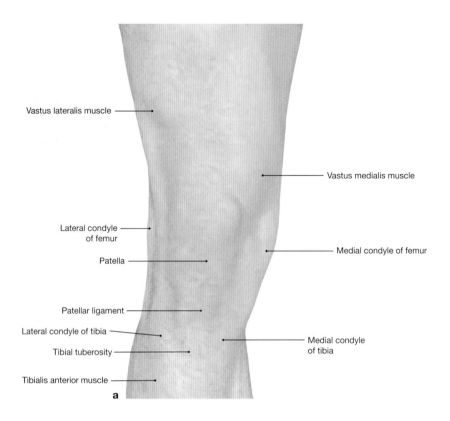

Vastus lateralis muscle

Vastus medialis muscle

Lateral condyle of femur

Medial condyle of femur

Patella

Patellar ligament

Lateral condyle of tibia

Medial condyle of tibia

Tibial tuberosity

Tibialis anterior muscle

a

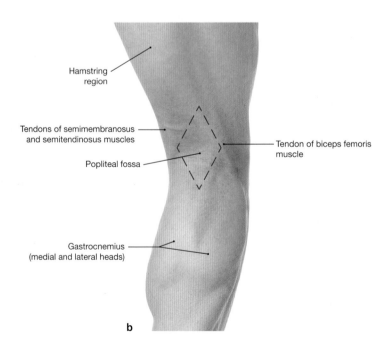

Hamstring region

Tendons of semimembranosus and semitendinosus muscles

Tendon of biceps femoris muscle

Popliteal fossa

Gastrocnemius (medial and lateral heads)

b

Fig. 4.31a and b Surface anatomy of the knee, right side; anterior view **(a),** posterior view **(b).** a [S002-8], b [K340]

Palpation of the key bony and muscular attachments around the knee should be included as part of a thorough and complete musculoskeletal examination.

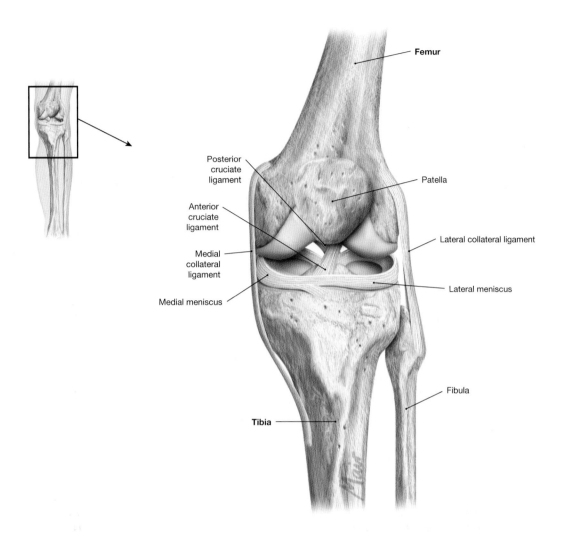

Fig. 4.32 The knee, left side; anterior view. [L127]

The knee is one of the largest and most complex joints of the human body. It is formed by the **articulation of the distal femur on the proximal tibia.** Because of the limited bone-on-bone contact between these two bones, knee joint stability is significantly influenced by the strength of muscles which cross the joint (primarily the quadriceps, hamstrings, and calf muscles), and ligamentous support provided by two cruciate ligaments (anterior and posterior), two collateral ligaments (medial and lateral) and two menisci (medial and lateral) located within the joint.

Clinical Remarks

Degenerative changes within the knee joint can occur secondarily to injury (e.g. following a torn anterior cruciate ligament or meniscus), or as the result of abnormalities in joint alignment. Knee osteoarthritis (OA) is most commonly diagnosed via plane radiography. The **KELLGREN and LAWRENCE classification system** is used to grade the degree of knee OA. Grade 0 (none, **a**) – no radiographic findings of OA; grade 1 (doubtful) – doubtful narrowing of joint space and possible osteophytic lipping; grade 2 (minimal OA) – definite osteophytes, definite narrowing of joint space; grade 3 (moderate OA) – moderate multiple osteophytes, definite narrowing of joint space, some sclerosis and possible deformity of bone contour; grade 4 (severe OA, **b**) – large osteophytes, marked narrowing of joint space, severe sclerosis, and definite deformity of bone contour.
b [M614]

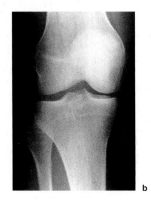
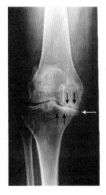

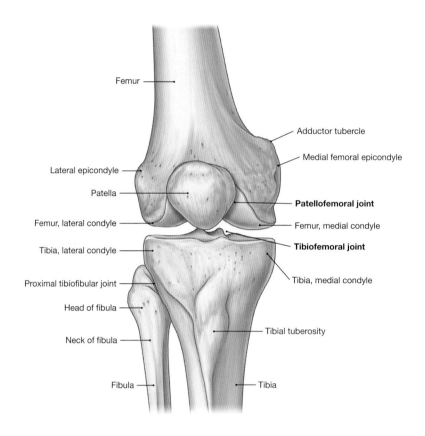

Fig. 4.33 Knee bones, right side; anterior view. [E460]
The knee is a **modified hinge type synovial joint,** in which, the femur articulates with both the tibia **(tibiofemoral joint)** and patella **(patellofemoral joint).** All bones are ensheathed by a common joint capsule. In the tibiofemoral joint, the femoral condyles constitute the head and the superior articular surface of both tibial condyles form the socket of the knee joint.

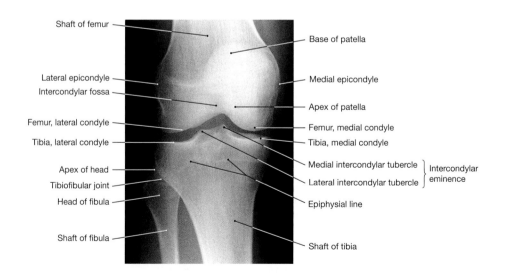

Fig. 4.34 Anteroposterior (A/P) radiograph of the knee, right side.

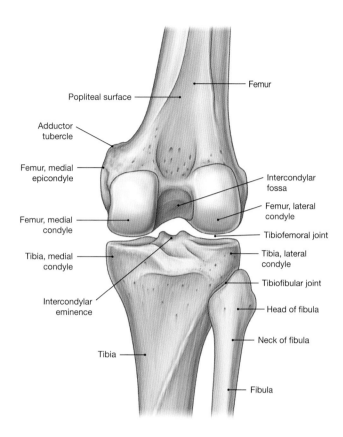

Femur

Popliteal surface

Adductor
tubercle

Femur, medial
epicondyle

Intercondylar
fossa

Femur, lateral
condyle

Femur, medial
condyle

Tibiofemoral joint

Tibia, medial
condyle

Tibia, lateral
condyle

Intercondylar
eminence

Tibiofibular joint

Head of fibula

Neck of fibula

Tibia

Fibula

Fig. 4.35 Knee bones, right side; posterior view. [E460]

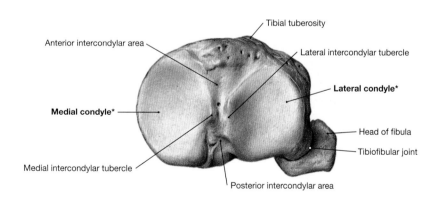

Tibial tuberosity

Anterior intercondylar area

Lateral intercondylar tubercle

Lateral condyle*

Medial condyle*

Head of fibula

Tibiofibular joint

Medial intercondylar tubercle

Posterior intercondylar area

Fig. 4.36 Tibia and fibula, right side; proximal view.

The **articular surfaces of the medial and lateral tibial condyles (*)**
are collectively referred to as **superior articular surface.**

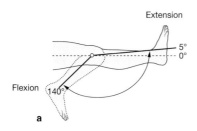

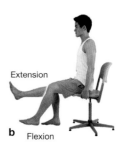

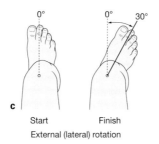

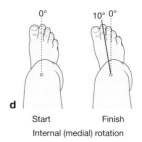

c

Start   Finish
External (lateral) rotation

d

Start   Finish
Internal (medial) rotation

Fig. 4.37a to d Range of motion of the knee. a, c, d [L126], b [L271]
Active knee flexion occurs up to 120°, but can be passively increased up to 160°, limited only by soft tissues. Active knee extension is possible up to 0°, but can be further increased passively by
5°–10°. Rotational movements are only possible when the knee
moves into a flexed position, because the tension of the collateral
ligaments during knee extension prevents rotational movements.

Lateral rotation is possible to a larger extent than medial rotation
because the cruciate ligaments twist around each other during medial rotation. Abduction and adduction movements of the joint are
prevented by the collateral ligaments.
a and b Extension – flexion: 5°–0°–140°
c Lateral rotation: 0°–30°
d Medial rotation: 0°–10°

Knee Movement	Muscles Active During Movements
Flexion	Hamstrings – biceps femoris, semitendinosus, semimembranosus, gastrocnemius, popliteus
Extension	Quadriceps femoris – rectus femoris, vastus lateralis, vastus intermedius, vastus medialis
Internal (medial) rotation	Semimembranosus, semitendinosus, popliteus
External (lateral) rotation	Biceps femoris

Clinical Remarks

The **Dial test** is an orthopedic maneuver used to examine for injury to the posterior cruciate ligament (PCL) and/or posterolateral corner of the knee joint. For the test, the patient is placed in a
prone lying position and their knees are flexed 90°. Keeping the
thighs together, the knees are then passively externally rotated.
Normally the range of knee external rotation will be bilaterally
symmetrical (i.e. the same on both sides). If one knee can be
externally rotated significantly more than the other, it is sugges-
tive of ligamentous instability in the posterolateral corner of the
joint.
[G052, G931]

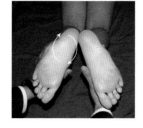

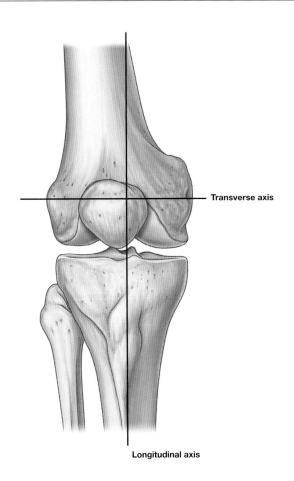

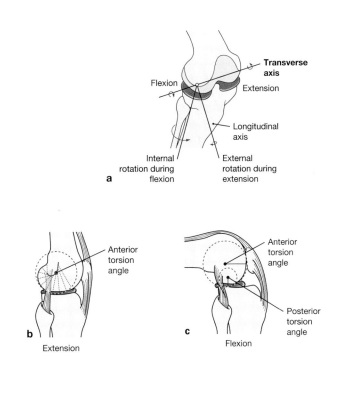

Fig. 4.38 Axes of the knee; anterior view. [E460]
The knee is a modified hinge type synovial joint that possesses two axes of movement. The **transverse axis** for extension and flexion movements extends horizontally through both femoral condyles. The **longitudinal axis** for rotational movements is positioned off center within the knee joint, and extends vertically through the medial intercondylar tubercle of the tibia.

Fig. 4.39a to c Knee, a modified hinge joint. a [L231], b, c [L126]
a The knee functions as a **pivot-hinge joint** about this two axes of movement.
b, c Because of radius curvature of the femoral condyles the transverse axis does not remain in a constant position, but moves posteriorly and superiorly during flexion on a convex line. Thus, knee flexion is a combined rolling and sliding movement in which the condyles roll up to 20° posteriorly. Since the shape of the medial and lateral condyles of the femur and tibia are not identical (the medial femoral condyle is larger than the lateral femoral condyle), it is the lateral femoral condyle that predominantly rolls (similar to a rocking chair) and the medial condyle remains in its position to rotate (similar to a ball-and-socket joint). At the same time the femur rotates slightly outwards. During terminal extension of the knee, the tension of the anterior cruciate ligament also causes a forced external rotation of 5°–10°. This rotation is referred to as the **screw home mechanism.**

Clinical Remarks

a Full terminal extension (beyond 0°) of the knee joint is achieved via a movement called the **'screw home mechanism'.**
b As the **medial condyle of femur is roughly 1 cm (0.4 in) longer than lateral condyle of femur,** subtle rotation of the tibia on the femur must occur in order for terminal extension or the initiation of knee flexion to occur.
c During terminal extension, the tibia externally rotates on the femur. This movement of the tibia on the femoral condyles adds a great deal of continuity to the joint surfaces and thus enhances joint stability and provides an energy efficient posture when standing.
d Knee flexion is initiated by contraction of the popliteus muscle which causes an internal rotation of the tibia on the femur, in essence unlocking the knee joint and allowing it to bend.
a [L231], b–d [L127]

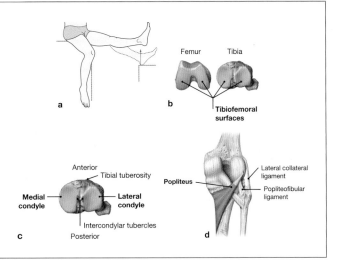

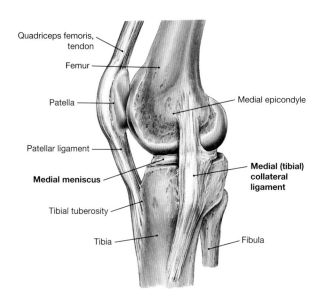

Quadriceps femoris, tendon
Femur
Patella
Patellar ligament
Medial meniscus
Tibial tuberosity
Tibia
Medial epicondyle
Medial (tibial) collateral ligament
Fibula

Fig. 4.40 Medial (tibial) collateral ligament in extension; medial view.

The **medial collateral ligament (MCL)** arises proximally from the medial epicondyle of the femur and attaches distally to the medial condyle of the tibia. It functions to stabilize the medial side of the joint against abduction movements of the lower leg (i.e. valgus forces). It is a flat, broad membranous band that serves to reinforce the joint capsule on the medial side of the knee, and has direct attachment through the joint capsule and synovial lining to the **medial meniscus.**

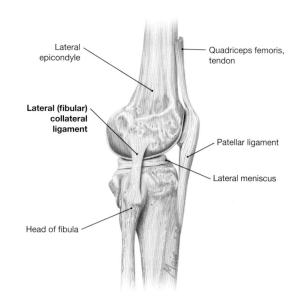

Lateral epicondyle
Quadriceps femoris, tendon
Lateral (fibular) collateral ligament
Patellar ligament
Lateral meniscus
Head of fibula

Fig. 4.41 Lateral (fibular) collateral ligament in extension; lateral view. [L127]

The **lateral collateral ligament (LCL)** arises proximally from the lateral epicondyle of the femur and attaches distally to the head of the fibula (which is also the distal attachment point for the biceps femoris muscle of the hamstrings). It functions to stabilize the lateral side of the joint against adduction movements of the lower leg (i.e. varus forces). While the LCL helps to reinforce the joint capsule on the lateral side of the knee, it is smaller, and narrower than the MCL, and has no direct attachment to the lateral meniscus.

Clinical Remarks

The collateral ligaments serve to reinforce the joint capsule on both the medial and lateral sides of the knee. Because of the large radius of curvature of the femoral condyles, the collateral ligaments are under greatest tension when the knee is in a fully extended or 'locked-out' position. This ligamentous tension diminishes as the knee 'unlocks' and moves into a flexed position, thus allowing rotational movements of the joint to occur.

a The application of a **valgus load** (a force directed to the lateral side of the knee) to the fully extended knee commonly results in injury or a 'sprain' of the MCL. The severity of sprain (mild/moderate/severe) is dependent upon the extent to which the medial side of the joint gaps open when the valgus load is applied.

b Conversely, the application of a **varus load** (a force applied to the medial side of the knee) can result in damage to the LCL. Epidemiology data suggest that MCL sprains occur much more frequently than LCL sprains.
[L271]

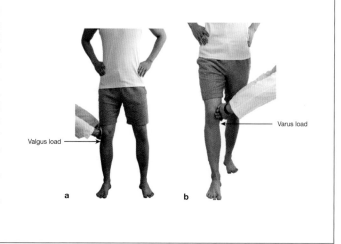

Valgus load
Varus load
a
b

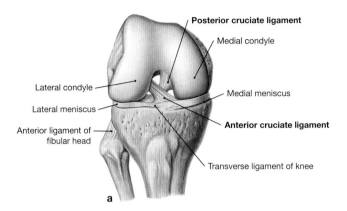

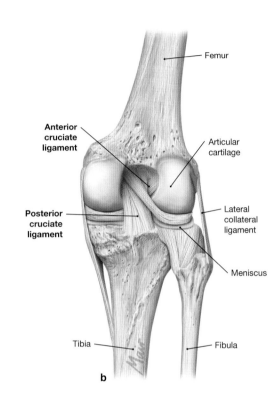

Fig. 4.42a and b Anterior and posterior cruciate ligaments; anterior **(a)** and posterior **(b)** views. b [L127]

The cruciate ligaments are intercapsular ligaments, but are positioned outside the synovial joint cavity – they are surrounded by a thin, vascularized envelope formed by the synovial lining within the knee. The **anterior cruciate ligament (ACL)** arises from the anterior intercondylar area of the tibia (just posterior to the attachment of the medial meniscus) and courses upwards in an **a**nterior to **p**osterior direction, winding **ex**ternally (or outwards) to attach to the medial wall of the lateral condyle of the femur (it is referred to

as the **APEX ligament).** The **posterior cruciate ligament (PCL)** arises from the posterior intercondylar area of the tibia, and courses upwards in a **p**osterior to **a**nterior direction, winding **in**wards to attach to the lateral wall of the medial condyle of femur (it is referred to as the **PAIN ligament).** Together, the cruciate ligaments serve as the primary restraint for translation of the tibia on the femur (anterior translation is restricted by the ACL; posterior translation is restricted by the PCL), as well as to provide restraint against excessive rotation of the tibia on the femur.

Clinical Remarks

a The anterior cruciate ligament (ACL) is the most commonly injured ligament of the knee, and injury is frequently associated with damage to other structures of the knee joint such as the collateral ligaments, menisci, or articular surfaces.
b While a torn ACL can be easily detected through physical examination, MR imaging is frequently used to determine the extent of damage to associated joint structures, as well as to evaluate the integrity of the joint surfaces. Once torn, the ACL is not capable of regeneration. Surgical reconstruction is frequently used to re-establish joint stability and enhance joint function. Unfortunately, longitudinal data suggests that after an ACL injury the knee is at significant risk for premature joint degeneration, with one in two patients developing knee osteoarthritis within 20 years of their initial ACL injury.
a [L126], b [R333]

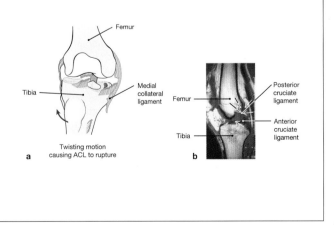

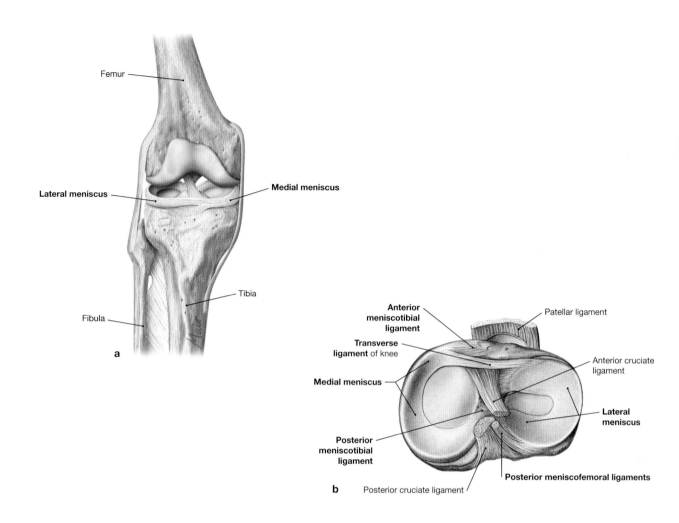

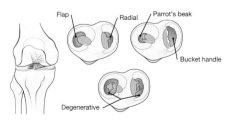

Fig. 4.43a and b Menisci of the knee joint, right side; frontal **(a)** and superior **(b)** views. b [L127]

The menisci of the knee joint are disc-like structures that are comprised of fibrous cartilage on the inside and dense connective tissue on the outside. They function to deepen the tibial articular surface and enhance joint stability; serve as a shock absorber; help control rotational and gliding movements of the tibiofemoral joint; and facilitate the circulation of synovial fluid throughout the entire joint. The 'open c-shaped' **medial meniscus** is larger (to accommodate the larger femoral condyle) and anchored via the **anterior and posterior meniscotibial ligaments** to the respective intercondylar area of the tibia. In addition, the medial meniscus is also fixed on its periphery to the medial collateral ligament. In contrast, the 'closed c-shaped' **lateral meniscus** is smaller and is anchored via the **anterior** (not depicted) and **posterior meniscofemoral ligaments** to the medial femoral condyle. It has no direct connection to the lateral collateral ligament because it is separated by the tendon of the popliteus muscle. Anteriorly, both menisci are connected by the **transverse ligament of knee.**

Clinical Remarks

Injuries of the menisci are common. The medial meniscus is more frequently affected due to its 'open c-shape' and its connection through the joint capsule to the medial collateral ligament. Acute injuries can occur as a result of sudden rotational movements of a weighted and flexed knee (i.e. pivoting or cutting maneuvers often associated with change of direction in sports), while chronic degenerative changes are frequently associated with malalignment (genu varum/valgum) or chronic loading of the knee joint in extreme ranges of flexion (i.e. often associated with occupations that involve prolonged kneeling). While the peripheral regions of the menisci receive some blood supply through a perimenisceal network of blood vessels (from the genicular arteries of the knee), the internal portions are devoid of blood vessels and thus require surgical (arthroscopic) resection/removal of the torn parts should a lesion occur. [L126]

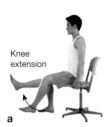

Knee extension

a

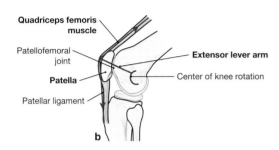

Quadriceps femoris muscle

Patellofemoral joint

Patella

Patellar ligament

Extensor lever arm

Center of knee rotation

b

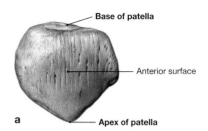

Base of patella

Anterior surface

Apex of patella

a

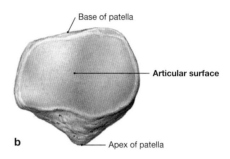

Base of patella

Articular surface

Apex of patella

b

Fig. 4.44a and b Knee extension. a [L271], b [L126]
The **patella** serves as the centerpiece of the extensor mechanism, acting as a 'pulley' to enhance the ability of the **quadriceps femoris muscle** to generate force because it helps to increase the length of the **extensor lever arm** and increase the force generated by the muscle as it crosses the knee joint.

Fig. 4.45a and b Patella, right side; anterior **(a)** and posterior **(b)** views.
The patella is a triangular sesamoid bone found within the patellar ligament of the quadriceps femoris muscle. The anterior surface is convex, with a thick superior base (which provides attachment for the quadriceps tendon), that extends inferiorly to form the apex (which provides attachment for the patellar ligament). The smooth articular surface is divided into articular facets by a vertical ridge.

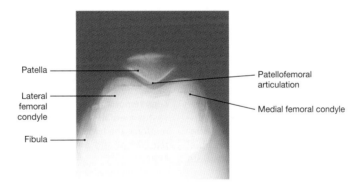

Patella

Lateral femoral condyle

Fibula

Patellofemoral articulation

Medial femoral condyle

Fig. 4.46 A 'skyline' or 'sunrise' view of the patella. [G366, E712]
In extension, only a small contact area exists between the patella and femur. As the degree of knee flexion increases, so do the contact area and compressive forces. The skyline (or sunrise) view is used when a patellar fracture is suspected, to assess patellar dislocation, or to detect patellofemoral compartment osteoarthritis. The axial view requires the patient to be able to flex their knee 45 degrees.

Structure/Function

Radiologically, **patella alta** (or a high-riding patella) describes a situation where the position of the patella is considered high (the INSALL-SALVATI ratio is greater than 1.2–1.5); **patella baja** (or **patella infera**) is an abnormally low lying patella (INSALL-SALVATI ratio is less than 0.8). The INSALL-SALVATI ratio is considered normal between 0.8 and 1.2. Both patella alta and patella baja are frequently associated with restricted range of motion of the knee joint, crepitus and retropatellar pain.
From left to right: [G198, G729, F905-002]

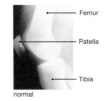

Femur

Patella

Tibia

normal

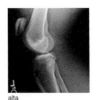

alta

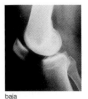

baja

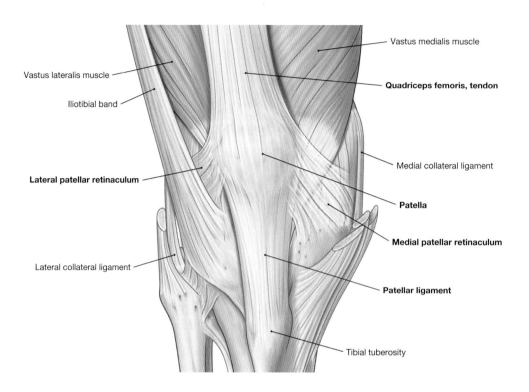

Fig. 4.47 Patellofemoral joint, right side; anterior view. [E460]
The patella is a **sesamoid bone** within the tendon of the quadriceps femoris muscle. It articulates with the femur to form the **patellofemoral joint (PFJ).** The PFJ is stabilized superiorly by the **quadriceps tendon,** inferiorly by the **patellar ligament** (which is a continuation of the quadriceps tendon and attaches distally to the tibial tuberosity), and the **medial** and **lateral patellar retinaculum.** Both patellar retinacula have superficial longitudinal and deep circular fibers and appear as distal expansions of the tendon of the quadriceps femoris. Medially and laterally, they connect fibers from the vastus medialis and vastus lateralis muscles to the tibia; serve to reinforce the two collateral ligaments (MCL/LCL), as well as the anteromedial and anterolateral aspects of the joint capsule of the knee.

Clinical Remarks

The **Q angle** is defined as the angle of intersection between one line connecting the anterior superior iliac spine (ASIS) and the midpoint of the patella, and another line connecting the midpoint of the patella and the tibial tuberosity. When measured in the frontal plane with the knee in extension, it is believed to provide a reasonable estimate of the force vector formed between the quadriceps muscle group and the patellar ligament. This measurement is routinely used by clinicians to describe the line of pull of the quadriceps muscle through the PFJ. In general practice, goniometer measurements of greater than 13° for males, and 18° for females are considered to be indicative of malalignment, and believed to serve as a contributing factor in the development of PFJ pathology.

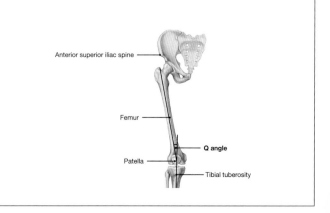

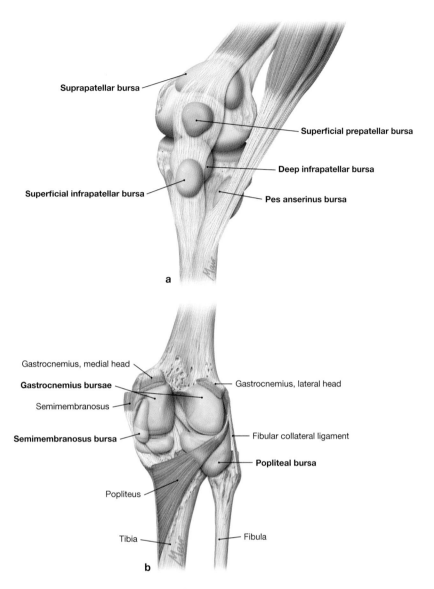

Fig. 4.48a and b Knee joint with bursae, right side; medial **(a)** and posterior **(b)** views. [L127]

The knee joint is surrounded by up to 30 **synovial bursae.** Some bursae communicate with the joint capsule, such as the **suprapatellar bursa** (anterior superior) beneath the tendon of the quadriceps femoris. Other bursae are positioned in places with exposure to higher pressure (e. g. when kneeling) such as the **prepatellar bursa** or the **superficial infrapatellar bursa.** Others serve as a glid-ing surface for tendons where they cross bone (**deep infrapatellar bursa**), or where they cross other tendons (**pes anserinus bursa**). This region also represents the area of distal attachment for the tendons of the sartorius (anterior thigh), gracilis (medial thigh), and semitendinosus (posterior thigh) muscles.

The mnemonic '**S**ay **G**race before **t**ea' is often used to remember the order of tendinous insertion of these muscles within the pes anserinus region.

Clinical Remarks

a, b With blunt force trauma, or extensive mechanical stress (activities in kneeling position), inflammation of the bursae may occur **(bursitis).**

c In the case of chronic inflammatory diseases (e. g. rheumatoid arthritis), enlargement and fusion of bursae may occur which appear as swelling in the popliteal fossa. A fusion of the semimembranosus bursa with the medial subtendinous bursa of the gastrocnemius is referred to as **BAKER's cyst.**

a [L126], b [E989], c [M614]

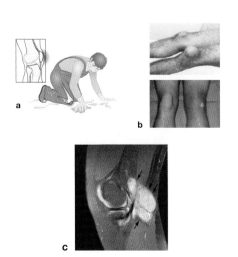

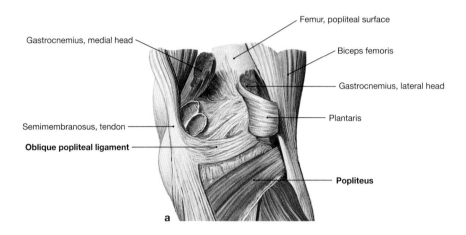

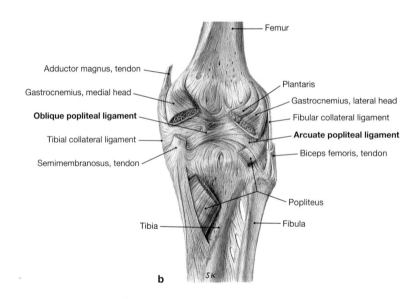

Fig. 4.49a and b Knee joint, right side; posterior view, superficial **(a)** with closed joint capsule, and posterior view, deep **(b).**
After removal of the superficial knee flexors, the deep muscles of the posterior knee (popliteal fossa) are visible. The **popliteus** muscle originates from the lateral femoral condyle and the posterior horn of the lateral meniscus. The muscle courses in an inferomedial direction to insert on the posterior aspect of the tibia, just proximal to the soleal line. Its primary function is to power internal (medial) rotation of the tibia on the femur, thus unlocking the fully extended knee (or initiating knee flexion). It is innervated by the tibial nerve (L5–S1). The posterior joint capsule is also reinforced by two major external ligaments which help prevent hyperextension of the knee joint. The **oblique popliteal ligament** projects medially and inferiorly from the lateral femoral condyle, and the **arcuate popliteal ligament** courses in the opposite direction, thus, crossing the popliteus muscle.

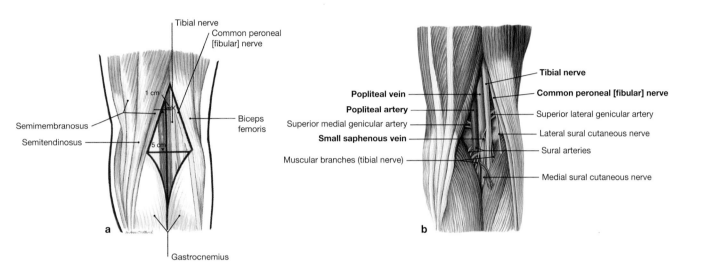

Fig. 4.50a and b Neurovasculature of the popliteal fossa, right side; posterior views. a [G730]

a The **popliteal fossa** is a diamond-shaped space located in the posterior knee that contains important vessels and nerves of the leg. Its boundaries include: semimembranosus and semitendinosus (superomedial); biceps femoris (superolateral); lateral head of gastrocnemius (inferolateral); and medial head of gastrocnemius (inferomedial). The roof of the fossa is formed by skin, and a superficial fascia (that contains the small saphenous vein, the terminal branch of the posterior cutaneous nerve of the thigh, and the pos-

terior division of the medial cutaneous nerve of leg). The floor is made up of the popliteal surface of the femur, the popliteus muscle, and the oblique popliteal ligament.

b Key neurovascular structures found within the popliteal fossa include: **1. popliteal artery, 2. popliteal vein, 3. tibial nerve, 4. common peroneal [fibular] nerve; 5. popliteal lymph nodes and lymphatic vessels** (not displayed). The subcutaneous tissue overlying the fossa contains fat. A deep popliteal fascia forms a strong protective covering around the vascular structures as they pass from the medial thigh through the adductor hiatus into the popliteal region.

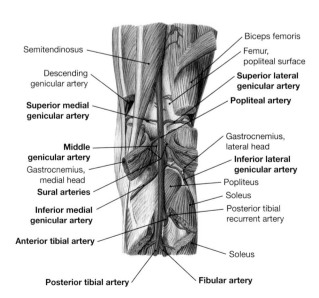

Fig. 4.51 Arteries of the popliteal fossa, right side; posterior view. **The popliteal artery** supplies the knee joint and forms arterial networks with its branches above **(superior medial and lateral genicular arteries)** and below **(inferior medial and lateral genicular arteries)** the joint cavity. These arterial networks contribute to the genicular anastomosis on the anterior side of the knee. At the level of the joint, the **middle genicular artery** branches off to supply the knee joint. The tibial arteries supply the muscles of the calf. Below the popliteal fossa, the popliteal artery descends between the two heads of the gastrocnemius and divides into two terminal branches – the **anterior and posterior tibial arteries.**

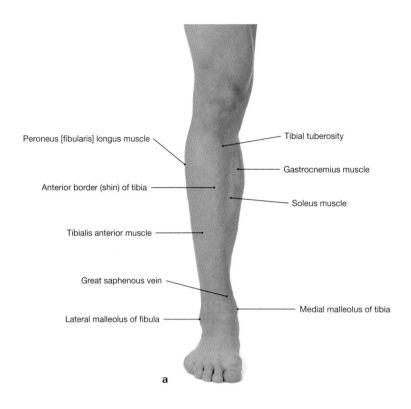

Peroneus [fibularis] longus muscle

Tibial tuberosity

Anterior border (shin) of tibia

Gastrocnemius muscle

Soleus muscle

Tibialis anterior muscle

Great saphenous vein

Medial malleolus of tibia

Lateral malleolus of fibula

a

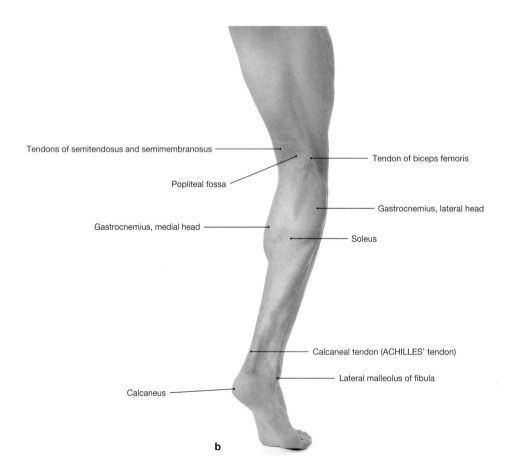

Tendons of semitendosus and semimembranosus

Tendon of biceps femoris

Popliteal fossa

Gastrocnemius, lateral head

Gastrocnemius, medial head

Soleus

Calcaneal tendon (ACHILLES' tendon)

Lateral malleolus of fibula

Calcaneus

b

Fig. 4.52a and b Surface anatomy of the lower leg, right side; anterior **(a)** and posterior **(b)** views. [K340]
Many of the key bony and muscular landmarks of the lower leg and ankle regions are located superficially and can be easily palpated and observed when performing a musculoskeletal examination of the region. Asymmetries from side-to-side may be indicative of underlying pathologies.

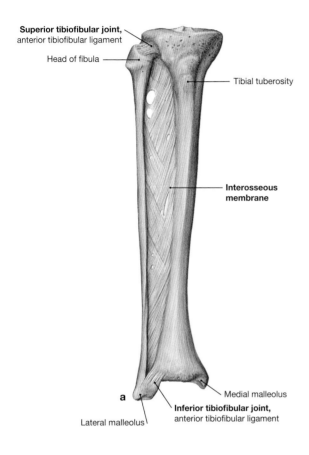

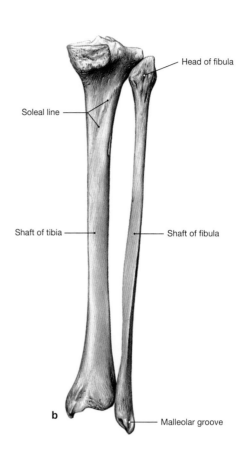

Fig. 4.53a und b Tibia and fibula, right side; anterior **(a)** and posterior **(b)** views.

The alignment of the lower leg is determined by the orientation of the tibia and fibula. These bones are connected by **superior and inferior tibiofibular joints** (plane type synovial joints) that are reinforced by anterior and posterior ligaments. Between both bones, the **interosseous membrane** serves as an additional stabilizer with dense connective tissue and collagen fibers, which predominantly course obliquely downwards from the tibia to the fibula. The inferior articular surfaces of the tibia and the fibula are referred to as **medial malleolus and lateral malleolus.** Together they form the socket of the ankle joint (malleolar mortise).

⌐ Clinical Remarks ──────────────────────────────────

The tibia is the most commonly fractured long bone in the body and is a frequent site of compound fracture – the bone is broken into more than two pieces. Complex bony fractures of the lower leg are routinely stabilized through the use of surgical fixation. Research suggests that these methods of stabilization (intramedullary nails or open reduction and internal fixation) result in faster fracture healing, but can increase the likelihood of infection.
[P489]

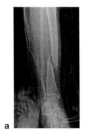

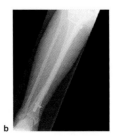

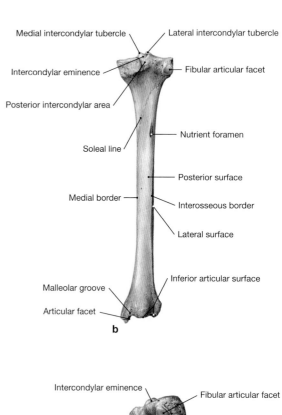

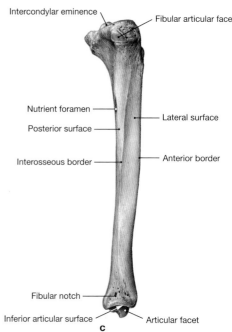

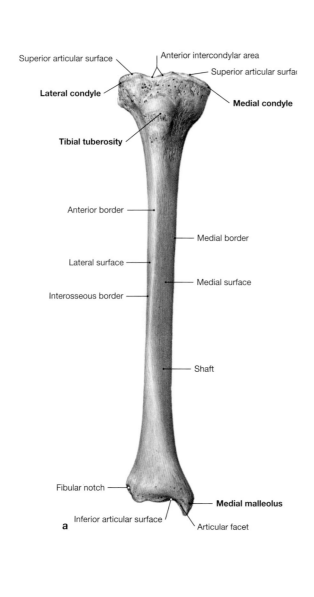

Fig. 4.54a to c Tibia, right side; anterior **(a)**, posterior **(b)** and lateral **(c)** views.
The superior articular surface of the tibia sits in a dorsally shifted position in relation to the long axis of the tibial shaft (retroposi-tion). Beyond this, the articular surface is also tilted dorsally. This retroverted position is more pronounced on the **medial condyle** than on the **lateral condyle.**

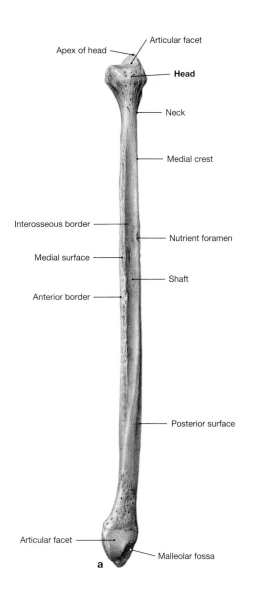

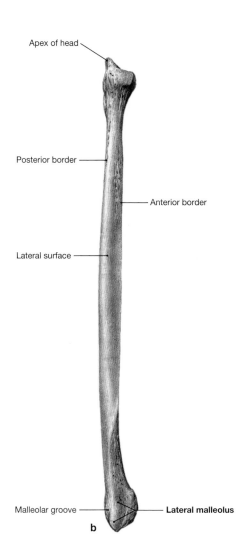

Fig. 4.55a and b Fibula, right side; medial **(a)** and lateral **(b)** views.
The fibula supports only approximately one-sixth of body weight during weight bearing activities. In the case of an isolated fibula, orientation is determined by the fact that the articular surfaces of the **head of fibula** and of the **lateral malleolus** both point medially.

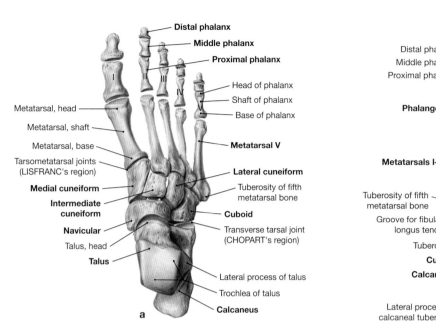

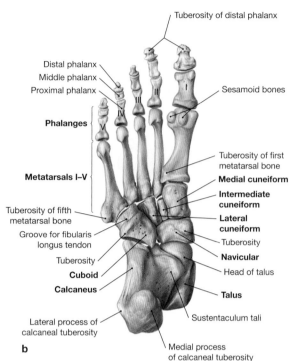

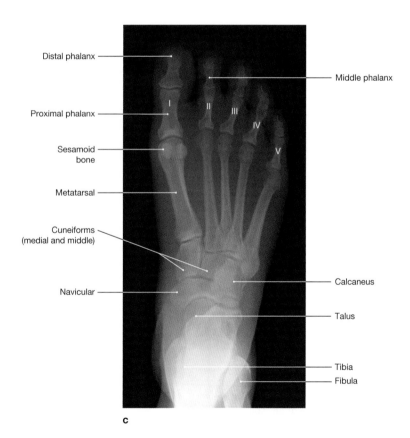

Fig. 4.56a to c Bones of the foot, right side; dorsal **(a)** and plantar **(b)** views; anteroposterior radiograph **(c)**. c [G731]
The foot is organized into three regions: tarsal, metatarsal, and phalangeal (toe) regions. The tarsal region is comprised of the ta- lus, the calcaneus, the navicular, the cuboid, and the three cunei- form bones. Clinically, the forefoot is distinguished from the rear foot by an articular line that runs through the tarsometatarsal joints (LISFRANC's region).

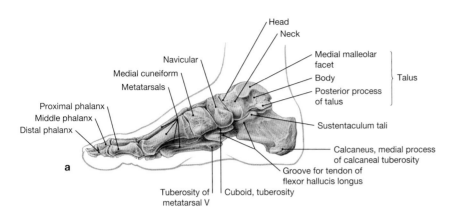

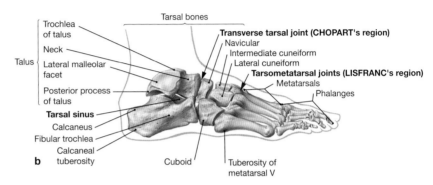

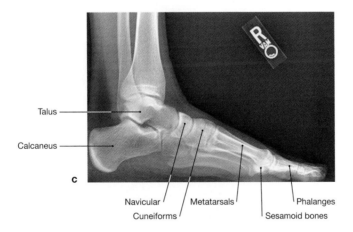

Fig. 4.57a to c Bones of the foot, right side; medial **(a)** and lateral **(b)** views; sagittal radiograph **(c)**. c [G729]

The **tarsal sinus** is a hollow space on the lateral side of the foot which is formed by the calcaneal sulcus and the sulcus tali.

Clinical Remarks

The base of the 5th metatarsal is a common site of injury – stress fracture; avulsion fracture; **JONES' fracture.** First described by Sir Robert JONES in 1902, a JONES' fracture refers to a **transverse fracture at the base of the 5th metatarsal,** 1.5–3.0 cm (0.6–1.2 in) distal to the proximal tuberosity at the metadiaphyseal junction, without distal extension. It is believed to occur as a result of a significant adduction (inversion) force to the forefoot and ankle region, when the ankle joint is in a position of plantarflexion. In contrast to avulsion fractures, a JONES' fracture is prone to nonunion (with rates as high as 30–50%), and routinely takes much longer to heal (> 2 months).
[E890]

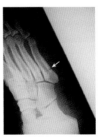

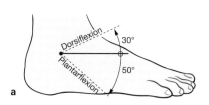

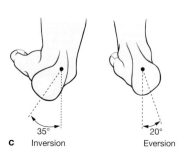

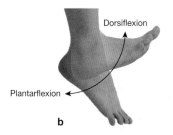

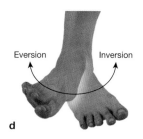

Fig. 4.58a to d Range of motion at the ankle. a, c [L126], b, d [L271]
a and **b** Talocrural joint: dorsiflexion (extension) – plantarflexion:
30°–0°–50°.

c and **d** Talocalcaneal (or subtalar) joint: eversion – inversion: 20°–0°–35°

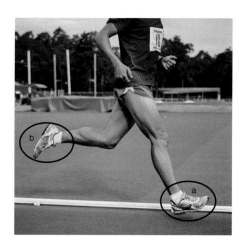

Fig. 4.59 Movement at the ankle joint during running. [J787]
The **ankle joint (talocrural joint)** is a classical **hinge joint** allowing for **dorsiflexion (extension, a)** and **plantarflexion (b)** movements.

The **subtalar or talocalcaneal joint** is an **atypical pivot joint** which enables **inversion** (sole moving inwards) and **eversion** (sole moving outwards) of the foot.

Ankle Movement	Muscles Active During Movements
Dorsiflexion	Tibialis anterior, extensor digitorum longus, extensor hallucis longus, peroneus tertius
Plantarflexion	Gastrocnemius, soleus, plantaris, tibialis posterior, flexor digitorum longus, flexor hallucis longus
Inversion	Tibialis posterior, flexor digitorum longus, flexor hallucis longus
Eversion	Peroneus [fibularis] longus, peroneus [fibularis] brevis

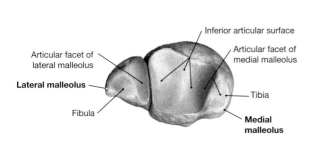

Fig. 4.60 Distal ends of the tibia and fibula, right side; inferior view.

Fig. 4.61 Talus, right side; superior view.
The trochlea is broader anteriorly, as compared to its posterior aspect.

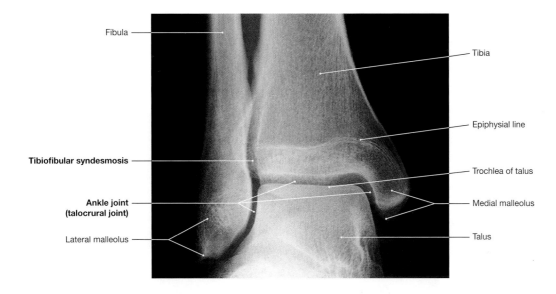

Fig. 4.62 Talocrural (ankle) joint, right side; anteroposterior (A/P) radiograph.
The distal ends of the tibia and fibula are connected via the **tibiofibular syndesmosis.** Together they form the malleolar mortise – or socket of the ankle joint – which articulates with the proximal aspect of the talus to form the **talocrural joint** of the ankle joint.

Clinical Remarks

On an A/P radiograph of the ankle or malleolar mortise, the space between the articular surfaces of the talus and the medial malleolus is referred to as the **medial clear space (MCS).**
a This space should be approximately equal to the space between the articular surfaces of the tibia and the talus (superior clear space).

b If the width of the MCS is greater than 5 mm, it suggests a lateral shift of the talus, and is indicative of pathology in the ankle region.
b [S008-3]

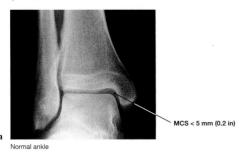

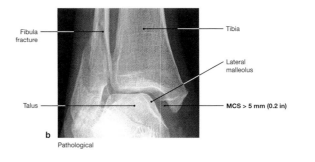

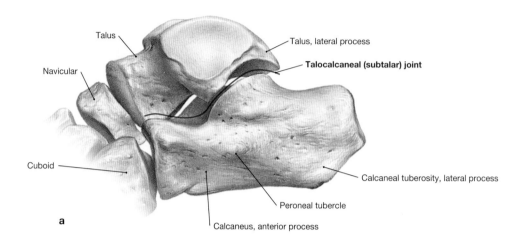

Talus

Talus, lateral process

Talocalcaneal (subtalar) joint

Navicular

Cuboid

Calcaneal tuberosity, lateral process

Peroneal tubercle

a

Calcaneus, anterior process

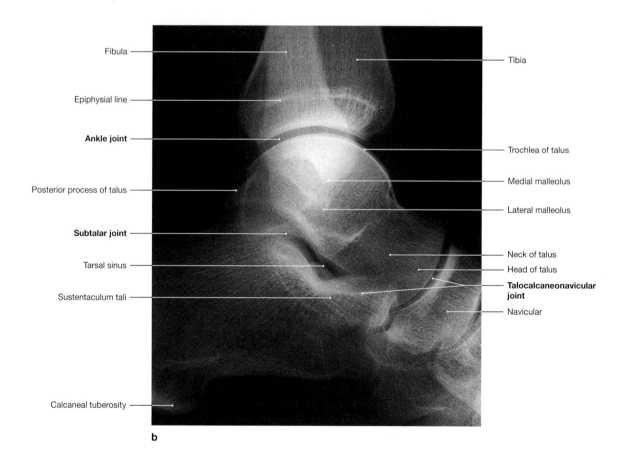

Fibula

Tibia

Epiphysial line

Ankle joint

Trochlea of talus

Medial malleolus

Posterior process of talus

Lateral malleolus

Subtalar joint

Neck of talus

Tarsal sinus

Head of talus

Talocalcaneonavicular joint

Sustentaculum tali

Navicular

Calcaneal tuberosity

b

Fig. 4.63a and b Subtalar (talocalcaneal) joint, right side; lateral view **(a)** and radiograph in medial beam projection **(b)**.
The **subtalar joint** is formed by an articulation of the inferior aspect of the talus and the superior aspect of the calcaneus. It is considered a plane type of synovial joint. It allows **inversion and eversion** **movements** of the ankle joint to take place, but plays no role in the movements of plantar- or dorsiflexion. In combination with the navicular bone, it helps form the **talocalcaneonavicular joint** – the region of the foot responsible for the pronation and supination movements of the foot.

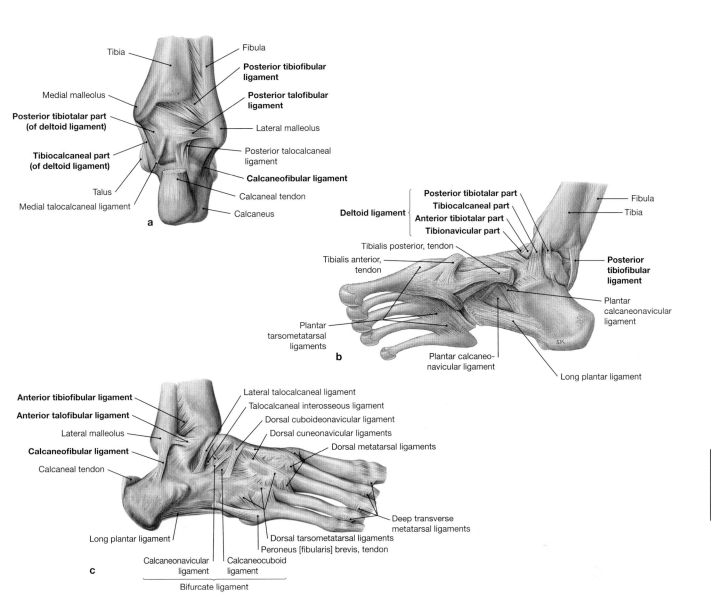

Tibia
Fibula
Posterior tibiofibular ligament
Medial malleolus
Posterior talofibular ligament
Posterior tibiotalar part (of deltoid ligament)
Lateral malleolus
Posterior talocalcaneal ligament
Tibiocalcaneal part (of deltoid ligament)
Calcaneofibular ligament
Talus
Calcaneal tendon
Medial talocalcaneal ligament
Calcaneus

a

Posterior tibiotalar part
Fibula
Tibiocalcaneal part
Tibia
Anterior tibiotalar part
Deltoid ligament {
Tibionavicular part
Tibialis posterior, tendon
Posterior tibiofibular ligament
Tibialis anterior, tendon
Plantar calcaneonavicular ligament
Plantar tarsometatarsal ligaments
Plantar calcaneonavicular ligament
Long plantar ligament

b

Anterior tibiofibular ligament
Lateral talocalcaneal ligament
Anterior talofibular ligament
Talocalcaneal interosseous ligament
Lateral malleolus
Dorsal cuboideonavicular ligament
Dorsal cuneonavicular ligaments
Calcaneofibular ligament
Dorsal metatarsal ligaments
Calcaneal tendon
Deep transverse metatarsal ligaments
Long plantar ligament
Dorsal tarsometatarsal ligaments
Peroneus [fibularis] brevis, tendon
Calcaneonavicular ligament
Calcaneocuboid ligament
Bifurcate ligament

c

Fig. 4.64a to c Ankle ligaments (talocrural joint), right side;
posterior **(a)**, medial **(b)** and lateral **(c)** views.
The distal connection of the tibia and fibula is reinforced by the **anterior and posterior tibiofibular ligaments**. They stabilize the inferior tibiofibular syndesmosis and reinforce the malleolar mortise (i.e. socket of the ankle joint). On the medial aspect, the ankle is stabilized by a fan-shaped radiation of ligaments that is collective-

ly referred to as the **deltoid ligament** complex. It consists of four parts **(anterior tibiotalar, posterior tibiotalar, tibiocalcaneal, and tibionavicular ligaments)** and functions to restrict eversion movements of the ankle joint. The lateral aspect of the ankle is stabilized by three separate and distinct ligaments **(anterior talofibular, posterior talofibular, and calcaneofibular ligaments)** which all function to restrict inversion movements of the ankle joint.

Clinical Remarks

A **sprained ankle joint** is one of the most common injuries observed in the lower limb. Lateral ankle injuries occur more frequently than medial injuries because the lateral ligaments are weaker than those on the medial side of the joint, and the fibula extends more distally than does the tibia (providing a bony block to excessive eversion movements).
a The position for inversion sprains is plantarflexion and inversion (the trochlea of the talus is wider in the anterior than the posterior part, thus secure guidance of the bones is only guaranteed in dorsiflexion), and the **anterior talofibular ligament (ATFL)** is the most frequently injured ligament.
b Following injury, patients typically complain of pain on the lateral side of their ankle and present with various degrees of swelling, bruising (ecchymosis) and diminished range of movement.
a [G123], b [J787]

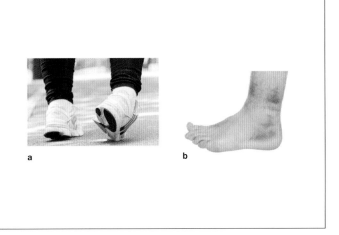

a

b

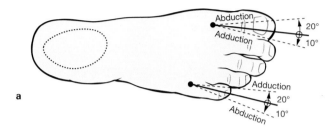

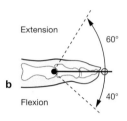

Fig. 4.65a and b Range of motion in joints of the foot. [L126]
a The **metatarsophalangeal (MTP) joints** are condyloid joints which are limited to two axes of movement (flexion/extension and adduction/abduction). Adduction – abduction: 20°–0°–10° (adduction is the movement towards the midline of the foot).

b The proximal and distal interphalangeal joints are hinge joints and only allow flexion/extension movements. Toe extension – flexion: 60°–0°–40°.

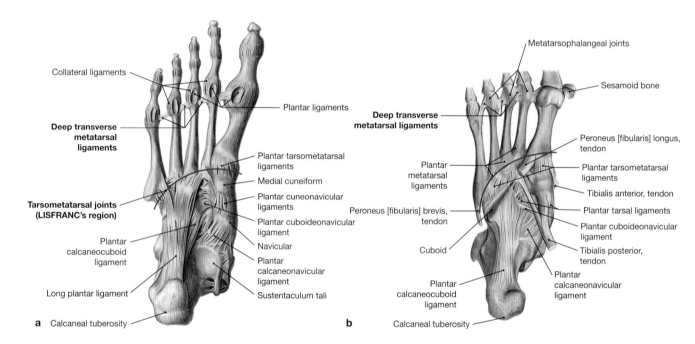

Fig. 4.66a and b Joints of the foot, right side, plantar surface with ligaments; superficial **(a)** and deep **(b)** views.
In the tarsal region (rear foot) there are several important articulations that contribute significantly to supination and pronation movements of the foot. The talonavicular and the calcaneocuboid joints form the transverse tarsal joint region of the foot. The **tarsometatarsal joints** (identified by the red line) are often referred to as

LISFRANC's region, and separates the rear and midfoot. The metatarsal bones articulate in several separates joints – they are connected proximally by the intermetatarsal joints and distally by the **deep transverse metatarsal ligaments**. The joints of forefoot and midfoot are linked by strong plantar, dorsal, and interosseous ligaments.

Clinical Remarks

The most common deformity in the first metatarsophalangeal joint is the **hallux valgus** – in which the head of the first metatarsal bone deviates and protrudes medially, causing the distal aspect of the big toe (hallux) to adduct laterally. This condition can lead to severe pain in the metatarsophalangeal joint and may cause soft tissue swelling. In cases of severe deformity and dysfunction, it may require surgical realignment.
[M614]

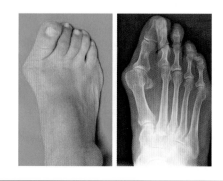

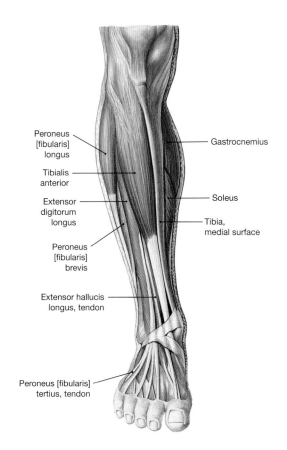

Peroneus [fibularis] longus

Tibialis anterior

Extensor digitorum longus

Peroneus [fibularis] brevis

Extensor hallucis longus, tendon

Peroneus [fibularis] tertius, tendon

Gastrocnemius

Soleus

Tibia, medial surface

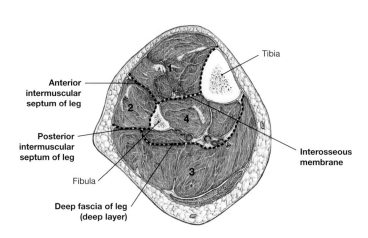

Anterior intermuscular septum of leg

Posterior intermuscular septum of leg

Deep fascia of leg (deep layer)

Fibula

Tibia

Interosseous membrane

Fig. 4.67 Anterior and lateral muscles of the lower leg, ankle and foot, right side; anterior view.

Fig. 4.68 Lower leg, right side; transverse section at the mid-leg level with illustration of the osteofibrous compartments; distal view.

The muscles of the lower leg are organized into four distinct compartments by strong, thick layers of fascia which originate from the long bones of tibia and fibula. The anterior (extensor) compartment (1) is separated from the lateral (peroneal) compartment (2) by the **anterior intermuscular septum.** The lateral compartment is separated from the superficial posterior (plantarflexor) compartment (3) by the **posterior intermuscular septum.** The superficial posterior compartment is isolated from the deep posterior compartment (4) by a **deep layer of the deep fascia of leg.**

Clinical Remarks

A **compartment syndrome** can develop in the anterior compartment of the lower leg following acute trauma (fracture, blunt force, etc).

a Posttraumatic swelling of the extensor muscles can lead to constriction of the blood vessels and nerves in the region, and result in significant pain and loss of function. If left untreated, the compression can lead to a loss of palpable arterial pulse of the dorsalis pedis artery in the foot, and cause a lesion of the deep peroneal (fibular) nerve with resulting functional deficits including the inability to extend the toes and dorsiflex the ankle joint, as well as result in a loss of sensory innervation within the first interdigital space.

b In severe cases, injury management requires immediate decompression of the anterior compartment by surgical incision of the fascia **(fasciotomy)** surrounding the anterior compartment.
a [E993], b [E475]

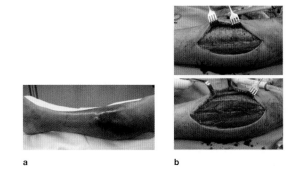

a

b

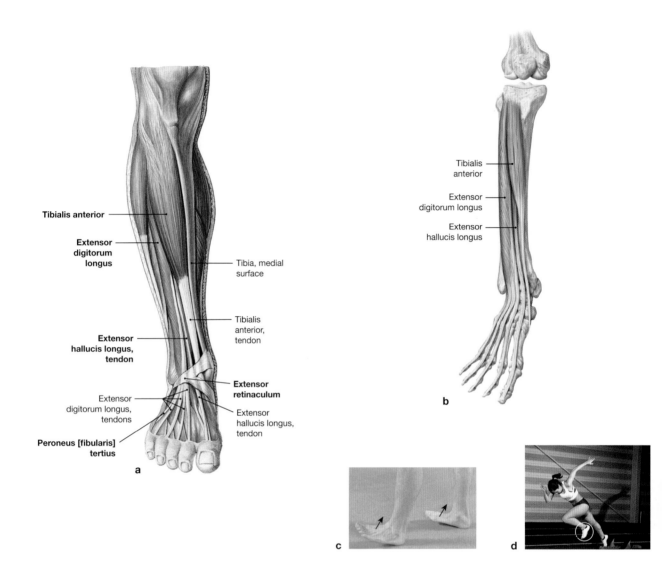

Fig. 4.69a to d Anterior muscles of the lower leg, right side; anterior views **(a** and **b).** b [L127], c [E563], d [J787]

The anterior (or extensor) compartment of the lower leg is comprised of four muscles that cross the front of the ankle joint. They are held in place by a fascial reinforcement called the **extensor retinaculum,** which prevents the tendons from lifting off the bones during dorsiflexion and toe extension movements. Together these muscles function to power movements such as tapping your foot on the ground – up phase **(c),** and the 'toe-up' position of the foot and ankle during the swing phase of the gait cycle when walking/running **(d).**

Muscle	Attachments (P = proximal, D = distal)	Action/Function	Innervation
Tibialis anterior	**P:** Lateral condyle and upper $^1/_2$ of lateral surface of the tibia; interosseous membrane **D:** Medial cuniform and 1st metatarsal bones of the foot	Dorsiflexion of ankle	Deep peroneal [fibular] nerve – from common fibular nerve (L4 and L5)
Extensor digitorum longus	**P:** Lateral condyle of tibia; interosseous membrane, and superior $^2/_3$ of medial surface of fibula **D:** Middle and distal phalanges of the four lateral digits	Extension of four lateral toes; assists with dorsiflexion of ankle	Deep peroneal [fibular] nerve – from common fibular nerve (L5–S1)
Extensor hallucis longus	**P:** Interosseous membrane, and anterior surface of the middle portion of the fibula **D:** Distal phalanx of big toe	Extension of big toe, assists with dorsiflexion of ankle	Deep peroneal [fibular] nerve – from common fibular nerve (L5–S1)
Peroneus [fibularis] tertius	**P:** Interosseous membrane, and lower third of anterior surface of the fibula **D:** Dorsal surface of the base of the 5th metatarsal	Assists with dorsiflexion and eversion of ankle	Deep peroneal [fibular] nerve – from common fibular nerve (L5–S1)

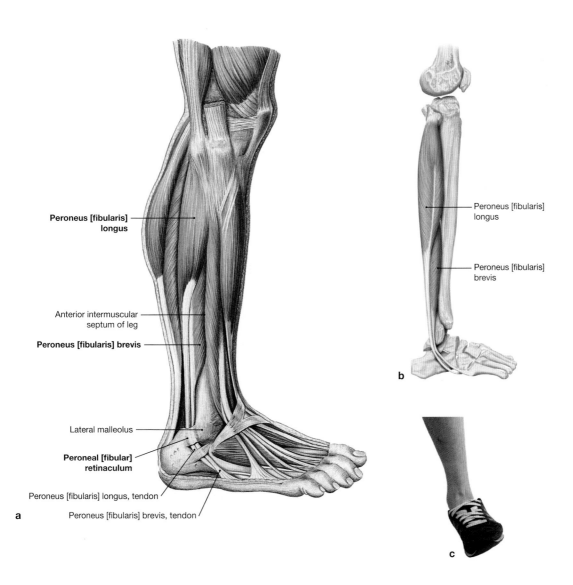

Peroneus [fibularis] longus

Anterior intermuscular septum of leg

Peroneus [fibularis] brevis

Lateral malleolus

Peroneal [fibular] retinaculum

Peroneus [fibularis] longus, tendon

a

Peroneus [fibularis] brevis, tendon

Peroneus [fibularis] longus

Peroneus [fibularis] brevis

b

c

Fig. 4.70a to c Lateral muscles of the lower leg, right side; lateral views **(a** and **b).** b [L127], c [L271]

The muscles of the **lateral (peroneal) compartment** of the lower leg are held in place by the **peroneal [fibular] retinaculum** as they pass posterior and inferior to the lateral malleolus. The distal attachments of both peroneus [fibularis] muscles (base of 5th metatarsal – brevis; base of 1st metatarsal – longus) are on the plantar surface of the foot, thus allowing them to play an important role in actively supporting the medial and lateral longitudinal plantar arches of the foot. Both peroneal muscles' primary function is to power **eversion** movements of the ankle joint; such as you might experience when walking on the inside edge (medial side) of your feet **(c)**.

Muscle	Attachments (P = proximal, D = distal)	Action/Function	Innervation
Peroneus [fibularis] longus	**P:** Head and superior $^2/_3$ of lateral surface of fibula **D:** Base of 1st metatarsal and medial cuniform bones (plantar surfaces)	Eversion of ankle, assists weakly with plantarflexion	Superficial peroneal [fibular] nerve – branch of the common fibular nerve (L5–S2)
Peroneus [fibularis] brevis	**P:** Inferior $^2/_3$ of lateral surface of fibula **D:** Base of 5th metatarsal (lateral aspect)	Eversion of ankle, assists weakly with plantarflexion	Superficial peroneal [fibular] nerve – branch of the common fibular nerve (L5–S2)

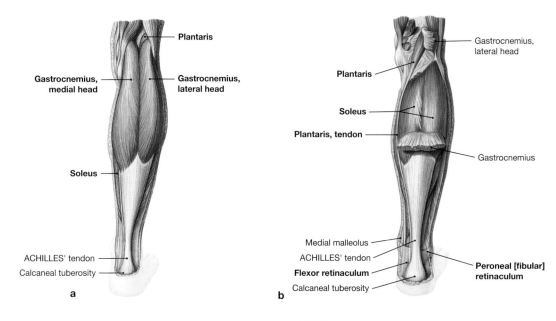

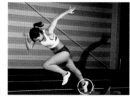

a

b

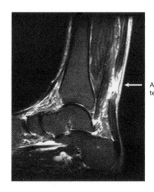

c

Fig. 4.71a to c Superficial muscles of the posterior compartment of the lower leg, right side; superficial view **(a),** with superior aspect of gastrocnemius muscle reflected **(b).** c [J787]
The **triceps surae** (group of three muscles of the superficial posterior compartment) is a strong **plantarflexor** of the ankle joint. After folding the **gastrocnemius** inferiorly, the **plantaris** is visible proxi-

mal to the soleus. The bellies of the deep flexor muscles are located distally and are visible on both sides of the ACHILLES' tendon after removal of the fascia of leg. Their tendons are guided by the **flexor retinaculum** at the medial malleolus. The triceps surae function to power the **'toe-off' phase** of the gait cycle when walking/running/jumping **(c).**

Muscle	Attachments (P = proximal, D = distal)	Action/Function	Innervation
Gastrocnemius	**P:** Posterior aspect of lateral (lateral head) and medial (medial head) femoral condyles **D:** Posterior calcaneus via the ACHILLES' tendon	Plantarflexion of ankle; weak flexor of knee	Tibial division of sciatic nerve (S1 – S2)
Soleus	**P:** Posterior surface of: upper ¼ of fibula, interosseous membrane and middle ⅓ of tibia **D:** Posterior calcaneus via the ACHILLES' tendon	Plantarflexion of ankle	Tibial division of sciatic nerve (L5 – S2)
Plantaris	**P:** Lateral supracondylar ridge of posterior femur, just superior to lateral head of gastrocnemius **D:** Posterior calcaneus via the ACHILLES' tendon	Weak plantarflexion of ankle; weak flexor of knee	Tibial division of sciatic nerve (S1–S2)

Clinical Remarks

An **ACHILLES' tendon rupture** can occur as a result of forceful eccentric loading of the triceps surae muscle complex during sudden movements which force the ankle joint into dorsiflexion (i.e. the triceps surae is being lengthened at the same time it is being loaded). Clinically, an ACHILLES' tendon rupture is suspected when there is an absence of plantarflexion of the ankle joint when the middle part of the triceps surae muscle complex is squeezed (THOMPSON's test). MR imaging is typically used to confirm the diagnosis and to plan the method of treatment (surgical or conservative).
[G729]

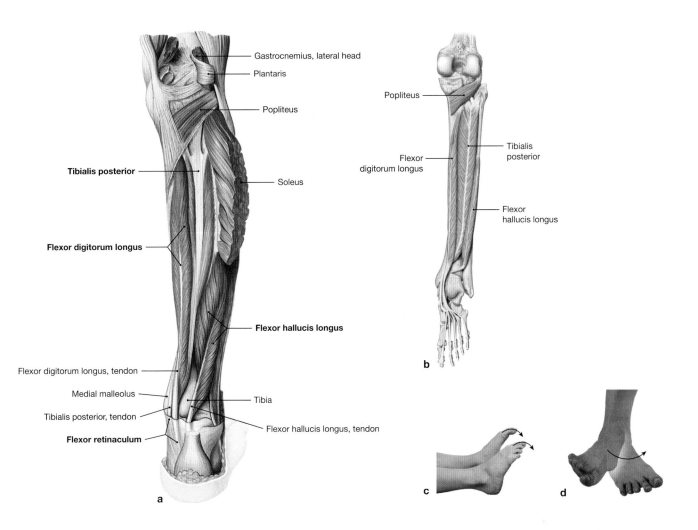

Gastrocnemius, lateral head
Plantaris
Popliteus
Tibialis posterior
Soleus
Flexor digitorum longus
Flexor hallucis longus
Flexor digitorum longus, tendon
Medial malleolus
Tibia
Tibialis posterior, tendon
Flexor retinaculum
Flexor hallucis longus, tendon

a

Popliteus
Flexor digitorum longus
Tibialis posterior
Flexor hallucis longus

b

c   d

Fig. 4.72a to d Deep muscles of the posterior compartment of the leg, right side; posterior view; after removal of the superficial flexors **(a** and **b).** b [L127], c, d [L271]

The three tendons of the deep muscles of the posterior compartment all cross behind and below the medial malleolus and are held in place by a **flexor retinaculum.** In their course, the tendon of the **flexor digitorum longus** crosses the tendon of the **tibialis posterior.** These muscles function to support the medial longitudinal arch of the foot, and are active when performing movements such as **flexing or 'curling' your toes (c),** and rolling the soles of your feet in towards one another – **inversion of the ankle (d).**

Muscle	Attachments (P = proximal, D = distal)	Action/Function	Innervation
Tibialis posterior	**P:** Posterior surface of the tibia (inferior to the soleal line); interosseous membrane; posterior surface of fibula **D:** Tuberosity of navicular; cuboid; cuniform; sustentaculum tali of calcaneus; bases of 2nd, 3rd, and 4th metatarsals	Inversion of ankle; assists with plantarflexion of the ankle	Tibial division of sciatic nerve (L4 and L5)
Flexor digitorum longus	**P:** Medial part of posterior surface of the tibia (inferior to the soleal line); broad tendon to fibula. **D:** Bases of distal phalanges of lateral four digits.	Flexes lateral four digits; assists with inversion and plantarflexion of the ankle; supports medial longitudinal arch of the foot	Tibial division of sciatic nerve (S2 and S3)
Flexor hallucis longus	**P:** Inferior ⅔ of posterior surface of the tibia; inferior part of interosseous membrane. **D:** Base of distal phalanx of big toe	Flexes big toe; assists with plantarflexion and inversion of ankle; supports medial longitudinal arch of the foot.	Tibial division of sciatic nerve (S2 and S3)

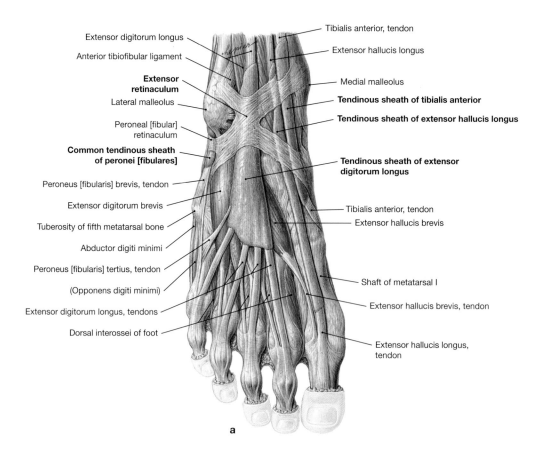

Extensor digitorum longus

Anterior tibiofibular ligament

Extensor retinaculum

Lateral malleolus

Peroneal [fibular] retinaculum

Common tendinous sheath of peronei [fibulares]

Peroneus [fibularis] brevis, tendon

Extensor digitorum brevis

Tuberosity of fifth metatarsal bone

Abductor digiti minimi

Peroneus [fibularis] tertius, tendon

(Opponens digiti minimi)

Extensor digitorum longus, tendons

Dorsal interossei of foot

Tibialis anterior, tendon

Extensor hallucis longus

Medial malleolus

Tendinous sheath of tibialis anterior

Tendinous sheath of extensor hallucis longus

Tendinous sheath of extensor digitorum longus

Tibialis anterior, tendon

Extensor hallucis brevis

Shaft of metatarsal I

Extensor hallucis brevis, tendon

Extensor hallucis longus, tendon

a

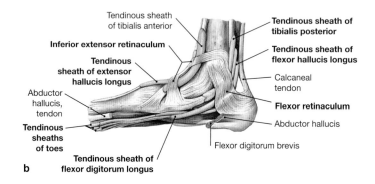

Tendinous sheath of tibialis anterior

Inferior extensor retinaculum

Tendinous sheath of extensor hallucis longus

Abductor hallucis, tendon

Tendinous sheaths of toes

Tendinous sheath of flexor digitorum longus

Tendinous sheath of tibialis posterior

Tendinous sheath of flexor hallucis longus

Calcaneal tendon

Flexor retinaculum

Abductor hallucis

Flexor digitorum brevis

b

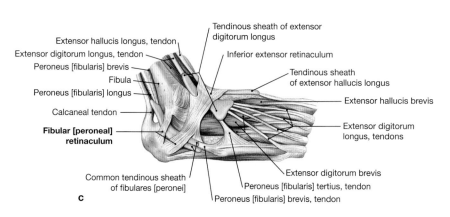

Extensor hallucis longus, tendon

Extensor digitorum longus, tendon

Peroneus [fibularis] brevis

Fibula

Peroneus [fibularis] longus

Calcaneal tendon

Fibular [peroneal] retinaculum

Common tendinous sheath of fibulares [peronei]

Tendinous sheath of extensor digitorum longus

Inferior extensor retinaculum

Tendinous sheath of extensor hallucis longus

Extensor hallucis brevis

Extensor digitorum longus, tendons

Extensor digitorum brevis

Peroneus [fibularis] tertius, tendon

Peroneus [fibularis] brevis, tendon

c

Fig. 4.73a to c Synovial sheaths of the ankle and foot regions, right side; anterior **(a)**, medial **(b)** and lateral **(c)** views.
The **retinacula** of the foot serve as retaining straps and prevent the tendons from lifting off the bones during muscle contractions. Tendinous sheaths surround the tendons of all three muscle groups of the leg, particularly where the tendons are fixed to the bones by the retinacula. Each extensor muscle has its own tendinous sheath which encloses all tendons of the respective muscle and serves as a guide, as well as gliding surface. In contrast, the tendons of the peroneus [fibularis] longus and brevis muscles share a common tendinous sheath.

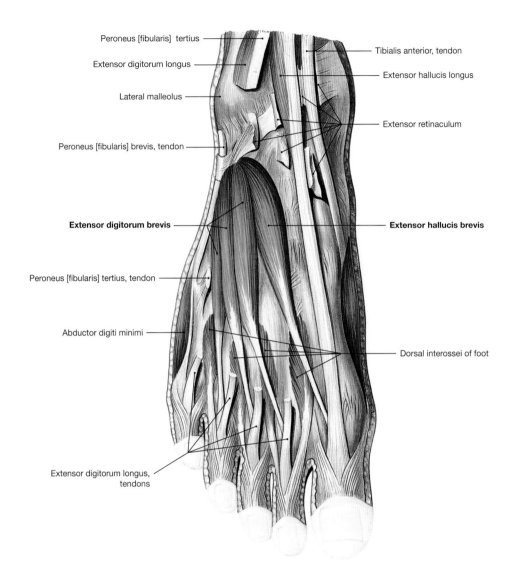

Peroneus [fibularis] tertius
Extensor digitorum longus
Lateral malleolus
Peroneus [fibularis] brevis, tendon
Extensor digitorum brevis
Peroneus [fibularis] tertius, tendon
Abductor digiti minimi
Extensor digitorum longus, tendons

Tibialis anterior, tendon
Extensor hallucis longus
Extensor retinaculum
Extensor hallucis brevis
Dorsal interossei of foot

Fig. 4.74 Muscles on the dorsal surface of the foot, right side; anterior view.
Beneath the tendons of the long extensor muscles (whose muscle bellies are located on the anterior surface of the lower leg) there are two short extensor muscles that comprise the short extensor muscles of the four lateral toes and the big toe.

Muscle	Attachments (P = proximal, D = distal)	Action/Function	Innervation
Extensor hallucis brevis	**P:** Dorsal surface of anterior calcaneus **D:** Proximal phalanx of big toe	Extends proximal phalanx of big toe	Deep peroneal [fibularis] nerve (L5, S1)
Extensor digitorum brevis	**P:** Dorsal surface of anterior calcaneus **D:** Proximal aspect of middle phalanx of 2nd, 3rd and 4th digit	Helps extend 2nd, 3rd and 4th digit when the foot is fully dorsiflexed	Deep peroneal [fibularis] nerve (L5, S1)

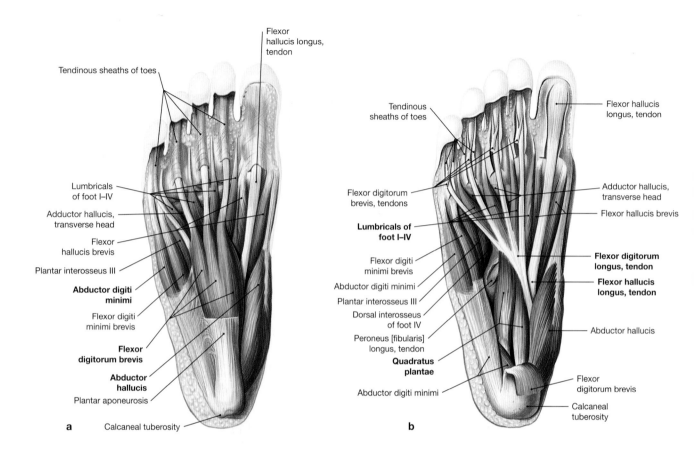

Fig. 4.75a and b **1ˢᵗ and 2ⁿᵈ layer of muscles on the plantar surface of the foot, right side;** plantar view **(a)**; after removal of the plantar aponeurosis **(b)**.
The muscles on the sole of foot can be organized into **four layers,** which all function as one muscular unit that helps maintain the arches of the foot and enables the foot to adjust to uneven surfaces/ground when walking or running. The 1ˢᵗ layer of the foot is comprised of **abductor hallucis, flexor digitorum brevis** and **abductor digiti minimi.** The 2ⁿᵈ layer is formed by **quadratus plantae** and the **lumbricals,** as well as the tendons of flexor digitorum longus and flexor hallucis longus (➤ Fig. 4.72)

Muscle	Attachments (P = proximal, D = distal)	Action/Function	Innervation
Abductor hallucis	**P:** Medial tubercle of tuberosity of calcaneus; flexor retinaculum; and plantar aponeurosis **D:** Medial side of base of proximal phalanx of big toe	Abducts and flexes big toe	Medial plantar nerve (S2 and S3)
Flexor digitorum brevis	**P:** Medial tubercle of calcaneal tuberosity; intermuscular septa; and plantar aponeurosis **D:** Both sides on middle phalanges of the lateral four digits	Flexes lateral four digits	Medial plantar nerve (S2 and S3)
Abductor digiti minimi	**P:** Medial and lateral tubercles of calcaneal tuberosity; intermuscular septa; and plantar aponeurosis **D:** Lateral side of base of proximal phalanx of 5ᵗʰ digit	Abducts and flexes little toe (5ᵗʰ digit)	Lateral plantar nerve (S2 and S3)
Quadratus plantae	**P:** Medial surface and lateral margin of plantar surface of the calcaneus **D:** Posterolateral margin of the flexor digitorum longus tendon	Assists flexor digitorum longus in flexing lateral four digits	Lateral plantar nerve (S2 and S3)
Lumbricals	**P:** Tendons of flexor digitorum longus **D:** Medial aspect of expansions over lateral four digits	Flex metatarsophalangeal joint and extends the interphalangeal joints of the four digits	Medial lumbricals: medial plantar nerve (S2 and S3) Lateral three lumbricals: lateral plantar nerve (S2 and S3)

Information for the flexor digitorum longus and flexor hallucis longus muscles is located on p. 205.

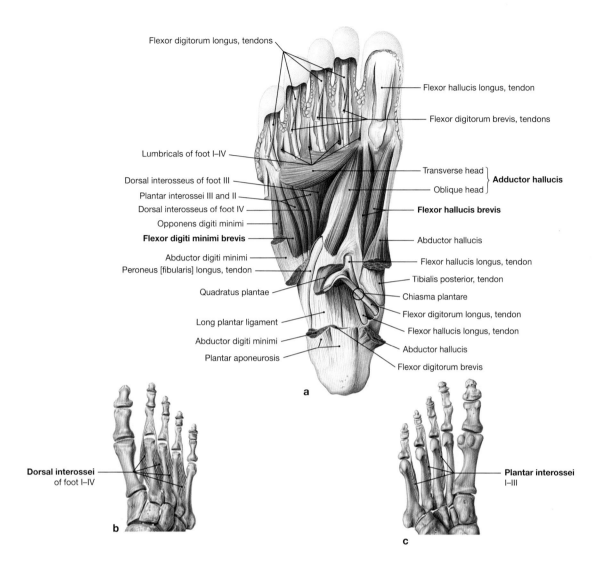

Flexor digitorum longus, tendons

Flexor hallucis longus, tendon

Flexor digitorum brevis, tendons

Lumbricals of foot I–IV

Dorsal interosseus of foot III

Plantar interossei III and II

Dorsal interosseus of foot IV

Opponens digiti minimi

Flexor digiti minimi brevis

Abductor digiti minimi

Peroneus [fibularis] longus, tendon

Quadratus plantae

Long plantar ligament

Abductor digiti minimi

Plantar aponeurosis

Transverse head
Oblique head
} **Adductor hallucis**

Flexor hallucis brevis

Abductor hallucis

Flexor hallucis longus, tendon

Tibialis posterior, tendon

Chiasma plantare

Flexor digitorum longus, tendon

Flexor hallucis longus, tendon

Abductor hallucis

Flexor digitorum brevis

a

Dorsal interossei
of foot I–IV

b

Plantar interossei
I–III

c

Fig. 4.76a to c 3rd and 4th Layer of Muscles on the Plantar Surface of Foot, right side; plantar view.
The 3rd layer of muscles on the sole of the foot is comprised of the **flexor hallucis brevis, adductor hallucis,** and **flexor digiti minimi**

brevis muscles. The 4th and **deepest layer** is comprised of the three **plantar interossei (c)** and four **dorsal interossei (b)** muscles.

Muscle	Attachments (P = proximal, D = dorsal)	Action/Function	Innervation
Flexor hallucis brevis	**P:** Plantar surface of cuboid and lateral cuneiforms **D:** Both sides of base of proximal phalanx of big toe	Flexes proximal phalanx of big toe	Medial plantar nerve (S2 and S3)
Adductor hallucis	**P:** Oblique head: base of metatarsals II–IV; transverse head: plantar ligament of metatarsophalangeal joints **D:** Lateral side of base of proximal phalanx of big toe	Adducts big toe; assists in maintenance of transverse arch of foot	Deep branch of lateral plantar nerve (S2 and S3)
Flexor digiti minimi brevis	**P:** Base of metatarsal V **D:** Base of proximal phalanx of 5th digit	Flexes proximal phalanx of little toe (5th digit)	Superficial branch of lateral plantar nerve (S2 and S3)
Plantar interossei (three muscles)	**P:** Bases and medial sides of metatarsals III–V **D:** Medial sides of proximal phalanges of 3rd, 4th and 5th digits	Adduct digits II–IV, and flex metatarsophalangeal joints	Lateral plantar nerve (S2 and S3)
Dorsal interossei (four muscles)	**P:** Sides of metatarsal I–V **D:** Interosseus I: medial side of proximal phalanx of 2nd digit; interossei II to IV: lateral sides of 2nd to 4th digits	Abduct digits II–IV, and flex metatarsophalangeal joints	Lateral plantar nerve (S2 and S3)

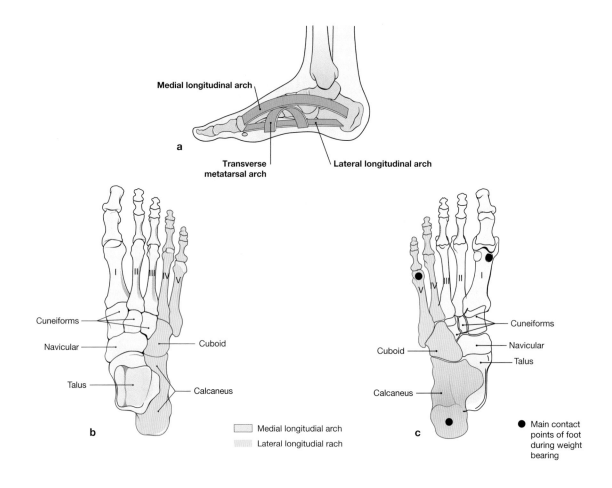

Fig. 4.77a to c Plantar arches of the foot, right side; medial **(a)**, dorsal **(b)** and plantar **(c)** views. [L126]

a The ligaments and bony alignment of the foot passively maintain three plantar arches: **medial longitudinal arch, lateral longitudinal arch,** and **transverse metatarsal arch.**

b The arches are actively supported by the long tendons of muscles from the deep posterior and lateral compartments of the lower leg, along with the short muscles that comprise the four layers of mus-

cle on the sole of the foot. These supporting structures create a tension band system that absorbs body weight on foot strike and allows the foot to become a rigid lever during the push-off phase of gait.

c In a healthy foot, the arches allow the foot to have three main contact points with the floor during weight bearing activities: at the heads of the 1st and 5th metatarsal bones, and at the calcaneal tuberosity.

Clinical Remarks

The arches of the foot serve as an adaptable, supportive base for the entire body. They can impact the normal biomechanics of the lower limb and deviations in their normal structure (such as **pes cavus** – high arched foot or **pes planus** – flat foot) can result in excessive foot pronation or supination which leads to muscular imbalances and functionally unstable conditions of the foot. [L126]

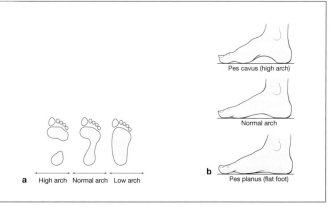

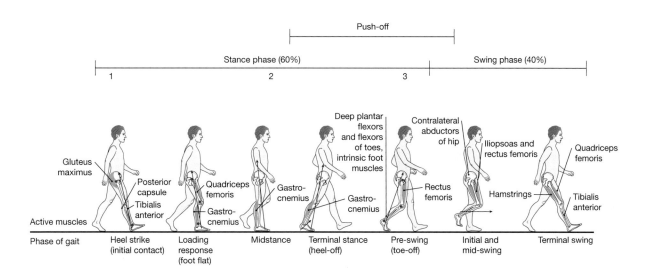

Push-off

Stance phase (60%) | Swing phase (40%)

1 | 2 | 3

| Phase of gait | Heel strike (initial contact) | Loading response (foot flat) | Midstance | Terminal stance (heel-off) | Pre-swing (toe-off) | Initial and mid-swing | Terminal swing |

Fig. 4.78 Normal gait. [L126]
During normal gait, one limb provides support while the other limb is advanced in preparation for its role as the support limb. The **gait cycle** (GC) in its simplest form is comprised of **stance and swing phases.** The stance phase can be further subdivided into three segments, including 1. initial double stance, 2. single limb stance,

and 3. terminal double limb stance. Gait velocity will influence the duration of stance and swing phases – each aspect of stance decreases as walking velocity increases. The transition from walking to running is marked by elimination of the periods of double support.

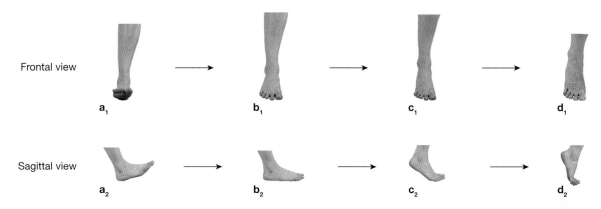

Fig. 4.79 Foot pronation and supination, frontal (**a₁–d₁**) and sagittal (**a₂–d₂**) views. [L271]
The foot serves two main functions: 1. It acts as a mobile adaptor to adjust to varying terrain. 2. It acts as a rigid lever for forward propulsion in locomotion. During walking and running, the movements of foot pronation and supination normally occur. **Pronation** is important for optimal movement and shock absorption. At heel strike **(a),** the foot begins to pronate – with dorsiflexion of the ankle joint the foot rolls inward, everts slightly, and the plantar arches flatten. This is a normal action – one that occurs with every step of a healthy foot. The purpose of this motion is to loosen the

foot so it can adapt to the surface, especially on uneven terrain **(b).** As the foot continues through the gait cycle and into the toe-off (or lift-off) phase **(c and d), supination** occurs – with plantarflexion of the ankle joint, the foot inverts, and the arches become higher, thus enabling the foot to properly roll over the big toe. Supination allows the foot to change from a flexible, shock-absorbing structure to a rigid lever which transmits force to the ground and propels the body forward. During normal gait, these two functions (pronation vs. supination) are time specific – when the foot spends too much time being a mobile adapter (over-pronation), it cannot spend enough time being a rigid lever and vice versa.

Clinical Remarks

Lesions of the common peroneal (fibular) nerve are among the most common nerve injuries of the lower limb. Potential causes of injury include fractures of the proximal fibula and anterior compartment syndrome within the lower leg. Nerve injury may lead to a **'drop foot disability'** that causes patients to adopt compensatory gait patterns, in order to avoid dragging the foot of the affected leg during the swing phase of gait.
[L231]

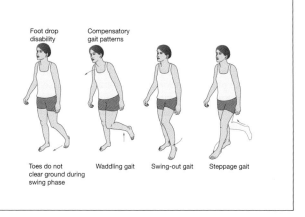

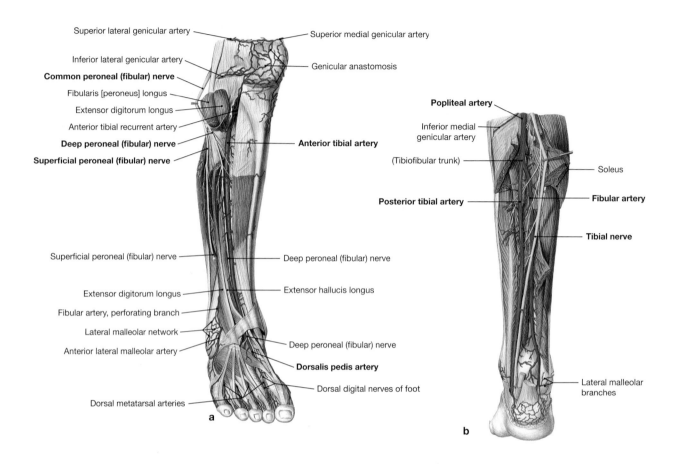

Superior lateral genicular artery

Inferior lateral genicular artery

Common peroneal (fibular) nerve

Fibularis [peroneus] longus

Extensor digitorum longus

Anterior tibial recurrent artery

Deep peroneal (fibular) nerve

Superficial peroneal (fibular) nerve

Superior medial genicular artery

Genicular anastomosis

Anterior tibial artery

Popliteal artery

Inferior medial genicular artery

(Tibiofibular trunk)

Posterior tibial artery

Soleus

Fibular artery

Tibial nerve

Superficial peroneal (fibular) nerve

Deep peroneal (fibular) nerve

Extensor digitorum longus

Extensor hallucis longus

Fibular artery, perforating branch

Lateral malleolar network

Anterior lateral malleolar artery

Deep peroneal (fibular) nerve

Dorsalis pedis artery

Dorsal digital nerves of foot

Dorsal metatarsal arteries

Lateral malleolar branches

a

b

Fig. 4.80a and b Arteries and nerves of the lower leg and ankle, right side; anterior view **(a)**; posterior view **(b)**; after removal of the deep fascia of leg.

Below the popliteal fossa, the **popliteal artery** descends between the two heads of the gastrocnemius and divides into two terminal branches: 1. **posterior tibial artery** continues its course; 2. **anterior tibial artery** traverses the interosseous membrane of leg to enter the anterior compartment. The anterior tibial artery descends between the extensor digitorum longus and tibialis anterior muscles and continues as **dorsalis pedis artery** on the dorsum of the foot. Shortly after passing through the tendinous arch of the soleus, the posterior tibial artery gives rise to its most important branch, the

fibular artery, which descends to the lateral malleolus. The posterior tibial artery descends together with the **tibial nerve** between the superficial and deep flexor muscles of the leg to the medial malleolus and continues through the **malleolar canal** beneath the flexor retinaculum to the plantar side of the foot. The **common peroneal (fibular) nerve** winds laterally around the head of fibula, enters the fibular compartment, and then divides into its two terminal branches: 1. **superficial peroneal (fibular) nerve** provides innervation within the peroneal compartment; 2. **deep peroneal (fibular) nerve** passes over to the extensor compartment and descends adjacent to the anterior tibial artery.

┌ Clinical Remarks

The word **Claudication** comes from the Latin word 'claudicare' meaning to limp. It refers to a pain and/or cramping in the **lower leg** due to inadequate blood flow to the muscles. The most common cause of claudication is peripheral artery disease, which is especially common at branching points of the arteries in the legs. The area of impairment is frequently identified via the use of medical imaging such as DOPPLER guided ultrasound. [T824]

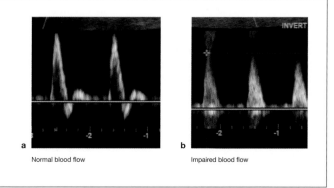

a Normal blood flow

b Impaired blood flow

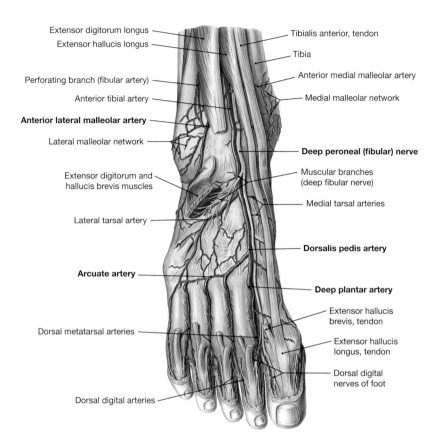

Extensor digitorum longus
Extensor hallucis longus
Perforating branch (fibular artery)
Anterior tibial artery
Anterior lateral malleolar artery
Lateral malleolar network
Extensor digitorum and hallucis brevis muscles
Lateral tarsal artery
Arcuate artery
Dorsal metatarsal arteries
Dorsal digital arteries

Tibialis anterior, tendon
Tibia
Anterior medial malleolar artery
Medial malleolar network
Deep peroneal (fibular) nerve
Muscular branches (deep fibular nerve)
Medial tarsal arteries
Dorsalis pedis artery
Deep plantar artery
Extensor hallucis brevis, tendon
Extensor hallucis longus, tendon
Dorsal digital nerves of foot

Fig. 4.81 Arteries and nerves on the dorsum of foot, right side; anterior view after removal of the tendons of the extensor digitorum longus and the short extensor muscles of the toes. After innervating the extensor muscles of the leg and dorsum of foot, the **deep peroneal (fibular) nerve** divides into terminal sensory branches which supply the first interdigital space. At the level of the malleoli, the **anterior tibial artery** supplies the **anterior medial and lateral malleolar arteries** for the arterial networks around the malleoli (medial and lateral malleolar networks). The anterior tibial artery continues on the dorsum of foot as the **dorsalis pedis artery.** It provides several smaller medial tarsal arteries and one lateral tarsal artery to the tarsus and then continues to supply the **arcuate artery.** It arches to the lateral margins of the foot and gives rise to the dorsal metatarsal arteries which continue as dorsal digital arteries to supply the toes. The **deep plantar artery** participates in the perfusion of the sole of foot by supplying the deep plantar arch.

Fig. 4.82 Arteries and nerves on the plantar surface of the foot, right side; plantar view. The **medial and lateral plantar nerves** are accompanied by the corresponding branches of the **posterior tibial artery.** The blood vessels continue beneath the flexor digitorum brevis to reach the intermediate layer of the neurovascular structures of the toes. The **deep plantar arch** continues the **lateral plantar artery** and receives blood from the deep branch of the medial plantar artery and from the deep plantar artery which derives from the dorsalis pedis artery. Together with the deep branch of the lateral plantar nerve it arches over the interossei of the sole of foot in the deep layer of the neurovascular structures.

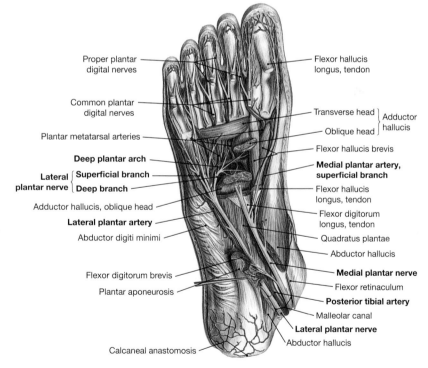

Proper plantar digital nerves
Common plantar digital nerves
Plantar metatarsal arteries
Deep plantar arch
Lateral plantar nerve { **Superficial branch** / **Deep branch** }
Adductor hallucis, oblique head
Lateral plantar artery
Abductor digiti minimi
Flexor digitorum brevis
Plantar aponeurosis
Calcaneal anastomosis

Flexor hallucis longus, tendon
Transverse head } Adductor hallucis
Oblique head
Flexor hallucis brevis
Medial plantar artery, superficial branch
Flexor hallucis longus, tendon
Flexor digitorum longus, tendon
Quadratus plantae
Abductor hallucis
Medial plantar nerve
Flexor retinaculum
Posterior tibial artery
Malleolar canal
Lateral plantar nerve
Abductor hallucis

Structure/Function

The most distal and palpable pulse in the lower extremity is the dorsalis pedis artery on the dorsum of foot. Examination of the arterial pulse reveals many clues about the frequency of the heartbeat, differences of blood flow between upper and lower limbs, and offers general clues about the circulation system. [L126]

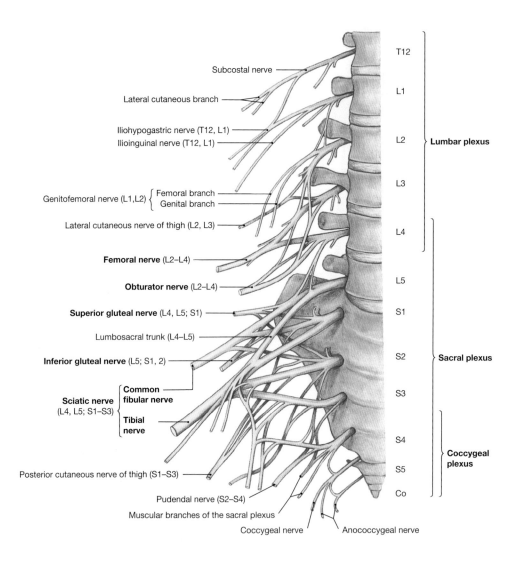

Subcostal nerve

Lateral cutaneous branch

Iliohypogastric nerve (T12, L1)
Ilioinguinal nerve (T12, L1)

Genitofemoral nerve (L1,L2) { Femoral branch / Genital branch

Lateral cutaneous nerve of thigh (L2, L3)

Femoral nerve (L2–L4)

Obturator nerve (L2–L4)

Superior gluteal nerve (L4, L5; S1)

Lumbosacral trunk (L4–L5)

Inferior gluteal nerve (L5; S1, 2)

Sciatic nerve (L4, L5; S1–S3) { **Common fibular nerve** / **Tibial nerve**

Posterior cutaneous nerve of thigh (S1–S3)

Pudendal nerve (S2–S4)

Muscular branches of the sacral plexus

Coccygeal nerve   Anococcygeal nerve

T12

L1

L2 } **Lumbar plexus**

L3

L4

L5

S1

S2 } **Sacral plexus**

S3

S4

S5 } **Coccygeal plexus**

Co

Fig. 4.83 Lumbosacral plexus (T12–S5, Co1): segmental organization of the nerves, right side.

The lower extremity is innervated by the lumbosacral plexus. The plexus is composed of anterior branches of the spinal nerves which originate from the lumbar (L), sacral (S), and coccygeal (Co) segments of the spinal cord and combine to form the **lumbar plexus** (T12–L4) and the **sacral plexus** (L4–S5, Co1). The segments S4 to Co1 are also referred to as **coccygeal plexus.** Most importantly, the lumbosacral plexus supplies **five key nerves** that are imperative for normal musculoskeletal function of the lower extremity:

1. The **femoral nerve** innervates the anterior thigh or 'quads' region. It powers the movements of hip flexion and knee extension.

2. The **obturator nerve** supplies the medial thigh or adductor ('groin') region. It powers the movement of hip adduction.

3. The **superior gluteal nerve** innervates the deep gluteal muscles within the buttocks region, and is responsible for powering internal rotation and abduction movements of the hip.

4. The **inferior gluteal nerve** innervates the superficial region of the buttocks, and powers extension and external rotation of the hip.

5. The largest and longest branch of the lumbosacral plexus is the **sciatic nerve.** It innervates the posterior thigh and everything below the knee. Its two main divisions **(tibial and common peroneal nerves)** power knee flexion, as well as all movements of the ankle, foot and toes.

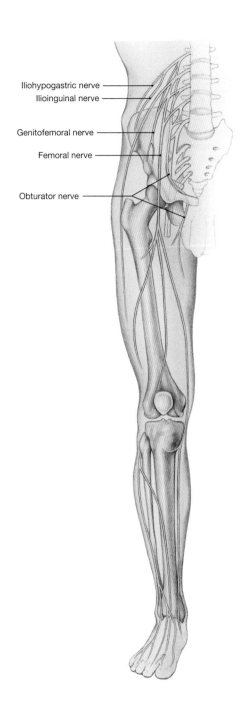

Iliohypogastric nerve

Ilioinguinal nerve

Genitofemoral nerve

Femoral nerve

Obturator nerve

Fig. 4.84 Lumbar plexus (T12–L4): nerves of the lower extremity, right side; anterior view.
The nerves of the **lumbar plexus** (T12–L4; ➤ Fig. 12.72, ➤ Fig. 12.73, ➤ Fig. 12.74) course anterior to the hip joint and innervate the inferior part of the anterolateral abdominal wall and the anterior and medial aspects of the thigh.

Lumbar Plexus – Motor Innervation of the Lower Extremity

- Motor branches to the iliopsoas and quadratus lumborum muscles (T12–L4)

- Iliohypogastric nerve (T12, L1): provides motor innervation to the inferior aspect of transversus abdominis and internal oblique muscles

- Ilioinguinal nerve (T12, L1): provides motor innervation to the inferior aspect of transversus abdominis and internal oblique muscles

- Genitofemoral nerve (L1, L2): divides into two branches (lateral femoral branch and medial genital branch). The medial genital branch provides motor fibers to the cremaster muscle in men

- Femoral nerve (L2–L4): the muscular branches provide motor fibers to the anterior muscles of the hip (iliacus) and the thigh (sartorius and quadriceps femoris) and in part to the pectineus muscle

- Obturator nerve (L2–L4): one of its branches reaches the obturator externus. It then divides into anterior and posterior branches which convey motor fibers to the muscles of the adductor region

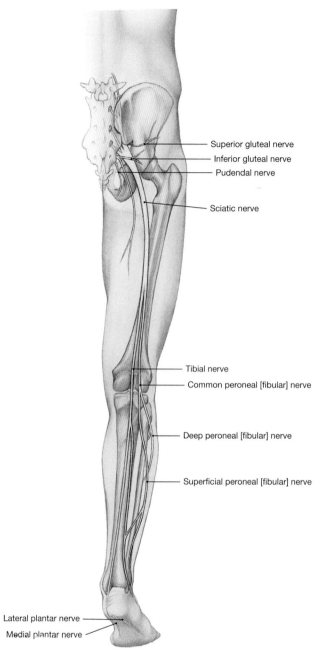

— Superior gluteal nerve
— Inferior gluteal nerve
— Pudendal nerve

— Sciatic nerve

— Tibial nerve
— Common peroneal [fibular] nerve

— Deep peroneal [fibular] nerve

— Superficial peroneal [fibular] nerve

Lateral plantar nerve —
Medial plantar nerve —

Fig. 4.85 Sacral plexus (L4–S5, Co1): nerves of the lower extremity, right side; posterior view.

The branches of the sacral plexus course posterior to the hip joint. They innervate muscles in the buttocks region, the posterior and lateral thigh and all muscles in the lower leg, ankle and foot (➤ Fig. 12.72, ➤ Fig. 12.73, ➤ Fig. 12.74).

Sacral Plexus – Motor Innervation of the Lower Extremity

- Motor branches to the deep posterior muscles of the hip – obturator internus, gemellus superior, gemellus inferior, quadratus femoris, piriformis muscles (L4–S2)

- Superior gluteal nerve (L4–S1): provides motor innervation to the small gluteal muscles (most important abductors and medial rotators of the hip joint) and the tensor fasciae latae muscle and the iliotibial band

- Inferior gluteal nerve (L5–S2): innervates the gluteus maximus, the strongest extensor and external rotator muscle of the hip joint

- Sciatic nerve (L4–S3): consists of two divisions – tibial and common fibular nerves that are combined as one common nerve over a variable distance in the posterior thigh. The tibial nerve provides motor innervation to the hamstring muscles and the posterior head of the adductor magnus. The fibular nerve innervates the short head of the biceps femoris. Both portions of the sciatic nerve together innervate all muscles below the knee.

- Pudendal nerve* (S2–S4): innervates the external anal sphincter and all muscles of the perineum

- Pelvic splanchnic nerves* (S2–S4)

- Motor branches to the pelvic floor* – levator ani and ischiococcygeus muscles (S3, S4)

* denotes nerves/branches from the sacral plexus which innervate structures within the pelvic region, not the lower extremity

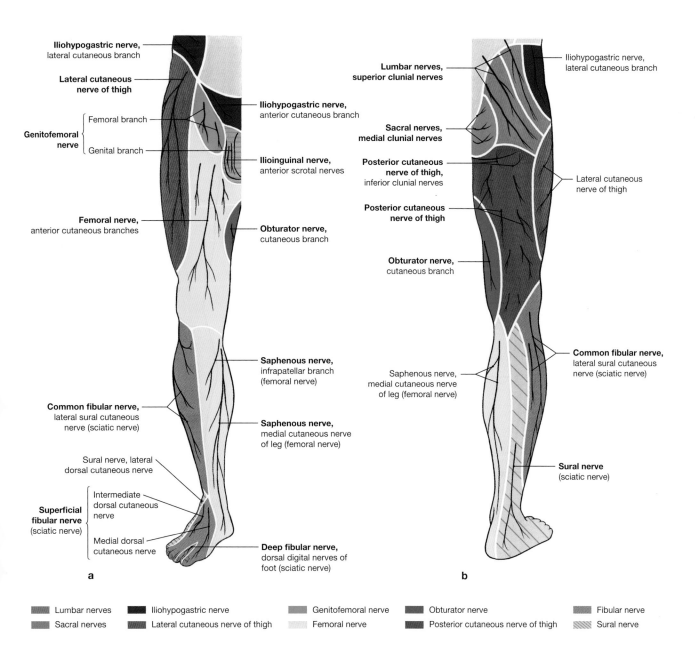

Iliohypogastric nerve,
lateral cutaneous branch

Lateral cutaneous
nerve of thigh

Genitofemoral
nerve
  Femoral branch
  Genital branch

Femoral nerve,
anterior cutaneous branches

Common fibular nerve,
lateral sural cutaneous
nerve (sciatic nerve)

Sural nerve, lateral
dorsal cutaneous nerve

Superficial
fibular nerve
(sciatic nerve)
  Intermediate
  dorsal cutaneous
  nerve
  Medial dorsal
  cutaneous nerve

Iliohypogastric nerve,
anterior cutaneous branch

Ilioinguinal nerve,
anterior scrotal nerves

Obturator nerve,
cutaneous branch

Saphenous nerve,
infrapatellar branch
(femoral nerve)

Saphenous nerve,
medial cutaneous nerve
of leg (femoral nerve)

Deep fibular nerve,
dorsal digital nerves of
foot (sciatic nerve)

a

Lumbar nerves,
superior clunial nerves

Sacral nerves,
medial clunial nerves

Posterior cutaneous
nerve of thigh,
inferior clunial nerves

Posterior cutaneous
nerve of thigh

Obturator nerve,
cutaneous branch

Saphenous nerve,
medial cutaneous nerve
of leg (femoral nerve)

Iliohypogastric nerve,
lateral cutaneous branch

Lateral cutaneous
nerve of thigh

Common fibular nerve,
lateral sural cutaneous
nerve (sciatic nerve)

Sural nerve
(sciatic nerve)

b

Lumbar nerves	Iliohypogastric nerve
Sacral nerves	Lateral cutaneous nerve of thigh

Genitofemoral nerve	Obturator nerve
Femoral nerve	Posterior cutaneous nerve of thigh

Fibular nerve	
Sural nerve	

Fig. 4.86a and b Cutaneous nerves of the lower extremity, right side; anterior **(a)** and posterior **(b)** views.
All peripheral nerves of the **lumbar plexus** contribute to the sensory innervation of the **inguinal region** and the **anterior and medial surfaces of the thigh**. The **lateral aspect of the leg** and the **dorsal aspect of the foot** are supplied by branches of the sacral plexus.

The **gluteal region** is innervated by **posterior branches** from the lumbar (superior clunial nerves) and sacral (medial clunial nerves) spinal nerves. The posterior aspect of the whole lower extremity and the sole (plantar surface) of the foot are innervated by branches of the sacral plexus.

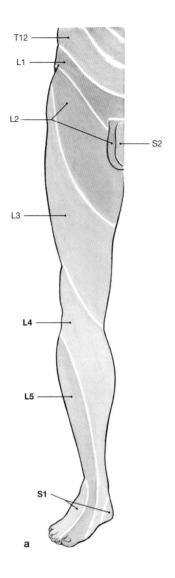

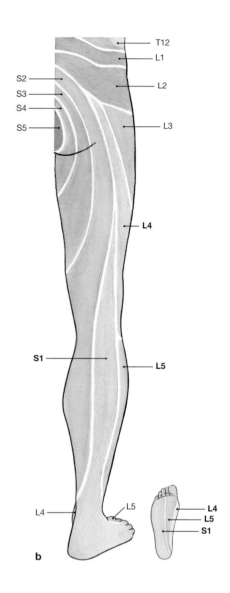

Fig. 4.87a and b **Dermatomal patterns of the lower extremity, right side;** anterior (a) and posterior (b) views.

Distinct areas of the skin are supplied by a single spinal cord segment. These cutaneous areas are referred to as **dermatomes** (➤ Fig. 12.75). Since peripheral nerves of the lower extremity convey sensory fibers from several spinal cord segments, the borders of the dermatomes do not correspond to the cutaneous area supplied by each specific peripheral nerve. In contrast to the circular pattern of the dermatomes of the trunk, dermatomes on the **anterior surface of the lower extremity are obliquely oriented** in a lateral superior to medial inferior direction. On the **posterior surface they are oriented in a nearly longitudinal direction.**

Clinical Remarks

The localization of dermatomes is clinically important in the diagnosis of **spinal cord/nerve or disc injury.** Disc herniation/prolapse commonly occurs in the lower lumbar vertebral column and may compress the roots of the spinal nerves L4–S1. The specific level of the lesion can be ascertained through an evaluation of the dermatomal patterns: Fibers from the L4 segment innervate the medial margin of the foot/L5 supplies the big toe and the second toe/S1 supplies the lateral side of the foot, including the little toe (5th digit).
[E402]

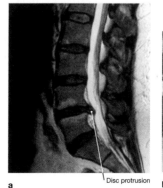

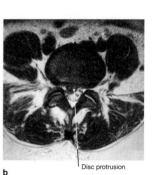

Disc protrusion a   Disc protrusion b

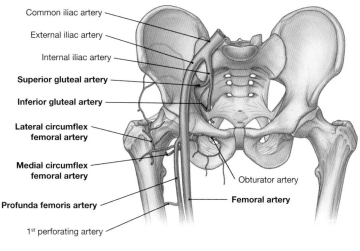

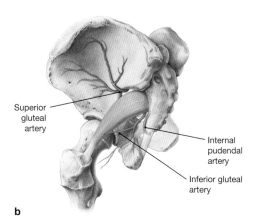

Fig. 4.88a und b Arteries of the pelvic girdle, right side; anterior **(a)** and posterior **(b)** views. a [E402], b [L285]

The **femoral artery** is the main branch of the anterior thigh and arises from the external iliac artery (➤ Fig. 6.133). Approximately 3–6 cm (1.2–2.4 in) below the inguinal ligament, it gives rise to the **profunda femoris artery** (deep artery of thigh), which supplies the posterior thigh and a portion of the adductor region. The profunda femoris artery then divides into the **lateral and medial circumflex** femoral arteries. In the adult, the **femoral head** is almost exclusively supplied by the **medial circumflex femoral artery.** The **superior and inferior gluteal arteries** are branches of the **internal iliac artery.** They exit the pelvis via the **greater sciatic foramen,** and are named in relation to the **piriformis muscle** – the superior gluteal artery exits above the piriformis muscle, the inferior exits below the piriformis muscle. Both arteries supply the gluteal region.

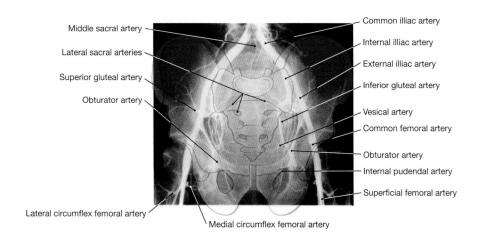

Fig. 4.89 Angiogram of pelvic arteries; anterior view. [L126, G198]

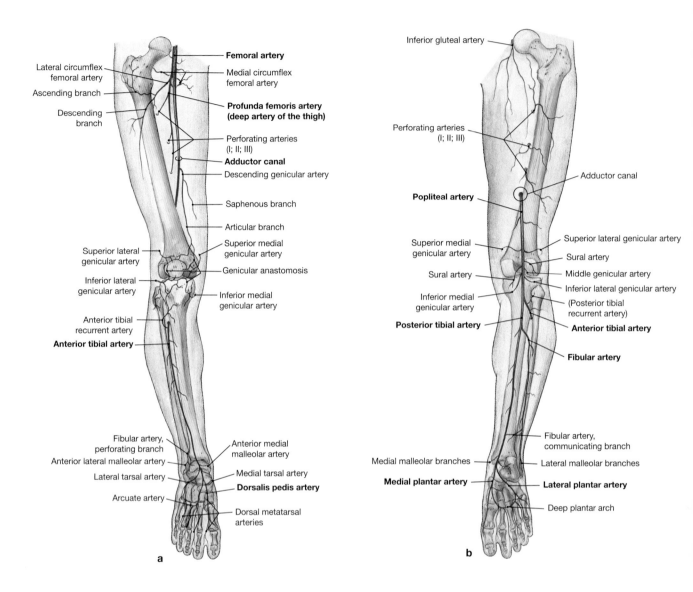

Fig. 4.90a and b Arteries of the lower extremity, right side; anterior **(a)** and posterior **(b)** views.

The external iliac artery branches off the common iliac artery anterior to the sacroiliac joint and continues beneath the inguinal ligament in the vascular space as **femoral artery.** Following the passage through the **adductor canal** it is then referred to as **popliteal artery** (supplying the knee joint). The popliteal artery descends underneath the tendinous arch of the soleus between the superficial and deep flexors of the leg and divides into two main branch-

es: 1. the **anterior tibial artery** pierces the interosseous membrane of leg to reach the anterior extensor compartment, and continues distally as the **dorsalis pedis artery** on the dorsum of the foot; 2. the **posterior tibial artery** descends on the posterior aspect of the leg. In the superior aspect of the leg, the strong **fibular artery** courses on the outside of the leg, before passing through the malleolar canal around the medial malleolus to reach the sole of foot, where it provides two terminal branches (**medial** and **lateral plantar arteries**).

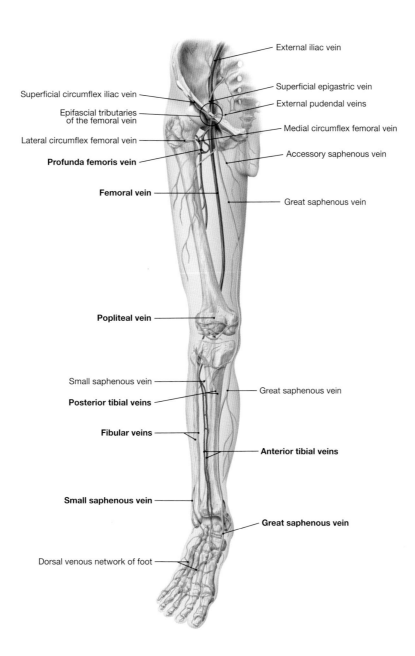

- External iliac vein
- Superficial epigastric vein
- External pudendal veins
- Medial circumflex femoral vein
- Accessory saphenous vein
- Great saphenous vein

- Superficial circumflex iliac vein
- Epifascial tributaries of the femoral vein
- Lateral circumflex femoral vein
- **Profunda femoris vein**
- **Femoral vein**

- **Popliteal vein**

- Small saphenous vein
- **Posterior tibial veins**
- Great saphenous vein
- **Fibular veins**
- **Anterior tibial veins**
- **Small saphenous vein**
- **Great saphenous vein**
- Dorsal venous network of foot

Fig. 4.91 Veins of the lower extremity, right side; anterior view. [L127]

The **deep veins** (dark blue) accompany the corresponding arteries. In the leg, usually two veins course together with the respective artery, whereas in the regions of the thigh and popliteal fossa only one concomitant vein is found. The **superficial venous system** (light blue) consists of **two main veins** which collect the blood from the dorsum and the sole of foot. The **great saphenous vein** originates anterior to the medial malleolus and ascends on the medial side of the leg and thigh to the saphenous opening. Here, the great

saphenous vein receives tributaries (superficial epigastric vein, superficial circumflex iliac vein, accessory saphenous vein, external pudenal veins) from several veins of the inguinal region and enters the femoral vein at the femoral triangle (> Fig. 7.126).

On the posterior side, the **small saphenous vein** originates from the lateral margin of the foot posterior to the lateral malleolus and ascends on the middle of the calf to the popliteal fossa to enter the popliteal vein. The great saphenous vein and small saphenous vein communicate through variable branches.

Clinical Remarks

Deep vein thrombosis (or DVT) refers to the formation of a blood clot (i.e. thrombus) within a deep vein (most commonly in the legs). Signs of a DVT may include pain, swelling, redness, and engorged superficial veins. If the clot becomes detached, it can lead to an embolism – a potentially life threatening complication in which the clot travels to the lungs. [E288]

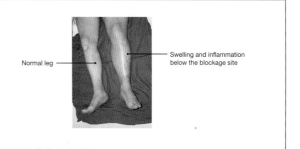

Normal leg

Swelling and inflammation below the blockage site

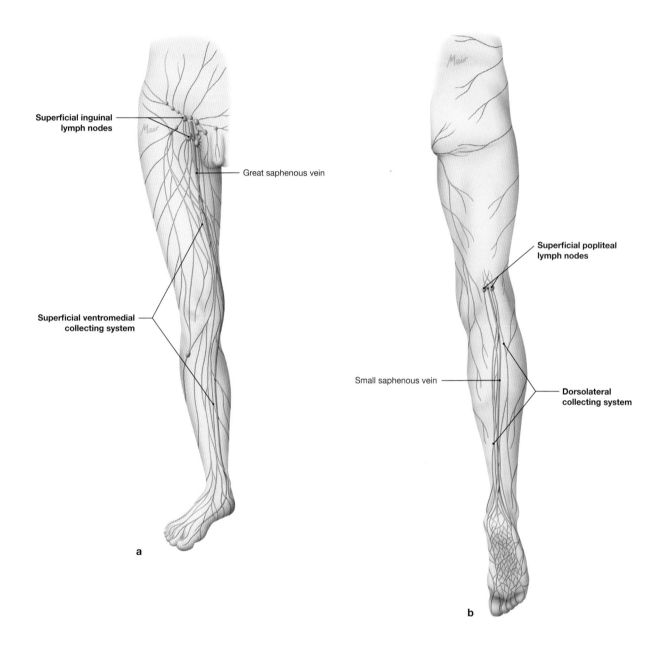

Superficial inguinal
lymph nodes

Great saphenous vein

Superficial ventromedial
collecting system

Superficial popliteal
lymph nodes

Small saphenous vein

Dorsolateral
collecting system

a

b

Fig. 4.92a and b Superficial lymphatic vessels of the lower extremity, right side; anterior **(a)** and posterior **(b)** views. [L127]
Alongside the veins there are a superficial and a deep system of collecting lymphatic vessels with incorporated lymph nodes. The **superficial ventromedial system** runs alongside the great saphenous vein and is the main lymphatic drainage of the lower extremity. It drains into the **superficial inguinal lymph nodes.** The smaller **dorsolateral collecting system** parallels the small saphenous vein

and drains into the lymph nodes of the popliteal fossa (**superficial and deep popliteal lymph nodes**) and continues into the deep inguinal lymph nodes (not depicted). The deep collecting systems directly drain into the deep popliteal and inguinal lymph nodes. While most of the venous drainage from the lower extremity occurs via the deep veins, the major part of the lymph is drained by the superficial lymphatic vessels.

Thorax

Surface Anatomy 225

Cutaneous Innervation 229

Mammary Gland 230

Mammary Gland – Blood Supply ... 231

Ribs and Costovertebral Joints 234

Intercostal Muscles 235

Diaphragm 236

Muscles of Respiration 238

Thoracic Wall 239

Pleural Cavities 242

Lungs 245

Mediastinum 250

Surface Projection of the Heart 254

Pericardium 255

Heart 257

Cardiac Valves 261

Great Vessels and Heart 264

Coronary Arteries 266

Cardiac Veins 269

Conducting System of the Heart 270

5

Innervation of the Heart 272

Prenatal and Postnatal
Blood Circulation 273

Superior Mediastinum 274

Posterior Mediastinum 278

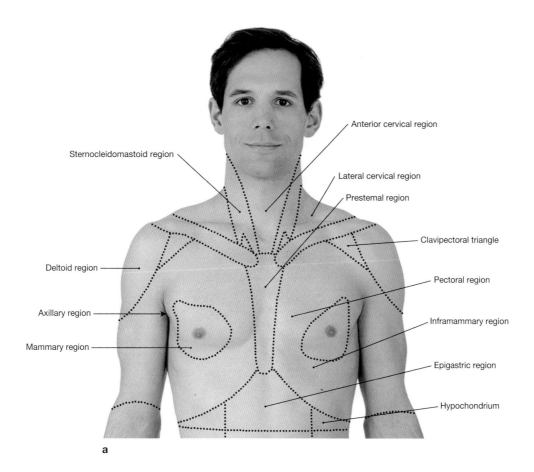

Anterior cervical region

Sternocleidomastoid region

Lateral cervical region

Prestemal region

Clavipectoral triangle

Deltoid region

Pectoral region

Axillary region

Inframammary region

Mammary region

Epigastric region

Hypochondrium

a

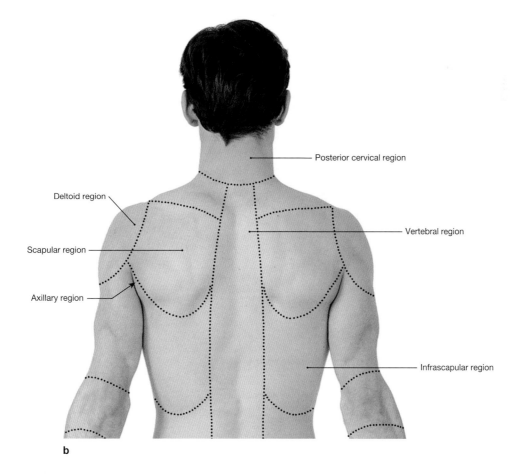

Posterior cervical region

Deltoid region

Vertebral region

Scapular region

Axillary region

Infrascapular region

b

Fig. 5.1a and b Regions of the thorax. [K340]

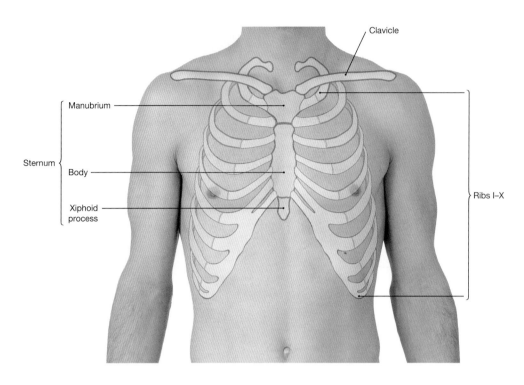

Fig. 5.2 Projection of the rib cage onto the thoracic wall. [L126, L271]

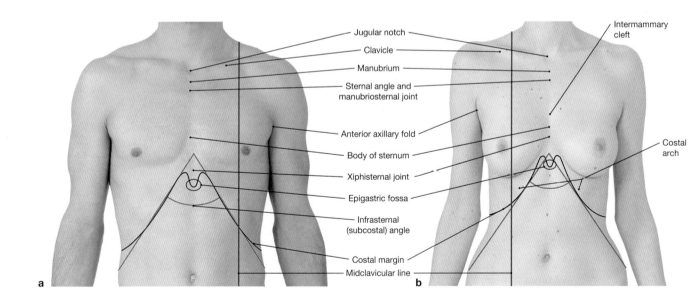

Fig. 5.3a and b Surface landmarks of the anterior thoracic wall;
in the male **(a)** and female **(b)**. [K340]

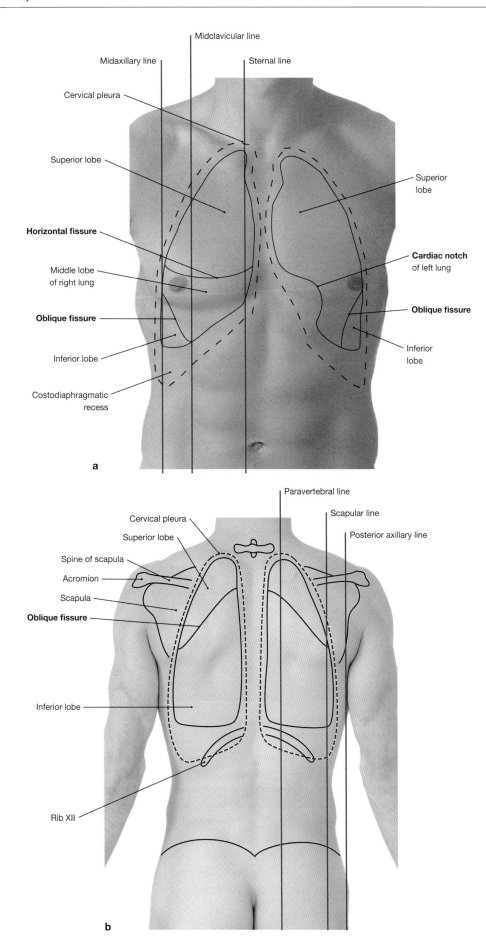

Fig. 5.4a and b Projections of the borders of the lungs and pleura onto the anterior (a) and posterior thoracic (b) walls. b [L126, K340]
The **horizontal fissure** separates the superior and middle lobes of the right lung and projects along rib IV on the anterior chest wall.
The **oblique fissure** separates the middle from the inferior lobe of

the right lung and the superior from the inferior lobe of the left lung. It projects mainly to the posterior thoracic wall.
The **cardiac notch** leaves a pleura-free area on the left side of the sternum from rib IV to rib VII.

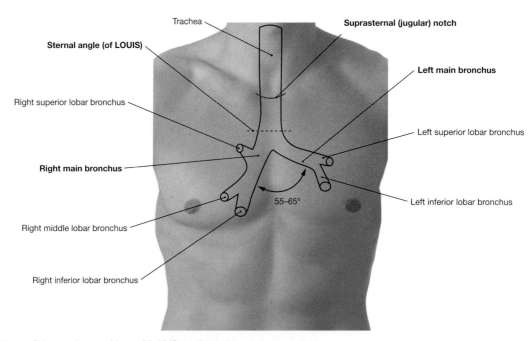

Fig. 5.5 Projections of the trachea and bronchial bifurcation onto the thoracic wall.

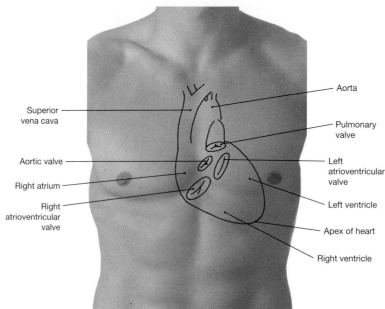

Fig. 5.6 Projections of the heart and the cardiac valves onto the thoracic wall.

Surface Landmarks and Projections to Vertebral Levels			
Surface Landmark	**Ribs/Intercostal Space (ICS)**	**Vertebral Projection**	**Orientation**
Suprasternal (jugular) notch	Between upper sternoclavicular joints	Level T2/T3	Trachea entering mediastinum; inferior thyroid veins, thyroid ima artery
Manubrium of sternum	Rib I	Level T3/T4	Aortic arch; superior vena cava; thymus
Sternal angle (of LOUIS); manubriosternal joint	Rib II	Level T4/T5	Marks transition from superior to inferior mediastinum, and the articulation with the second costal cartilage
Nipple (male)	ICS IV		
Body of sternum	Ribs II–VI (false ribs VIII–X)	Level T5–T9	Tricuspid valve (5th costal cartilage); right ventricle
Infrasternal angle		Level T9/T10 Xiphisternal plane (T9)	Central tendon of diaphragm with attachment of fibrous pericardium

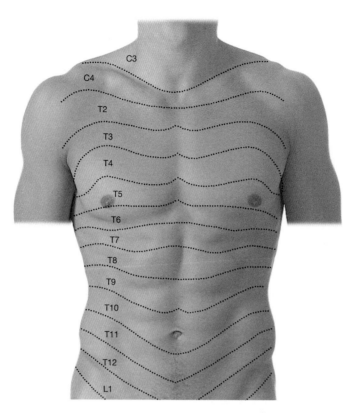

Fig. 5.7 Dermatomes of the anterior thoracoabdominal wall. The structure of the intercostal nerves is shown in ➤ chapter 12 (Neuroanatomy).

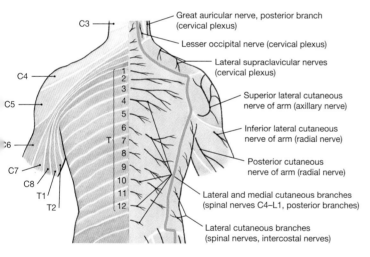

Fig. 5.8 Segmental innervation of the skin and corresponding cutaneous nerves of the posterior thoracic wall.
The dark blue line on the right side indicates the demarcation between the cutaneous innervation by the posterior and anterior rami of the spinal nerves (➤ Fig. 12.74, ➤ Fig. 12.75).

Labels in Fig. 5.8:
- Great auricular nerve, posterior branch (cervical plexus)
- Lesser occipital nerve (cervical plexus)
- Lateral supraclavicular nerves (cervical plexus)
- Superior lateral cutaneous nerve of arm (axillary nerve)
- Inferior lateral cutaneous nerve of arm (radial nerve)
- Posterior cutaneous nerve of arm (radial nerve)
- Lateral and medial cutaneous branches (spinal nerves C4–L1, posterior branches)
- Lateral cutaneous branches (spinal nerves, intercostal nerves)

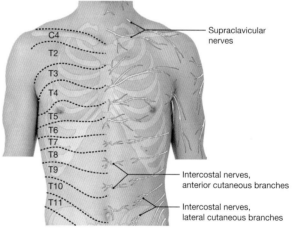

Fig. 5.9 Segmental innervation of the skin and corresponding cutaneous nerves of the anterior thoracic wall (➤ Fig. 12.75).
[L126, K340]

Labels in Fig. 5.9:
- Supraclavicular nerves
- Intercostal nerves, anterior cutaneous branches
- Intercostal nerves, lateral cutaneous branches

Clinical Remarks

Following a varicella-zoster virus infection (chicken pox), the virus may reside dormant in neurons of the dorsal root ganglion. Upon reactivation a painful cutaneous eruption occurs, known as **shingles,** that is confined to the respective dermatome. [E545]

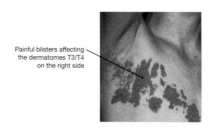

Painful blisters affecting the dermatomes T3/T4 on the right side

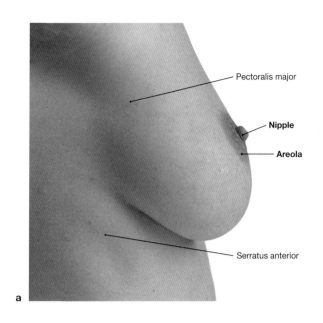
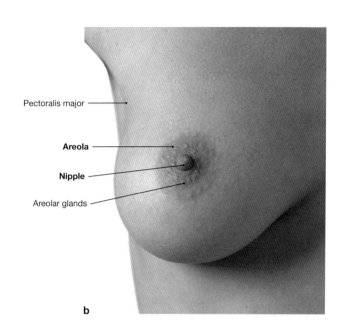

Fig. 5.10a and b Breast, right side; lateral **(a)** and anterior **(b)** views.

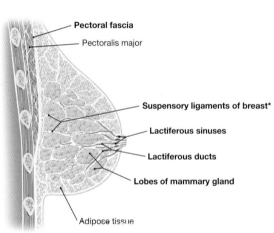

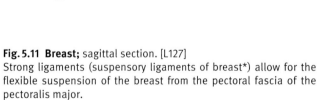

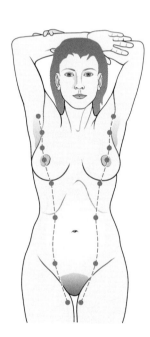

Fig. 5.11 Breast; sagittal section. [L127]
Strong ligaments (suspensory ligaments of breast*) allow for the flexible suspension of the breast from the pectoral fascia of the pectoralis major.

* clin. term: COOPER's ligaments

Fig. 5.12 Milk line. [L126]
Mammary gland development initiates in the milk line **(mammary ridge),** a strip of thickened surface ectoderm formed in embryonic week 6 that extends from the axillary pit to the inguinal region. Except for the area above the pectoralis major, the location for the development of the future breast, the rest of the milk line normally regresses.

┌ Clinical Remarks

The absence of the nipples **(athelia)** or breasts **(amastia, mammary aplasia)** are rare congenital anomalies that can occur uni- or bilaterally. Supernumerary nipples or breasts are called **polythelia** or **polymastia,** respectively. This is usually hereditary and can also affect males. When breast growth occurs in males (possibly due to hormonal disorders), this condition is called **gynecomastia.**

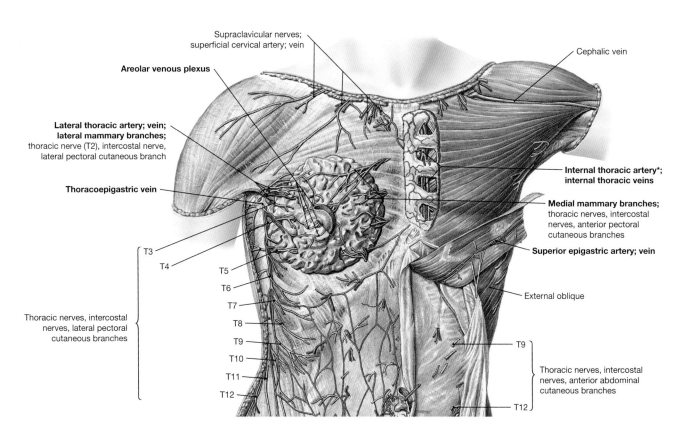

Supraclavicular nerves;
superficial cervical artery; vein

Cephalic vein

Areolar venous plexus

**Lateral thoracic artery; vein;
lateral mammary branches;**
thoracic nerve (T2), intercostal nerve,
lateral pectoral cutaneous branch

Thoracoepigastric vein

Internal thoracic artery*;
internal thoracic veins

Medial mammary branches;
thoracic nerves, intercostal
nerves, anterior pectoral
cutaneous branches

Superior epigastric artery; vein

T3
T4

External oblique

T5
T6
T7
T8
T9
T10
T11
T12

Thoracic nerves, intercostal
nerves, lateral pectoral
cutaneous branches

T9

Thoracic nerves, intercostal
nerves, anterior abdominal
cutaneous branches

T12

Fig. 5.13 Epifascial blood vessels of the thorax.
The mammary gland develops from the ectoderm and has an epifascial position in the subcutaneous tissue of the anterior thoracic wall. The epifascial **lateral** and **medial mammary branches** are connected to the lateral thoracic and to the internal thoracic blood vessels.

* Internal mammary artery and vein

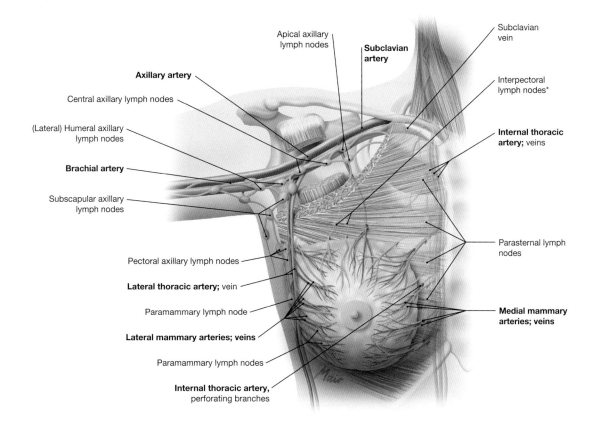

Apical axillary
lymph nodes

**Subclavian
artery**

Subclavian
vein

Axillary artery

Central axillary lymph nodes

(Lateral) Humeral axillary
lymph nodes

Brachial artery

Subscapular axillary
lymph nodes

Interpectoral
lymph nodes*

**Internal thoracic
artery;** veins

Parasternal lymph
nodes

Pectoral axillary lymph nodes

Lateral thoracic artery; vein

Paramammary lymph node

Lateral mammary arteries; veins

Paramammary lymph nodes

Internal thoracic artery,
perforating branches

**Medial mammary
arteries; veins**

Fig. 5.14 Arteries and veins of the mammary gland. Arteries are labelled and corresponding veins are shown. [L127]

* clin. term: ROTTER's lymph nodes

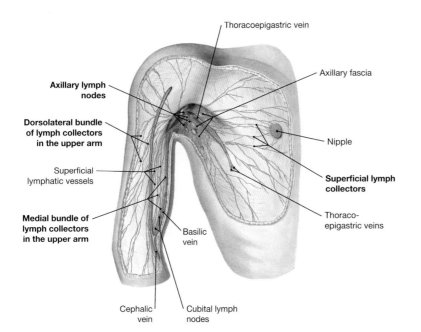

Fig. 5.15 Superficial axillary lymph vessels and nodes in the axillary fossa; anterior view.
The axillary lymph nodes collect lymph from the arm and serve as regional lymph nodes in the wall of the upper quadrants of the trunk and back.

Clinical Remarks

Surgery for breast cancer is performed either as removal of the whole breast (**mastectomy**) or as breast-conserving surgery only removing the tumor with some normal tissue around it (**lumpectomy**) followed by radiation therapy.

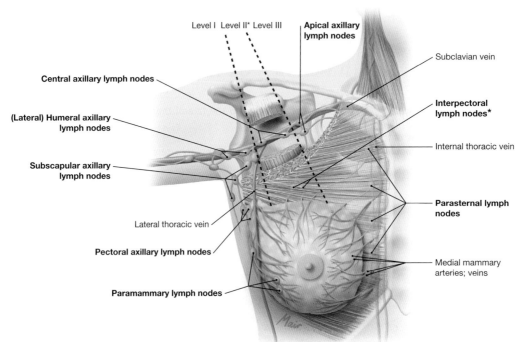

Fig. 5.16 Lymphatic drainage, regional lymph nodes and blood supply of the female breast. [L127]
The approximately 40 axillary lymph nodes do not just filter the lymph of almost the entire upper limb but take on also two thirds of the lymph from the breast and the major part of the lymph fluids derived from the thoracic and upper abdominal wall. The **subclavian lymph trunk** collects the lymph of the axillary nodes and drains into the **right lymphatic duct** and the **thoracic duct** (not shown) on the right and left side, respectively.
* clin. term: ROTTER's lymph nodes

Structure/Function

Lymph nodes of the female breast are categorized into **three hierarchical levels.** The pectoralis minor muscle acts as a boundary:
- **Level I** lies lateral to the pectoralis minor.
- **Level II** lies inferior to the pectoralis minor.
- **Level III** lies medial to the pectoralis minor.

The parasternal lymph nodes of both sides are interconnected. Level I lymph nodes are referred to as **sentinel** (= the one that keeps guard) **nodes** which are usually also the first lymph nodes of metastatic colonization. The number of affected lymph nodes in the three hierarchical levels is directly related to the survival rate. Breast carcinoma of the medial quadrants can metastasize via the interconnected parasternal lymph nodes to the contralateral side.

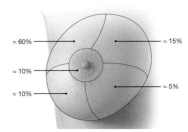

Frequency of mammary carcinoma in relation to the location in percentage.

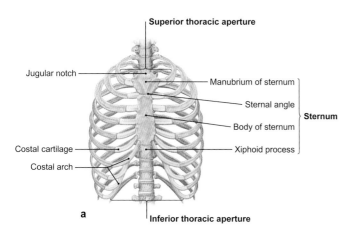

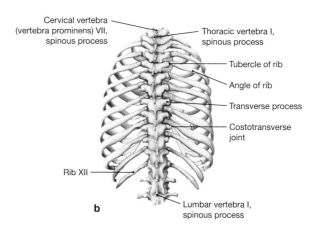

Fig. 5.17a and b Thoracic skeleton; anterior (a) and posterior (b) views. [L127]

The rib cage (➤ Fig. 2.39) consists of the sternum, 12 pairs of ribs and costal cartilages, and 12 thoracic vertebrae. The costal cartilages of ribs I–VII directly articulate with the sternum **(true ribs),** whereas ribs VIII–X are indirectly connected via the costal cartilages of the next upper rib **(false ribs),** and ribs XI and XII lack an anterior connection **(floating ribs).** The medial aspect of the clavicle is anterior to the 1st rib.

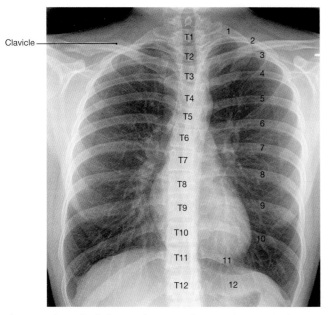

Fig. 5.18 Thoracic skeleton. Chest X-ray in posterior-anterior beam projection. The ribs are numbered on their posterior aspects. [T975]

Fig. 5.19a and b Sternum; anterior (a) and lateral (b) views.

The sternum (➤ Fig. 3.11) comprises the manubrium, body and xiphoid process. The **jugular notch** is a palpable surface landmark for the ventral upper margin of the superior thoracic aperture (clin. term: thoracic outlet). The sternum articulates with the clavicles and with the upper ribs (I–VII). The manubrium and body of sternum are connected by the manubriosternal symphysis (*clin. term: angle of LOUIS). The xiphoid process may be divided.

Structure/Function

The first rib is not palpable as it is covered by the clavicle and the associated muscles.

The **angle of LOUIS (sternal angle)** is a palpable surface landmark for the:

- transition from superior to inferior mediastinum;
- articulation with the 2nd costal cartilage;
- horizontal thoracic level of vertebra T4/T5;
- tracheal bifurcation.

The sternum (similar to the iliac bone) contains red bone marrow in adults and is accessible for **bone marrow aspiration** (biopsy).

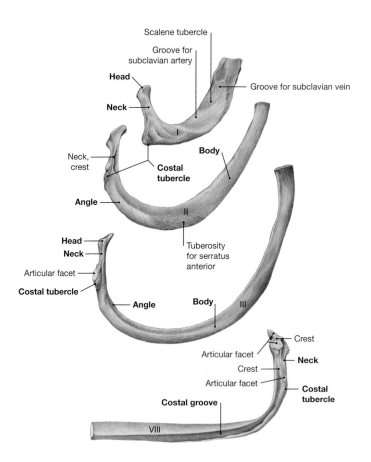

Fig. 5.20 Ribs; ribs I–III: superior view; rib VIII: inferior view.
Ribs III to X have the typical rib shape with head, neck, costal tubercle and body. The head of rib is wedge-shaped and has two joint facets. The costal tubercle has one joint and articulates with the corresponding transverse process of the thoracic vertebra. The intercostal artery, vein and nerve course in close proximity to the costal groove.

Clinical Remarks

Supernumerary or accessory ribs are common in the cervical region **(cervical ribs),** mostly C7, and can occur uni- or bilaterally. Cervical ribs may connect to the first thoracic rib or to the sternum and may cause a compression of the brachial plexus and the subclavian artery **(thoracic outlet syndrome: TOS).**

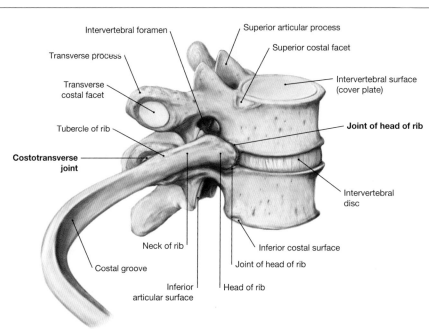

Fig. 5.21 Costovertebral joints; shown for vertebrae T7 and T8. [L266]
Both costovertebral joints (➤ Fig. 2.39), the **joint of head of rib** and the **costotransverse joint,** are synovial plane joints. Their small gliding and rotational movements facilitate the elevation and depression movements of the lateral and anterior parts of the ribs.

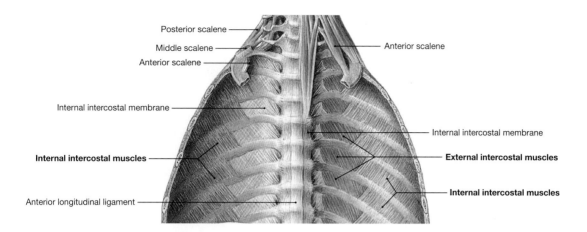

Fig. 5.22 Muscles of the posterior thoracic wall; anterior view with anterior part of the thoracic cage removed.
The **external intercostal muscles** project from posterior cranial to anterior caudal. They **elevate the ribs** during inspiration. The **internal** intercostal muscles project from posterior caudal to anterior cranial. They act during expiration by **depressing the ribs.** Not shown are the subcostal muscles which stretch across multiple segments and serve the same function as the internal intercostal muscles.

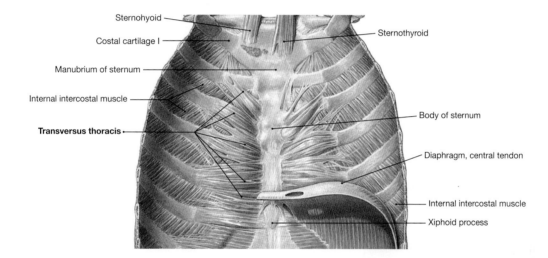

Fig. 5.23 Muscles of the anterior thoracic wall; posterior view with posterior part of the thoracic cage removed.
The view onto the inner side of the anterior thoracic wall displays the sternum and the muscular bundles of the **transversus thoracis.** They originate from the lateral side of the sternum and of the xiphoid process and insert on the inside of the costal cartilages of ribs II–VI. The transversus thoracis supports expiration.

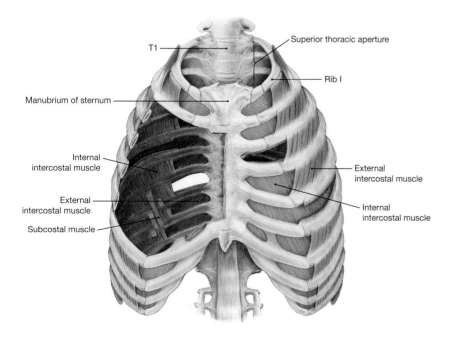

Fig. 5.24 Superior thoracic aperture and intercostal muscles; anterior view. [L285]
The superior thoracic aperture is bordered by the vertebra T1, the first ribs and the superior border of the manubrium. Intercostal muscles of the posterior thorax wall (right side) and the anterior thorax wall (left side) are shown.

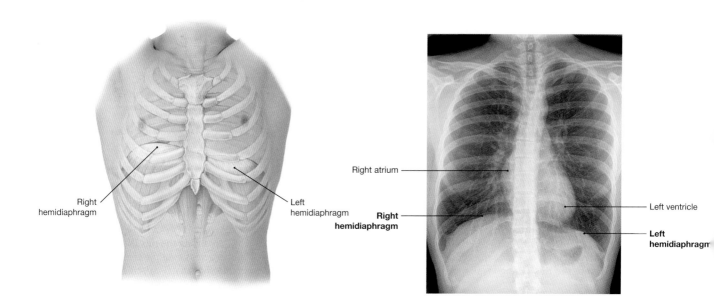

Fig. 5.25 Diaphragm. [L285]
The diaphragm originates from the margins of the inferior thoracic aperture. The central tendon is the aponeurosis of the diaphragm.

Fig. 5.26 Chest X-ray in posterior-anterior (P/A) projection. The right dome of the diaphragm projects higher than its left dome.

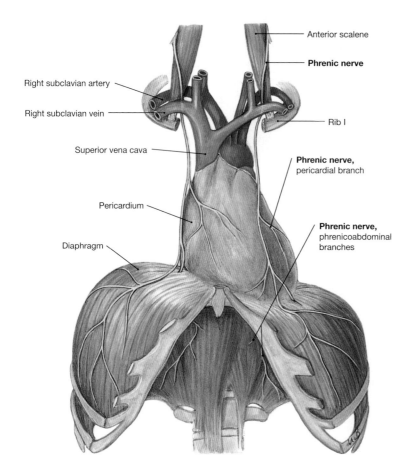

Fig. 5.27 Innervation of the diaphragm: phrenic nerve.
The phrenic nerve originates from the C3, C4, C5 spinal cord segments of the cervical plexus and descends **anterior to the anterior scalene muscle** (landmark!) in the neck. It enters the mediastinum posterior to the subclavian vein and descends **anterior to the root of the lung** together with the pericardiacophrenic blood vessels between the pericardium and the mediastinal pleura to the diaphragm. The phrenic nerves provide motor innervation to the diaphragm and sensory innervation to the pericardium (pericardial branch), the diaphragmatic pleura, and the parietal peritoneum at the abdominal side of the diaphragm (phrenicoabdominal branches).

Structure/Function

Due to the size of the liver the dome of the **right hemidiaphragm** reaches further cranially and projects to the level of thoracic vertebra **T8** as seen in a chest X-ray or axial CT or MRI scans. The **left dome** of the diaphragm projects to the level of **T9.**

Clinical Remarks

Injury to the phrenic nerve may occur in the neck or the mediastinum where it courses in close proximity to the hilum of the lung. Phrenic nerve lesions cause unilateral **diaphragmatic paralysis** which usually remains asymptomatic during normal daily activity.

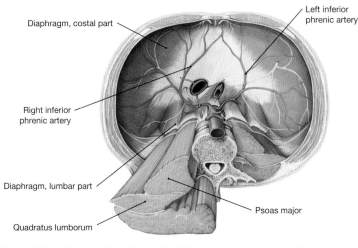

Left inferior phrenic artery

Diaphragm, costal part

Right inferior phrenic artery

Diaphragm, lumbar part

Quadratus lumborum

Psoas major

Fig. 5.28 Blood supply of the diaphragm; inferior view. [L285]
In addition to the right and left superior phrenic arteries (not shown) branching off the thoracic aorta, the right and left inferior phrenic arteries supply the diaphragm as first paired branches of the abdominal aorta.

Blood Supply of the Diaphragm

Origin of Artery	Arterial Branch	Supply to
Internal thoracic artery (branch of subclavian artery)	Pericardiacophrenic artery (courses with phrenic nerve)	Domes of diaphragm
	Musculophrenic artery	Costal parts of diaphragm
	Phrenicoabdominal branch	Sternal parts of diaphragm
Thoracic aorta	Superior phrenic arteries	Lumbar part of diaphragm
Abdominal aorta	Inferior phrenic arteries	Major blood supply to diaphragm

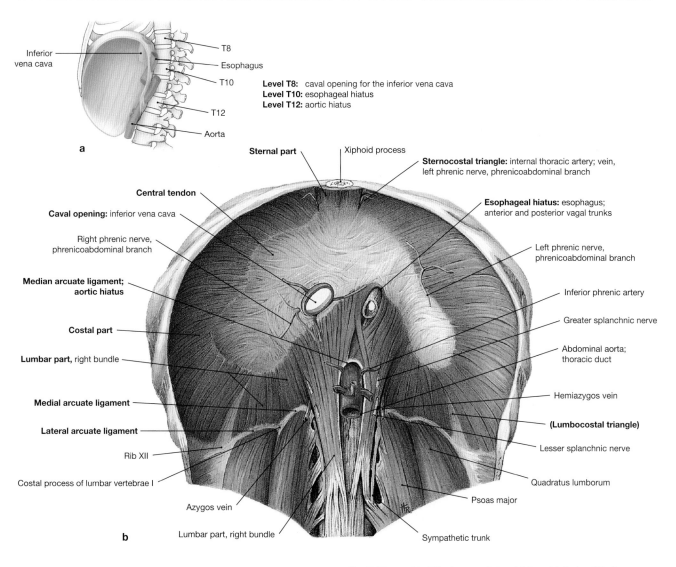

Inferior vena cava — T8

Esophagus

T10

Level T8: caval opening for the inferior vena cava
Level T10: esophageal hiatus
Level T12: aortic hiatus

T12

Aorta

a

Sternal part — Xiphoid process

Sternocostal triangle: internal thoracic artery; vein, left phrenic nerve, phrenicoabdominal branch

Central tendon

Caval opening: inferior vena cava

Esophageal hiatus: esophagus; anterior and posterior vagal trunks

Right phrenic nerve, phrenicoabdominal branch

Left phrenic nerve, phrenicoabdominal branch

Median arcuate ligament; aortic hiatus

Inferior phrenic artery

Costal part

Greater splanchnic nerve

Lumbar part, right bundle

Abdominal aorta; thoracic duct

Medial arcuate ligament

Hemiazygos vein

Lateral arcuate ligament

(Lumbocostal triangle)

Rib XII

Lesser splanchnic nerve

Costal process of lumbar vertebrae I

Quadratus lumborum

Azygos vein

Psoas major

b   Lumbar part, right bundle

Sympathetic trunk

Fig. 5.29a und b Diaphragm; lateral **(a)** and inferior **(b)** views.
a [L285]

Structure/Function

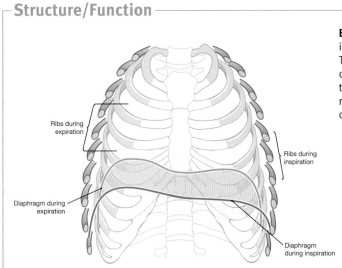

Excursions of the thorax during respiration; schematic drawing. [L126]
The driving force for respiration at rest is the contraction of the diaphragm resulting in an increased vertical dimension of the thorax. In forced respiration, the inspiratory muscles of the thoracic wall contribute to increased transverse and anteroposterior dimensions of the thorax.

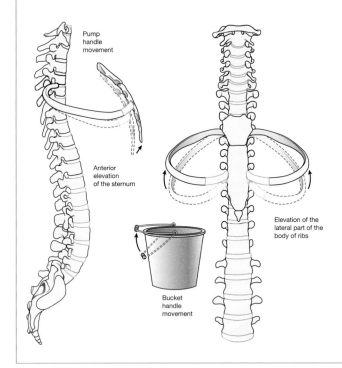

Pump handle and bucket handle movements of the rib cage during respiration; schematic drawings. [L126]
The pump handle movement represents the elevation of the ribs resulting in an increased anteroposterior (A/P) dimension of the inferior thorax. The bucket handle movement reflects the lateral elevation of the middle part of the lower ribs which increases the transverse dimension of the thorax.

Muscles of Respiration		
Muscle	**Innervation**	**Action**
Scalene muscles (anterior, middle and posterior scalene)	Muscular branches of cervical and brachial plexus (C3–C6)	Inspiration (auxiliary) Elevation of 1st rib (anterior and middle scalene muscles) and of 2nd rib (posterior scalene muscle)
External intercostal muscles	Intercostal nerves	Inspiration (elevation of ribs)
Internal intercostal muscles	Intercostal nerves	Expiration (depression of ribs)
Innermost intercostal muscles	Intercostal nerves	Expiration (depression of ribs)
Transversus thoracis muscle	Intercostal nerves	Expiration (depression of ribs)
Subcostal muscle (inconsistent)	Intercostal nerves	Expiration (depression of ribs)
Diaphragm	Phrenic nerve (C3–C5)	Inspiration
Latissimus dorsi muscle (➤ chapter 2)	Thoracodorsal nerve (C6–C8)	Forced expiration (coughing) Compresses lower rib cage when arms are fixed

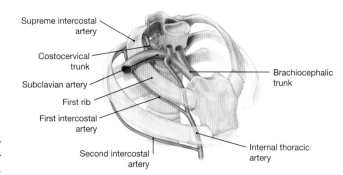

Fig. 5.30 Arteries of the superior two intercostal spaces. [L285]
The first two posterior intercostal arteries derive from the subclavian artery via the costocervical trunk and anastomose with the respective anterior intercostal arteries of the internal thoracic artery.

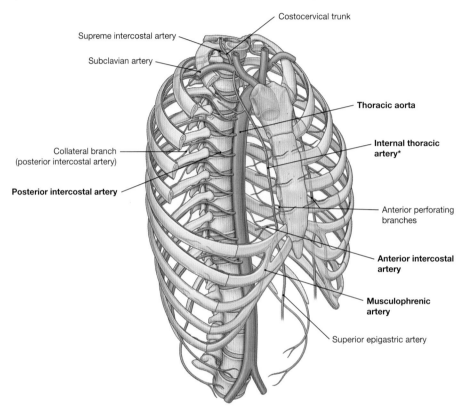

Fig. 5.31 Arteries of the thoracic wall. [E402]
The **posterior intercostal arteries** branch off the thoracic aorta and anastomose with the **anterior intercostal branches** of the **internal thoracic (internal mammary) artery.** The **musculophrenic artery,** a branch of the internal thoracic artery, courses beneath the costal arch.

* clin. term: internal mammary artery

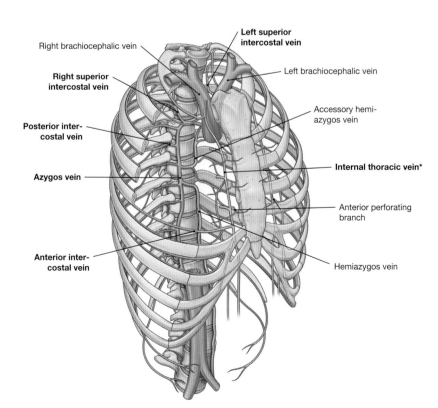

Fig. 5.32 Veins of the thoracic wall. [E402]
Superior and inferior venae cavae are connected by the lumbar, hemiazygos and azygos veins. Additional anastomoses exist between the azygos system and the internal thoracic vein through the **anterior and posterior intercostal veins.** They drain the venous blood of the thoracic and abdominal walls.

* clin. term: internal mammary vein

239

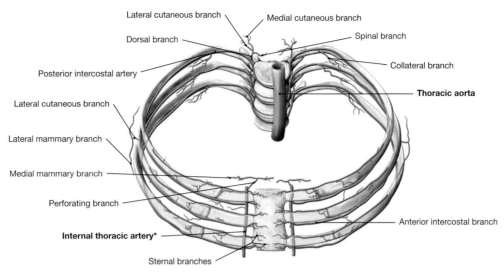

Fig. 5.33 Intercostal arteries. [L266]

The intercostal arteries create anastomoses between the internal thoracic artery (anterior intercostal arteries) and the thoracic aorta (posterior intercostal arteries).

* clin. term: internal mammary artery

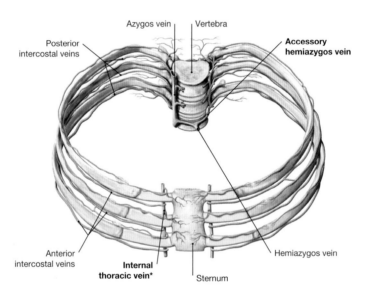

Fig. 5.34 Intercostal veins. [L127]

The intercostal veins connect the internal thoracic vein and the azygos venous system.

* clin. term: internal mammary vein

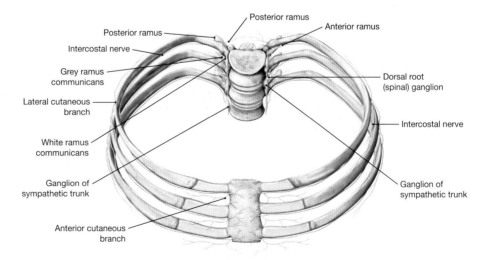

Fig. 5.35 Intercostal nerves. [L127]

Intercostal nerves are the anterior branches (anterior rami) of the thoracic nerves T1–T11.

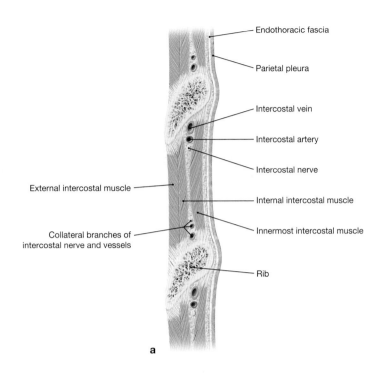

Endothoracic fascia

Parietal pleura

Intercostal vein

Intercostal artery

Intercostal nerve

External intercostal muscle

Internal intercostal muscle

Innermost intercostal muscle

Collateral branches of
intercostal nerve and vessels

Rib

a

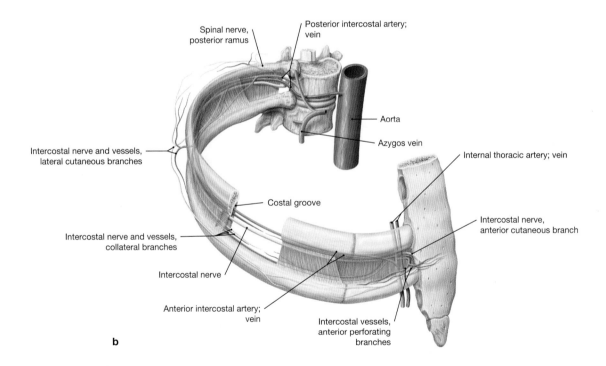

Spinal nerve,
posterior ramus

Posterior intercostal artery;
vein

Aorta

Azygos vein

Intercostal nerve and vessels,
lateral cutaneous branches

Internal thoracic artery; vein

Costal groove

Intercostal nerve,
anterior cutaneous branch

Intercostal nerve and vessels,
collateral branches

Intercostal nerve

Anterior intercostal artery;
vein

Intercostal vessels,
anterior perforating
branches

b

**Fig. 5.36a and b Position of the intercostal neurovascular struc-
tures;** longitudinal section **(a)** and schematic illustration **(b).** The
collateral branches appear near the costal angle. [L285]

Structure/Function

The intercostal neurovascular structures course between the internal and innermost intercostal muscles with a typical topography from superior to inferior: **vein – artery – nerve (VAN).** Thus,
the intercostal nerve is the least protected by the costal groove.

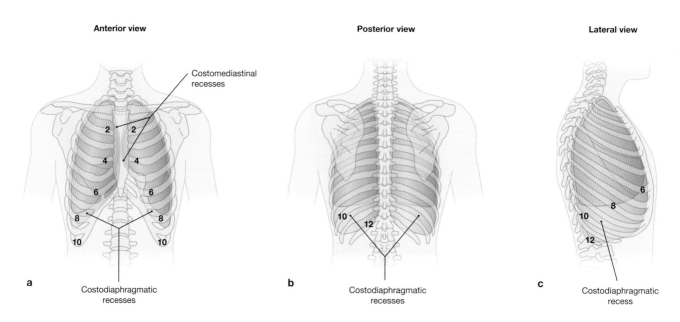

Anterior view

Posterior view

Lateral view

Costomediastinal recesses

a

Costodiaphragmatic recesses

b

Costodiaphragmatic recesses

c

Costodiaphragmatic recess

Fig. 5.37a to c Projection of lungs and pleura; schematic drawings anterior (**a**), posterior (**b**) and lateral (**c**) views. [L127]
Visceral pleura covering the lungs is represented in brown color; extension of the parietal pleura is shown in blue color. Selected ribs are numbered. Each lung resides in a separate pleural cavity.

The **costodiaphragmatic** and **costomediastinal recesses** are pleural spaces in which the lungs can extend during forced inspiration.

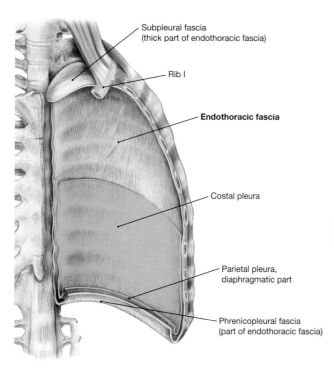

Subpleural fascia (thick part of endothoracic fascia)

Rib I

Endothoracic fascia

Costal pleura

Parietal pleura, diaphragmatic part

Phrenicopleural fascia (part of endothoracic fascia)

Fig. 5.38 Thoracic cavity, left side; view from inside after removal of the left lung. [L285]
The inner thoracic wall is lined by the **endothoracic fascia.** The **costal pleura** (a part of the parietal pleura) is tightly adjacent to the endothoracic fascia.

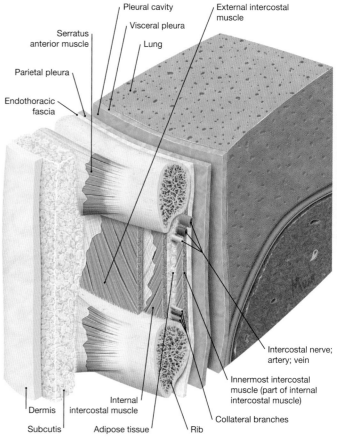

Pleural cavity

External intercostal muscle

Serratus anterior muscle

Visceral pleura

Lung

Parietal pleura

Endothoracic fascia

Dermis

Subcutis

Internal intercostal muscle

Adipose tissue

Rib

Intercostal nerve; artery; vein

Innermost intercostal muscle (part of internal intercostal muscle)

Collateral branches

Fig. 5.39 Layers of the thoracic wall. [L127]

Clinical Remarks

The apex of lung and the **cervical pleura** extend up to 5 cm above the level of the superior thoracic aperture. Thus, with placement of a central venous catheter (central line) via the subclavian or internal jugular veins, injury to the cervical pleura may cause a **pneumothorax** with resulting collapse of the lung.

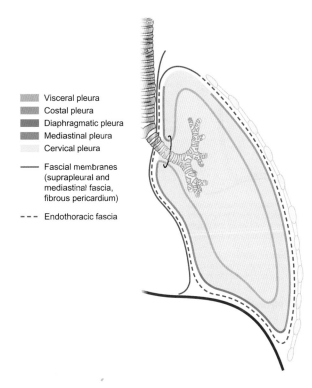

Visceral pleura
Costal pleura
Diaphragmatic pleura
Mediastinal pleura
Cervical pleura

—— Fascial membranes
(suprapleural and
mediastinal fascia,
fibrous pericardium)

--- Endothoracic fascia

Fig. 5.40 Pleural cavity; schematic drawing. [L126]
The right and left pleural cavities are separate spaces. The **visceral pleura** covers the lungs and is continuous with the parietal pleura at the hilum of lung. The **parietal pleura** has several parts referred to as costal, diaphragmatic, mediastinal and cervical pleura. The narrow space between the visceral and parietal pleura is the pleural cavity.

Clinical Remarks

During a physical examination, the expansion of the lung into the costodiaphragmatic recess can be assessed by auscultation and percussion during deep inspiration and expiration. If air enters the pleural cavity the capillary force between the pleural layers is abolished and the lung collapses **(pneumothorax)** due to the elastic recoil of the lung tissue. This causes a loud (hypersonorous) sound during percussion with concurrent lack of breath sounds upon auscultation. With a pneumothorax the lung cannot follow the respiratory movements of the thoracic wall resulting in lack of ventilation for the respective lung.
a [T975], b [L126]

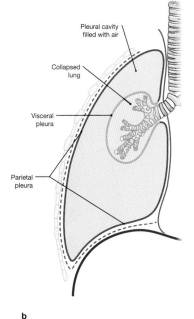

Pleural cavity
filled with air

Collapsed
lung

Visceral
pleura

Parietal
pleura

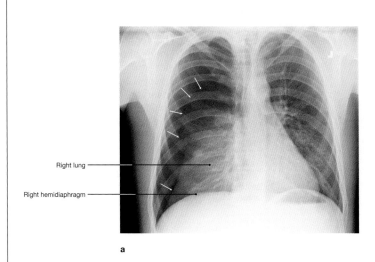

Right lung

Right hemidiaphragm

a

b

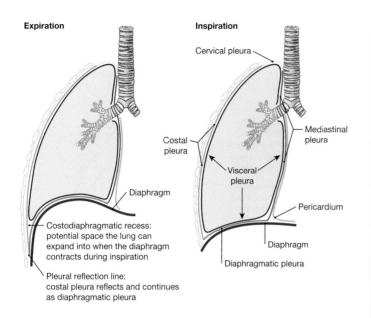

Expiration

Inspiration

Cervical pleura

Costal pleura

Mediastinal pleura

Visceral pleura

Diaphragm

Pericardium

Costodiaphragmatic recess: potential space the lung can expand into when the diaphragm contracts during inspiration

Diaphragm

Diaphragmatic pleura

Pleural reflection line: costal pleura reflects and continues as diaphragmatic pleura

Fig. 5.41 Pleural movements during respiration; schematic drawings. [L126]

The pleural cavity contains a capillary film of serous fluid produced by the pleura which reduces friction during respiration. Importantly, this capillary fluid film forces the visceral pleura of the lungs to follow the movements of the parietal pleura and thus, is the driving force of lung expansions with movements of the thoracic wall and diaphragm.

Clinical Remarks

Increased fluid in the pleural cavity **(pleural effusion)** will collect in the costodiaphragmatic recess when the patient is in the upright position. Needle insertion through the intercostal space for thoracocentesis may be required to drain the fluid in the case of a large pleural effusion. Pain during breathing usually derives from the pleura and shows involvement of the somatically innervated parietal pleura. [T975]

Fluid of a pleural effusion

Sensory Innervation of the Pleura	
Visceral pleura: autonomic innervation	
Parietal pleura: somatic innervation	
Cervical pleura (yellow)	
Mediastinal pleura (red)	Phrenic nerve
Diaphragmatic pleura (central part) (green)	
Diaphragmatic pleura (peripheral part) (green)	Intercostal nerves
Costal pleura (blue)	

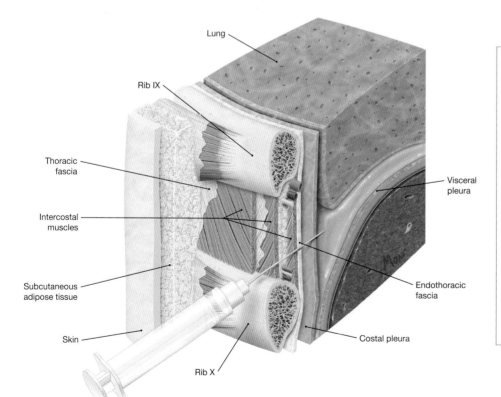

Lung

Rib IX

Thoracic fascia

Intercostal muscles

Subcutaneous adipose tissue

Skin

Rib X

Visceral pleura

Endothoracic fascia

Costal pleura

Structure/Function

To access pleural fluids for diagnostic reasons a **thoracocentesis** is performed: the needle is inserted in the 8th or 9th intercostal space closer to the upper border of the lower rib to avoid injury of the major neurovascular structures near the costal groove. The collateral branches near the lower rib are much smaller. The needle penetrates the following structures:

*   Skin and subcutaneous fascia
*   Thoracic fascia
*   External intercostal muscles
*   Internal and innermost intercostal muscles
*   Endothoracic fascia
*   Parietal (costal) pleura

Fig. 5.42 Structures of the intercostal space; schematic drawing. [L127]

Layers of the thoracic wall pierced by the needle when performing a thoracocentesis. The main intercostal neurovascular structures and their much smaller collaterals are shown.

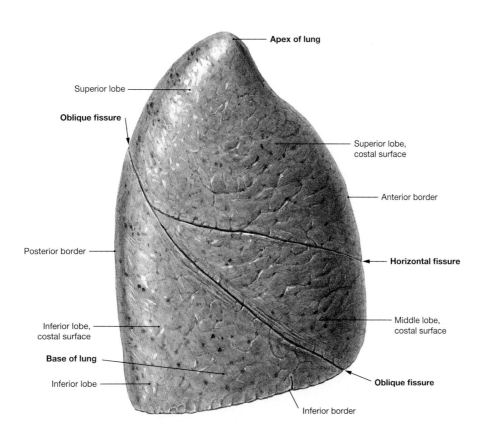

Fig. 5.43 Right lung; lateral view.
The right lung has three lobes (superior, middle and inferior lobes) which are separated by the **oblique** and the **horizontal fissures.**

The apex of lung is the superior part, the broad base of lung is the inferior part. The visceral pleura covers the surface of the lung and follows into the fissures.

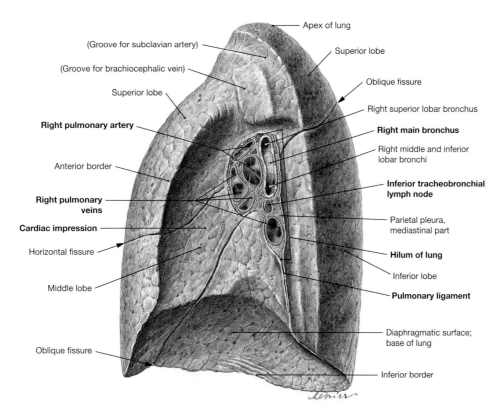

Fig. 5.44 Right lung; medial view.
The **hilum of lung** (root of the lung) is the medially positioned entry for the main bronchi and the neurovascular structures to the lungs. At the hilum, the visceral pleura blends into the parietal pleura. This pleural fold extends inferiorly into the **pulmonary ligament.**
The topographical orientation of the main bronchi in relation to the great blood vessels at the hilum is different for both lungs. At the

right lung, the main bronchus is the most superior structure and the pulmonary artery is positioned anteriorly. The pulmonary veins are positioned anteriorly and inferiorly within the hilum. The **tracheobronchial lymph nodes** are located at the hilum (clin. term: hilar nodes).

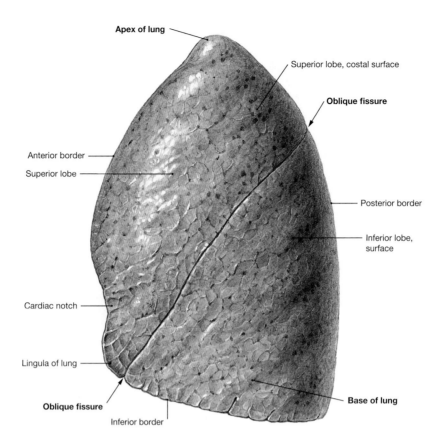

Apex of lung

Superior lobe, costal surface

Oblique fissure

Anterior border

Superior lobe

Posterior border

Inferior lobe, surface

Cardiac notch

Lingula of lung

Oblique fissure

Inferior border

Base of lung

Fig. 5.45 Left lung; lateral view.
The left lung has only two lobes (superior and inferior lobes) separated by the **oblique fissure.** The apex of lung is the superior part,

the broad base of lung is the inferior part. The visceral pleura covers the surface of the lungs and follows into the fissures.

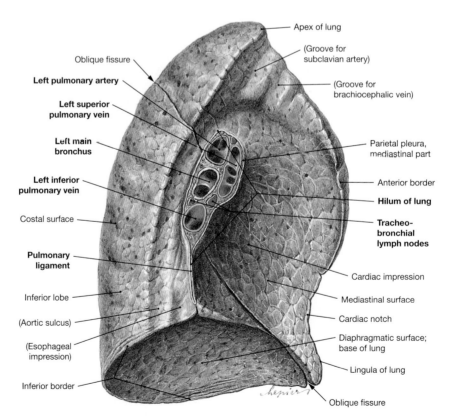

Apex of lung

(Groove for subclavian artery)

Oblique fissure

(Groove for brachiocephalic vein)

Left pulmonary artery

Left superior pulmonary vein

Left main bronchus

Parietal pleura, mediastinal part

Anterior border

Hilum of lung

Left inferior pulmonary vein

Tracheo-bronchial lymph nodes

Costal surface

Pulmonary ligament

Cardiac impression

Mediastinal surface

Inferior lobe

Cardiac notch

(Aortic sulcus)

Diaphragmatic surface; base of lung

(Esophageal impression)

Lingula of lung

Inferior border

Oblique fissure

Fig. 5.46 Left lung; medial view.
The **hilum of lung** is the medially positioned entry for the main bronchi and the neurovascular structures to the lungs. At the hilum, the visceral pleura blends into the parietal pleura. This pleural fold extends inferiorly into the **pulmonary ligament.** In contrast to

the right lung, the main bronchus of the left lung is positioned below the pulmonary artery. The pulmonary veins are positioned anteriorly and inferiorly within the hilum. The **tracheobronchial lymph nodes** are located at the hilum (clin. term: hilar nodes).

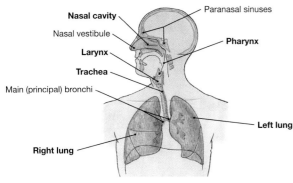

Fig. 5.47 Respiratory tract: upper and lower airways; overview.

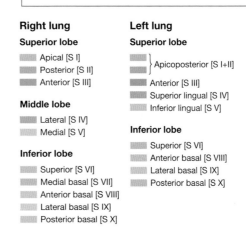

Fig. 5.48 Trachea and bronchial tree.

Right main bronchus

Right superior lobar bronchus
   1 = Apical segmental bronchus [B I]
   2 = Posterior segmental bronchus [B II]
   3 = Anterior segmental bronchus [B III]

Right middle lobar bronchus
   4 = Lateral segmental bronchus [B IV]
   5 = Medial segmental bronchus [B V]

Right inferior lobar bronchus
   6 = Superior segmental bronchus [B VI]
   7 = Medial basal segmental bronchus [B VII]
   8 = Anterior basal segmental bronchus [B VIII]
   9 = Lateral basal segmental bronchus [B IX]
   10 = Posterior basal segmental bronchus [B X]

Left main bronchus

Left superior lobar bronchus
   1, 2 = Apicoposterior segmental bronchus [B I+II]
   3 = Anterior segmental bronchus [B III]
   4 = Superior lingular bronchus [B IV]
   5 = Inferior lingular bronchus [B V]

Left inferior lobar bronchus
   6 = Superior segmental bronchus [VI]
   8 = Anterior basal segmental bronchus [VIII]
   9 = Lateral basal segmental bronchus [IX]
   10 = Posterior basal segmental bronchus [X]

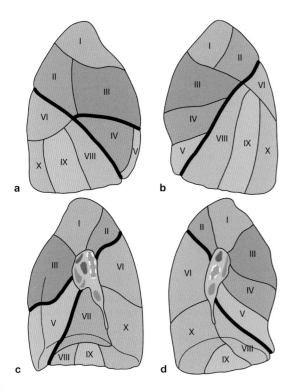

Fig. 5.49a to d Bronchopulmonary segments of the right and left lungs.

Clinical Remarks

The volume of the airways of the respiratory tract (from the nose to the terminal bronchioles in the lungs) is referred to as **anatomical dead space** (150–170 ml [5–5.7 fl oz]) due to the lack of gas exchange capacity. Thus, artificial ventilation is more effective when performed with low frequency and with larger volumes.

The right main bronchus is a relatively straight continuation from the trachea. Therefore, **foreign body aspiration** occurs more frequently in the right main bronchus.

Right lung

Superior lobe
- Apical [S I]
- Posterior [S II]
- Anterior [S III]

Middle lobe
- Lateral [S IV]
- Medial [S V]

Inferior lobe
- Superior [S VI]
- Medial basal [S VII]
- Anterior basal [S VIII]
- Lateral basal [S IX]
- Posterior basal [S X]

Left lung

Superior lobe
- } Apicoposterior [S I+II]
- Anterior [S III]
- Superior lingual [S IV]
- Inferior lingual [S V]

Inferior lobe
- Superior [S VI]
- Anterior basal [S VIII]
- Lateral basal [S IX]
- Posterior basal [S X]

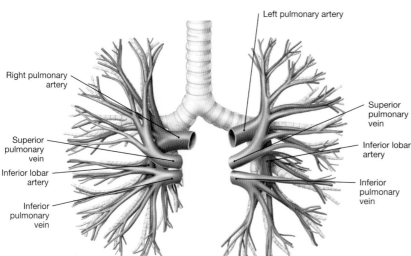

Fig. 5.50 Pulmonary circulation; overview. [L275]
At each hilum one pulmonary artery (deoxygenated blood) enters the lung and two pulmonary veins (oxygenated blood) leave the lung to reach the left atrium of the heart. Branches of the pulmonary artery course in close proximity to the bronchi.

Clinical Remarks

In cases of secondary lung metastases or primary lung cancer the affected lobe **(lobectomy)** or segment **(segment resection)** can be surgically removed.

The **bronchopulmonary segment** is the smallest surgically resectable subdivision of the lobes of the lungs. Each segment contains a segmental bronchus and accompanying blood vessels. The base of the cone-shaped segments is positioned towards the peripheral surface of the lung.

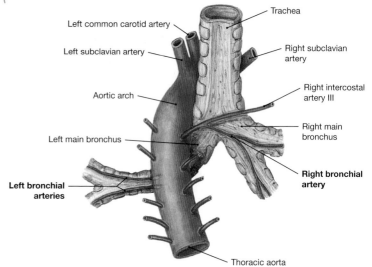

Fig. 5.51 Bronchial blood vessels; posterior view.
The small bronchial arteries supply the lung tissue with oxygenated blood. They derive directly from the thoracic aorta on the left side, but usually branch off the third intercostal artery on the right side. The bronchial veins are highly variable and drain into the azygos system (not shown here).

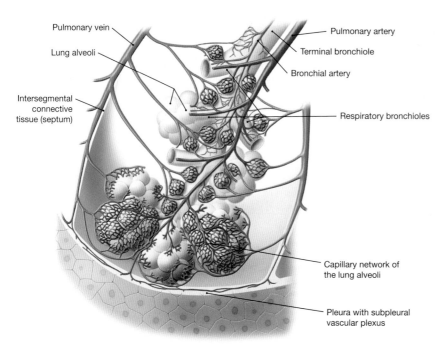

Fig. 5.52 Bronchopulmonary segment and pulmonary vasculature; schematic drawing. [L238]
The bronchopulmonary segment is the smallest functional unit of the lungs. Branches of the pulmonary artery (shown in red) accompany the bronchial tree and continue in capillary networks around the alveoli of the lung. The pulmonary veins (shown in blue) course in the intersegmental connective tissue septa.

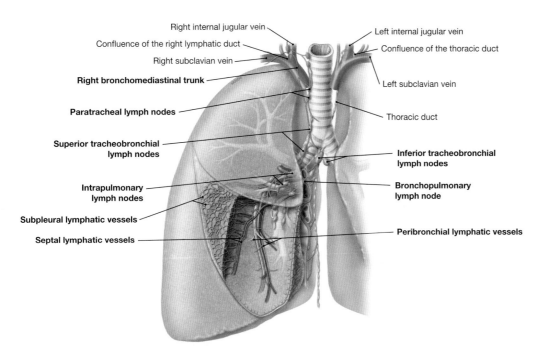

Fig. 5.53 Lymphatic vessels and lymph nodes of the lung; schematic drawing; anterior view. [L238]

The lung has two lymphatic systems which converge at the hilum. The peribronchial system follows the bronchi and feeds into several lymph node stations. The first station are the **intrapulmonary lymph nodes** at the transition from segmental to lobar bronchi. The second station comprises the **bronchopulmonary lymph nodes** at the hilum of lung (clin. term: hilar lymph nodes). The subsequent **tracheobron-**

chial lymph nodes are located above and below the tracheal bifurcation and near the extrapulmonary bronchi. From here the lymph passes on to the paratracheal lymph nodes or to the bronchomediastinal trunk on both sides. The subpleural and septal lymph systems drain into the tracheobronchial lymph nodes as the first station. Their delicate lymphatic vessels form a polygonal network at the surface of the lung.

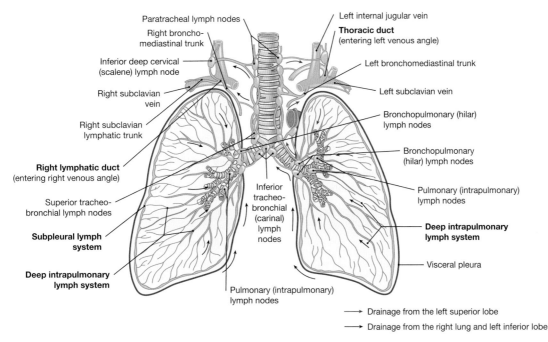

→ Drainage from the left superior lobe
→ Drainage from the right lung and left inferior lobe

Fig. 5.54 Lymphatic drainage of the lungs; schematic drawing. [L126]

The **intrapulmonary peribronchial** and the **subpleural lymph systems** converge at the bronchopulmonary lymph nodes (hilar nodes). The subsequent tracheobronchial lymph nodes drain via the right

and left bronchomediastinal trunks into the **right lymphatic duct** and **thoracic duct,** respectively. Importantly, the majority of the lymph from the lower lobe of the left lung drains via the right tracheobronchial lymph nodes into the right lymphatic duct.

Clinical Remarks

Determining the involvement of lymph nodes in cancer cell spreading is an important factor in clinical staging of lung cancer. **Pulmonary embolism** is the obstruction of one or more pulmonary arteries with a blot clot, most commonly derived from a

deep venous thrombosis (DVT) in the leg. The acute cardiovascular signs include an increased respiratory rate (tachypnea) and increased heart rate (tachycardia).

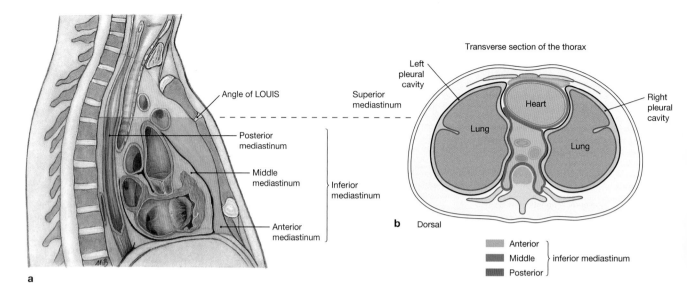

Fig. 5.55a and b Partitions of the mediastinum; schematic drawings, sagittal **(a)** and horizontal **(b)** views. b [L126]

The mediastinum is the space of the thoracic cavity that is located between the two pleural cavities.

Clinical Remarks

The manubriosternal angle (angle of LOUIS) is a palpable surface landmark for the separation between superior and inferior mediastinum.

Structure/Function

The thymus usually comprises two lobes and is positioned in the superior mediastinum behind the sternum. After puberty, the specific thymus parenchyma is gradually substituted by adi-

pose tissue and the residual functional thymus is hardly visible in the adult.

Major Anatomical Structures in the Mediastinum	
Superior Mediastinum	**Inferior Mediastinum**
<ul><li>Thymus</li><li>Great vessels</li><li>Brachiocephalic vein</li><li>Superior vena cava</li><li>Arch of Aorta:<ul><li>– Brachiocephalic trunk</li><li>– Left common carotid artery</li><li>– Left subclavian artery</li></ul></li><li>Vagus and phrenic nerves</li><li>Left recurrent laryngeal nerve</li><li>Sympathetic trunks</li><li>Cardiac nerve plexus</li><li>Trachea</li><li>Esophagus</li><li>Thoracic duct</li></ul>	Anterior Mediastinum (➤ Fig. 5.55b; green)<ul><li>Internal thoracic artery and vein</li><li>Thymus</li></ul>Middle Mediastinum (➤ Fig. 5.55b; blue)<ul><li>Heart and pericardium</li><li>Hilum of the lungs</li><li>Phrenic nerves and pericardiacophrenic vessels</li></ul>Posterior Mediastinum (➤ Fig. 5.55b; red)<ul><li>Thoracic aorta</li><li>Vagus nerve (right and left vagal trunks)</li><li>Azygos and hemiazygos veins</li><li>Esophageal nerve plexus</li><li>Thoracic sympathetic trunks and splanchnic nerves</li><li>Intercostal neurovascular structures</li><li>Esophagus</li><li>Thoracic duct</li><li>Posterior mediastinal lymph nodes</li></ul>

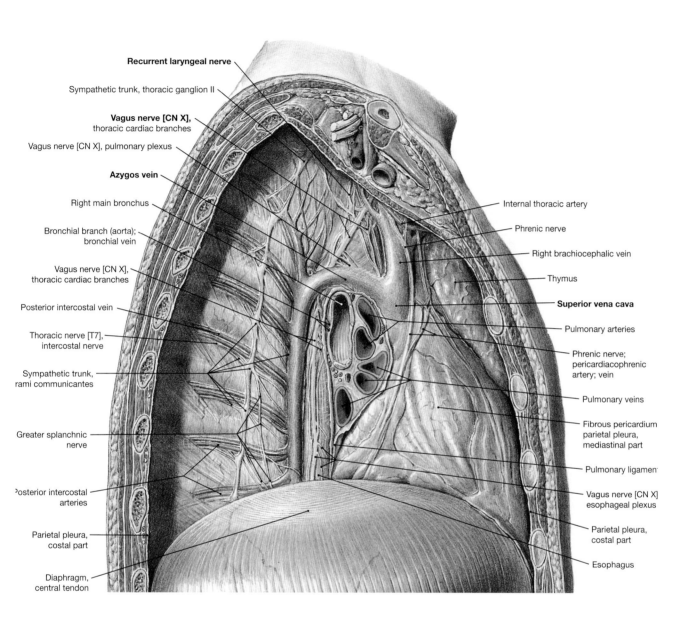

Recurrent laryngeal nerve

Sympathetic trunk, thoracic ganglion II

Vagus nerve [CN X], thoracic cardiac branches

Vagus nerve [CN X], pulmonary plexus

Azygos vein

Right main bronchus

Bronchial branch (aorta); bronchial vein

Vagus nerve [CN X], thoracic cardiac branches

Posterior intercostal vein

Thoracic nerve [T7], intercostal nerve

Sympathetic trunk, rami communicantes

Greater splanchnic nerve

Posterior intercostal arteries

Parietal pleura, costal part

Diaphragm, central tendon

Internal thoracic artery

Phrenic nerve

Right brachiocephalic vein

Thymus

Superior vena cava

Pulmonary arteries

Phrenic nerve; pericardiacophrenic artery; vein

Pulmonary veins

Fibrous pericardium parietal pleura, mediastinal part

Pulmonary ligamen

Vagus nerve [CN X] esophageal plexus

Parietal pleura, costal part

Esophagus

Fig. 5.56 Mediastinum and pleural cavity of an adolescent; view from the right side; after removal of the lateral thoracic wall and the right lung and pleura.

The azygos vein crosses the root of the right lung superiorly and enters the superior vena cava from posterior at the level of the thoracic vertebrae T4/T5. The vagus nerve [CN X] descends posterior and the phrenic nerve courses anterior to the root of the lung.

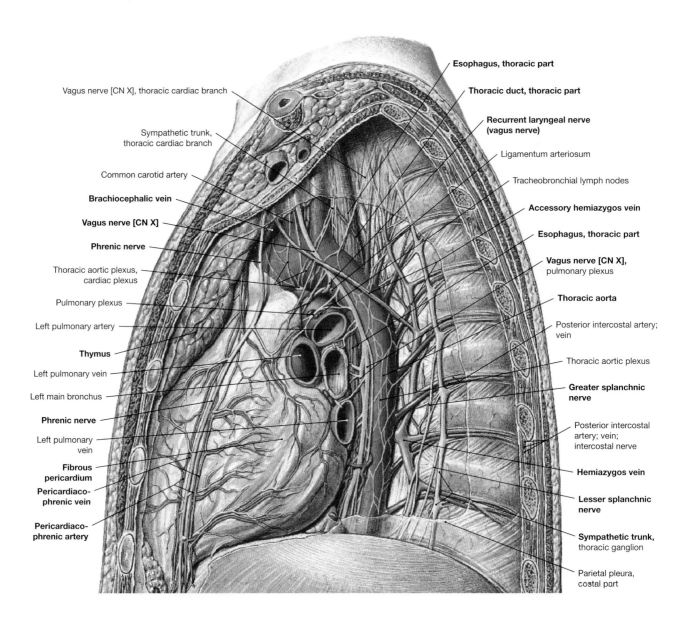

Vagus nerve [CN X], thoracic cardiac branch

Sympathetic trunk, thoracic cardiac branch

Common carotid artery

Brachiocephalic vein

Vagus nerve [CN X]

Phrenic nerve

Thoracic aortic plexus, cardiac plexus

Pulmonary plexus

Left pulmonary artery

Thymus

Left pulmonary vein

Left main bronchus

Phrenic nerve

Left pulmonary vein

Fibrous pericardium

Pericardiaco-phrenic vein

Pericardiaco-phrenic artery

Esophagus, thoracic part

Thoracic duct, thoracic part

Recurrent laryngeal nerve (vagus nerve)

Ligamentum arteriosum

Tracheobronchial lymph nodes

Accessory hemiazygos vein

Esophagus, thoracic part

Vagus nerve [CN X], pulmonary plexus

Thoracic aorta

Posterior intercostal artery; vein

Thoracic aortic plexus

Greater splanchnic nerve

Posterior intercostal artery; vein; intercostal nerve

Hemiazygos vein

Lesser splanchnic nerve

Sympathetic trunk, thoracic ganglion

Parietal pleura, costal part

Fig. 5.57 Mediastinum and pleural cavity of an adolescent; view from the left side; after removal of the lateral thoracic wall and the left lung and pleura.
The hemiazygos vein takes the blood from the accessory hemiazygos vein and drains into the azygos vein at the level of the thoracic vertebrae T7 to T10. The ganglia of the sympathetic trunk course near the heads of ribs and branch off the greater (major) splanchnic nerve and the lesser (minor) splanchnic nerve. The vagus nerve [CN X] descends next to the esophagus posterior to the root of lung. The phrenic nerve, accompanied by the pericardiacophrenic blood vessels, courses between the fibrous pericardium and mediastinal pleura (removed).

Clinical Remarks

The esophagus is posteriorly adjacent to the left atrium and just separated by the pericardium. Left atrial enlargement, such as in **mitral valve stenosis** leads to compression of the esophagus resulting in difficulty of swallowing **(dysphagia)**. **Transesophageal echocardiography** also utilizes the close proximity of the esophagus to the left atrium to obtain detailed information on the posterior aspect of the heart or the aorta.
[G198]

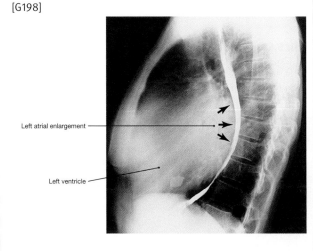

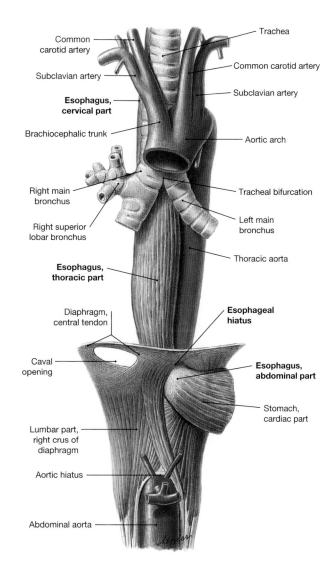

Fig. 5.58 Thoracic part of esophagus; anterior view.
The thoracic part of the esophagus courses in the posterior mediastinum. The aortic arch and the left main bronchus cause a physiological constriction of the esophagus at the level of T4/T5.

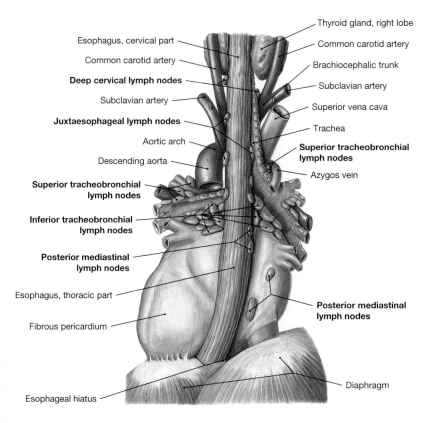

Fig. 5.59 Lymph nodes of the posterior mediastinum; dorsal view.
The lymph of the esophagus drains into lymph nodes directly adjacent to the esophagus (juxtaesophageal lymph nodes):
- **Cervical part:** deep cervical lymph nodes;
- **Thoracic and abdominal parts:** lymph nodes of the mediastinum (posterior mediastinal lymph nodes, tracheobronchial and paratracheal lymph nodes) and of the peritoneal cavity (inferior phrenic lymph nodes on the abdominal side of the diaphragm, gastric lymph nodes on the lesser curvature of the stomach).

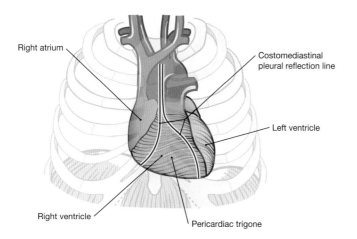

Right atrium

Costomediastinal pleural reflection line

Left ventricle

Right ventricle

Pericardiac trigone

Fig. 5.60 Projection of the heart onto the thorax; anterior view. [L126]
The apex of the heart is directed anteriorly and to the left side. The right ventricle is located behind the sternum.

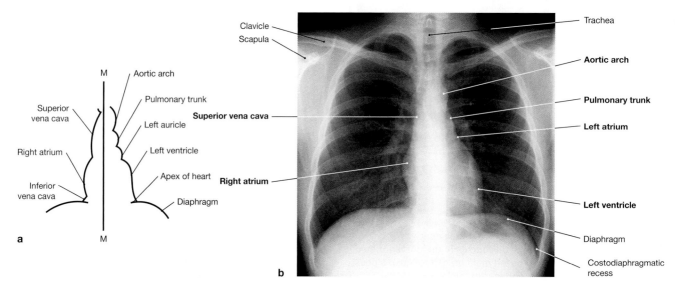

M

Aortic arch

Pulmonary trunk

Superior vena cava

Left auricle

Left ventricle

Right atrium

Apex of heart

Inferior vena cava

Diaphragm

a

M

Clavicle

Scapula

Trachea

Aortic arch

Pulmonary trunk

Superior vena cava

Left atrium

Right atrium

Left ventricle

Diaphragm

Costodiaphragmatic recess

b

Fig. 5.61a and b Chest X-ray with heart silhouette; posterior-anterior (P/A) beam projection.
The right ventricle is located behind the sternum and the left atrium is positioned posteriorly. The right ventricle does not partici-

pate in the formation of the cardiac borders in the P/A chest X-ray and the left atrium just forms a small contour through its auricle.

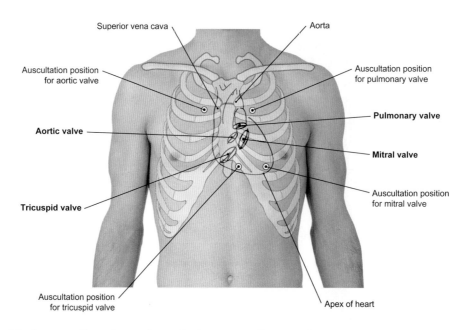

Superior vena cava

Aorta

Auscultation position for aortic valve

Auscultation position for pulmonary valve

Pulmonary valve

Aortic valve

Mitral valve

Tricuspid valve

Auscultation position for mitral valve

Auscultation position for tricuspid valve

Apex of heart

Fig. 5.62 Contours of the heart, cardiac valves and auscultation sites projected onto the anterior thoracic wall. [L126, K340]
*   The base of heart with all four cardiac valves has an oblique and posteriorly oriented position behind the sternum.

*   The apex of heart is positioned towards the anterior chest wall in the midclavicular line in the 5th intercostal space.

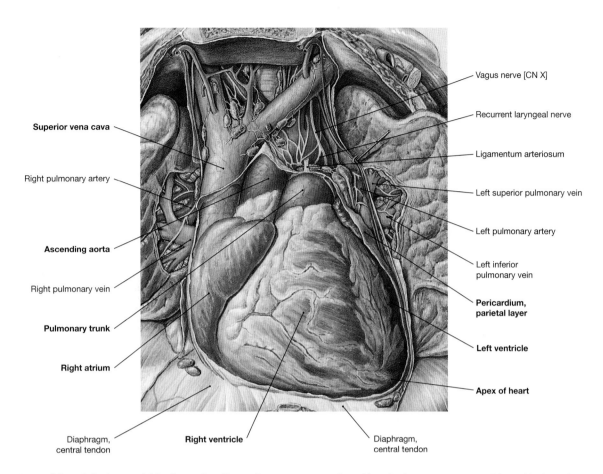

Superior vena cava

Right pulmonary artery

Ascending aorta

Right pulmonary vein

Pulmonary trunk

Right atrium

Vagus nerve [CN X]

Recurrent laryngeal nerve

Ligamentum arteriosum

Left superior pulmonary vein

Left pulmonary artery

Left inferior
pulmonary vein

Pericardium,
parietal layer

Left ventricle

Apex of heart

Diaphragm,
central tendon

Right ventricle

Diaphragm,
central tendon

Fig. 5.63 Position of the heart within the pericardium; after opening of the pericardium; anterior view.
The heart is positioned within the pericardial cavity in the middle mediastinum. The apex of heart points to the inferior left side and anteriorly. The right ventricle is located behind the body of sternum. The pericardium surrounds the heart, stabilizes its position and enables the heart to contract without friction. The roots of the great vessels are located within the pericardial sac: the inferior part of the superior vena cava, and the superior part of the inferior vena cava, ascending aorta, pulmonary trunk. The fibrous pericardium is adherent to the central tendon of the diaphragm.

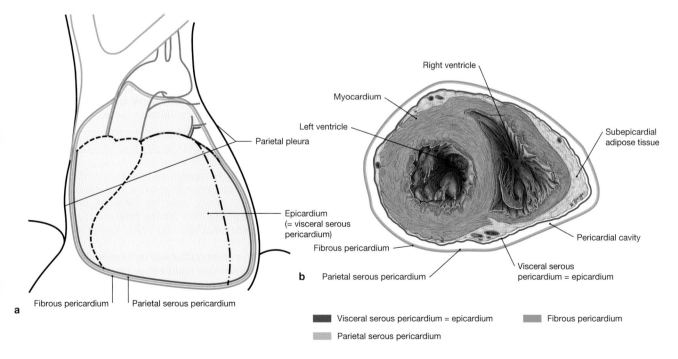

Parietal pleura

Epicardium
(= visceral serous
pericardium)

Fibrous pericardium

Parietal serous pericardium

Fibrous pericardium

Parietal serous pericardium

Right ventricle

Myocardium

Left ventricle

Subepicardial
adipose tissue

Pericardial cavity

Visceral serous
pericardium = epicardium

a

b

■ Visceral serous pericardium = epicardium   ■ Fibrous pericardium

▨ Parietal serous pericardium

Fig. 5.64a and b Layers of the pericardium; schematic drawings; anterior view **(a)**; cross-section of the heart **(b)**. a [L231]
The outer layer of the pericardium is the dense connective tissue of the **fibrous pericardium.** The **serous pericardium** comprises the visceral pericardial layer, referred to as **epicardium,** and the **parietal serous pericardium** that is adjacent to the fibrous pericardium. Both serous layers are continuous to form the **pericardial cavity** and produce a serous fluid film for friction-free movements of the heart. The epicardium (shaded blue in **a** and marked with a blue line in **b**) covers the myocardium of the heart, the coronary blood vessels and the epicardial adipose tissue.

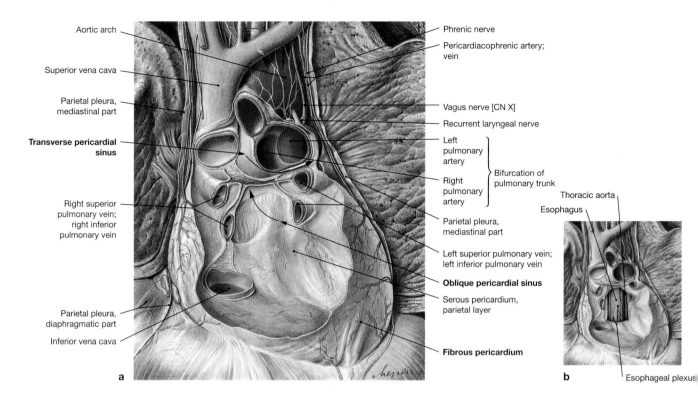

Aortic arch
Superior vena cava
Parietal pleura, mediastinal part
Transverse pericardial sinus
Right superior pulmonary vein; right inferior pulmonary vein
Parietal pleura, diaphragmatic part
Inferior vena cava

Phrenic nerve
Pericardiacophrenic artery; vein
Vagus nerve [CN X]
Recurrent laryngeal nerve
Left pulmonary artery
Right pulmonary artery
Bifurcation of pulmonary trunk
Thoracic aorta
Esophagus
Parietal pleura, mediastinal part
Left superior pulmonary vein; left inferior pulmonary vein
Oblique pericardial sinus
Serous pericardium, parietal layer
Fibrous pericardium

a
b
Esophageal plexus

Fig. 5.65a and b Pericardium; anterior view; after removal of the anterior part of the pericardium and the heart.
The outer fibrous pericardium and the adjacent parietal serous pericardium constitute the outer wall of the pericardial sac. The parietal serous layer is a continuation of the visceral layer of the pericardium (= epicardium).
a The pericardial reflection creates two sinuses of the pericardial cavity at the posterior side (pericardial sinuses, arrows):

Transverse pericardial sinus: above the horizontal fold between the superior vena cava (posterior) and the aorta and pulmonary trunk (anterior).
Oblique pericardial sinus: below the horizontal fold between the pulmonary veins on both sides.
b The posterior aspect of the pericardium is adjacent to the esophagus as demonstrated here by fenestrating the pericardial sac behind the left atrium.

Structure/Function

The **fibrous pericardium** is connected to:
* the central tendon of the diaphragm
* the posterior aspect of the sternum (sternopericardial ligaments)
* the tracheal bifurcation (bronchopericardial membrane)
At the outer side, the fibrous pericardium is covered by the mediastinal pleura. The phrenic nerve and the pericardiacophrenic blood vessels course between these two layers.

Clinical Remarks

The pericardial cavity usually contains 15–35 ml (0.5–1.2 fl oz) of serous fluid. The pericardium has a total volume of 700–1,100 ml (23.7–37.2 fl oz), including the heart. Inflammatory reactions of the pericardium **(pericarditis)** can cause fluid accumulation **(pericardial effusion)** which may impede cardiac function.
Following rupture of the cardiac wall or the ascending aorta due to injury (stab wounds) or rupture of an aneurysm, blood rapidly accumulates in the pericardial cavity and inhibits the cardiac contraction resulting in death **(pericardial tamponade).**
[H043-001]

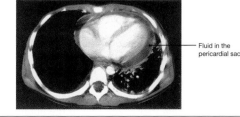

Fluid in the pericardial sac

Ascending aorta
Superior vena cava
Finger placed in the transverse pericardial sinus
Right atrium
Pulmonary trunk
Right ventricle

Fig. 5.66 Transverse pericardial sinus; schematic drawing; anterior view. [L238]
The transverse pericardial sinus is located behind the ascending aorta and pulmonary trunk and marks the separation between the arteries of the heart and the superior vena cava.

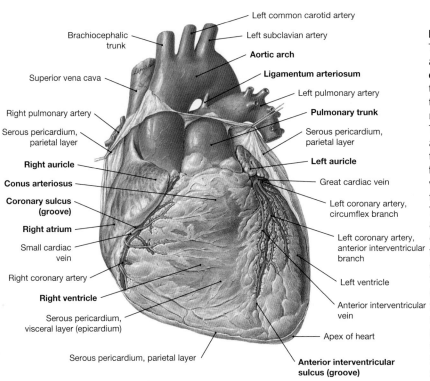

Brachiocephalic trunk
Left common carotid artery
Left subclavian artery
Aortic arch
Superior vena cava
Ligamentum arteriosum
Left pulmonary artery
Right pulmonary artery
Pulmonary trunk
Serous pericardium, parietal layer
Serous pericardium, parietal layer
Right auricle
Left auricle
Conus arteriosus
Great cardiac vein
Coronary sulcus (groove)
Left coronary artery, circumflex branch
Right atrium
Small cardiac vein
Left coronary artery, anterior interventricular branch
Right coronary artery
Left ventricle
Right ventricle
Anterior interventricular vein
Serous pericardium, visceral layer (epicardium)
Apex of heart
Serous pericardium, parietal layer
Anterior interventricular sulcus (groove)

Fig. 5.67 Heart; anterior view.
The **apex** of heart is a part of the left ventricle and is directed to the inferior left side. The **coronary sulcus** (aka coronary groove, atrioventricular groove) on the outer surface separates the atria from the ventricles. The **base** of heart represents the position of the **coronary sulcus.** The heart consists of four chambers, a ventricle and an atrium on the right and left side, respectively. At the anterior surface **(sternocostal surface)**, the **anterior interventricular sulcus** is visible. It depicts the position of the interventricular septum.

The **right ventricle** locates behind the sternum and does not form a border of the heart silhouette in a chest X-ray. Prior to the transition into the pulmonary trunk, the right ventricle is dilated as **conus arteriosus.** The origin of the aorta from the left ventricle is not visible from the outer surface due to its spiral course behind the pulmonary trunk. The aorta appears on the right side of the pulmonary trunk. The **aortic arch** is connected with the **pulmonary trunk** through the **ligamentum arteriosum.**

Both atria have an anterior muscular pouch which is referred to as **left and right auricles.**

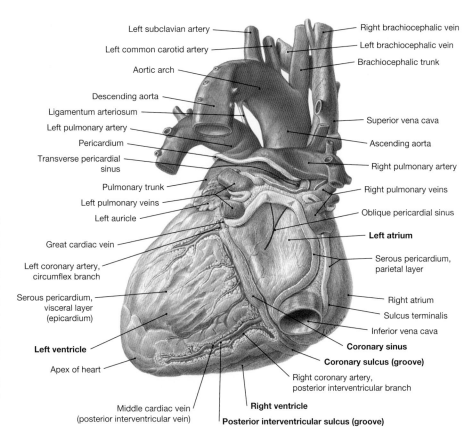

Left subclavian artery
Right brachiocephalic vein
Left common carotid artery
Left brachiocephalic vein
Aortic arch
Brachiocephalic trunk
Descending aorta
Ligamentum arteriosum
Left pulmonary artery
Superior vena cava
Pericardium
Ascending aorta
Transverse pericardial sinus
Right pulmonary artery
Pulmonary trunk
Right pulmonary veins
Left pulmonary veins
Oblique pericardial sinus
Left auricle
Left atrium
Great cardiac vein
Serous pericardium, parietal layer
Left coronary artery, circumflex branch
Serous pericardium, visceral layer (epicardium)
Right atrium
Sulcus terminalis
Inferior vena cava
Left ventricle
Coronary sinus
Apex of heart
Coronary sulcus (groove)
Right coronary artery, posterior interventricular branch
Middle cardiac vein (posterior interventricular vein)
Right ventricle
Posterior interventricular sulcus (groove)

Fig. 5.68 Heart; posterior view.
The inferior surface **(diaphragmatic surface)** is formed by both ventricles and rests on the diaphragm. The border between the two ventricles is marked by the **posterior interventricular sulcus** which contains the posterior interventricular coronary artery and the middle cardiac vein. The **coronary sinus** collects venous blood from the great, middle and small cardiac veins, locates in the posterior coronary sulcus and drains directly into the right atrium. The superior and inferior venae cavae enter the right atrium, the four pulmonary veins enter the left atrium.

Structure/Function

Veins are defined as the blood vessels transporting blood towards the heart, independent of the oxygenation status. Pulmonary veins carry oxygenated blood from the lungs to the left atrium and the superior and inferior venae cavae bring deoxygenated blood from the systemic circulation to the right atrium. Arteries transport blood away from the heart. The pulmonary trunk brings deoxygenated blood from the right ventricle to the lungs and the aorta brings oxygenated blood from the left ventricle to the systemic circulation.

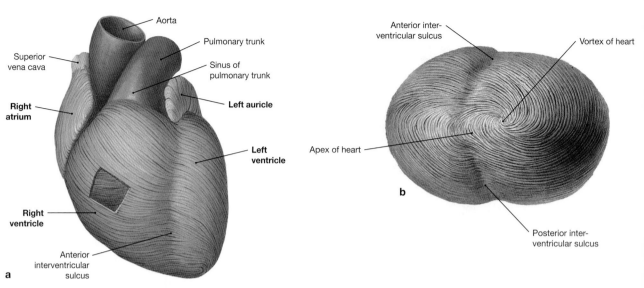

a

Fig. 5.69a and b Cardiac muscle, myocardium; anterior view **(a),** view from the apex **(b).**
The cardiac muscle fibers consist of cardiomyocytes and have a spiral arrangement within the cardiac wall. In the wall of the atria and the right ventricle they form two layers, in the wall of the left ventricle they even form three layers. Thus, the myocardium and the cardiac wall are much thicker in the region of the left ventricle (8–12 mm thick) reflecting the higher pressure required in the left ventricle to pump the blood into the systemic circulation.

Fig. 5.70 Structure of the cardiac wall; cross-section; superior view.
The wall of the heart is composed of three layers:
- **Endocardium:** inner surface consisting of endothelium and connective tissue
- **Myocardium:** cardiac muscle with cardiomyocytes
- **Epicardium:** serous layer and subserous connective tissue at the outer surface of the heart, representing the visceral layer of the serous pericardium. The subserous layer contains plenty of white adipose tissue in which the coronary blood vessels and nerves are embedded.

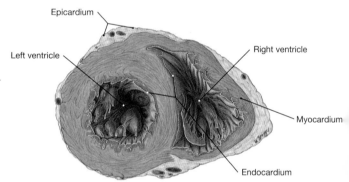

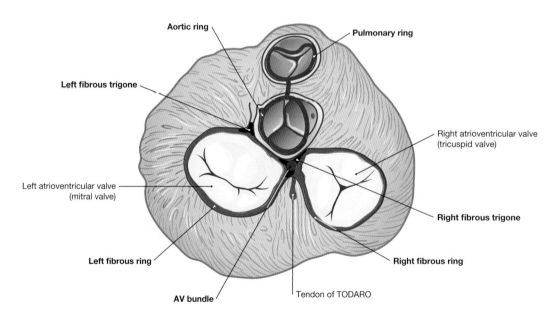

Fig. 5.71 Fibrous skeleton of the heart; schematic drawing; view from the base of the heart. [L126]
The valves are anchored to the cardiac skeleton which consists of connective tissue forming the right and left fibrous ring around the atrioventricular valves and a fibrous ring around the semilunar valves. At the fibrous trigone the atrioventricular bundle (**AV bundle** of HIS), a part of the conducting system of the heart, passes over from the right atrium to the interventricular septum. The fibrous skeleton stabilizes the valves and serves as an electrical insulator between the atria and the ventricles. The electrical impulse reaches the ventricles exclusively through the AV bundle. The tendon of TODARO is the connection between the valve of the inferior vena cava to the central fibrous skeleton.

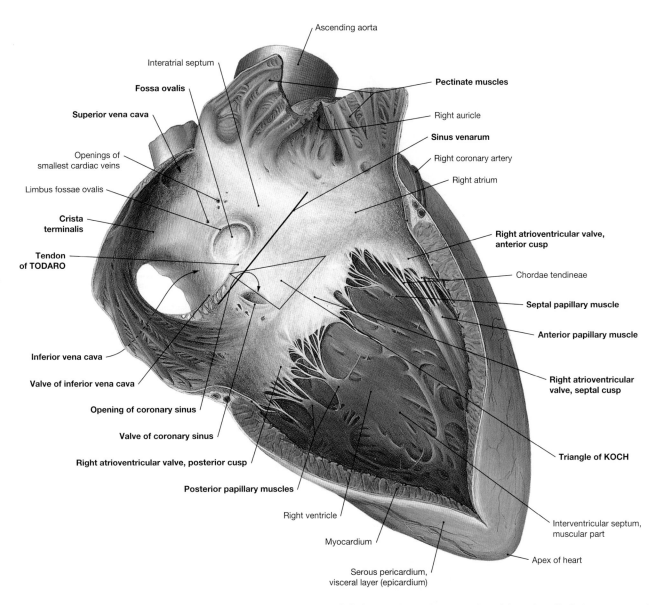

Fig. 5.72 Right atrium and right ventricle; anterior view.
The **right atrium** is separated by the **crista teminalis** into the smooth **sinus venarum** and the muscular part with a rough inner surface consisting of the **pectinate muscles.** The interatrial septum shows a remnant of the former foramen ovale, the **fossa ovalis** with its rim, the limbus fossae ovalis. The opening of the **coronary sinus,** the largest cardiac vein, is demarcated by the valve of coronary sinus, and the opening of the inferior vena cava by the **valve of**

inferior vena cava. An extension of the valve of inferior vena cava is the **tendon of TODARO,** a tendinous structure connecting the valve of the inferior vena cava ostium to the posterior wall of the atrium. In the right ventricle, the three cusps of the right atrioventricular valve are attached via tendinous cords (chordae tendineae) to the three papillary muscles **(anterior, posterior and septal papillary muscles).** Of the interventricular septum only the muscular part is visible in this illustration.

Structure/Function

Three major veins open into the right atrium: superior vena cava, inferior vena cava and the coronary sinus.
The **triangle of KOCH** is demarcated by the tendon of TODARO, the opening of the coronary sinus and the tricuspid valve (septal cusp). It serves as an anatomical landmark for the location of the atrioventricular node **(AV node)** during electrophysiology procedures.

The subepicardial sinuatrial node **(SA node)** is positioned near the opening of superior vena cava and the tip of the sulcus terminalis, the external mark for the crista terminalis.
Starting from the interventricular septum, specific fibers of the cardiac conducting system **(moderator band** described by LEONARDO DA VINCI, not visible here) course to the anterior papillary muscle. This connection is referred to as the **septomarginal trabecula (➤ Fig. 5.91).**

Clinical Remarks

Patent foramen ovale: approximately 20 % of the adult population have a remaining opening in the area of the foramen ovale. Usually, this has no functional relevance. In some cases, how-

ever, this opening may facilitate ascending emboli dislodged from crural thrombi to reach the systemic circulation and cause an organ infarction or stroke.

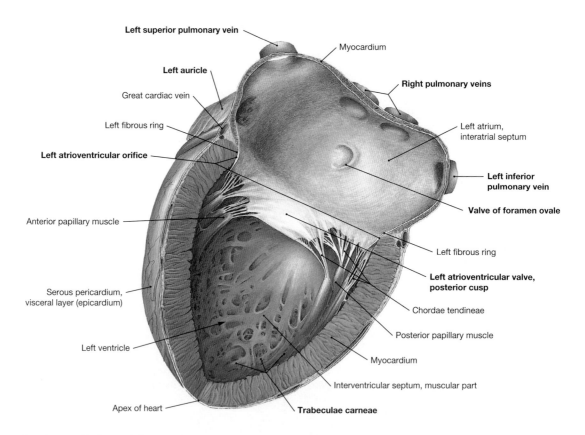

Fig. 5.73 Left atrium and left ventricle; lateral view.
The **left auricle** represents the muscular part of the left atrium. The four pulmonary veins enter the smooth-walled part of the left atrium. The **valve of foramen ovale** is a remnant of the septum primum during the development of the heart. The left atrioventricular orifice is the junction to the left ventricle and contains the left atrioventricular valve **(mitral valve).** The wall of the left ventricle is structured by trabeculae of the ventricular myocardium **(trabeculae carneae).**

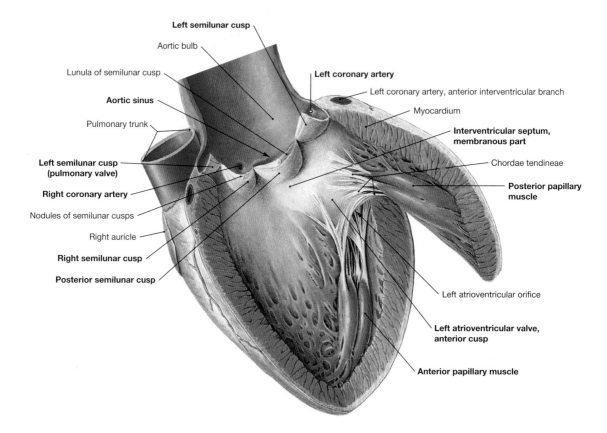

Fig. 5.74 Left ventricle; lateral view.
The **mitral valve** (left atrioventricular valve) consists of two cusps. Thus, only two papillary muscles are required **(anterior and posterior papillary muscles).** Blood from the left ventricle is pumped through the aortic valve into the dilated part of the aorta (aortic bulb). The three **semilunar cusps of the aortic valve** cover the **aortic sinuses** from which the **right and left coronary** arteries originate.

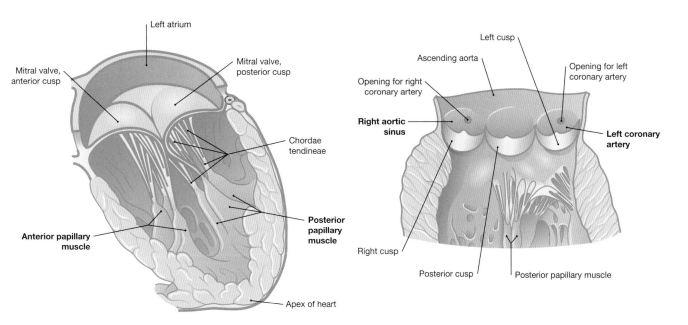

Fig. 5.75 Atrioventricular (AV) valve; example of the mitral valve. [L126]
The **anterior and posterior papillary muscles** connect via tendinous cords (chordae tendineae) to the two cusps of the left atrioventricular valve (mitral valve).

Fig. 5.76 Semilunar valve; example of the aortic valve. [L 126]
The **right and left coronary arteries** originate at the **right and left aortic sinuses,** respectively. Their openings are closed during systole when the aortic valve is open.

Structure/Function

Semilunar valves open passively during ventricular contraction (systole) when the increased intraventricular pressure pushes the blood into the systemic and pulmonary circulation. They close passively during ventricular relaxation (diastole) when the backflow of blood towards the ventricle fills the cusps.
Atrioventricular valves open passively during diastole when blood is sucked into the ventricles from the atria. During early systole contraction (shortening) of the papillary muscles via tendinous cords actively pulls the atrioventricular cusps towards the apex of heart. This closes the AV valves during high systolic pressure in the ventricles to prevent regurgitation of blood into the atria.

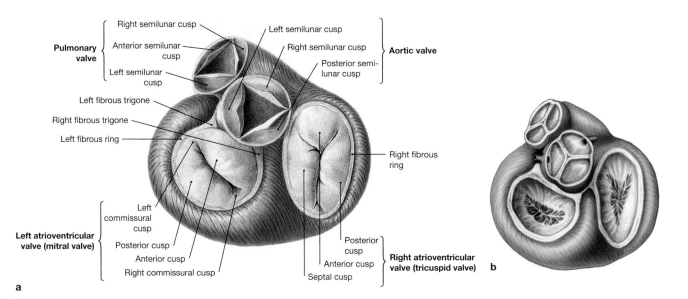

Fig. 5.77a and b Valves during systole (a) and during diastole (b).

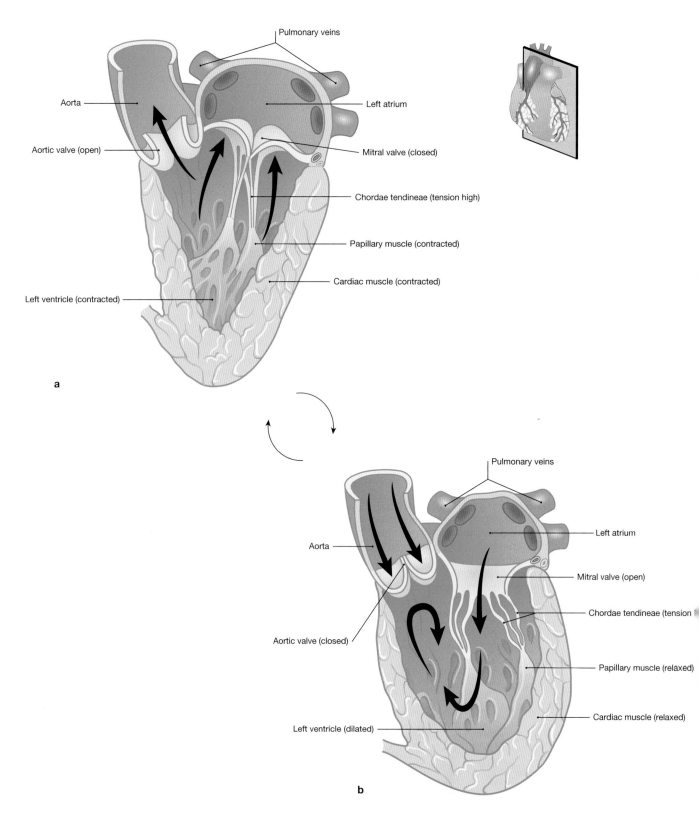

Pulmonary veins

Aorta

Left atrium

Aortic valve (open)

Mitral valve (closed)

Chordae tendineae (tension high)

Papillary muscle (contracted)

Cardiac muscle (contracted)

Left ventricle (contracted)

a

Pulmonary veins

Aorta

Left atrium

Aortic valve (closed)

Mitral valve (open)

Chordae tendineae (tension

Papillary muscle (relaxed)

Cardiac muscle (relaxed)

Left ventricle (dilated)

b

Fig. 5.78a and b Ventricular action, blood flow and valve position during systole (a) and diastole (b); schematic drawing; section through the apex of heart and perpendicular to the base of heart. Arrows depict the direction of the blood flow. [L126]

Structure/Function

Diastole: ventricular relaxation draws blood passively from the atria into the ventricles. Contractions of the atrial pectinate muscles empty the remaining blood from the atria at the end of diastole. Ventricular relaxation also leads to a reflux of blood from the outgoing arteries of the heart which fills the semilunar valves causing passive closure of the semilunar valves.

Systole: with increasing ventricular filling and the beginning of myocardial contraction the cusps of the AV valves are first passively closed. Later in systole, the increasing intraventricular pressure necessitates contraction of the papillary muscles to keep the AV valves closed. Peak systolic ventricular pressure passively opens the semilunar valves allowing ejection of blood into the great arteries (pulmonary trunk and aorta).

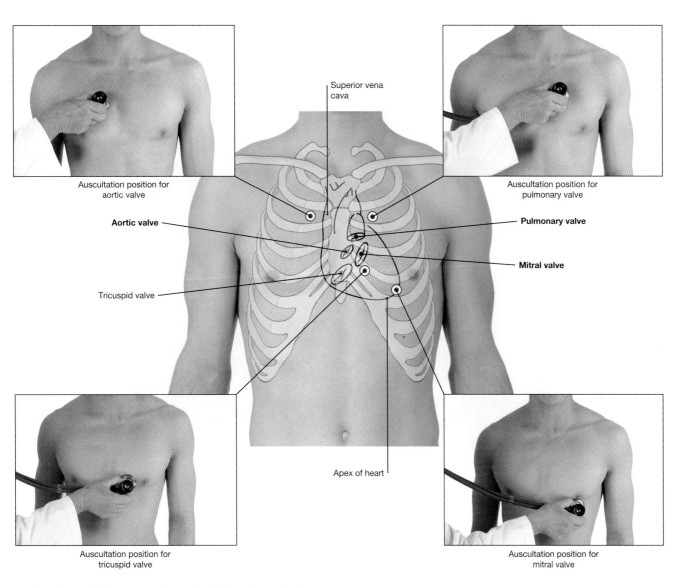

Superior vena cava

Auscultation position for aortic valve

Aortic valve

Tricuspid valve

Auscultation position for pulmonary valve

Pulmonary valve

Mitral valve

Apex of heart

Auscultation position for tricuspid valve

Auscultation position for mitral valve

Fig. 5.79 Auscultation sites for the cardiac valves. [L126, K340, L271]

Auscultation Sites for the Cardiac Valves		
	Surface Projection	**Auscultation Site**
Pulmonary valve	Left (!) sternal border, 3rd costal cartilage	Parasternal left 2nd ICS
Aortic valve	Left sternal border, 3rd ICS	Parasternal right 2nd ICS
Mitral valve	Left 4th to 5th costal cartilages	In the midclavicular line 5th ICS
Tricuspid valve	Retrosternal 5th costal cartilage	Parasternal left 5th ICS*

* ICS = intercostal space; depending on the individual position of the heart the tricuspid valve may be auscultated in the 5th ICS on the right side of the sternum

Clinical Remarks

If the valves are constricted (stenosis) or do not close properly (insufficiency), **heart murmurs** develop. These are most noticeable at the auscultation sites of the respective valves (> Fig. 5.79). A systolic murmur is detected with insufficiency of the AV valves or stenosis of the semilunar valves. A diastolic murmur points to an insufficiency of semilunar valves or steno-sis of AV valves. Valvular stenoses are either congenital or acquired (rheumatic diseases, bacterial endocarditis). Valvular insufficiencies are mostly acquired.

A **myocardial infarction** (MI) affecting the papillary muscles leads to AV valve insufficiency with resulting regurgitation of blood into the atria during systole.

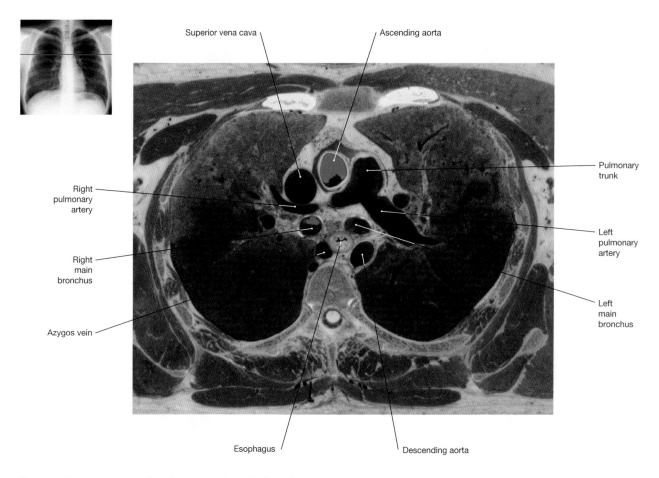

Fig. 5.80 Thorax cross-sectional anatomy, level T5. [X338]

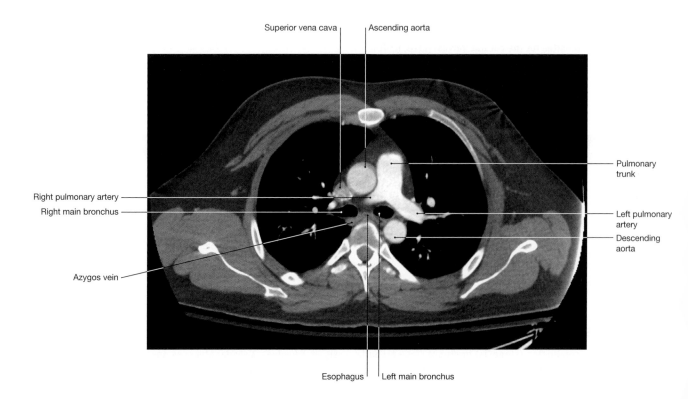

Fig. 5.81 Thorax CT cross-section, level T5. [T975]

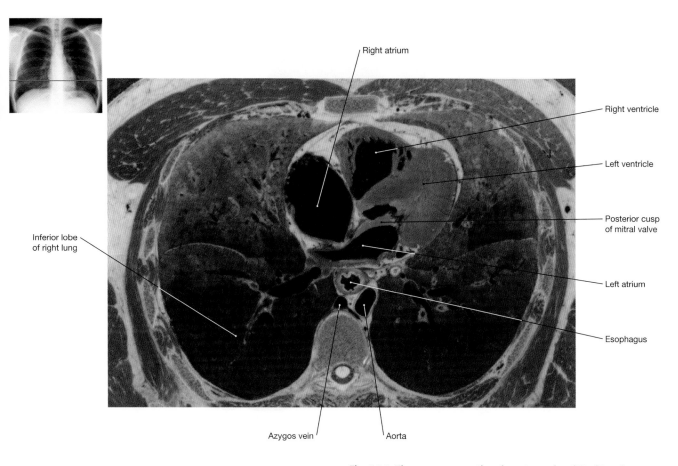

Right atrium

Right ventricle

Left ventricle

Posterior cusp
of mitral valve

Left atrium

Inferior lobe
of right lung

Esophagus

Azygos vein   Aorta

Fig. 5.82 Thorax cross-sectional anatomy, level T7. [X338]

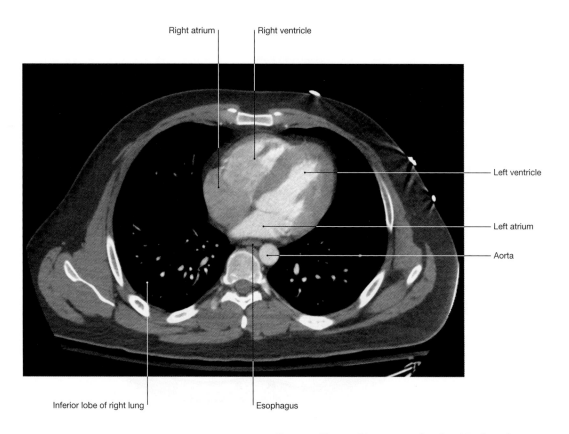

Right atrium   Right ventricle

Left ventricle

Left atrium

Aorta

Inferior lobe of right lung   Esophagus

Fig. 5.83 Thorax CT cross-section, level T7. [T975]

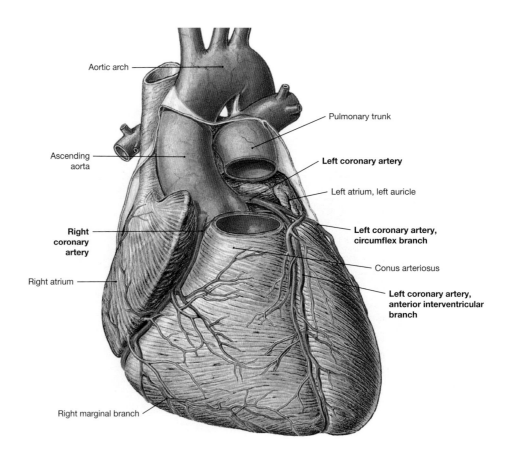

Fig. 5.84 Coronary arteries; anterior view.

The **right coronary artery** courses in the coronary sulcus to the inferior margin (right margin). It continues to the diaphragmatic surface and branches off the posterior interventricular branch in most cases as its terminal branch.

The **left coronary artery** courses behind the pulmonary trunk and divides after 1cm to form the **anterior interventricular branch,** which courses to the apex of heart, and the **circumflex branch.** The latter courses in the coronary sulcus around the left cardiac margin to reach the posterior aspect of the heart.

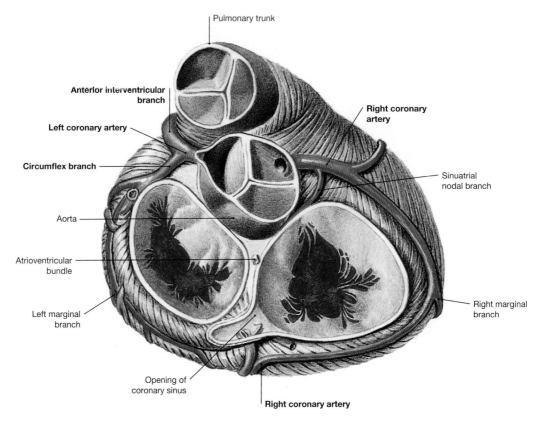

Fig. 5.85 Coronary arteries; superior view.

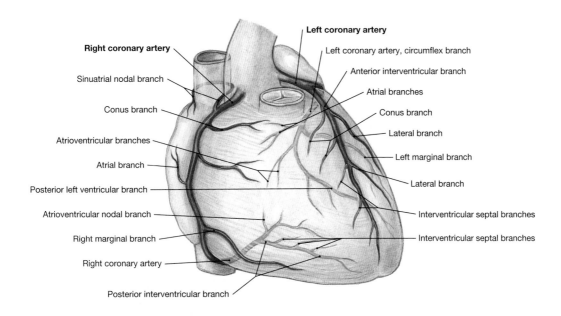

Right coronary artery

Sinuatrial nodal branch

Conus branch

Atrioventricular branches

Atrial branch

Posterior left ventricular branch

Atrioventricular nodal branch

Right marginal branch

Right coronary artery

Posterior interventricular branch

Left coronary artery

Left coronary artery, circumflex branch

Anterior interventricular branch

Atrial branches

Conus branch

Lateral branch

Left marginal branch

Lateral branch

Interventricular septal branches

Interventricular septal branches

Fig. 5.86 Coronary arteries of the anterior (red) and posterior (purple) region of the heart. The major branches of the right and left coronary artery are shown.

Structure/Function

Important Branches of the Right Coronary Artery (RCA)
- Conus branch to conus arteriosus
- Sinuatrial nodal branch (⅔ of all cases): to the SA node
- Right marginal branch
- Right posterolateral branch
- Atrioventricular nodal branch: to the AV node (if "right dominant")
- Posterior interventricular branch [posterior descending artery = PDA] (if "right dominant") with interventricular septal branches, supplying the atrioventricular bundle

Important Branches of the Left Coronary Artery (LCA)
Anterior interventricular artery [left anterior descending artery = LAD]:

- Conus branch
- Lateral branch (clin. term: diagonal branch)
- Interventricular septal branches

Circumflex branch (artery):
- Sinuatrial nodal branch (⅓ of all cases): to the SA node
- Left marginal branch
- Posterior left ventricular branch

Coronary dominance is determined by the artery that supplies the posterior descending artery (PDA) and the diaphragmatic surface of the heart. In 75% of cases the PDA derives from the RCA (right dominant perfusion type). Left coronary dominance: PDA derives from circumflex artery; co-dominance: RCA and LCA contribute to PDA.

Clinical Remarks

The **coronary artery disease** (CAD) is caused by a stenosis of the coronary arteries resulting from arteriosclerosis. Due to insufficient myocardial perfusion this may cause pain in the chest **(angina pectoris)** which may radiate into the arm (mostly the left arm) or into the neck. Total occlusion of an artery results in necrosis of the dependent myocardium **(myocardial infarction, MI).** Functionally, coronary arteries are terminal arteries and a distinct infarction pattern results from the occlusion of the supplying arteries. These patterns may be detected in various leads of electrocardiography (ECG). The most definitive evidence is provided by coronary catheterization using radiocontrast agents **(coronary angiography).** Due to the low pressure system of the right heart, the myocardium of the right ventricle requires less oxygen when compared to the left ventricle. Thus, even a proximal occlusion of the right coronary artery may only result in an isolated posterior myocardial infarction. In this case, however the bradycardia may be severe due to the insufficient perfusion of the SA node. Coronary dominance determines the severity of a proximal MI. Since the coronary perfusion occurs during ventricular relaxation in diastole, a tachycardia can critically reduce myocardial perfusion in CAD.
[H081]

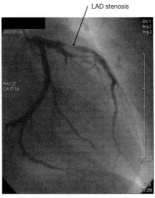

LAD stenosis

Coronary angiogram of LCA

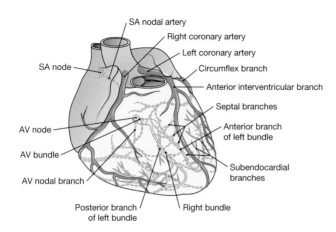

Fig. 5.87 Blood supply of the conducting system of the heart. Yellow: parts of the conducting system, red: coronary arteries and branches. [L126]
The sinuatrial node (SA node) and the atrioventricular node (AV node) are usually supplied by branches of the right coronary artery. The right and left bundles are predominantly supplied by the anterior septal branches of the anterior interventricular artery (LAD).

Clinical Remarks

Severe **bradycardia** may occur from a proximal occlusion of the right coronary artery due to the insufficient perfusion of the SA node. Posterior myocardial infarction (PMI) is often accompanied by arrhythmias (bradycardia) because the artery supplying the AV node originates near the posterior interventricular branch. [L126]

Common myocardial infarction (MI) zones (shaded green):

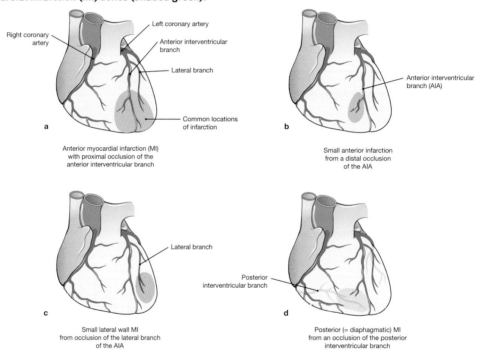

In **coronary bypass surgery** a part of an artery or vein is connected to the ascending aorta or the coronary artery proximal to the occlusion and to the coronary artery distal of the occlusion. Commonly, either the internal mammary artery and/or radial artery or the great saphenous vein of the leg are used as graft. [L266]

Options for arterial (a) or venous (b) coronary bypass grafting:

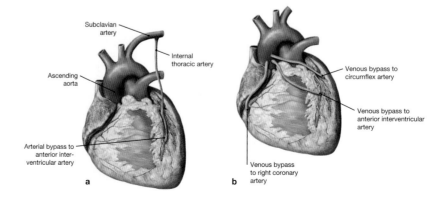

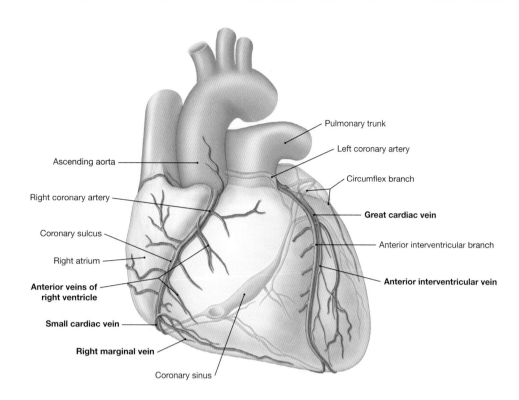

Fig. 5.88 Cardiac veins;
anterior view. [L238]

Labels (Fig. 5.88):
- Pulmonary trunk
- Left coronary artery
- Circumflex branch
- **Great cardiac vein**
- Anterior interventricular branch
- **Anterior interventricular vein**
- Ascending aorta
- Right coronary artery
- Coronary sulcus
- Right atrium
- **Anterior veins of right ventricle**
- **Small cardiac vein**
- **Right marginal vein**
- Coronary sinus

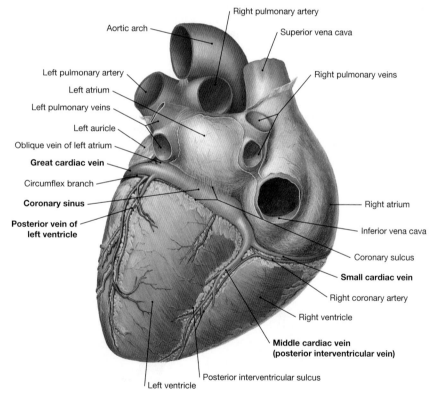

Fig. 5.89 Cardiac veins;
posterior view.

Labels (Fig. 5.89):
- Right pulmonary artery
- Aortic arch
- Superior vena cava
- Left pulmonary artery
- Right pulmonary veins
- Left atrium
- Left pulmonary veins
- Left auricle
- Oblique vein of left atrium
- **Great cardiac vein**
- Circumflex branch
- **Coronary sinus**
- **Posterior vein of left ventricle**
- Right atrium
- Inferior vena cava
- Coronary sulcus
- **Small cardiac vein**
- Right coronary artery
- Right ventricle
- **Middle cardiac vein (posterior interventricular vein)**
- Posterior interventricular sulcus
- Left ventricle

Structure/Function

Cardiac Veins
75 % of the venous blood are collected in the **coronary sinus** which collects blood from the **great, middle and small cardiac veins** and drains directly into the right atrium.

Coronary sinus system
- **Great cardiac vein:** corresponds to the perfusion area of the left coronary artery
  - Anterior interventricular vein
  - Left marginal vein
  - Posterior veins of the left ventricle
- **Middle cardiac vein:** in the posterior interventricular sulcus
- **Small cardiac vein:** in the right coronary sulcus, present in 50 %
- Oblique vein of the left atrium

The remaining 25% of the venous blood drain into the atria and ventricles directly via small transmural and endomural veins.

Transmural system
- Right anterior ventricular veins
- Atrial veins

Endomural system
- Smallest cardiac veins (THEBESIAN veins)

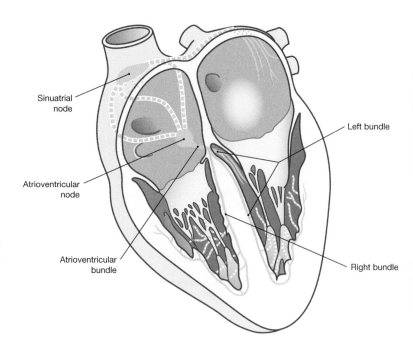

Fig. 5.90 Conducting system of heart. [L126]
The stimulating and conducting system of the heart consists of modified cardiomyocytes. This system is divided into the following parts:

- **sinuatrial node** (SA node; node of KEITH-FLACK)
- **atrioventricular node** (AV node, node of TAWARA)
- **atrioventricular bundle** (AV bundle of HIS)
- **right and left bundle branches**

Structure/Function

The electrical stimulation is initiated within the SA node by spontaneous depolarisation in the specialised myocardial cells with a frequency of about 70/min. The SA node is located within the wall of the right atrium in a groove (sulcus terminalis) between the entry of the superior vena cava and the right auricle. It is supplied by the sinuatrial nodal branch which derives from the right coronary artery in most cases. The electrical signal spreads from the SA node through the myocardium of both atria (myogenic conduction) and reaches the AV node which slows down the frequency of the signal to allow a sufficient filling of the ventricles.

The AV node is embedded within the myocardium of the atrioventricular septum at the triangle of KOCH (➤ Fig. 5.72,

➤ Fig. 5.90). The AV node is supplied by the atrioventricular nodal branch which in most cases derives from the right coronary artery near the origin of the posterior interventricular branch. From the AV node the electrical signal is conveyed by the AV bundle (bundle of HIS) through the right fibrous trigone to the interventricular septum. The AV bundle divides into the right and left bundle branches. The left bundle branch splits into the anterior, septal and posterior subendocardial fascicles to the respective parts of the myocardium including the papillary muscles and the apex of heart. The right bundle branch descends subendocardially in the septum to the apex of heart and reaches the anterior papillary muscle via the septomarginal trabecula (➤ Fig. 5.91).

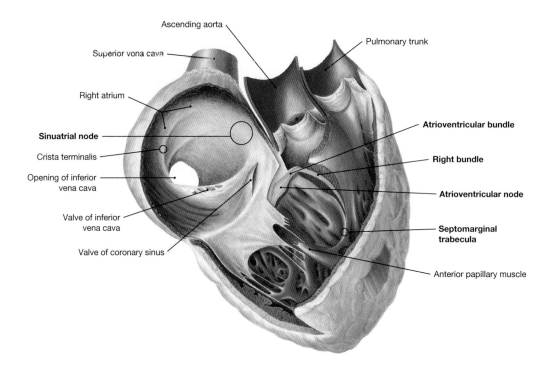

Fig. 5.91 Stimulating and conducting system of heart.

A part of the right bundle branch **(moderator band)** reaches the right anterior papillary muscle via the **septomarginal trabecula**.

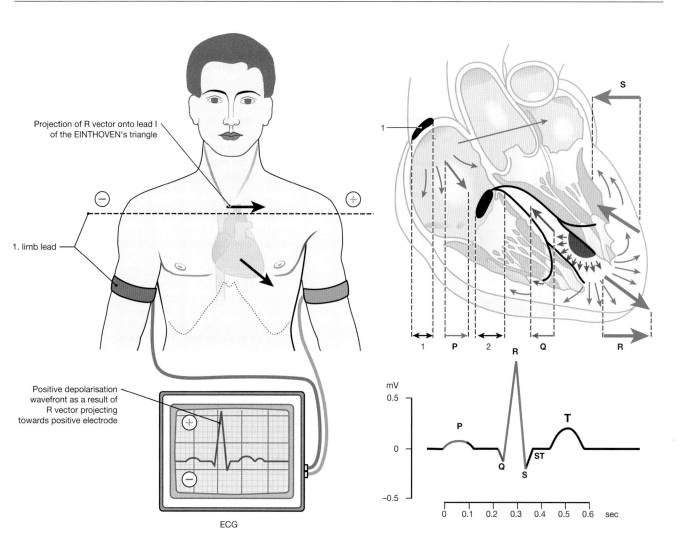

Projection of R vector onto lead I
of the EINTHOVEN's triangle

1. limb lead

Positive depolarisation
wavefront as a result of
R vector projecting
towards positive electrode

ECG

1	Sinus node depolarisation (no ECG signal)	Q	Depolarisation of the interventricular septum	ST	Complete depolarisation of ventricles (no potential difference = isoelectric)
2	Depolarisation delay in AV node (PQ interval)	R	Depolarisation of the distal third of the interventricular septum (vector in longitudinal cardiac axis)	T	Repolarisation of ventricles
P	Atrial depolarisation	S	Depolarisation of remaining parts of the ventricles		

Fig. 5.92 Anatomical principles of the electrocardiography (ECG).
[L126]
The electrical signal spreads from the SA node to the AV node which causes a delay in conduction before reaching the interventricular septum via the AV bundle. The right and left bundle branches then divide to reach the ventricular myocardium. This conduction of impulses within the heart can be detected by electrodes on the surface of the body. If the electrical signal travels towards the electrode at the surface of the body, it results in a positive (upward) amplitude of the baseline voltage. Because of the small volume of the SA node, the SA excitation is not detectable in the ECG. The depolarization of the atria is represented by the **P wave.** The depolarization delay by the AV node occurs during the **PQ segment.** The rapid retrograde direction of the depolarisation of the

interventricular septum is illustrated by the **Q wave.** Depolarisation of the ventricular myocardium towards the apex of heart is represented by the ascending limb of the **R wave,** whereas the propagation of the depolarisation away from the apex results in the descending limb of the R wave and in the **short S wave.** During the **ST segment** the entire ventricular myocardium is depolarised. Since the repolarization of the ventricular myocardium occurs in the same direction as the depolarization, the **T wave** also shows a positive (upward) amplitude. Usually, three limb leads are recorded to determine the electrical axis of the heart according to the largest amplitude of the R wave. However, this electrical axis is influenced by the thickness of the myocardium in both ventricles and by the excitability of the tissue and is therefore not identical with the anatomical axis of the heart.

Clinical Remarks

The **electrocardiography** (ECG) is used to detect cardiac arrhythmias, for example if the heart beats too fast (**tachycardia,** > 100/min), too slow (**bradycardia,** < 60/min), or in an irregular way (**arrhythmia**). The ECG is of particular importance for the identification of myocardial infarction.

If atrial fibers bypass the AV node and directly link to the AV bundle of HIS or the ventricular myocardium, cardiac arrhythmias are the result (**WOLFF-PARKINSON-WHITE syndrome**). If these arrhythmias cause severe symptoms and resist pharmacological treatment, it may be necessary to interrupt the accessory bundles using a cardiac catheter device.

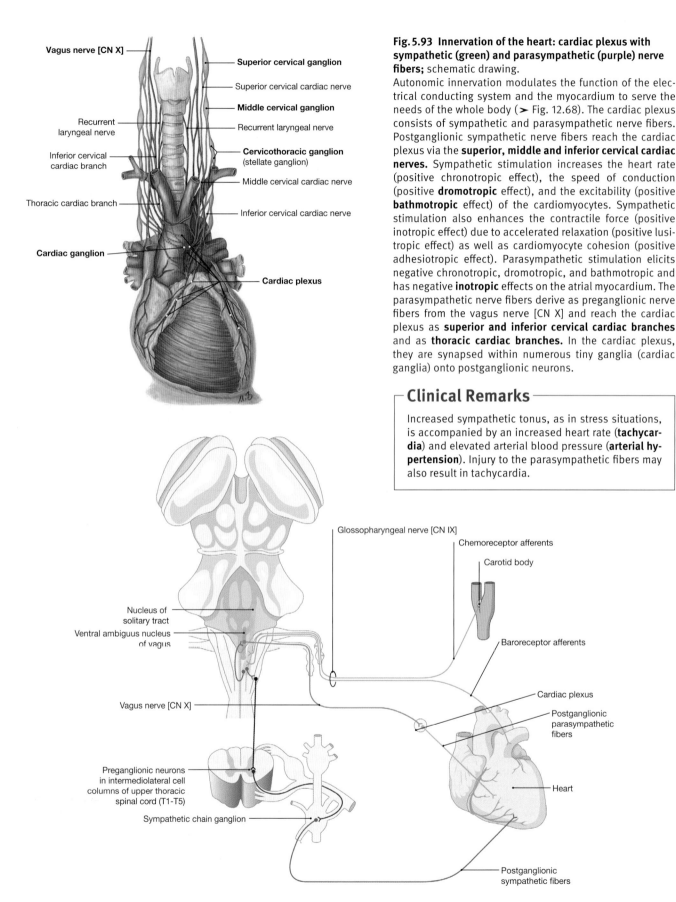

Fig. 5.93 Innervation of the heart: cardiac plexus with sympathetic (green) and parasympathetic (purple) nerve fibers; schematic drawing.

Autonomic innervation modulates the function of the electrical conducting system and the myocardium to serve the needs of the whole body (➤ Fig. 12.68). The cardiac plexus consists of sympathetic and parasympathetic nerve fibers. Postganglionic sympathetic nerve fibers reach the cardiac plexus via the **superior, middle and inferior cervical cardiac nerves.** Sympathetic stimulation increases the heart rate (positive chronotropic effect), the speed of conduction (positive **dromotropic** effect), and the excitability (positive **bathmotropic** effect) of the cardiomyocytes. Sympathetic stimulation also enhances the contractile force (positive inotropic effect) due to accelerated relaxation (positive lusitropic effect) as well as cardiomyocyte cohesion (positive adhesiotropic effect). Parasympathetic stimulation elicits negative chronotropic, dromotropic, and bathmotropic and has negative **inotropic** effects on the atrial myocardium. The parasympathetic nerve fibers derive as preganglionic nerve fibers from the vagus nerve [CN X] and reach the cardiac plexus as **superior and inferior cervical cardiac branches** and as **thoracic cardiac branches.** In the cardiac plexus, they are synapsed within numerous tiny ganglia (cardiac ganglia) onto postganglionic neurons.

Clinical Remarks

Increased sympathetic tonus, as in stress situations, is accompanied by an increased heart rate (**tachycardia**) and elevated arterial blood pressure (**arterial hypertension**). Injury to the parasympathetic fibers may also result in tachycardia.

Fig. 5.94 Regulatory circuitry of the autonomic heart innervation; schematic drawing. [L127]

Preganglionic parasympathetic cardiac (C-)fibers of the vagus nerve [CN X] synapse in the cardiac plexus and the postganglionic fibers innervate the SA node, the AV node and atrial muscle. Vagal innervation for the ventricular myocardium is sparse. Spinal cord segments T1–T5 harbor the sympathetic neurons for the innervation of the heart. Preganglionic sympathetic fibers synapse in the cervical ganglia of the sympathetic chain and descend to the heart. Sensory fibers of the glossopharyngeus nerve [CN IX] connect chemo- and baroreceptors with the nucleus of solitary tract (NST). The NST connects vagal parasympathetic and sympathetic systems.

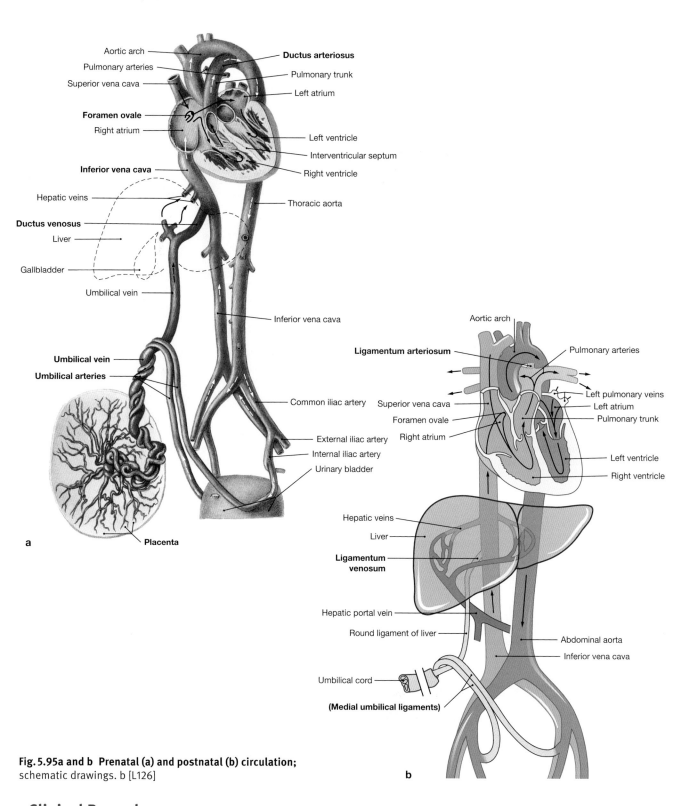

Fig. 5.95a and b Prenatal (a) and postnatal (b) circulation; schematic drawings. b [L126]

Clinical Remarks

Patent ductus arteriosus: Since prostaglandin E₂ dilates the ductus, prostaglandin synthesis inhibitors may be successfully applied to close this vessel and prevent surgical intervention. However, their use as anti-inflammatory agents in pregnant women may result in premature closure of the ductus arteriosus in the fetus.

Patent foramen ovale: Approximately 20 % of the adult population have a remaining opening in the area of the foramen ovale. Usually, this has no functional relevance. In some cases, however, this opening may facilitate ascending emboli dislodged from crural thrombi to reach the systemic circulation and cause an organ infarction or stroke.

Aortic coarctation: If the closure of the ductus arteriosus extends to the adjacent parts of the aortic arch this may cause an aortic coarctation. As a result, a left ventricular hypertrophy develops with concomitant arterial hypertension in the upper body and low arterial blood pressure in the lower body. Physical examination reveals a systolic heart murmur between both scapulae. Radiological findings may include notching of the ribs due to a strong collateral circulation from the internal thoracic artery via the intercostal arteries. The stenosis is treated surgically or with dilation to prevent heart failure or strokes which occur already at a young age.

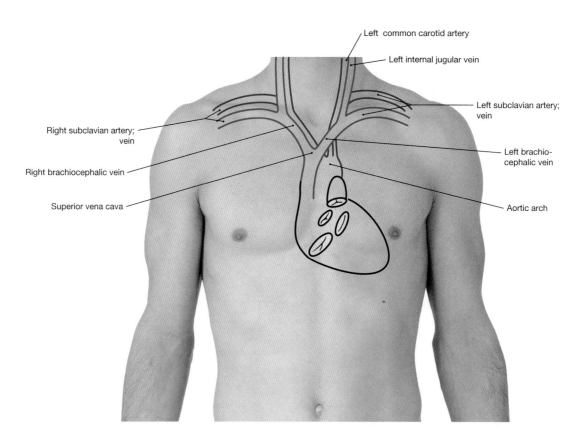

Fig. 5.96 Surface projection of major blood vessels of the superior mediastinum. [L126, K340]

The left brachiocephalic vein crosses the anterior superior mediastinum behind the manubrium to join the superior vena cava.

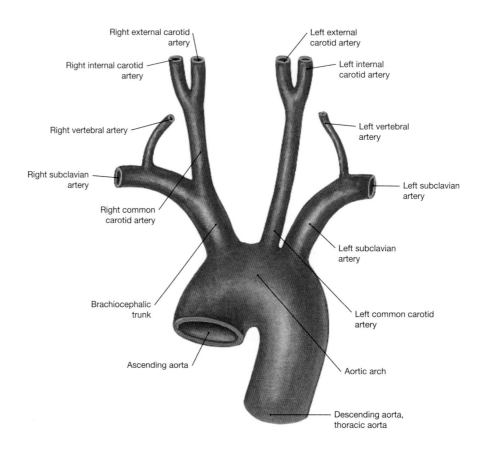

Fig. 5.97 Arterial branches of the aortic arch; schematic drawing.

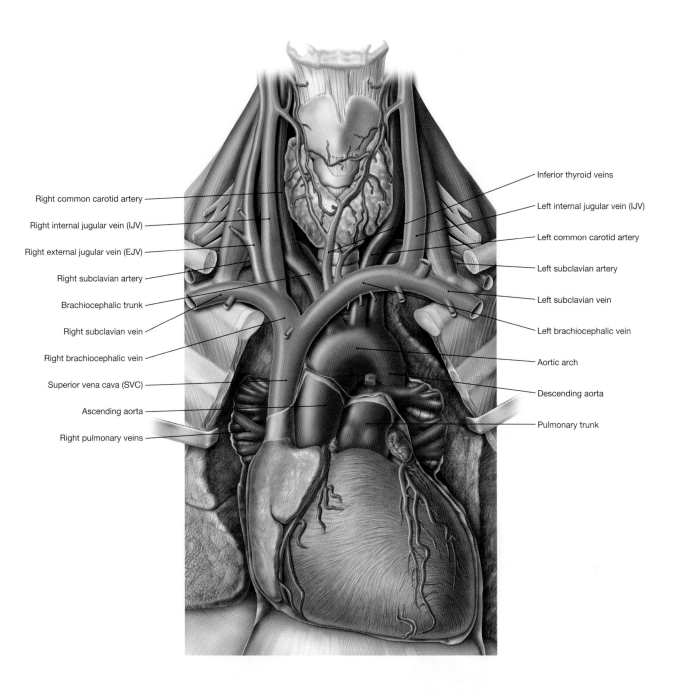

Right common carotid artery

Right internal jugular vein (IJV)

Right external jugular vein (EJV)

Right subclavian artery

Brachiocephalic trunk

Right subclavian vein

Right brachiocephalic vein

Superior vena cava (SVC)

Ascending aorta

Right pulmonary veins

Inferior thyroid veins

Left internal jugular vein (IJV)

Left common carotid artery

Left subclavian artery

Left subclavian vein

Left brachiocephalic vein

Aortic arch

Descending aorta

Pulmonary trunk

Fig. 5.98 Blood vessels in the superior mediastinum and superior thoracic aperture (thoracic outlet); ventral view. [L238]

Clinical Remarks

Anatomical variations in the region of the scalene gap (cervical rib [cervical rib syndrome], narrow scalene hiatus, accessory scalenus minimus, or aberrant muscular fibers [collectively called scalenus anticus syndrome], or narrowing of the space between rib I and clavicle [costoclavicular syndrome]) are the cause for the **thoracic outlet syndrome (TOS).** TOS can result in the compression of the brachial plexus and the subclavian artery.
The scalene hiatus is also the site for the administration of an **interscalene brachial plexus block.**
[E402]

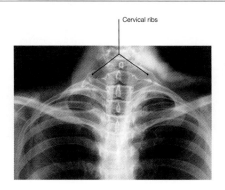

Cervical ribs

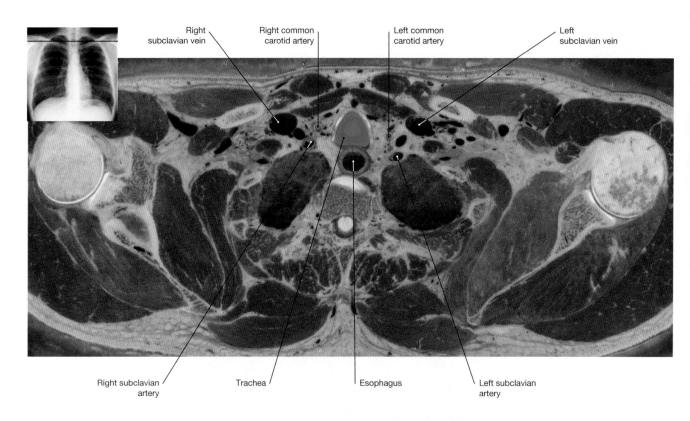

Fig. 5.99 Cross-sectional anatomy, level T2. [X338]

The horizontal section just above the jugular notch shows the apex of lungs as they reach above the superior thoracic aperture.

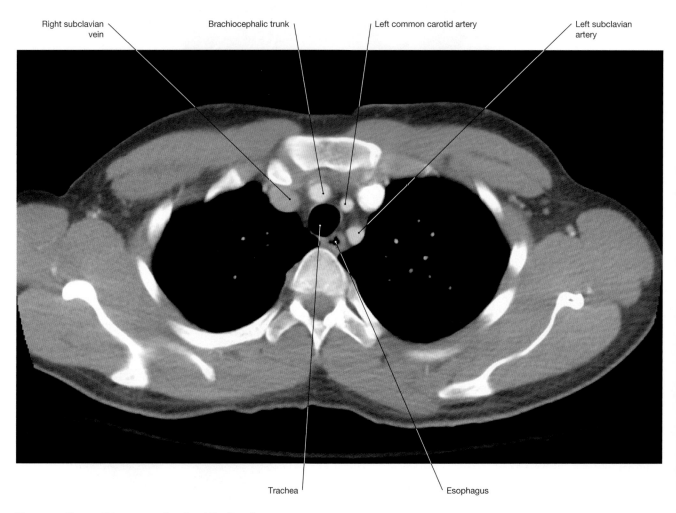

Fig. 5.100 Thorax CT cross-section, level T2. [T975]

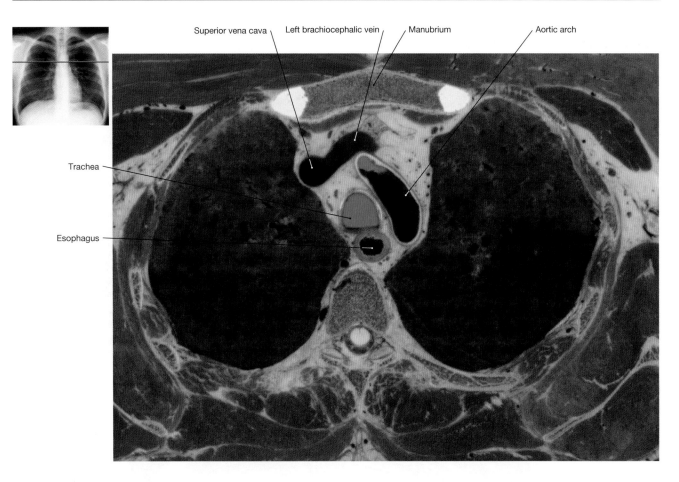

Fig. 5.101 Cross-sectional anatomy, level T4. [X338]

The horizontal section behind the manubrium of sternum shows the left brachiocephalic vein crossing over to the right side and features the aortic arch.

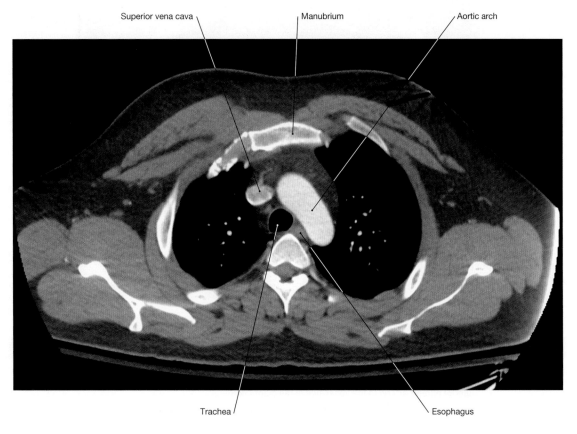

Fig. 5.102 Thorax CT cross-section, level T4. [T975]

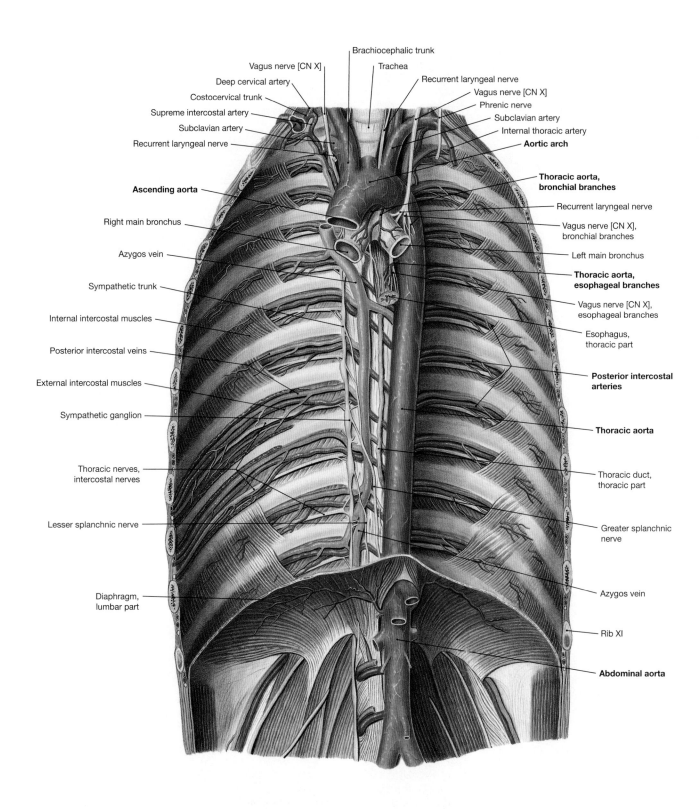

Fig. 5.103 Arteries of the posterior wall of the trunk; after removal of the diaphragm.

Branches of the Thoracic Aorta	
Parietal branches to the wall of the trunk	• **Posterior intercostal arteries:** 9 pairs (the first two are branches of the costocervical trunk from the subclavian artery) • **Subcostal artery:** the last pair below rib XII • **Superior phrenic artery:** to the upper side of the diaphragm
Visceral branches to the thoracic viscera	• **Bronchial branches:** vasa privata of the lung (on the right side mostly from the third right posterior intercostal artery) • **Esophageal branches:** 3–6 branches to the esophagus • **Mediastinal branches:** small branches to mediastinum and pericardium

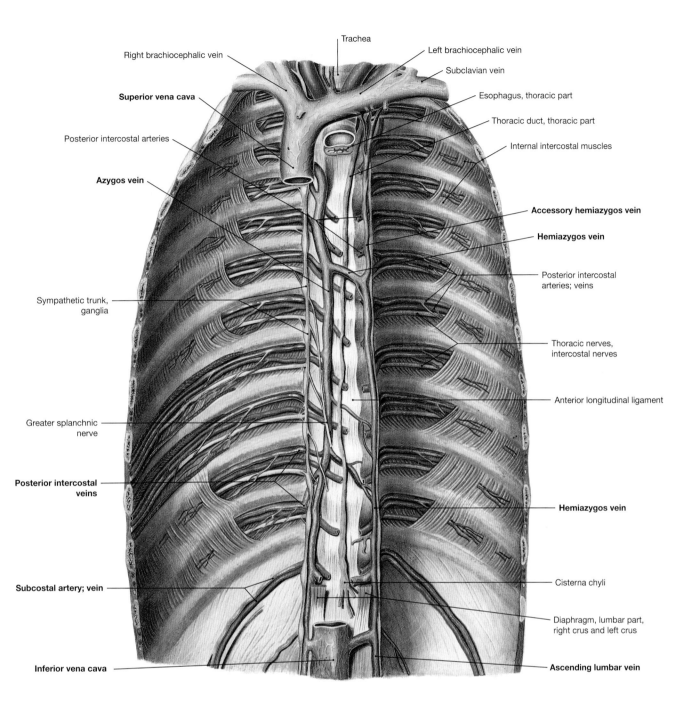

Right brachiocephalic vein

Superior vena cava

Posterior intercostal arteries

Azygos vein

Sympathetic trunk,
ganglia

Greater splanchnic
nerve

**Posterior intercostal
veins**

Subcostal artery; vein

Inferior vena cava

Trachea

Left brachiocephalic vein

Subclavian vein

Esophagus, thoracic part

Thoracic duct, thoracic part

Internal intercostal muscles

Accessory hemiazygos vein

Hemiazygos vein

Posterior intercostal
arteries; veins

Thoracic nerves,
intercostal nerves

Anterior longitudinal ligament

Hemiazygos vein

Cisterna chyli

Diaphragm, lumbar part,
right crus and left crus

Ascending lumbar vein

Fig. 5.104 Veins of the azygos system; anterior view onto the posterior wall of the trunk; after removal of the diaphragm.
The azygos system connects the superior and inferior venae cavae.
The **azygos vein** ascends on the right side of the vertebral column, loops posteriorly around the hilum of the right lung and drains into the superior vena cava from dorsal at the level of the T4/5 thoracic vertebrae. The equivalent blood vessel on the left side is the **hemiazygos vein** which merges with the azygos vein at the level of T7 to T10. Blood from the upper intercostal veins drains into the **acces-** sory hemiazygos vein. Beneath the diaphragm, the ascending lumbar vein on each side continues the course of the azygos vein and connects to the inferior vena cava.

Tributaries:

• **Mediastinal veins:** from the mediastinal organs (esophageal, bronchial, and pericardial veins)
• **Posterior intercostal veins and subcostal vein:** from the posterior wall of the trunk

┌─ **Structure/Function** ─────────────────────────

The structure, course and composition of the azygos system
is highly variable between individuals.

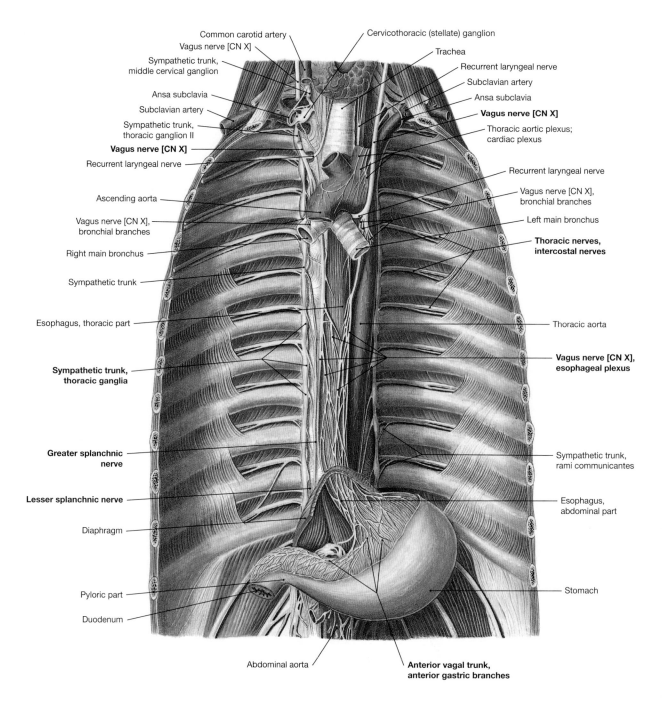

Common carotid artery
Vagus nerve [CN X]
Sympathetic trunk, middle cervical ganglion
Ansa subclavia
Subclavian artery
Sympathetic trunk, thoracic ganglion II
Vagus nerve [CN X]
Recurrent laryngeal nerve
Ascending aorta
Vagus nerve [CN X], bronchial branches
Right main bronchus
Sympathetic trunk
Esophagus, thoracic part
Sympathetic trunk, thoracic ganglia
Greater splanchnic nerve
Lesser splanchnic nerve
Diaphragm
Pyloric part
Duodenum
Abdominal aorta

Cervicothoracic (stellate) ganglion
Trachea
Recurrent laryngeal nerve
Subclavian artery
Ansa subclavia
Vagus nerve [CN X]
Thoracic aortic plexus; cardiac plexus
Recurrent laryngeal nerve
Vagus nerve [CN X], bronchial branches
Left main bronchus
Thoracic nerves, intercostal nerves
Thoracic aorta
Vagus nerve [CN X], esophageal plexus
Sympathetic trunk, rami communicantes
Esophagus, abdominal part
Stomach
Anterior vagal trunk, anterior gastric branches

Fig. 5.105 Nerves of the posterior mediastinum; anterior view; after removal of the diaphragm.

The posterior mediastinum contains the intercostal nerves of the somatic nervous system and parts of the sympathetic (**sympathic trunk**) and parasympathetic systems (**vagus nerve [X]**) as components of the autonomic nervous system. The sympathetic trunk forms a paravertebral chain of twelve thoracic ganglia which are connected via interganglionary branches. The preganglionic sympathetic neurons originate in the lateral horns (C8–L3) of the spinal cord and exit the vertebral canal with the spinal nerves, course as white rami communicantes to the ganglia of the sympathetic trunk where they are synapsed to postganglionic neurons. Axons of the postganglionic neurons join the spinal nerves and their branches via the grey rami communicantes. Some preganglionic fibers continue as **greater and lesser splanchnic nerves** to the nerve plexus around the abdominal aorta. Preganglionic fibers of the vagus nerve [X] course behind the root of the lung adjacent to the esophagus and form the esophageal plexus. The latter is the origin of the two vagal trunks (**anterior and posterior vagal trunks**) which traverse the diaphragm together with the esophagus to reach the autonomic nerve plexus of the abdominal aorta.

Structure/Function

Postganglionic sympathetic fibers travel with the cutaneous branches of the intercostal nerves to the skin where they innervate the smooth muscle cells of the cutaneous blood vessels (thermoregulation), the sweat glands and the arrector pili muscles associated with hair follicles ("goose bumps"). The **phrenic nerves** originate from the cervical plexus (C2–C4) and descend in the middle mediastinum between the fibrous pericardium and the mediastinal pleura (not shown here).

Abdomen

Surface Anatomy 283

Cutaneous Innervation 284

Abdominal Wall 285

Inguinal Region 291

Abdominal Peritoneal Cavity 297

Esophagus 306

Stomach 310

Small Intestines – Duodenum 317

Small Intestines –
Jejunum and Ileum 319

Large Intestines – Colon 321

Large Intestines –
Cecum and Appendix vermiformis . . 322

Intestines 323

Arteries of Abdominal Viscera 329

Liver 330

Gall Bladder and Bile Ducts 339

Pancreas 342

Spleen 346

Kidneys and Ureters 347

Suprarenal (Adrenal) Gland 357

Kidney, Ureter and
Suprarenal Gland 358

Branches of the Abdominal Aorta ... 359

Autonomic Innervation
of Abdominal Viscera 360

Lymphatic Drainage Pathways
in the Abdomen 361

Abdominal Regions	Clinical Importance
Right hypochondriac	Liver and gallbladder
Epigastric	Pain from gastric ulcer, heartburn
Left hypochondriac	Spleen
Right lumbar (flank)	Kidney, ascending colon
Umbilical	Visceral pain
Left lumbar (flank)	Kidney, descending colon
Right inguinal (groin)	Appendix
Hypogastric (pubic, suprapubic)	Urinary bladder, rectum
Left inguinal (groin)	Pain from intestinal gas

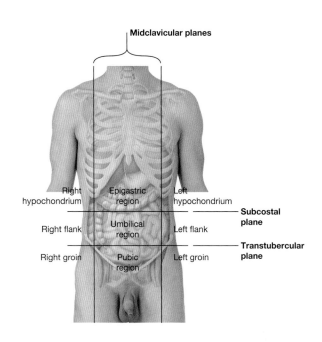

Fig. 6.1 Regions of the abdomen; anterior view. [L275, K340]

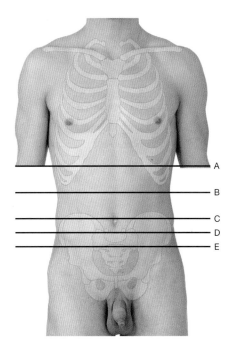

Fig. 6.2 Horizontal planes of the abdomen; anterior view. [L126, K340]

Horizontal Planes	Vertebral Level	Landmarks	Anatomical Structures
A: Transpyloric plane (plane of ADDISON)	L1	Midway between the superior borders of manubrium (jugular notch) and the upper border of the pubic symphysis:	Pylorus (usually at L1, but variable as viscera sag when in erect position), fundus of gallbladder, root of transverse mesocolon, neck of pancreas, origin of celiac trunk (L1), origin of hepatic portal vein, origin of superior mesenteric artery (SMA) (L1/L2), hilum of left kidney, origin of renal arteries (L1/L2), duodenojejunal junction
B: Subcostal plane	Lower **L2–L3**	Inferior border of the 10th rib	Origin of inferior mesenteric artery (IMA) at L3; third part of the duodenum
C: Transumbilical plane	**L3/L4**	Division in upper and lower abdominal regions	
Supracristal plane*	**L4**	Plane passing through the posterior aspects of the iliac crests	Bifurcation of the abdominal aorta, landmark for lumbar spinal tap
D: Transtubercular line	**L5**	Iliac tubercle: 5 cm (2 in) posterior to ASIS on the iliac crest	Origin of the inferior vena cava (IVC)
E: Interspinous plane	**Midsacrum**	At the level of the anterior superior iliac spine (**ASIS**)	Appendix vermiformis (depending on position)

* not shown here; used for orientation in posterior view

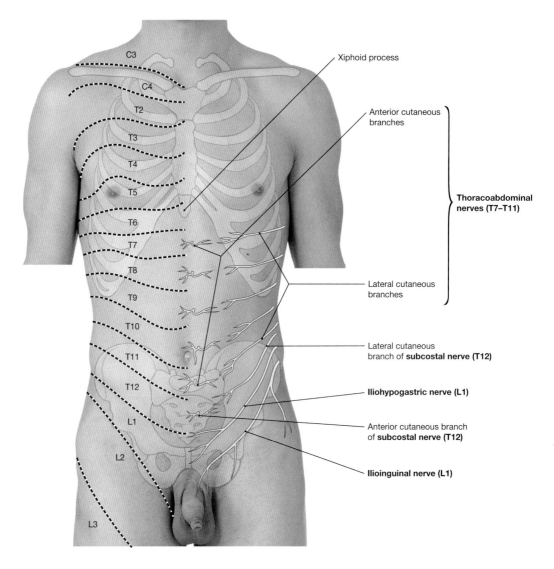

Fig. 6.3 Dermatomes of the anterior abdominal wall. [L126, K340]
The sensory innervation of the abdominal wall (➤ Fig. 12.75) is
conveyed by:

- **Thoracoabdominal nerves T7–T11:** the segmentally oriented anterior rami of the distal thoracic spinal nerves.
- **Subcostal nerve:** the anterior ramus of spinal nerve T12.

- **Iliohypogastric and ilioinguinal nerves:** anterior rami of the
  spinal nerves T12 and L1 from the lumbar plexus.

Abdomen surface orientation:

- Nipple area – dermatome T4/T5,
- Umbilical region – dermatome T10,
- Suprapubic region – dermatome L1,
- Inguinal region – dermatome L2.

Clinical Remarks

Pain sensation arising from an internal organ travels with autonomic nerves and is usually dull and poorly localized. Intense visceral pain may be projected to the dermatome of the same spinal
cord segment. This phenomenon is called **'visceral referred pain'.**
The current working hypothesis for this phenomenon is that
strong visceral pain afferents are 'interpreted' by our brain as
originating from the afferent somatic input from the periphery
(HEAD's zones) causing cutaneous hyperalgesia.

Examples: visceral pain from the stomach (peptic ulcer) is conveyed by the greater splanchnic nerve (T5–T9) and predominantly
projects to the T8/T9 dermatome on the ipsilateral side.

T7–T11: thoracoabdominal nerves;

T12: anterior cutaneous branch of the subcostal nerve (T12);

L1: ilioinguinal nerve.

*Note: the cutaneous innervation of the thorax region is shown in more details
in ➤ chapter 5 (Thorax).*

See also ➤ chapter 12 (Neuroanatomy) for referred pain.

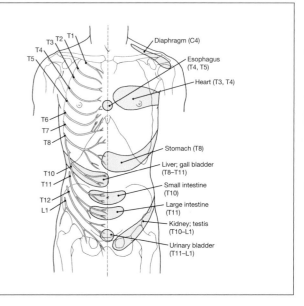

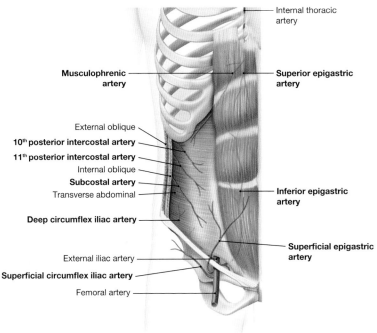

Fig. 6.4 Arteries of the anterior abdominal wall. [L275]

Arteries of the Anterior Abdominal Wall		
Origin	**Artery**	**Course and Distribution**
Aorta	Intercostal arteries 10 and 11	Between internal oblique and transverse abdominis muscles; supply wall of lateral abdominal region
	Subcostal artery	
Internal thoracic artery	Musculophrenic artery	Along costal margin; abdominal wall of hypochondriac region
	Superior epigastric artery	Posterior to rectus muscle within rectus sheath; rectus muscle above umbilicus
External iliac artery	Inferior epigastric artery	Posterior to rectus muscle within rectus sheath; rectus muscle below umbilicus
	Deep circumflex iliac artery	Parallel to inguinal ligament; deep inguinal and iliacus regions
Femoral artery	Superficial epigastric artery	Subcutaneous towards umbilicus; superficial pubic and inferior umbilical regions
	Superficial circumflex iliac artery	Subcutaneous along inguinal ligament; superficial inguinal region

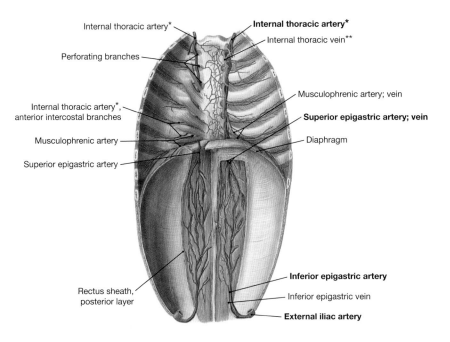

Fig. 6.5 Blood vessels at the posterior aspect of the anterior abdominal wall; view from posterior.

The internal thoracic artery originates from the subclavian artery. Its terminal branches are the musculophrenic and the superior epigastric artery. Superior and inferior epigastric arteries course and anastomose posterior to the rectus muscle within the rectus sheath.

* clin. term: internal mammary artery
** clin. term: internal mammary vein

Clinical Remarks

The **anastomoses between superior and inferior epigastric arteries** may serve as suitable bypass circulation for the perfusion of the lower extremities in cases of coarctation of the aorta (stenosis of the aortic isthmus, ➤ chapter 5 [Thorax], p. 273).
The internal thoracic (mammary) artery and the radial artery of the forearm may be used in **bypass surgery in cases of myocardial infarction**. The schematic to the right indicates potential anastomoses connecting the internal mammary arteries to the coronary arteries of the heart.
[L126]

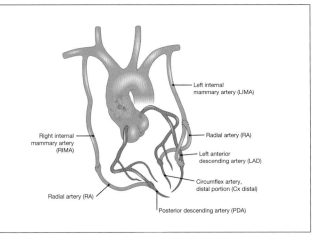

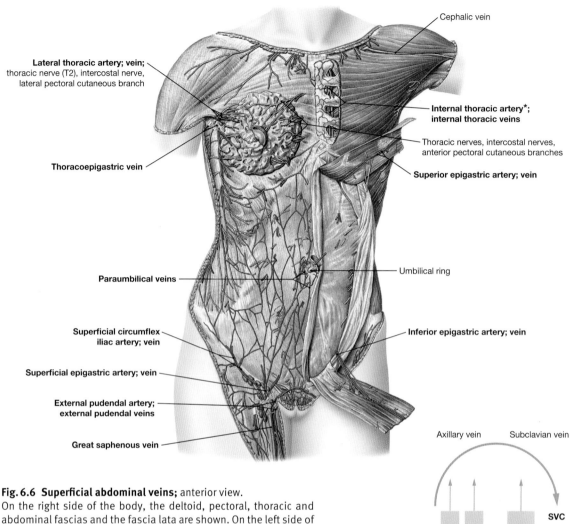

Cephalic vein

Lateral thoracic artery; vein;
thoracic nerve (T2), intercostal nerve,
lateral pectoral cutaneous branch

Internal thoracic artery*;
internal thoracic veins

Thoracic nerves, intercostal nerves,
anterior pectoral cutaneous branches

Thoracoepigastric vein

Superior epigastric artery; vein

Paraumbilical veins

Umbilical ring

Superficial circumflex
iliac artery; vein

Inferior epigastric artery; vein

Superficial epigastric artery; vein

External pudendal artery;
external pudendal veins

Great saphenous vein

Fig. 6.6 Superficial abdominal veins; anterior view.
On the right side of the body, the deltoid, pectoral, thoracic and
abdominal fascias and the fascia lata are shown. On the left side of
the body, the superficial fascia was removed to visualize the muscles. The rectus sheath is opened, the rectus muscle is cut and reflected up- and downward.

* clin. term: internal mammary artery and vein

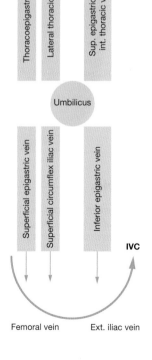

Axillary vein   Subclavian vein

SVC

Thoracoepigastric vein

Lateral thoracic vein

Sup. epigastric and
int. thoracic vein

Umbilicus

Superficial epigastric vein

Superficial circumflex iliac vein

Inferior epigastric vein

IVC

Femoral vein   Ext. iliac vein

Structure/Function

Superficial anastomoses between SVC and IVC: epifascial abdominal veins from the paraumbilical region drain into the axillary vein via thoracoepigastric and lateral thoracic veins or into
the femoral vein via superficial circumflex iliac and epigastric
veins. Obstruction of the blood flow in the IVC may cause substantial dilation of the epifascial veins of the abdominal wall
to facilitate venous drainage of the lower body.   [E273]

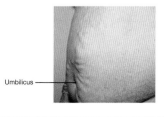

Umbilicus

Fig. 6.7 Superficial venous anastomoses; right side; schematic
illustration. [L231]
The tributaries to the superior vena cava (SVC) and inferior vena
cava (IVC) are shown.

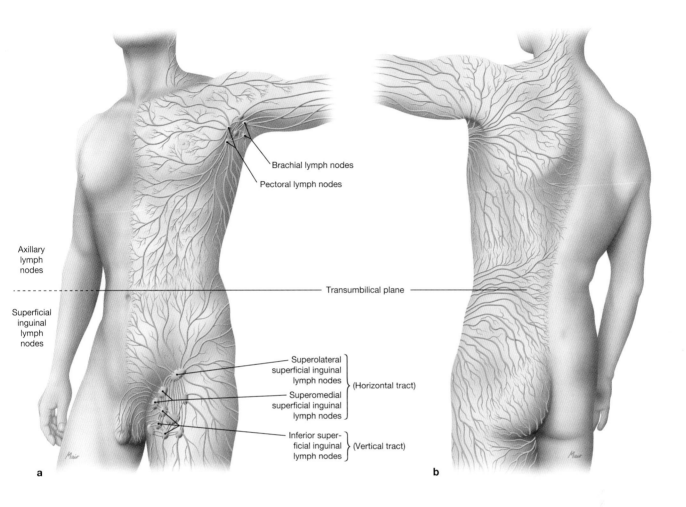

Fig. 6.8a and b Lymphatic drainage of the abdominal wall. [L127]
The **superficial inguinal lymph nodes** drain all superficial lymph below the umbilicus including:
- Lower abdominal wall,
- Buttocks,
- Penis and scrotum/labia majora (external genitalia),
- Perineum,
- Superficial lymphatic plexus of the lower limbs.

The axillary lymph nodes drain the lymph of the abdominal wall above the umbilicus.

Clinical Remarks

A complete physical exam includes the palpation of the superficial lymph nodes. Enlarged palpable lymph nodes may be a sign of an inflammatory reaction, a disease of the lymphatic system or a malignancy.

Lymph passes several consecutive lymph nodes before entering the venous system. **Sentinal lymph nodes,** the 'guardian' lymph nodes, are the first nodes a tumor drains to and are biopsied during cancer surgery for cancer staging. Cancer cells enter the node through one or more afferent lymphatic vessels. They may colonize the node and leave the node through the efferent vessels to spread to more distant regions of the body.
[L127]

* Reticular cells lining the sinus wall also reside within the sinus.

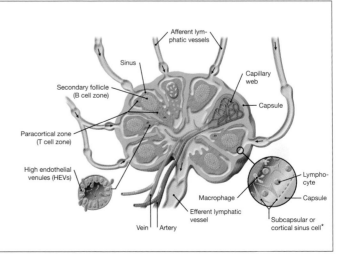

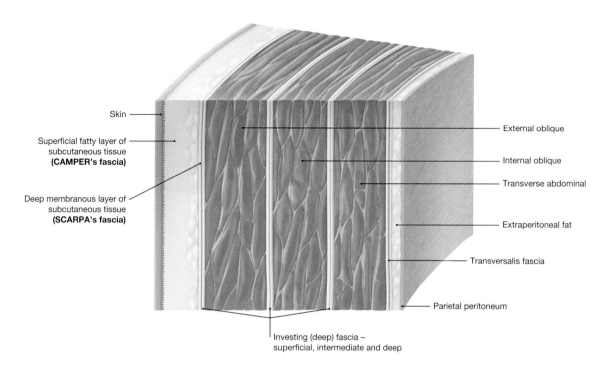

Fig. 6.9 Layers of the lateral abdominal wall; longitudinal section.
[L275]

Structure/Function

The deep membranous layer of the subcutaneous tissue at the anterior abdominal wall **(SCARPA's fascia)** is continuous inferiorly with the membranous layer of the perineal region **(COLLES' fas-** **cia).** It does not continue to the fascia lata of the thigh. Thus fluids (extravasated urine, blood) collecting underneath the COLLES' fascia can ascend to the anterior abdominal wall.

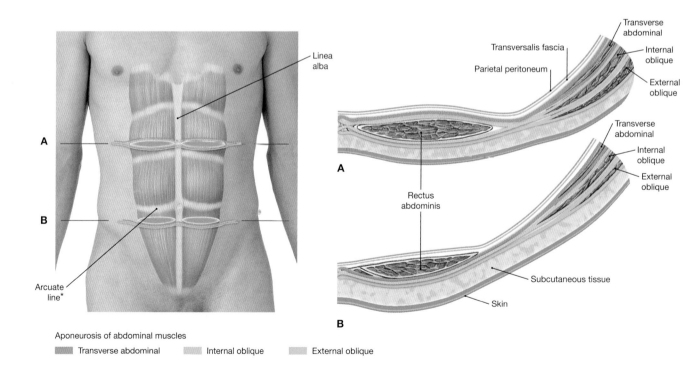

Fig. 6.10 Structure of the rectus sheath; cross-sections. Above the umbilicus **(A)** and below the arcuate line **(B).** [L275]
The **arcuate line** marks the border between the upper and lower sections of the rectus sheath (➤ Fig. 2.53) and usually projects to the level of the lower tendinous intersection of the rectus muscle (*). Below the arcuate line the aponeuroses of all three lateral abdomi- nal muscles (external oblique, internal oblique and transverse) contribute to the strong anterior layer of the sheath. The posterior layer of the sheath only consists of the transversalis fascia, extra- peritoneal adipose tissue and the parietal peritoneum.
Note: the muscles of the abdominal wall, their function and innervation are shown in ➤ chapter 2 (Trunk).

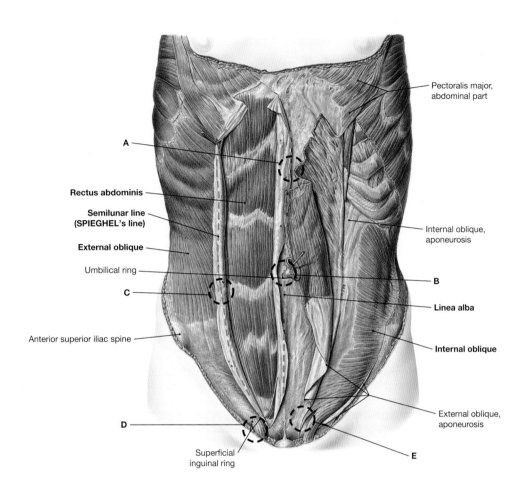

Pectoralis major, abdominal part

A

Rectus abdominis

Semilunar line (SPIEGHEL's line)

External oblique

Umbilical ring

C

Anterior superior iliac spine

Internal oblique, aponeurosis

B

Linea alba

Internal oblique

External oblique, aponeurosis

D

Superficial inguinal ring

E

Fig. 6.11 Muscle-free weak areas of the anterior abdominal wall.
The encircled areas A–E depict common locations for hernias of the anterior abdominal wall (➤ Fig. 2.54, ➤ Fig. 2.55).

Hernias of the anterior abdominal wall develop where the abdominal wall is weak and/or muscle-free.
A Epigastric hernia; **B** Umbilical hernia; **C** Semilunar (SPIGELIAN) hernia; **D** Indirect inguinal hernia; **E** Direct inguinal hernia. For inguinal hernias see ➤ Fig. 6.21.

Clinical Remarks

Abdominal surgical incisions:
Median or midline (dark blue) avoids nerves and blood vessels (➤ Fig. 6.4); may predistine to epigastric incisional hernias.
Pararectus (green) lateral to the rectus sheath.
Paramedian (red) rectus muscle is liberated from its sheath before posterior rectus sheath and peritoneum are opened.
Oblique and transverse: oriented to course of muscle fibers.
GRIDIRON (McBURNEY) (light blue): all abdominal muscle split with direction of muscle fibers; lateral one-third of the distance between ASIS and umbilicus.
Suprapubic (orange) **(PFANNENSTIEL):** pubic hairline; between inferior epigastric vessels.
Transverse (brown): through anterior rectus sheath and rectus abdominis muscle.
Subcostal (purple): 2.5 cm (1 in) below costal margin.
[L126, K340]

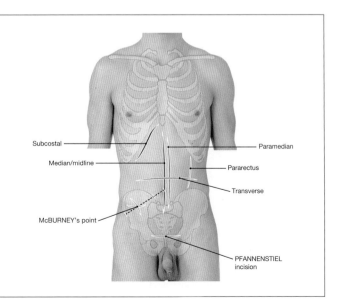

Subcostal

Median/midline

McBURNEY's point

Paramedian

Pararectus

Transverse

PFANNENSTIEL incision

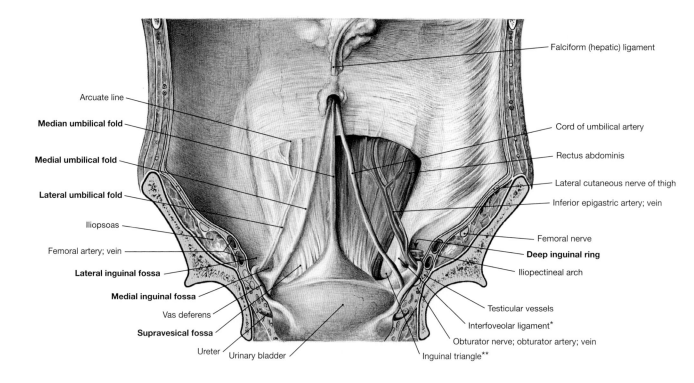

Arcuate line

Median umbilical fold

Medial umbilical fold

Lateral umbilical fold

Iliopsoas

Femoral artery; vein

Lateral inguinal fossa

Medial inguinal fossa

Vas deferens

Supravesical fossa

Ureter Urinary bladder

Falciform (hepatic) ligament

Cord of umbilical artery

Rectus abdominis

Lateral cutaneous nerve of thigh

Inferior epigastric artery; vein

Femoral nerve

Deep inguinal ring

Iliopectineal arch

Testicular vessels

Interfoveolar ligament*

Obturator nerve; obturator artery; vein

Inguinal triangle**

Fig. 6.12 Ventral abdominal wall; inside view. The inguinal and supravesical fossae are confined by the umbilical folds.

* clin. term: HESSELBACH's ligament
** clin. term: HESSELBACH's triangle

Abdominal Folds	Abdominal Fossae	Content
Median umbilical fold		Median umbilical ligament (obliterated urachus)
	Supravesical fossa	Reflection of peritoneum onto the bladder; horizontal position changes with filling of bladder
Medial umbilical fold		Medial umbilical ligament (obliterated umbilical artery)
	Medial inguinal fossa = HESSELBACH's triangle	Potential site for direct inguinal hernias
Lateral umbilical fold		Inferior epigastric blood vessels
	Lateral inguinal fossa	Includes the deep inguinal ring; potential site for indirect inguinal hernias

Structure/Function

The **HESSELBACH's triangle** comprises a muscle-free area of the anterior abdominal wall and constitutes a weak area in the abdominal wall. The anterior abdominal wall deep to the membra-nous layer (SCARPA's fascia of the subcutaneous abdominal tissue) here only consists of the transversalis fascia and the parietal peritoneum.

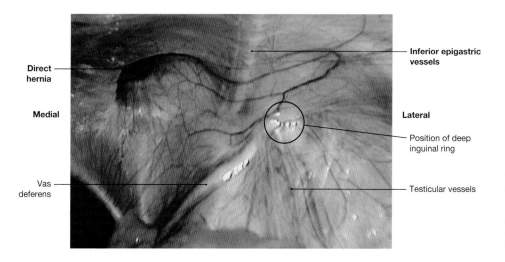

Direct hernia

Medial

Vas deferens

Inferior epigastric vessels

Lateral

Position of deep inguinal ring

Testicular vessels

Fig. 6.13 Laparoscopic image of the HESSELBACH's triangle with a direct inguinal hernia (hernia sac pulled back to show the opening); right side; inside view. [E402]

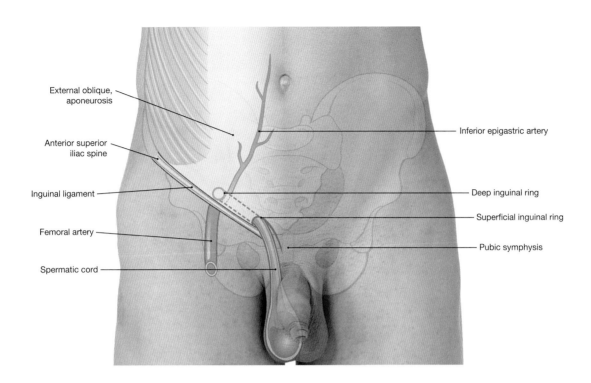

Fig. 6.14 Inguinal canal; surface anatomy; anterior view. [L126, K340]

Midinguinal point: midway between anterior superior iliac spine (ASIS) and pubic symphysis. It serves as landmark for femoral pulse (1.5 cm [0.6 in] below) and for the deep inguinal ring (1.5 cm [0.6 in] above) and is positioned just lateral to the origin of the inferior epigastric artery from the external iliac artery.

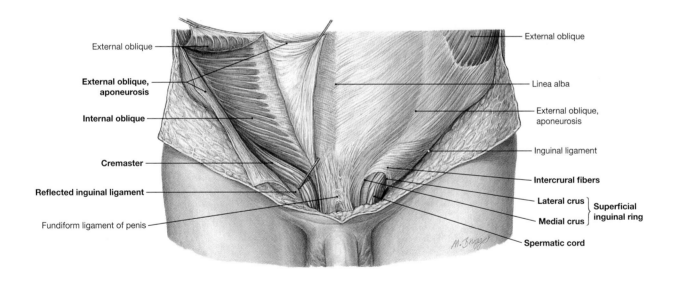

Fig. 6.15 Superficial inguinal ring; anterior view.
The **superficial inguinal ring** is confined by the **lateral and medial crus** of the external abdominal oblique aponeurosis and the **intercrural fibers** and serves as a passageway for the following structures:

- Male and female: ilioinguinal nerve;
- Female: round ligament of uterus;
- Male: spermatic cord, covered by cremaster muscle and fascia, and internal spermatic fascia.

Clinical Remarks

The **cremasteric reflex** is the contraction of the cremaster muscle and resulting elevation of the testicle on the same side when stroking the inside of the thigh. It is a physiological extrinsic reflex. The afferent fibers course in the femoral branch of the genitofemoral nerve (L1/L2) and the ilioinguinal nerve (L1), the efferent fibers project in the genital branch of the genitofemoral nerve.

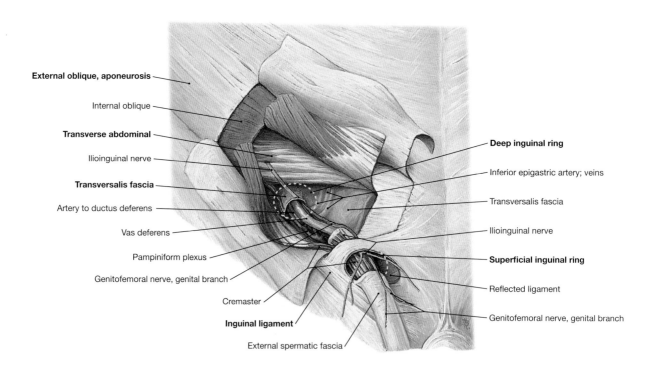

External oblique, aponeurosis

Internal oblique

Transverse abdominal

Ilioinguinal nerve

Transversalis fascia

Artery to ductus deferens

Vas deferens

Pampiniform plexus

Genitofemoral nerve, genital branch

Cremaster

Inguinal ligament

External spermatic fascia

Deep inguinal ring

Inferior epigastric artery; veins

Transversalis fascia

Ilioinguinal nerve

Superficial inguinal ring

Reflected ligament

Genitofemoral nerve, genital branch

Fig. 6.16 Walls and content of the inguinal canal; anterior view. [L240]

The deep and superficial inguinal rings are indicated with the yellow circles. The inguinal canal is 4–5 cm (2 in) long.

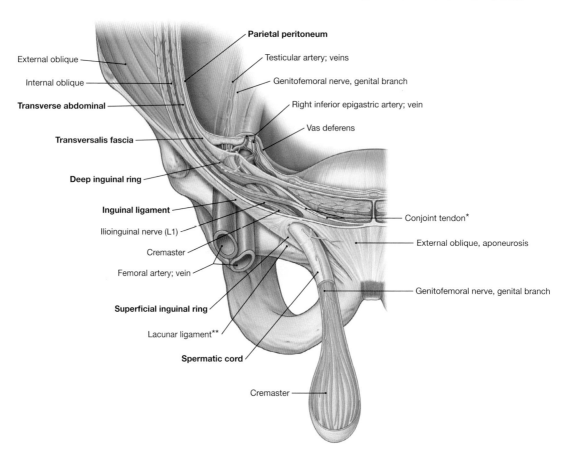

External oblique

Internal oblique

Transverse abdominal

Transversalis fascia

Deep inguinal ring

Inguinal ligament

Ilioinguinal nerve (L1)

Cremaster

Femoral artery; vein

Superficial inguinal ring

Lacunar ligament**

Spermatic cord

Cremaster

Parietal peritoneum

Testicular artery; veins

Genitofemoral nerve, genital branch

Right inferior epigastric artery; vein

Vas deferens

Conjoint tendon*

External oblique, aponeurosis

Genitofemoral nerve, genital branch

Fig. 6.17 Inguinal canal and spermatic cord; anterior view. The deep and superficial inguinal rings are indicated with yellow circles. [E460]

Borders of the inguinal canal:

Roof: muscular arches of transverse abdominis and internal oblique, medial crus of aponeurosis of external oblique;
Floor: inguinal ligament and lacunar ligament;

Anterior wall: aponeurosis of external oblique with lateral crus and intercrural fibers;
Posterior wall: transversalis fascia and reflected inguinal ligament (medially) and parietal peritoneum.

*   transversus tendinous arch, inguinal falx
** clin. term: GIMBERNAT's ligament

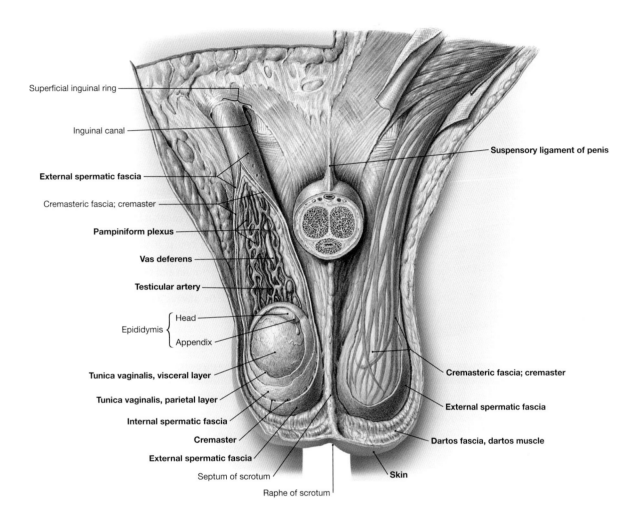

Fig. 6.18 Coverings of the spermatic cord and the testis; anterior view; scrotum opened.

Testis and spermatic cord have the following coverings:

- **Scrotal skin** (cutis);
- **Dartos fascia:** connective tissue of the scrotal skin with some smooth muscle cells;
- **External spermatic fascia:** continuation of the external oblique abdominal muscle;

- **Cremaster** with **cremasteric fascia:** Internal oblique abdominal muscle and its fascia;
- **Internal spermatic fascia:** continuation of the transversalis fascia;
- **Tunica vaginalis testis** (visceral and parietal layer): peritoneum.

Note: The anatomy of the testis, epididymis and vas deferens are shown in ➤ *chapter 7 (Pelvis).*

Structure/Function

Content of the spermatic cord:
- Vas deferens with artery of vas deferens (branch of the umbilical artery),
- Testicular artery (originates from the abdominal aorta),
- Pampiniform plexus of veins,
- Cremaster,
- Cremasteric artery (from the inferior epigastric artery),

- Genitofemoral nerve (genital branch) – innervation of cremaster,
- Lymph vessels,
- Autonomic nerves (testicular plexus).

Outside of the external spermatic fascia the ilioinguinal nerve passes through the superficial inguinal ring (sensory innervation of anterior scrotum – and labia majora in women).

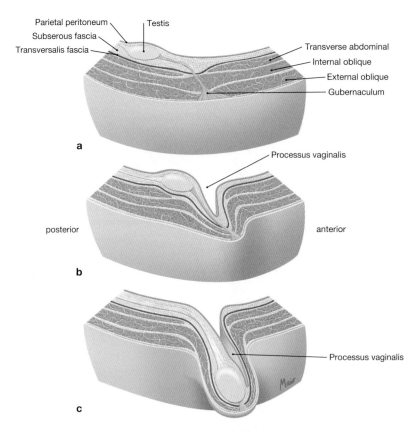

a

posterior   anterior

b

c

Fig. 6.19a to c Testicular descent; schematic illustrations. [L127]

a The gubernaculum, a mesenchymal condensation attached inferiorly to the labioscrotal swellings, is connected to the gonad and obliquely traverses the structures of the anterior abdominal wall at the site of the future inguinal canal.

b The processus vaginalis, a temporary evagination of the peritoneal cavity, forms and extends into the scrotal swellings anterior to the gubernaculum.

c The processus vaginalis is surrounded by the layers of the abdominal wall and forms the inguinal canal. It later obliterates and leaves only the tunica vaginalis testis directly surrounding the testis. If the processus vaginalis persists the remaining open connection between the scrotum and the peritoneal cavity promotes the formation of indirect inguinal hernias. **The testis always remains extraperitoneal during its descent.**

Coverings of the Spermatic Cord from Outside to Inside	
Coverings of the Spermatic Cord	**Layers of the Abdominal Wall**
Skin and subcutaneous tissue (dartos fascia and dartos muscle)	Skin and subcutaneous tissue (fatty and SCARPA's fascia)
External spermatic fascia	Fascia of external oblique
Cremaster	Internal oblique
Cremasteric fascia	Fascia of internal oblique
Internal spermatic fascia	Transversalis fascia
Tunica vaginalis testis (covering of testis and epididymis only)	Peritoneum

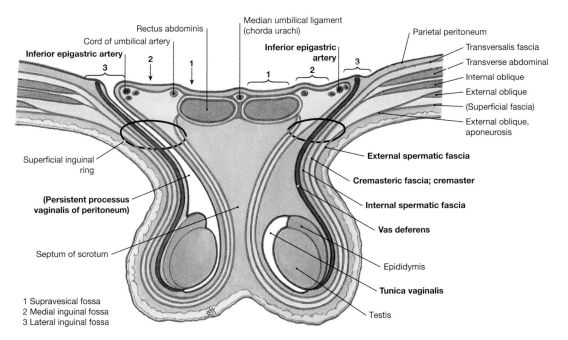

1 Supravesical fossa
2 Medial inguinal fossa
3 Lateral inguinal fossa

Fig. 6.20 Structure of the ventral abdominal wall and the coverings of the spermatic cord and testis; schematic illustration. [L240]

A persistent processus vaginalis is shown on the left side providing a communication between the tunica vaginalis of the testis and the peritoneal cavity of the abdomen.

Indirect Inguinal Hernia	Direct Inguinal Hernia (Congenital)
Enters the inguinal canal from the lateral inguinal fossa	Enters the hernia canal from the medial inguinal fossa (HESSELBACH's triangle)
Lateral to inferior epigastric artery and vein	Medial to inferior epigastric artery and vein
Passage through the deep inguinal ring	
Exits the inguinal canal through the superficial inguinal ring	Exits the hernial canal through the superficial inguinal ring
Position in the scrotum next to the spermatic cord	Position in the scrotum within the dilated spermatic cord
The hernial sac consists of parietal peritoneum and transversalis fascia and is positioned next to the spermatic cord, but within the external spermatic fascia in the scrotum.	With a persistent processus vaginalis the visceral peritoneum of the intestinal loop is next to the visceral layer of the tunica vaginalis testis. The peritoneal cavity extends into the scrotum; the hernia has all coverings of the spermatic cord.

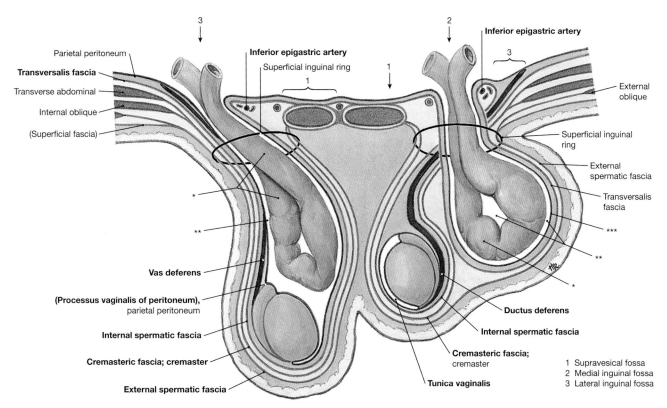

Fig. 6.21 Inguinal hernias; schematic illustration. [L240]
An indirect inguinal hernia is shown on the left side of the image, a direct inguinal hernia is shown on the right side.

*   intestinal loop in hernial sac
**   peritoneal cavity
*** newly formed peritoneal hernial sac

Clinical Remarks

Inguinal hernias always originate above the inguinal ligament and may reach into the scrotum in men or the labia majora in women. **Indirect inguinal hernia (a)** occur when content of the abdominal peritoneal cavity (greater omentum or intestinal loops) protrude into the inguinal canal or the scrotum. They are always positioned lateral to the inferior epigastric blood vessels (landmark!). **Direct inguinal hernias (b)** develop medial to the inferior epigastric blood vessels through the weak abdominal wall of HESSELBACH's triangle. In contrast, the hernial canal for femoral hernias is located inferior to the inguinal ligament (> p. 296). [L275]

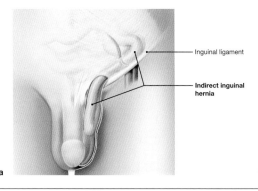

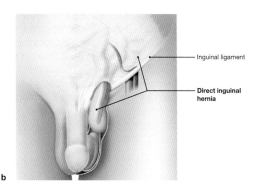

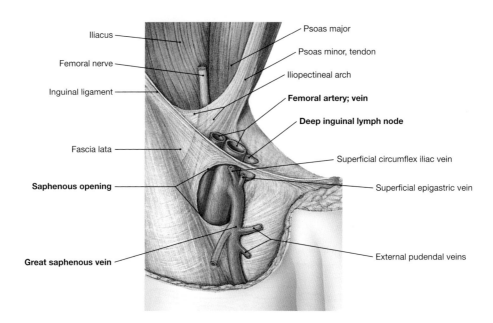

Iliacus
Femoral nerve
Inguinal ligament
Fascia lata
Saphenous opening
Great saphenous vein

Psoas major
Psoas minor, tendon
Iliopectineal arch
Femoral artery; vein
Deep inguinal lymph node
Superficial circumflex iliac vein
Superficial epigastric vein
External pudendal veins

Fig. 6.22 Hiatus saphenus and vascular compartment of retroinguinal space; right side; anterior view.
The iliopectinal arch separates the lateral muscular from the medial vascular compartment. The external iliac artery and vein transition into femoral artery and vein upon entering the femoral trian-

gle. The vascular compartment contains from lateral to medial: femoral artery, femoral vein and femoral canal. The deep inguinal lymph node, CLOQUET's node or ROSENMUELLER's node, is shown medial to the femoral vein in the femoral canal.

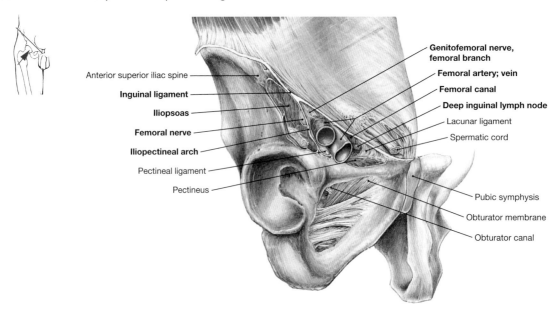

Anterior superior iliac spine
Inguinal ligament
Iliopsoas
Femoral nerve
Iliopectineal arch
Pectineal ligament
Pectineus

Genitofemoral nerve, femoral branch
Femoral artery; vein
Femoral canal
Deep inguinal lymph node
Lacunar ligament
Spermatic cord
Pubic symphysis
Obturator membrane
Obturator canal

Fig. 6.23 Muscular and vascular compartment of the retroinguinal space; right side; anterior view.

The femoral nerve travels in the muscular compartment. The **femoral canal** is positioned most medial in the vascular compartment and contains loose connective tissue and lymph vessels.

Clinical Remarks

Femoral hernias occur when content of the abdominal peritoneal cavity (greater omentum or intestinal loops) protrude into the femoral canal. The hernial canal for femoral hernias is located inferior to the inguinal ligament. **Femoral hernias** pass through the femoral ring and the femoral canal medial to the femoral vein and may surface through the saphenous opening of the fascia lata of the thigh. Femoral hernias are rare and occur more common in women than in men.
[L275]

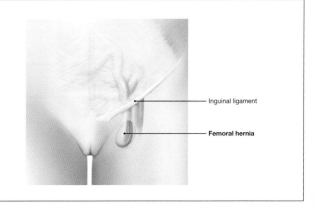

Inguinal ligament
Femoral hernia

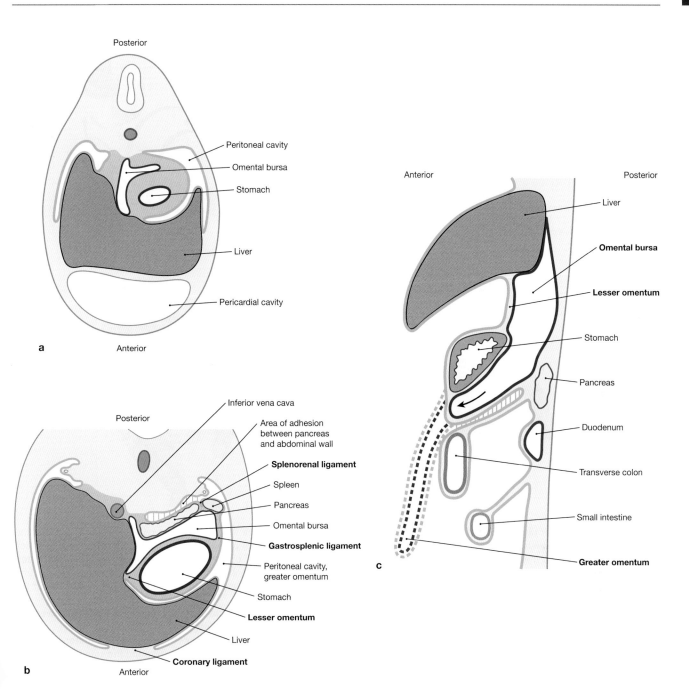

Fig. 6.24a to c Development of the upper abdominal situs at the beginning of week 5 (a), and at the beginning of week 7 (b and c); transverse sections **(a, b)** and paramedian section **(c)** of the upper abdomen. Peritoneum (green); peritoneum of the omental bursa (dark red). [L126]

The **primordial gut** derives from the endoderm and parts of the yolk sac. The mesoderm covering the primordial gut later forms the visceral peritoneum and, as parietal peritoneum, lines the abdominal cavity. The visceral peritoneum also forms the mesenteries which contain the neurovascular structures and serve as attachments. The dorsal mesentery connects the primordial gut with the dorsal wall of the trunk. The upper abdomen also contains a ventral mesentery.

An endodermal ventral outgrowth gives rise to the epithelial tissues of liver, gallbladder, bile ducts and pancreas. Subsequently, the following restructuring processes occur:

1. The liver expands into the ventral mesogastrium and, thus, creates a division into the ventral mesohepaticum (between ventral wall of the trunk and liver) and the dorsal mesohepaticum (between liver and stomach) **(a)**. The ventral mesohepaticum later forms the cranial **coronary ligament** and the caudal **falci-**

form ligament of liver. The **round ligament of liver** at the caudal margin is a remnant of the umbilical vein. The dorsal mesohepaticum becomes the **lesser omentum.**

2. In the dorsal mesogastrium a gap appears at the right side (pneumatoenteric recess) which later forms the **omental bursa (a).**
3. The stomach rotates **90°** in a **clockwise** direction (cranial view) and thus is located in a frontal position at the left side of the body **(b)**. The lesser omentum connects the liver and lesser curvature of the stomach also in a frontal plane and forms the ventral border of the omental bursa.
4. In the dorsal mesogastrium, the **pancreas** and the **spleen** develop. The pancreas subsequently acquires a retroperitoneal position, and the spleen remains intraperitoneal.

The dorsal mesogastrium eventually separates into the **gastrosplenic ligament** (from the greater curvature of the stomach to the spleen) and the **splenorenal ligament** (from the splenic hilum to the dorsal abdominal wall) and forms the greater omentum (apron-like at the greater curvature of the stomach; **c**). Therefore, due to its development and the neurovascular supply, the **greater omentum** is associated with the upper abdominal situs.

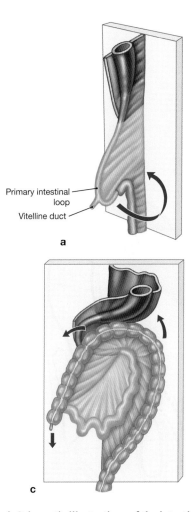

a

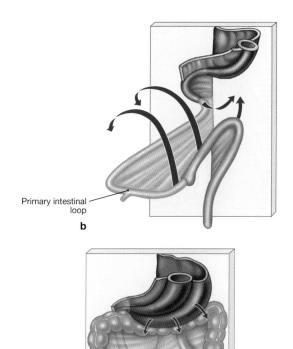

b

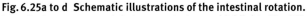

c

d

Fig. 6.25a to d Schematic illustrations of the intestinal rotation.
Intestinal segments and their mesenteries are highlighted in different colors: stomach and mesogastrium (purple), duodenum and mesoduodenum (blue), jejunum and ileum with associated mesenteries (orange), colon and mesocolon (brown). [L126]

Caused by the longitudinal growth of the primordial gut, a ventrally oriented loop forms **(primary intestinal loop).** The proximal (upper) limb of this loop develops into the major part of the small intestine, the distal (lower) limb develops into the colon including the transverse colon. The distal large intestine develops from the hindgut and, thus, differs in its neurovascular supply.

Due to a lack of space, the primary intestinal loop is temporarily located outside of the embryo in the umbilical cord **(physiological umbilical hernia)** and remains connected to the yolk sac via the vi-

telline duct. If the intestines fail to relocate entirely into the embryo, a congenital umbilical hernia **(omphalocele)** remains which contains portions of the intestinal segments and their mesenteries. Because this congenital hernia traverses through the later umbilical ring, it is covered by amnion only but not by muscles of the abdominal wall.

Remnants of the vitelline duct may remain as **MECKEL's diverticulum** located at the small intestine.

The elongation of the intestines initiates a **270° counter-clockwise rotation,** resulting in the colon to surround the small intestine like a frame.

Ascending colon and descending colon are secondarily relocated in a retroperitoneal position.

Clinical Remarks

Disturbances of the intestinal rotation can cause a **malrotation** (hyporotation and hyperrotation). These may result in intestinal obstruction (ileus) or an abnormal positioning of the respective intestinal segments, a condition that may impede the diagnosis

of an appendicitis. A **situs inversus** describes a condition where all organs are positioned mirror-inverted. Examples for **incomplete (a)** and **reversed (b)** secondary gut rotations are shown. [L275]

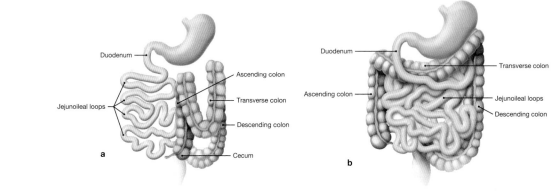

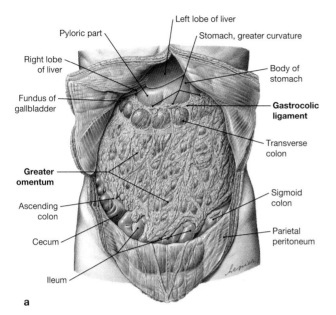

a

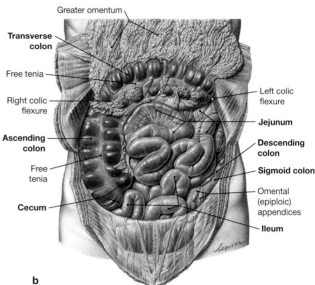

b

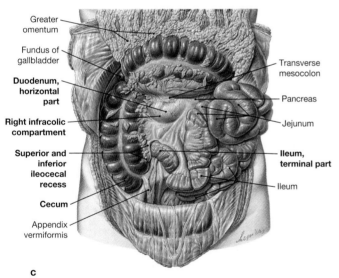

c

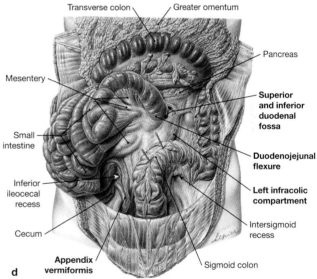

d

Fig. 6.26a to d Position of the viscera in the hypogastrium; anterior view.

a The transverse mesocolon divides the abdominal cavity into a **supracolic** (epigastrium) and an **infracolic** (hypogastrium) **compartment.** Viscera of the hypogastrium are almost completely covered by the greater omentum which is attached to the greater curvature of the stomach.

b After reflecting the greater omentum cranially the cecum, the ascending, transverse and sigmoid colon of the large intestine and the jejunum and ileum of the small intestine are visible.

c The loops of the small intestine are reflected to the left side to expose the retroperitoneal horizontal part of the duodenum. At the transition between the ileum and the cecum the vascular fold of the cecum (contains a branch of the ileocolic artery) creates two small peritoneal pouches: the **superior** and **inferior ileocecal recesses.**

d Reflecting the mesenteric root to the right side exposes the descending colon and the **superior** and **inferior duodenal recesses.** The **intersigmoid recess** is visible posterior to the sigmoid colon. The mesenteric root of the small intestines divides the hypogastrium into the **right (c)** and **left (d) infracolic compartment.**

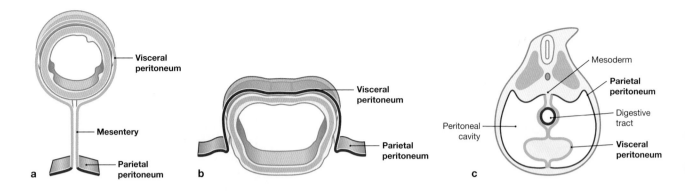

Fig. 6.27a to c Positions of abdominal viscera in relation to the peritoneum. [L126]

a Intraperitoneal viscera are surrounded by visceral peritoneum (green) which continues as mesentery, a peritoneal duplicature containing blood vessels, nerves and lymphatics. Mesenteries are attached to and continuous with the parietal peritoneum (purple).

b Primary retroperitoneal viscera are only covered with peritoneum on one surface. They lack mesenteries and are located outside the peritoneal cavity (retroperitoneal).

c The peritoneal abdominal cavity is lined by the visceral and parietal peritoneum (purple).

Structure/Function

The **parietal peritoneum** (purple in figure) comprises the inner lining of the abdominal wall and is continuous with the **visceral peritoneum** (green in figure) to line the abdomino pelvic peritoneal cavity. The **mesentery** comprises a double layer of visceral peritoneum which ensheathes the abdominal viscera and folds back to the posterior abdominal wall. It contains blood and lymph vessels and autonomic nerves.

Intraperitoneal abdominal organs are completely covered by visceral peritoneum and have a mesentery: stomach, spleen, liver and gallbladder cecum with appendix vermiformis, small intestines (but only superior part of duodenum), transverse and sigmoid colon.

Extraperitoneal abdominal organs lack a mesentery and are positioned towards the posterior abdominal wall (retroperitoneal) or inferior to the peritoneal cavity (subperitoneal):

- **Primary retroperitoneal organs:** kidneys, ureters, adrenal glands;
- **Secondary retroperitoneal organs** have lost their dorsal mesentery by its fusion to the posterior abdominal wall during development: pancreas, duodenum (except for superior part) ascending and descending colon, upper two-thirds of rectum;
- **Subperitoneal (infraperitoneal) organs:** cervix of uterus, urinary bladder, distal ureter, vagina, prostate, seminal vesicles, lower one-third of rectum.

Double-layered Peritoneal Folds

Mesentery:
- Provides continuity between the visceral and parietal peritoneum;
- Contains neurovascular structures and lymphatics;
- Connects the intraperitoneal organ with the posterior abdominal wall.

Omentum:
- **Lesser omentum*:** connects the lesser curvature of the stomach and the proximal duodenum to the liver (derived from the embryonic ventral mesogastrium);
- **Greater omentum*:** extends like an apron from the greater curvature of the stomach and the proximal duodenum to cover the viscera, then folds back to attach to the transverse colon (derived from the embryonic dorsal mesogastrium).

Peritoneal ligaments:
Connect intraperitoneal abdominal viscera to other organs or to the abdominal wall; examples:
- **Falciform ligament*** (derived from the embryonic ventral mesogastrium) from the liver to the anterior abdominal wall; contains the round ligament of the liver, the obliterated umbilical vein;
- **Hepatogastric ligament*** and hepatoduodenal ligament (together the lesser omentum);
- **Gastrophrenic ligament*** from the greater curvature of the stomach to the inferior diaphragm;
- **Gastrosplenic ligament*** from the greater curvature of the stomach to the hilum of the spleen (a part of the greater omentum);
- **Gastrocolic ligament** from the greater curvature of the stomach to the transverse colon (a part of the greater omentum);
- **Splenorenal ligament*** from the spleen to the posterolateral abdominal wall.

* shown in ➤ Fig. 6.28

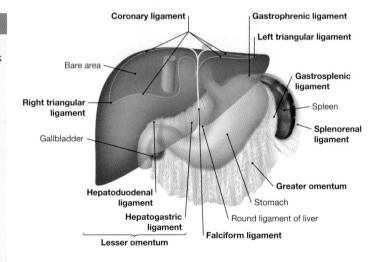

Fig. 6.28 Ligaments of the epigastrium; schematic illustration. [L275]

Clinical Remarks

Intense localized pain (e.g. with appendicitis) in the abdomen indicates the involvement of the **parietal peritoneum** that is innervated by **somatic nerves**: thoracoabdominal nerves T7–T11, subcostal nerve (T12) and iliohypogastric and ilioinguinal nerves (L1). Rigidity of the abdominal muscles results from muscle contraction over the affected peritoneum as a protective reflex. In contrast, the pain afferents of the visceral peritoneum travel with the autonomic nerves and usually produce a dull pain that is not well localized.

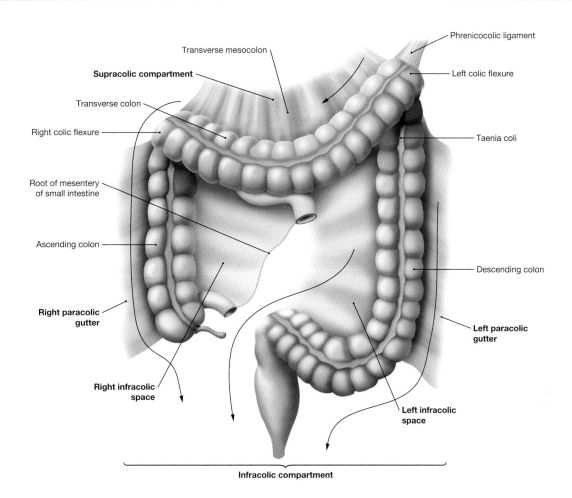

Transverse mesocolon

Phrenicocolic ligament

Supracolic compartment

Left colic flexure

Transverse colon

Right colic flexure

Taenia coli

Root of mesentery
of small intestine

Ascending colon

Descending colon

**Right paracolic
gutter**

**Left paracolic
gutter**

**Right infracolic
space**

**Left infracolic
space**

Infracolic compartment

Fig. 6.29 Compartments of the peritoneal cavity. [L275]
The transverse mesocolon divides the peritoneal cavity into a **supracolic** and an **infracolic compartment**. The mesenteric root divides the **right** and **left infracolic compartment**. The left infracolic space is continuous with the pelvic peritoneal cavity to the right of the sigmoid mesocolon. The right and left **paracolic gutters,** recesses lateral to the ascending and descending colon, communicate with the pelvic peritoneal cavity. The right paracolic gutter connects superiorly with the supracolic compartment up to the subphrenic space.
Supracolic compartment contains spleen, stomach, liver.
Infracolic compartment contains small intestines, ascending and descending colon.

The peritoneal compartments explain the movement of fluids (ascites, peritoneal infections) from the pelvic peritoneal cavity to the subphrenic peritoneal space under the diaphragm and vice versa. In an upright position (seldom in bedridden patients), inflammatory exudate or pus in cases of inflammatory events in the hypogastrium may accumulate in the most inferior extension of the peritoneal cavity, the rectovesical pouch in men, and the rectouterine pouch (pouch of DOUGLAS) in women (➤ Fig. 6.69) in the pelvic peritoneal cavity.

Clinical Remarks

The **hepatorenal recess (MORRISON's pouch),** the posterior right infrahepatic space that belongs to the supracolic compartment, is an important peritoneal space in which fluids collecting in the peritoneal cavity (e.g. ascites) can ascend to the right subphrenic space **(right subphrenic recess)** below the diaphragm. The hepatorenal recess is bordered posteriorly by the right kidney and the right adrenal gland, anteriorly by the right lobe of the liver and the gall bladder and superiorly by the coronary ligament of the liver.

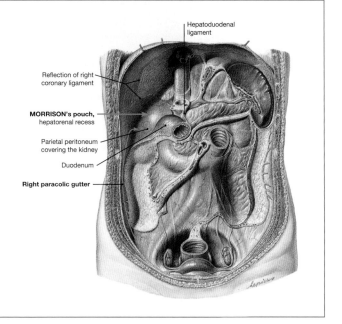

Hepatoduodenal ligament

Reflection of right
coronary ligament

MORRISON's pouch,
hepatorenal recess

Parietal peritoneum
covering the kidney

Duodenum

Right paracolic gutter

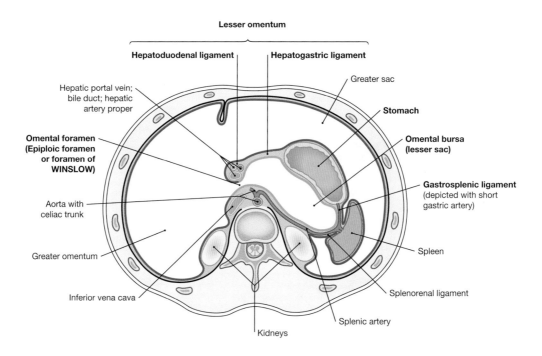

Fig. 6.30 Omental bursa, lesser sac; transverse section; schematic drawing. [L126]
The lesser sac is a subdivision of the peritoneal cavity located behind the lesser omentum and the stomach. It facilitates the friction-free movement of the stomach against the posterior struc-

tures. The only natural connection between the greater and the lesser sacs is the **omental foramen (epiploic foramen;** foramen of WINSLOW) located between the hepatoduodenal ligament and the peritoneal lining above the inferior vena cava.

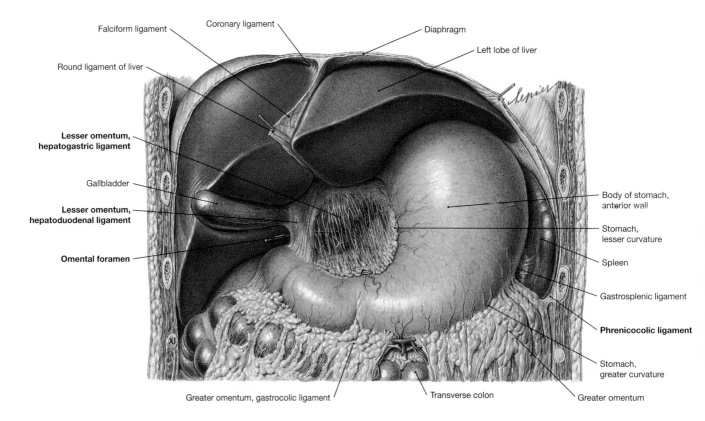

Fig. 6.31 Lesser omentum and omental foramen; anterior view.
The liver was reflected cranially to visualize the lesser omentum. It spans between the liver and the lesser curvature of the stomach and the superior part of the duodenum. The lesser omentum consists of the hepatogastric ligament and the hepatoduodenal ligament. The latter contains the common bile duct, the hepatic portal vein, and the hepatic artery proper to the hilum of the liver. The probe marks the **omental** or **epiploic foramen,** the natural entrance to the omental bursa behind the hepatoduodenal ligament.

The greater omentum is attached to the greater curvature of the stomach and to the omental taenia of the transverse colon. Below the transverse colon, the greater omentum comprises a four layered peritoneal fold. If these layers are not fused the space within the greater omentum is connected to the lesser sac and referred to as the **inferior recess of the omental bursa.** The spleen resides in the splenic niche and rests on the phrenicocolic ligament between the left colic flexure (splenic flexure) and the diaphragm.

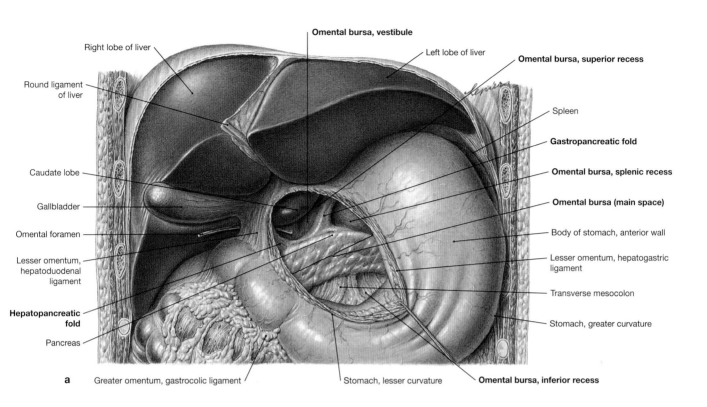

Omental bursa, vestibule

Right lobe of liver — Left lobe of liver

Round ligament of liver — Omental bursa, superior recess

Spleen

Caudate lobe — Gastropancreatic fold

Omental bursa, splenic recess

Gallbladder — Omental bursa (main space)

Omental foramen — Body of stomach, anterior wall

Lesser omentum, hepatoduodenal ligament — Lesser omentum, hepatogastric ligament

Hepatopancreatic fold — Transverse mesocolon

Pancreas — Stomach, greater curvature

a   Greater omentum, gastrocolic ligament   Stomach, lesser curvature   **Omental bursa, inferior recess**

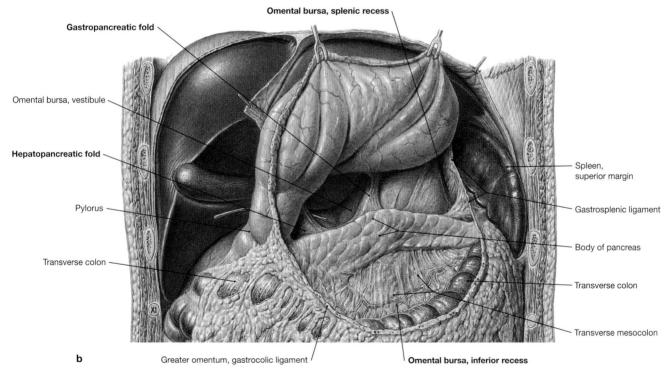

Omental bursa, splenic recess

Gastropancreatic fold

Omental bursa, vestibule — Spleen, superior margin

Hepatopancreatic fold — Gastrosplenic ligament

Pylorus — Body of pancreas

Transverse colon — Transverse colon

Transverse mesocolon

b   Greater omentum, gastrocolic ligament   **Omental bursa, inferior recess**

Fig. 6.32a and b Lesser sac; omental bursa; anterior view.
a The lesser omentum between the liver and the lesser curvature of the stomach was severed to show the omental bursa.
b The gastrocolic ligament was cut and the stomach reflected cranially to show the main space of the omental bursa.
The omental bursa is subdivided into four parts:
- **Omental (epiploic) foramen:** the entrance to the omental bursa is located at the free margin of the lesser omentum and is confined anteriorly by the hepatoduodenal ligament, cranially by the caudate lobe, caudally by the duodenal cap, and posteriorly by the inferior vena cava.
- **Vestibule:** the vestibule is confined by the lesser omentum ventrally and its **superior recess** extends behind the liver.

- **Isthmus:** the narrowing between vestibule and main space is confined by two peritoneal folds: on the right side by the hepatopancreatic fold which is created by the common hepatic artery, and on the left side by the gastropancreatic fold which marks the course of the left gastric artery.
- **Main space:** this space is located between the stomach (anterior) and the pancreas and the transverse mesocolon (posterior). On the left side, the **splenic recess** extends to the hilum of the spleen; the **inferior recess** lies behind the gastrocolic ligament and may extend inferiorly between the layers of the greater omentum to the origin of the mesocolon at the transverse colon.

303

Clinical Remarks

Similar to the other recesses of the peritoneal cavity, the omental bursa is of clinical relevance. Herniation of small intestinal loops **(internal hernia),** dissemination of malignant tumors **(peritoneal carcinosis),** or infections **(peritonitis)** can involve the omental bursa. Peptic ulcers of the posterior wall of the stomach may perforate and cause peritonitis in the lesser sac. Inflammation or injuries to the pancreas may also cause fluid accumulation in the omental bursa.

Common surgical access routes to the omental bursa:
1. **through the lesser omentum;**
2. **through the gastrocolic ligament;**
3. **through the transverse mesocolon.**

The inferior recess of the omental bursa may extend further into the greater omentum in cases where the anterior and posterior folds have not fused.
[L126]

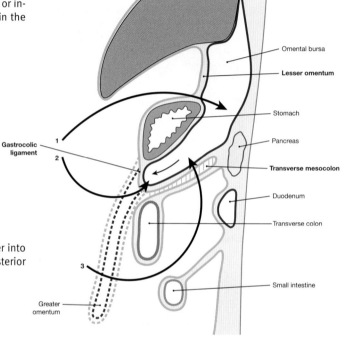

Boundaries of the Omental Bursa		
Boundary	**Constituents**	**Space/Recess**
Anterior	Lesser omentum, posterior surface of the stomach, gastrocolic ligament	
Posterior	Peritoneum covering the pancreas, aorta, celiac trunk, superior pole of left kidney and adrenal gland	
Posterior and left	Spleen, gastrosplenic ligament	Splenic recess
Inferior	Transverse mesocolon; Possible inferior extension between the layers of the greater omentum	Inferior recess
Superior	Liver (caudate lobe), posterior reflection of peritoneum to the diaphragm	Superior recess

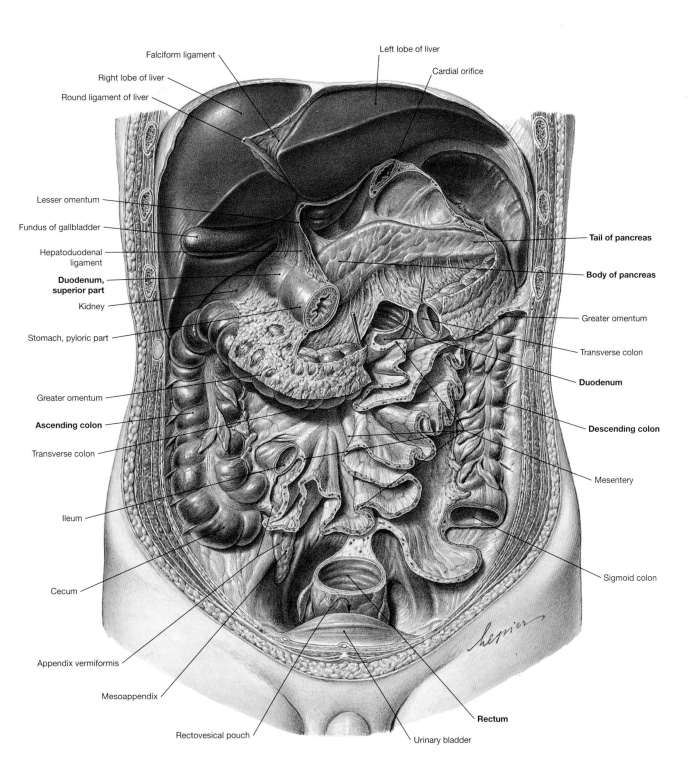

Falciform ligament

Left lobe of liver

Cardial orifice

Right lobe of liver

Round ligament of liver

Lesser omentum

Fundus of gallbladder

Hepatoduodenal ligament

Duodenum, superior part

Kidney

Stomach, pyloric part

Greater omentum

Ascending colon

Transverse colon

Ileum

Cecum

Appendix vermiformis

Mesoappendix

Rectovesical pouch

Tail of pancreas

Body of pancreas

Greater omentum

Transverse colon

Duodenum

Descending colon

Mesentery

Sigmoid colon

Rectum

Urinary bladder

Fig. 6.33 Position of secondary retroperitoneal abdominal organs; anterior view.
The stomach was removed, jejunum and ileum were resected at the mesentery, and transverse colon and sigmoid colon were cut. Most of the secondary retroperitoneal organs are now visible.
This peritoneal pouch is the most inferior part of the peritoneal cavity in men.

Secondary retroperitoneal organs:
- Duodenum (except for superior part),
- Pancreas,
- Ascending colon,
- Descending colon,
- Rectum to the sacral flexure.

Anterior to the rectum, the opening of the rectovesical pouch is visible.

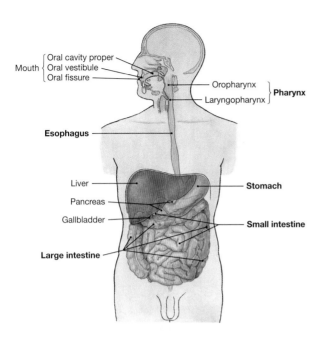

Fig. 6.34 **Overview of the alimentary tract.**

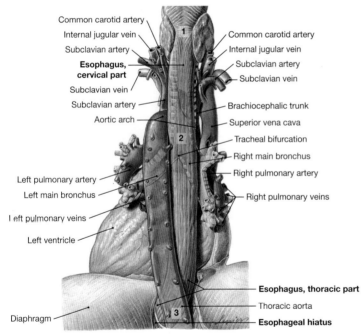

Fig. 6.36 **Esophagus, pericardium, and thoracic aorta;** posterior view.

The posterior view shows the close proximity of the thoracic part to the pericardium and to the left atrium (➤ Fig. 5.65b). The locations of the three constrictions of the esophagus are indicated.

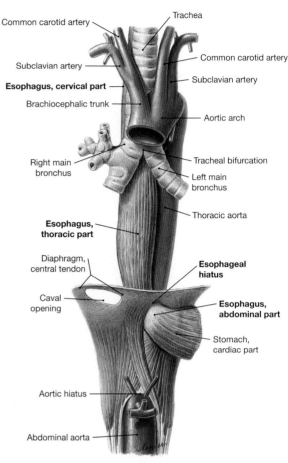

Fig. 6.35 **Esophagus, trachea, and thoracic aorta;** anterior view.

The esophagus is 25 cm long and is organized in three parts:

- Cervical part (5–8 cm / 2–3 in),
- Thoracic part (16 cm / 6.3 in),
- Abdominal part (1–4 cm / 0.5–1.5 in).

The **cervical part** is adjacent to the vertebral column. The **thoracic part** crosses the aortic arch which is adjacent on the dorsal left side. The esophagus courses along the left main bronchus and descends ventrally with increasing distance to the vertebral column. After traversing the esophageal hiatus of the diaphragm, the short intraperitoneal **abdominal part** begins.

Structure/Function

Anatomical constrictions of the esophagus

1. **Cervical (pharyngoesophageal) constriction:**
   Level of C6, pharyngoesophageal junction caused by cricopharyngeus muscle, 15 cm (6 in) from incisors.

2. **Thoracic (bronchoaortic) constriction:**
   Level of T4/T5, bronchoaortic constriction by arch of aorta, 22–23 cm (9 in) from incisors, visible in A/P views;

Level of T5, crossed by left main bronchus, 25–27 cm (10 in) from incisors, visible in lateral views.

3. **Diaphragmatic constriction:**
   Level of T10, esophageal hiatus, 40 cm (16 in) from incisors.

For cervical esophageal diverticula see ➤ *chapter 11 (Neck), p. 532.*

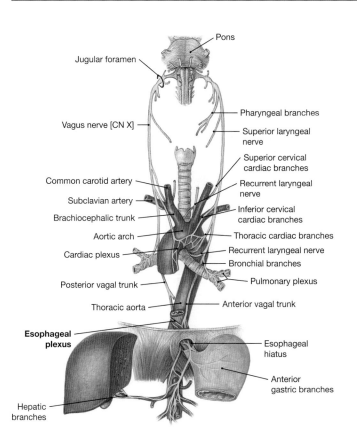

Fig. 6.37 Innervation of the esophagus; anterior view.
The parasympthathetic nerves of the posterior mediastinum are shown. **Parasympathetic fibers** travel with the right and left vagus nerves, continue as posterior and anterior vagal trunk, respectively, and traverse the diaphragm through the esophageal hiatus. Parasympathetic fibers to the esophagus synapse in ganglia of the esophageal nerve plexus. The presynaptic **sympathetic fibers** synapse in the T2–T6 sympathetic ganglia of the sympathetic trunk and join the esophageal plexus to reach the esophagus.
- **Parasympathetics:** increase peristalsis and secretory activity, and promote vasodilation;
- **Sympathetics:** decrease peristalsis and secretory activity and promote vasoconstriction.

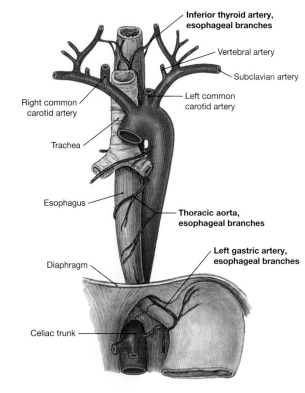

Fig. 6.38 Arteries of the esophagus; anterior view.
The three parts of the esophagus are supplied by surrounding arteries:
- **Cervical part:** inferior thyroid artery,
- **Thoracic part:** esophageal branches of the thoracic aorta,
- **Abdominal part:** left gastric artery and inferior phrenic artery.

Lymphatic Drainage of the Esophagus		
Esophagus	**Lymph Node Stations**	**Lymph Trunk**
Cervical	Deep cervical nodes	Jugular trunk
Thoracic (above tracheal bifurcation)	Paratracheal, tracheobronchial, posterior mediastinal nodes	Bronchomediastinal trunk
Thoracic (below tracheal bifurcation)	Gastric, celiac nodes	Intestinal trunk
Abdominal	Gastric, celiac nodes	Intestinal trunk
	Inferior phrenic nodes	Lumbar trunk

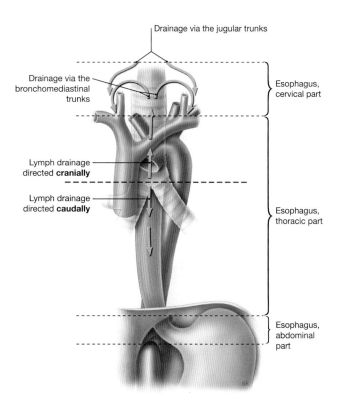

Fig. 6.39 Lymphatic drainage of the esophagus; anterior view.
[L238]

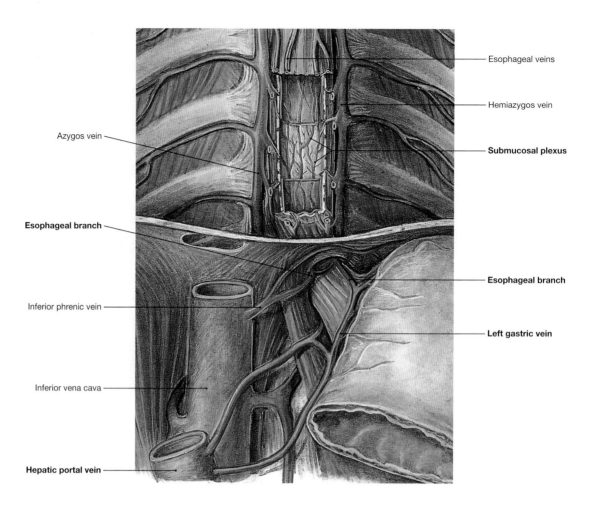

Esophageal veins

Hemiazygos vein

Submucosal plexus

Azygos vein

Esophageal branch

Inferior phrenic vein

Esophageal branch

Left gastric vein

Inferior vena cava

Hepatic portal vein

Fig. 6.40 Veins of the esophagus with illustration of the portocaval anastomoses between hepatic portal vein and superior vena cava; anterior view.

The extensive venous network in the adventitia is connected to the submucosal veins (submucosal venous plexus). The blood drains via azygos vein (right side) and hemiazygos vein (left side) upwards to the superior vena cava. The lower parts of the esophagus also connect to the hepatic portal vein via the veins at the lesser curvature of the stomach (left and right gastric vein).

Clinical Remarks

If pressure in the portal venous system increases **(portal hypertension)**, e.g. due to increased liver parenchymal resistance (cirrhosis of the liver), the venous blood is redirected to the superior vena cava and inferior vena cava via **portocaval anastomoses.** Clinically, the most important portocaval anastomosis is the connection of the esophagus to the gastric veins. This may result in dilations of the esophageal submucosal veins **(esophageal varices).** Rupture of these varices is associated with a mortality of approximately 50% and is, thus, the most frequent cause of death in patients with liver cirrhosis. Rupture into the lumen leads to the accumulation of darkened blood in the stomach, the rare external rupture results in bleeding into the peritoneal cavity. [G159, L126]

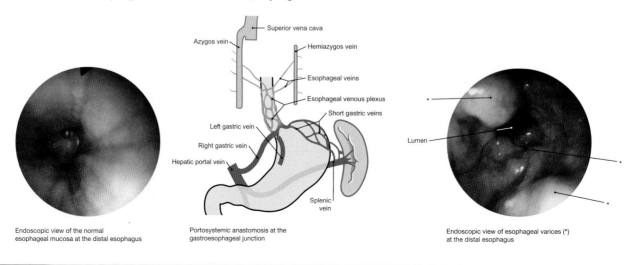

Superior vena cava

Azygos vein

Hemiazygos vein

Esophageal veins

Esophageal venous plexus

Short gastric veins

Left gastric vein

Right gastric vein

Hepatic portal vein

Splenic vein

Lumen

Endoscopic view of the normal
esophageal mucosa at the distal esophagus

Portosystemic anastomosis at the
gastroesophageal junction

Endoscopic view of esophageal varices (*)
at the distal esophagus

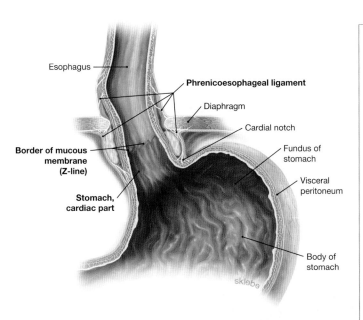

Fig. 6.41 Gastroesophageal junction; anterior view. [L238]
This junction is also referred to as esophagogastric junction. Attachments of the esophagus at the esophageal hiatus of the diaphragm are shown. The **Z-line** marks the transition between the gastric mucosa and the squamous epithelium of the esophageal mucosa.

Structure/Function

The **lower esophageal sphincter (LES)** is not a true sphincter muscle, but comprises a functional unit with several components:
Intrinsic components:
Esophageal muscle fibers with spiral orientation create longitudinal tension in the thoracic part and normally close the lumen. This intrinsic component is under neurohormonal influence. The lumen is widened locally with a peristaltic wave for the passage of food.
The **esophageal submucosal venous plexus** serves as mucosa cushion for a gas-tight closure of the lumen. The angle of 65° at the junction between cardia and fundus of the stomach is referred to as **cardial notch (angle of HIS)**. This angulation creates a mucosal fold which helps prevent reflux of gastric content into the cardia.
Extrinsic components:
Phrenicoesophageal ligaments anchor the abdominal part of the esophagus to the diaphragm and secure its position at the esophageal hiatus. It allows the esophagus to move independently from the diaphragm during respiration and swallowing. The contractions of the diaphragm muscle serve as functional external sphincter to the esophagus related to the movement during respiration.

Clinical Remarks

Insufficient lower esophageal sphincter components lead to **gastroesophageal reflux disease (GERD)**. Chronic acidic reflux causes inflammation of the esophageal mucosa and **BARRETT's esophagus** with epithelial metaplasia of the lower esophagus. This increases the risk for esophageal cancer.
A **hiatal gastric hernia** (sliding hernia) occurs when parts of the stomach are pushed through a widened esophageal hiatus into the thoracic cavity. Heartburn is the most common symptom, similar to GERD. Chronically increased abdominal pressure or being overweight are common risk factors for GERD and hiatal hernia.
A sliding hiatal hernia is detected during the course of a radiocontrast examination. The arrow marks a stricture resulting from reflux esophagitis. The area below shows the hiatal sliding hernia of the stomach, as marked by the hollow arrow. [E603]

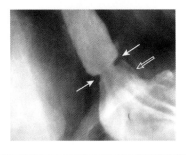

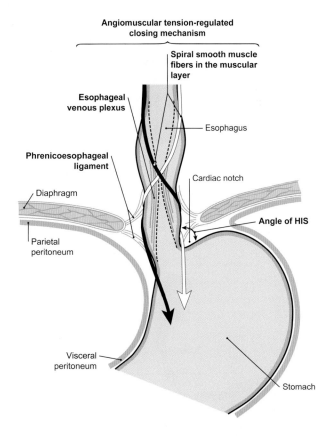

Fig. 6.42 Gastroesophageal junction; schematic illustration. [L126]
The course of the muscular fibers, the mucosa cushions and the supporting ligaments connecting to the esophageal hiatus in the diaphragm are shown.

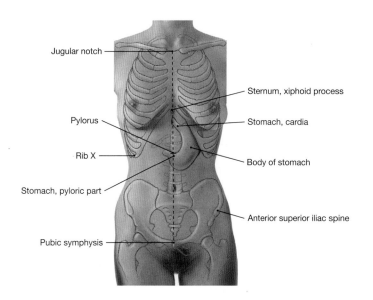

Jugular notch

Pylorus

Rib X

Stomach, pyloric part

Pubic symphysis

Sternum, xiphoid process

Stomach, cardia

Body of stomach

Anterior superior iliac spine

Fig. 6.43 Projection of the stomach onto the ventral body wall.
The cardia projects to the level of the T10 vertebra, ventrally just below the xiphoid process of the sternum. The position of the caudal part of the stomach is variable at the level of L2/L3 vertebra. The pylorus locates at the transpyloric plane (➤ Table on p. 283, bottom), projecting onto L1 vertebra.

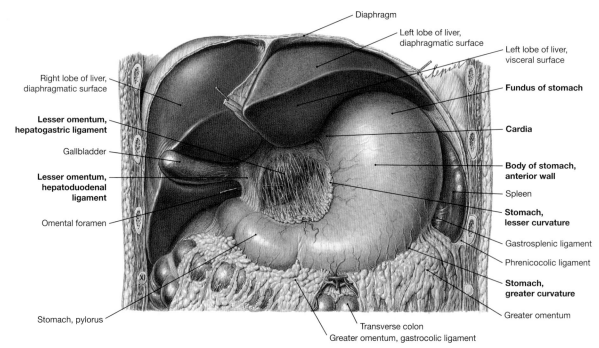

Diaphragm

Left lobe of liver, diaphragmatic surface

Left lobe of liver, visceral surface

Right lobe of liver, diaphragmatic surface

Fundus of stomach

Lesser omentum, hepatogastric ligament

Cardia

Gallbladder

Body of stomach, anterior wall

Lesser omentum, hepatoduodenal ligament

Spleen

Stomach, lesser curvature

Omental foramen

Gastrosplenic ligament

Phrenicocolic ligament

Stomach, greater curvature

Greater omentum

Stomach, pylorus

Transverse colon

Greater omentum, gastrocolic ligament

Fig. 6.44 Stomach in-situ; anterior view.
The abdominal wall was removed and the liver and gall bladder were lifted cranially to expose the stomach and the lesser and greater omentum.

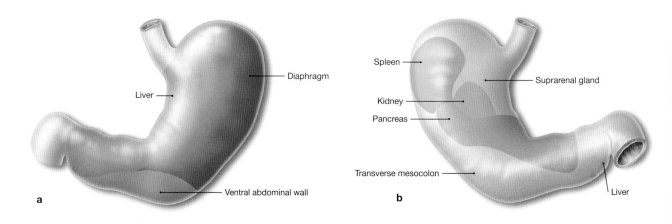

Diaphragm

Liver

Ventral abdominal wall

a

Spleen

Suprarenal gland

Kidney

Pancreas

Transverse mesocolon

Liver

b

Fig. 6.45a and b Spatial relations of the stomach; anterior wall **(a)** and posterior wall **(b)**. The posterior wall of the stomach faces the lesser sac (omental bursa) – ➤ p. 301, peritoneal cavity. [L238]

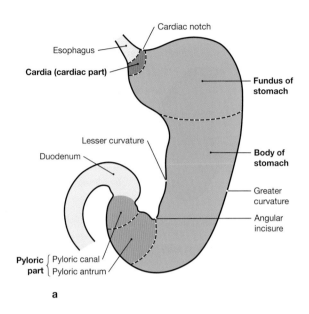

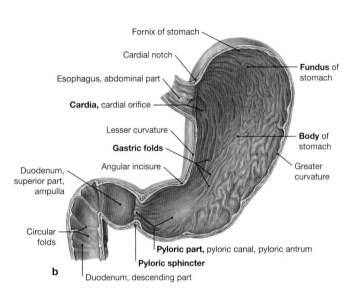

a

b

Fig. 6.46a and b Stomach; schematic illustration **(a)** and anterior view **(b).** a [L126]

The stomach has four parts:
- **Cardia:** entrance to the stomach
- **Fundus:** superior part below the left dome of the diaphragm
- **Body:** main part of the stomach
- **Pyloric part:** comprising the **pyloric antrum** and **pyloric canal** which is surrounded by the **pyloric sphincter.**

The lesser curvature is directed to the right side, the greater curvature to the left side. The kink in the lesser curvature (angular in-

cisure or angular notch) marks the beginning of the pyloric part. The greater curvature begins with an indentation (cardial notch) between the esophagus and the stomach. The gastric mucosa has a characteristic relief serving the enlargement of the inner surface. The macroscopically recognisable longitudinally oriented **gastric folds** form the functional **gastric canal** along the lesser curvature. At the exit of the stomach (pylorus), the circular muscle layer is thickened to form the **pyloric sphincter.**

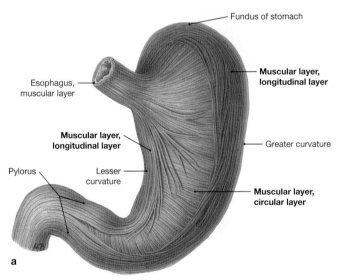

a

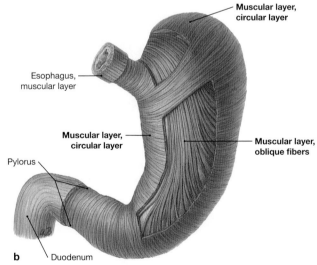

b

Fig. 6.47a and b Outer (a) and inner (b) muscular layers of the stomach; anterior view.

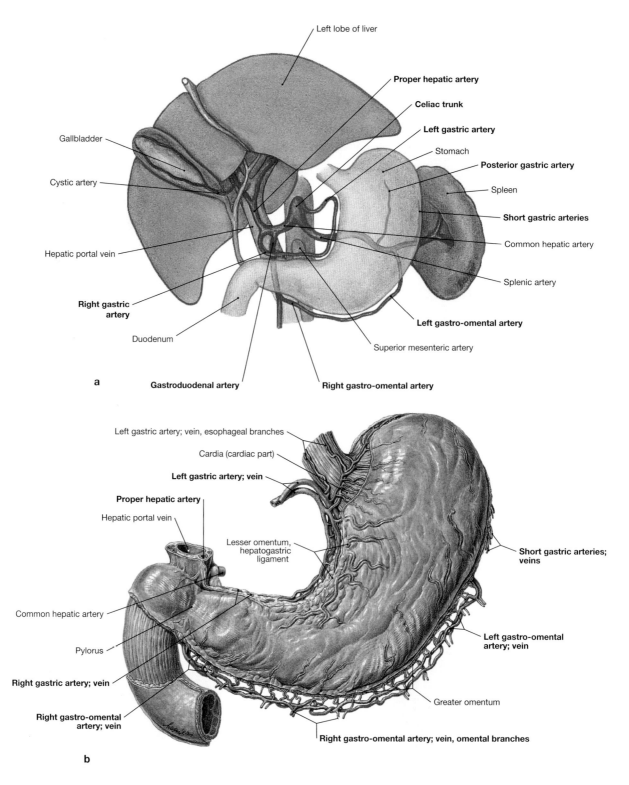

Fig. 6.48a and b Vascular supply of the stomach as schematic illustration **(a)** and their course along the curvatures of the stomach **(b)**; anterior view.

Region of Stomach	Arteries to the Stomach	Origin
Lesser curvature	**Left gastric artery**	Direct branch of the **celiac trunk**
	Right gastric artery	Branch of the **proper hepatic artery**
Greater curvature	Left gastro-omental artery*	Branch of the **splenic artery**
	Right gastro-omental artery*	**Gastroduodenal artery** of the common hepatic artery
Fundus	**Short gastric arteries**	Branches of the **splenic artery** near the splenic hilum
Posterior side	**Posterior gastric artery** (present in 30–60%)	Branches of the **splenic artery** behind the stomach

* These vessels also supply the greater omentum!

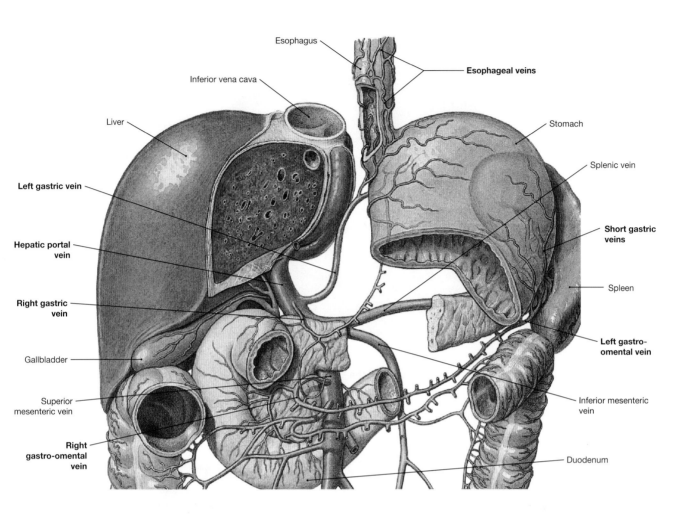

Esophagus

Esophageal veins

Inferior vena cava

Stomach

Liver

Splenic vein

Left gastric vein

Short gastric veins

Hepatic portal vein

Right gastric vein

Spleen

Gallbladder

Left gastro-omental vein

Superior mesenteric vein

Inferior mesenteric vein

Right gastro-omental vein

Duodenum

Fig. 6.49 Venous drainage of the stomach; anterior view.
The veins are corresponding to the arteries. Veins at the lesser curvature directly enter the portal vein, whereas the veins at the great-er curvature drain into the larger branches of the portal vein.
Note: The hepatic portal vein and the portal venous system are shown in more details with the liver later in this chapter.

Region of Stomach	Veins of the Stomach	Origin
Lesser curvature	**Left gastric vein**	Drain to the **hepatic portal vein;** anastomose via the esophageal veins with the **azygos system** (SVC)*
	Right gastric vein	
Greater curvature	**Left gastro-omental vein**	Drains to the **splenic vein**
	Right gastro-omental vein	drains to the **superior mesenteric vein**
Fundus	**Short gastric veins**	Drain to the **splenic vein**
Posterior side	**Posterior gastric veins** (present in 30–60 %)	Drain to the **splenic vein**

* Portocaval anastomoses

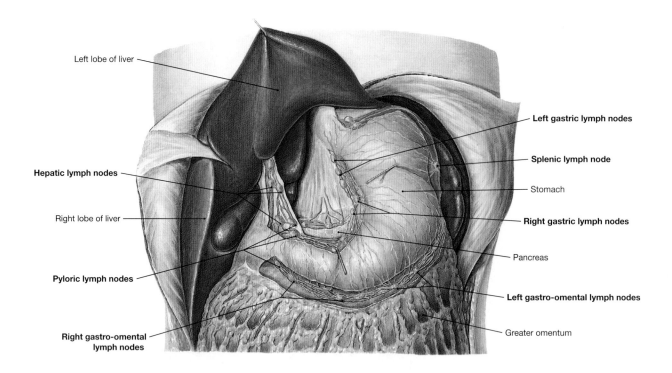

Fig. 6.50 Lymph vessels and lymph nodes of the stomach and the liver; anterior view.
The lymph vessels and lymph nodes of the stomach are located alongside both curvatures and around the pylorus: the lesser cur-vature shows the gastric nodes, the greater curvature harbors the splenic nodes and caudal thereof the gastro-omental nodes. The pyloric nodes in the region of the pylorus connect to the hepatic nodes at the hilum of the liver.

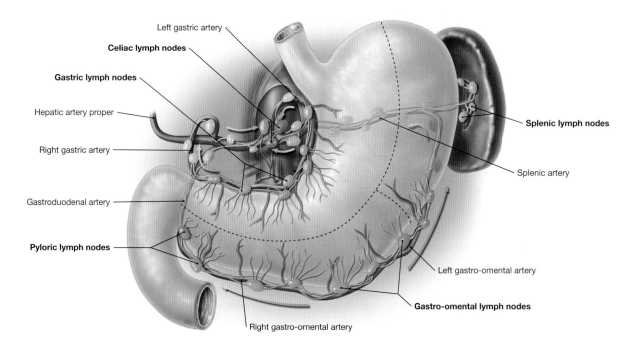

Fig. 6.51 Regional lymph nodes and lymphatic drainage stations of the stomach; anterior view. [L238]
There are three subsequent principal lymphatic drainage stations:
*   **First station (green):** lymph nodes along the curvatures;
*   **Second station (orange):** lymph nodes along the branches of the celiac trunk;
*   **Third station (blue):** lymph nodes at the origin of the celiac trunk (celiac nodes); from here the lymph is drained via the in-testinal trunk into the thoracic duct.

Clinical Remarks

The lymphatic drainage stations of the stomach are of clinical rel-evance in the surgical treatment of **gastric cancer.** The lymph nodes of the first (sentinel) and second stations are usually re-moved together with the stomach. If lymph nodes of the third sta-tion are also affected by metastatic cancer cells, curative therapy is not possible. In these cases, total gastrectomy will not be per-formed.

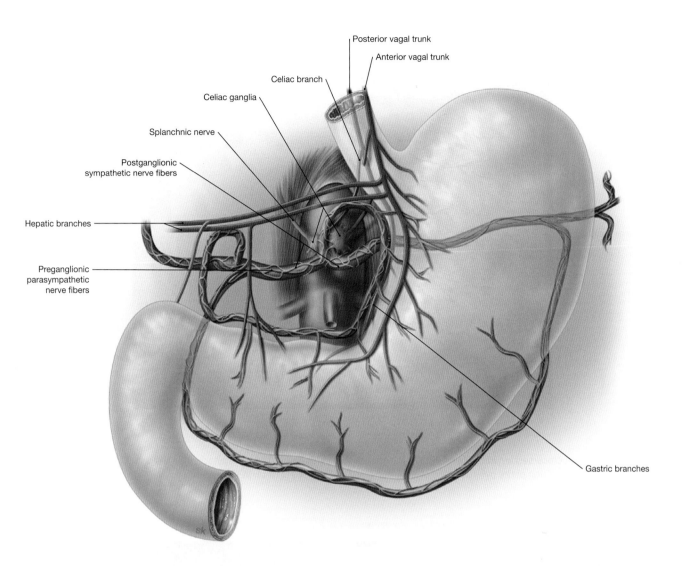

Fig. 6.52

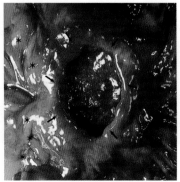

Fig. 6.52 Autonomic innervation of the stomach; semischematic illustration. Sympathetic innervation (green), parasympathetic innervation (purple). [L238]

Preganglionic parasympathetic (purple) fibers (gastric branches) reach the stomach as anterior and posterior vagal trunks descending along the esophagus and course along the lesser curvature. As a result of the gastric rotation during development, the anterior vagal trunk is predominantly derived from the left, the posterior vagal trunk from the right vagus nerve [CN X]. The pyloric part is innervated by separate branches **(hepatic branches)** of the vagal trunks.

The postganglionic neurons are located within the muscular layers of the stomach. The parasympathetic innervation stimulates the production of gastric acids and promotes the gastric peristalsis. Preganglionic sympathetic (green) fibers traverse the diaphragm on both sides **as greater and lesser splanchnic nerves** and are synapsed to the postganglionic sympathetic neurons in the **celiac ganglia** located at the origin of the celiac trunk. These postganglionic sympathetic fibers reach the stomach as periarterial nerve plexus. The sympathetic innervation reduces gastric acid production, peristalsis, and perfusion.

Clinical Remarks

Defects of the gastric mucosa occur as **peptic ulcers** and frequently are the result of a *Helicobacter pylori* infection in combination with reduced production of protective mucus and/or nonsteroidal anti-inflammatory antiphlogistic drugs (NSAID). Antibiotic treatment has almost completely replaced the **selective proximal vagotomy** (SPV) which aimed to reduce parasympathetic stimulation of the HCl-producing parietal cells in the gastric mucosa of the antrum. Frequent side effects of SPV are pyloric sphincter malfunction.
[R235]

Gastric ulcer; pylorus (*), arrows mark the rim of the ulcer

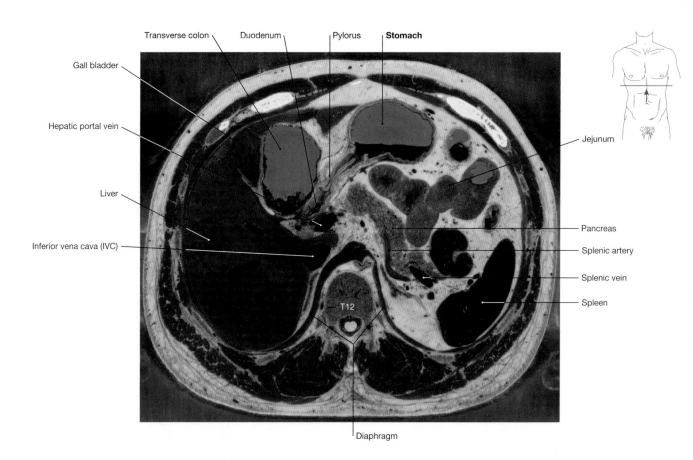

Fig. 6.53 Abdominal cross-section at the level of T12. This cross-section shows the transition of the pylorus of the stomach to the duodenum. The transpyloric plane is usually located at the transition of T12 to L1. [X338]

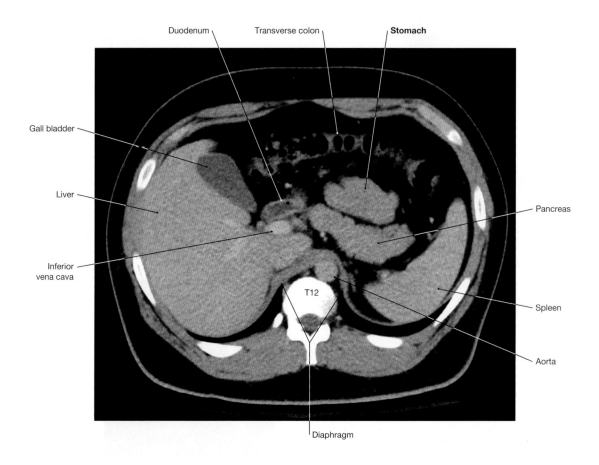

Fig. 6.54 Abdominal CT cross-section at the level of T12. [X338]

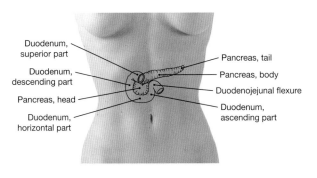

Fig. 6.55 Projection of duodenum and pancreas onto the body surface; anterior view.

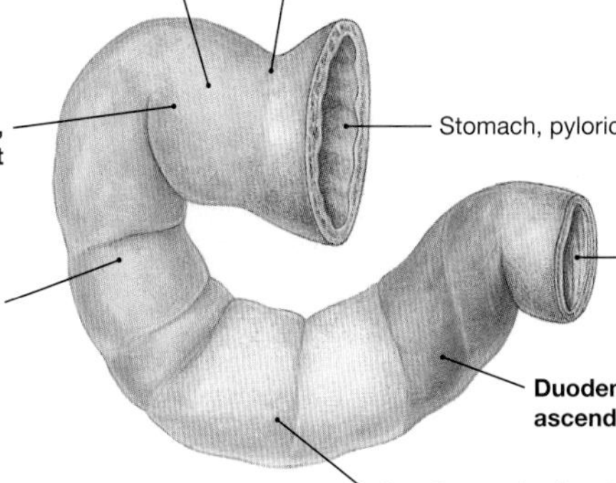

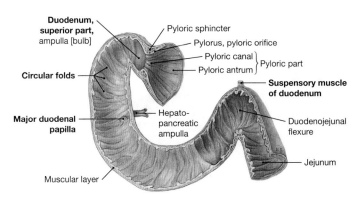

Fig. 6.57 Inner relief of the duodenum; frontal section; anterior view.

The inner relief of the duodenum shows circular mucosal folds **(KERCKRING's folds)** similar to other parts of the small intestine. The descending part contains the **major duodenal papilla** (ampulla of VATER) at the entrance of the pancreatic duct **(duct of WIRSUNG)** and the common bile duct (ductus choledochus), both of which usually merge to form the **hepatopancreatic ampulla** with its sphincter of ODDI.

Fig. 6.56 Divisions of the duodenum; anterior view.
The C-shaped duodenum surrounds the head of the pancreas. It extends from the pylorus to the duodenojejunal junction/flexure and has **four parts**:
* **Superior part,**
* **Descending part,**
* **Horizontal part,**
* **Ascending part.**

Only the superior part is intraperitoneal and its wider proximal lumen is referred to as **duodenal ampulla (duodenal cap).**

Parts of the Duodenum	Structural and Topographical Remarks
Superior	3–5 cm (1–2 in); projects to level of L1; duodenal ampulla = duodenal cap (first 2 cm [0.8 in]) is intra-peritoneal; attached to liver by hepatoduodenal ligament (free margin of lesser omentum)
Descending	7–10 cm (2.5–4 in); descends along L1–L3 vertebrae on right side of the midline; major duodenal papilla (VATER) separates blood supply and lymphatic drainage according to developmental origin from foregut and midgut; minor duodenal papilla above
Horizontal	6–8 cm (2–3 in); passes over IVC and aorta; is crossed anteriorly by the SMA and SMV and the mesenteric root; crosses vertebral column at level of L3
Ascending	Rises at inferior border of the pancreas to the level of L2 to enter the duodenojejunal junction 2–3 cm (1 in) left of midline

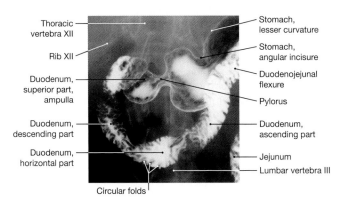

Fig. 6.58 Duodenum; radiograph in anteroposterior (A/P) beam projection after oral administration of a contrast material; patient in upright position; anterior view.

Structure/Function

The **duodenojejunal junction** is attached to the aorta near the origin of the superior mesenteric artery by a peritoneal fold, and some muscle fibers from the diaphragm and a fibromuscular band (suspensory muscle of duodenum), together referred to as **ligament of TREITZ**. It passes posterior to the pancreas and anterior to the left renal vein. The ligament of TREITZ serves as landmark for the duodenojejunal junction and is clinically associated with a potential barrier for endoscopic catheter advancement. **Upper gastrointestinal bleeding** (UGIB) originates from above the ligament of TREITZ.

The descending part of the duodenum receives secretions of the exocrine pancreas (**>** p. 345) and the bile produced by the liver (**>** p. 341).

Structure/Function

Developmental Origin	Parts of the Duodenum	Blood Supply	Lymphatic Drainage
Foregut	**Superior**	**Arteries: Celiac trunk:** right gastric and right gastro-epiploic artery. **Veins:** directly into hepatic portal vein.	Celiac nodes
	Descending, superior to major duodenal papilla	**Arteries: Celiac trunk:** superior pancreaticoduodenal artery (from gastroduodenal artery). **Veins:** superior pancreaticoduodenal vein via gastroduodenal vein into hepatic portal vein.	
Midgut	**Descending,** inferior to major duodenal papilla	**Arteries: Superior mesenteric artery (SMA):** inferior pancreaticoduodenal artery. **Veins:** inferior pancreaticoduodenal vein via superior mesenteric vein into hepatic portal vein.	Superior mesenteric nodes
	Horizontal		
	Ascending		

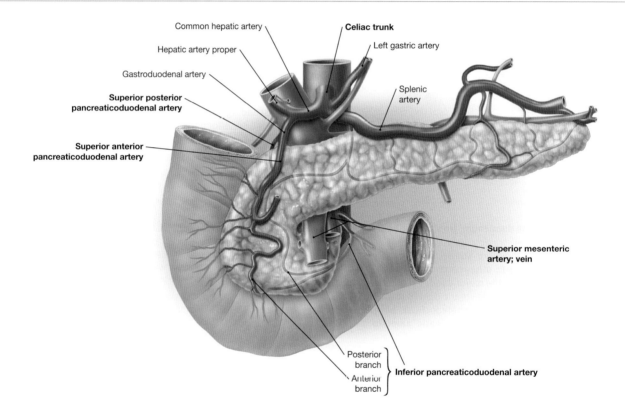

Fig. 6.59 Arteries of the duodenum; anterior view. [L238]
The blood supply of the duodenum is accomplished by a ventral and dorsal double arterial arch. This arch is supplied cranially by the superior anterior and posterior pancreaticoduodenal arteries which ultimately branch off the celiac trunk via the common hepat-ic and gastroduodenal arteries. Caudally, the arches are supplied by the inferior pancreaticoduodenal artery (anterior and posterior branch) of the superior mesenteric artery. Due to arterial anasto-moses, the vascular territories of the superior (shaded green) and inferior pancreaticoduodenal arteries (shaded blue) overlap.

Clinical Remarks

Superior mesenteric artery syndrome **(SMA syndrome),** also known as mesenteric root syndrome, is a rare vascular compression syndrome that affects the horizontal part of the duodenum. It is caused by a compression of the duodenum between the aorta and the SMA **(b).** The aortomesenteric angle is reduced to between 6° and 15° **(a,** normally between 25° and 60°). The compression of the duodenal lumen may cause nausea, vomiting and stabbing abdominal pain.
[L275]

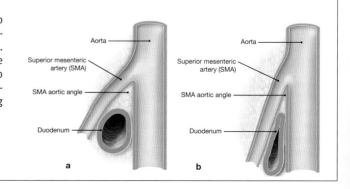

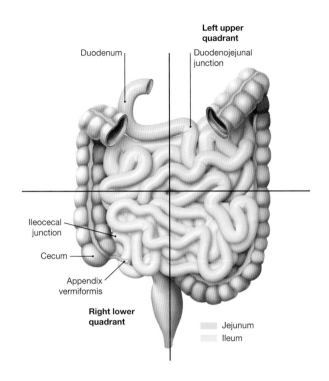

Duodenum

Duodenojejunal junction

Ileocecal junction

Cecum

Appendix vermiformis

Right lower quadrant

Jejunum

Ileum

Structure/Function

The long mesenteries of the small intestinal loops result in their relatively high mobility within the peritoneal cavity. Sectional imaging frequently shows small intestinal loops reaching into the pelvic peritoneal cavity. The anatomical cross-section shown here demonstrates the position of parts of the small intestines anterior and posterior to the uterus, e.g. in the rectouterine pouch of the peritoneal pelvic cavity.

Fig. 6.60 Position of jejunum and ileum; schematic illustration. [L275]
The intraperitoneal parts of the small intestines, jejunum and ileum, are framed by the colon. There is no clear external demarcation between the two parts. Intestinal loops may reach into the inferior recesses of the abdominopelvic peritoneal cavity: the rectouterine pouch (DOUGLAS) and vesicouterine pouch (in women) or the rectovesical pouch (in men).

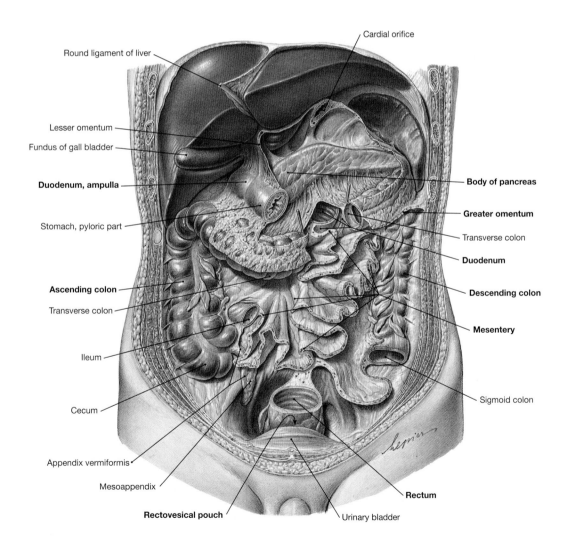

Cardial orifice

Round ligament of liver

Lesser omentum

Fundus of gall bladder

Duodenum, ampulla

Stomach, pyloric part

Ascending colon

Transverse colon

Ileum

Cecum

Appendix vermiformis

Mesoappendix

Rectovesical pouch

Body of pancreas

Greater omentum

Transverse colon

Duodenum

Descending colon

Mesentery

Sigmoid colon

Rectum

Urinary bladder

Fig. 6.61 Position of the mesenteric root; anterior view.
The intraperitoneal small intestinal convolute of jejunum and ileum was resected at the mesentery. The mesentery consists of a double layered peritoneal membrane, contains the neurovascular structures to supply the small intestine, and serves as mobile attachment of the small intestine to the posterior abdominal wall. The mesenteric root (about 15 cm [6 in] long) courses in the infracolic compartment from the left upper quadrant to the right lower quadrant of the abdomen.

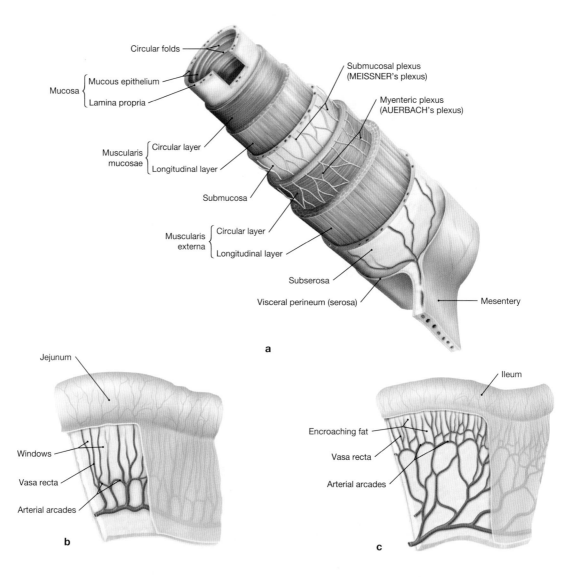

a

b

c

Fig. 6.62a to c Layers of the intestinal wall and distinctive structure of the mesentery; schematic illustrations. [L275]

The intraperitoneal small intestines are surrounded by visceral peritoneum which continues as double layered mesentery to guide neurovascular structures from the retroperitoneal space to the intraperitoneal intestines **(a)**. The arterial arcades are stronger in diameter and have larger loops in the jejunum **(b)** than the ileum **(c)**. The straight arteries (vasa recta) are longer and more numerous in the jejunum **(b)** versus the ileum **(c)**.

There are no arterial communications beyond the arcades and functionally the vasa recta are **terminal arteries**. Therefore, the obstruction of blood flow by emboli or any herniation and strangulation of intestinal loops will cause ischemia in the dependent part of the intestinal wall and will result in tissue death **(gangrene)** and obstruction of the intestine **(ileus)** if left untreated.

Note: Blood supply, innervation and lymphatic drainage of the small intestines are shown together with the large intestines on p. 324 and the following.

Clinical Remarks

MECKEL**'s diverticula** are remnants of the embryological omphalo-enteric duct. They are common (3% of the population) and are usually located in the part of the small intestine that is located approximately 100 cm (40 in) cranial of the iliocecal valve at the opposite side of the mesentery. Due to the fact that these diverticula frequently contain disseminated gastric mucosa, inflammation and subsequent bleeding thereof may mimic symptoms of an appendicitis.
[E347]

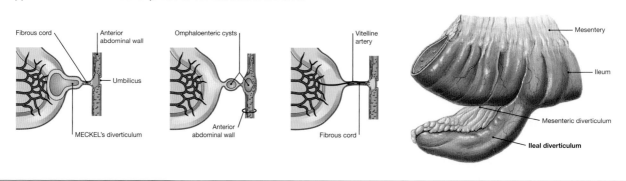

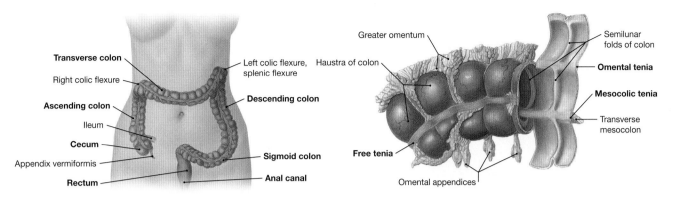

Fig. 6.63 Projection of the large intestine onto the anterior abdominal wall. [L126, K340]

Fig. 6.64 Structural characteristics of the large intestine, the transverse colon taken as an example; anterior caudal view.
The outer longitudinal muscle layer is reduced to three bands (teniae coli): the **free tenia** (tenia libera), the **omental tenia** with attached omental appendices, and the **mesocolic tenia** to which the transverse mesocolon attaches. Haustra are sacculations of the colic wall.

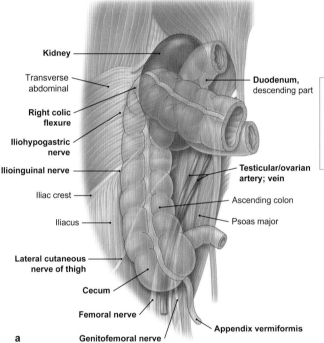

Structure/Function

The inferior mesenteric vein (IMV) courses behind the peritoneal lining of the left infracolic space. The IMV has close spatial relations to the left ureter and the left gonadal vessels. It continues superiorly adjacent to the ligament of TREITZ to join the splenic vein behind the pancreas.

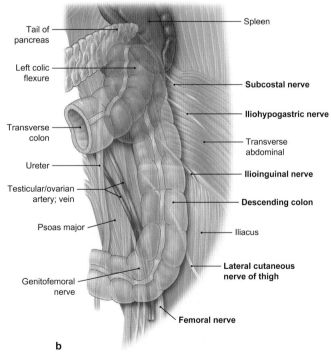

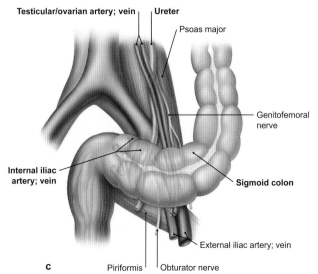

Fig. 6.65a to c Spatial relations of the colon. [G210]
a Cecum, ascending colon and right colic flexure;
b Left colic flexure and descending colon;
c Sigmoid colon.

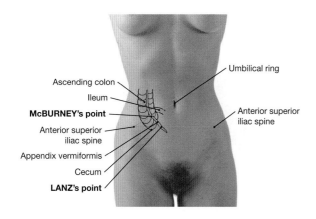

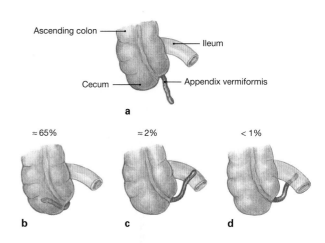

Fig. 6.66 Projection of the cecum and appendix vermiformis onto the anterior abdominal wall.
The base of the appendix vermiformis projects onto the **McBUR-NEY's point** (transition between the lateral third and the medial two-thirds on a line connecting the umbilicus with the anterior superior iliac spine (ASIS). The location of the tip of the appendix vermiformis is more variable. In 30% of cases it projects onto the **LANZ's point** (transition between the right third and the left two-thirds on a line connecting both ASIS).

Fig. 6.67a to d   Positional variants of the appendix vermiformis; anterior view.
a Descending into the small pelvis;
b Retrocecal (most common position);
c Preileal;
d Retroileal.

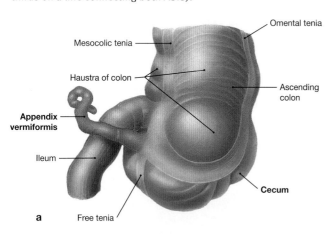

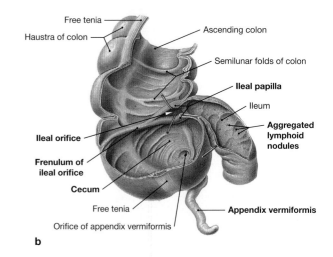

Fig. 6.68a and b   Cecum with appendix vermiformis and terminal ileum; posterior view **(a)** and anterior view **(b).**
a The cecum is approximately 7 cm (2.8 in) long. The teniae of the colon converge at the appendix vermiformis.
b The cecum is separated from the terminal ileum by the **ileocaecal valve (BAUHIN's valve).** Internally, the two lips of the valve form the

ileal papilla and confine the ileal orifice. Laterally, the lips continue in the frenulum of the ileal orifice. The terminal ileum contains aggregated lymphoid nodules, referred to as **PEYER's patches,** which are part of the mucosa-associated lymphoid tissue (MALT). Similarly, the appendix vermiformis contains large aggregated lymphoid nodules.

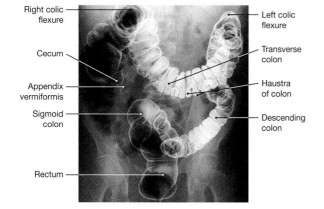

Fig. 6.69 Large intestine; radiograph in anteroposterior (A/P) beam projection after application of contrast medium and air (double contrast barium enema).

Clinical Remarks

A common cause of sudden abdominal pain is an acute inflammation of the appendix vermiformis **(appendicitis).** The pain is intense and localized to the right lower quadrant in a transmural inflammation when the parietal peritoneum is affected as it is innervated by somatic nerves. Abdominal rigidity is observed. The intense pain following the sudden release of pressure exerted at McBURNEY's point **(rebound tenderness)** is a classical sign for acute appendicitis. Intense localized pain (e.g. with appendicitis) in the abdomen indicates the involvement of the parietal peritoneum that is innervated by somatic nerves: thoracoabdominal nerves T7–T11, subcostal nerve (T12) and iliohypogastric and ilioinguinal nerves (L1). Rigidity of the abdominal muscles result from muscle contraction over the affected peritoneum as a protective reflex. In contrast, the pain afferents of the visceral peritoneum travel with the autonomic nerves and usually produce a dull pain that is not well localized.

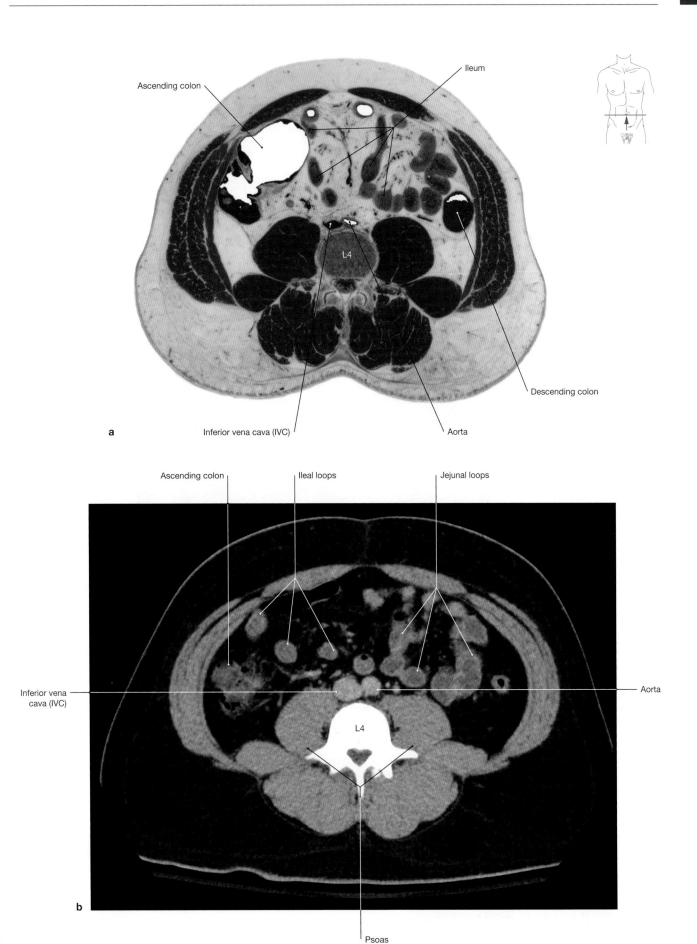

Fig. 6.70a and b Abdominal cross-section at the level of L4 (a; su-pracristal plane) and CT cross-section at the level of L4 (b). [X338]

The cross-sections show the small intestinal loops and the ascending and descending colon. The abdominal aorta seen just above its bifurcation into the common iliac arteries at the level of L4/L5.

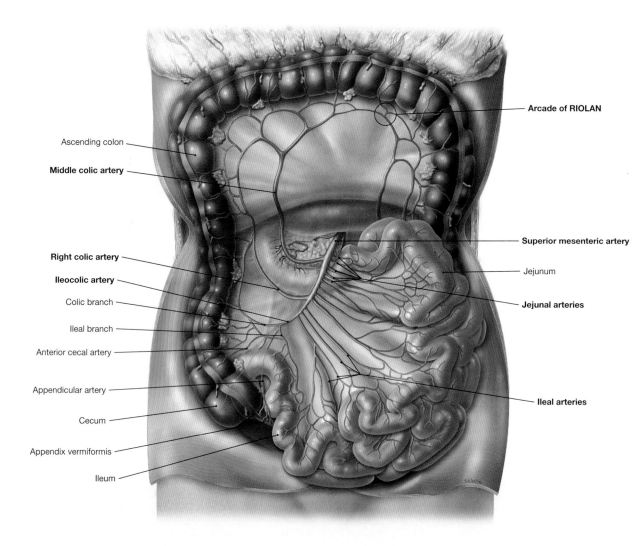

Ascending colon

Middle colic artery

Right colic artery

Ileocolic artery

Colic branch

Ileal branch

Anterior cecal artery

Appendicular artery

Cecum

Appendix vermiformis

Ileum

Arcade of RIOLAN

Superior mesenteric artery

Jejunum

Jejunal arteries

Ileal arteries

Fig. 6.71 Superior mesenteric artery (SMA); anterior view; transverse colon reflected cranially. [L238]

The unpaired superior mesenteric artery branches off the abdominal aorta directly below the celiac trunk at the **level of L1**, courses retroperitoneally behind the pancreas and then enters the mesentery. The SMA supplies parts of the pancreas and duodenum, the entire small intestine, and the large intestine up to the left colic flexure (splenic flexure).

Branches of the superior mesenteric artery:

- **Inferior pancreaticoduodenal artery:** branches off to the superior or right side; anterior and posterior branches anastomose with

the anterior and posterior superior pancreaticoduodenal arteries (➤ Fig. 6.103);
- **Jejunal arteries** (4–5) and **ileal arteries** (12): directed to the left side;
- **Middle colic artery:** originates on the right side and anastomoses with the right colic artery and with the left colic artery (RIOLAN's anastomosis);
- **Right colic artery:** courses to the ascending colon;
- **Ileocolic artery:** supplies the distal ileum, cecum and appendix vermiformis.

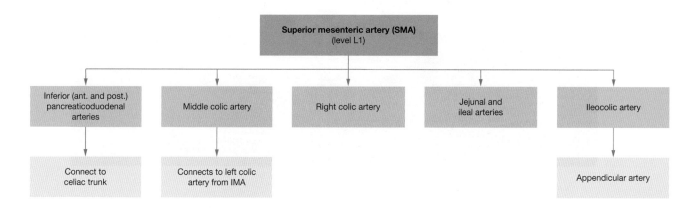

		Superior mesenteric artery (SMA) (level L1)		
Inferior (ant. and post.) pancreaticoduodenal arteries	Middle colic artery	Right colic artery	Jejunal and ileal arteries	Ileocolic artery
Connect to celiac trunk	Connects to left colic artery from IMA			Appendicular artery

Fig. 6.72 Branches of the superior mesenteric artery (SMA); schematic illustration. [L231]

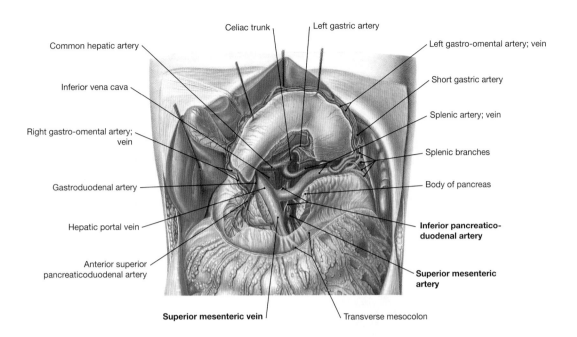

Common hepatic artery

Inferior vena cava

Right gastro-omental artery; vein

Gastroduodenal artery

Hepatic portal vein

Anterior superior pancreaticoduodenal artery

Superior mesenteric vein

Celiac trunk

Left gastric artery

Left gastro-omental artery; vein

Short gastric artery

Splenic artery; vein

Splenic branches

Body of pancreas

Inferior pancreatico-duodenal artery

Superior mesenteric artery

Transverse mesocolon

Fig. 6.73 Origin of superior mesenteric artery (SMA) and celiac trunk; anterior view; stomach reflected cranially and pancreas dissected.

The SMA branches off the abdominal aorta at the level of L1 – just inferior to the celiac trunk (level T12). The SMA descends behind the pancreas, then enters the mesentery to cross the duodenum anteriorly.

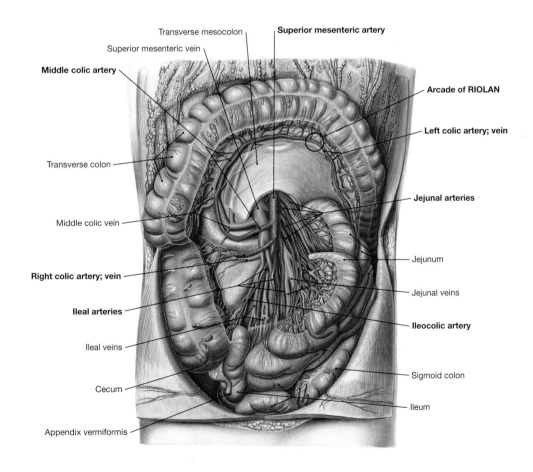

Transverse mesocolon

Superior mesenteric vein

Middle colic artery

Superior mesenteric artery

Arcade of RIOLAN

Left colic artery; vein

Transverse colon

Jejunal arteries

Middle colic vein

Jejunum

Right colic artery; vein

Jejunal veins

Ileal arteries

Ileocolic artery

Ileal veins

Cecum

Sigmoid colon

Ileum

Appendix vermiformis

Fig. 6.74 Course of the superior mesenteric artery and vein within the mesentery; anterior view; transverse colon reflected cranially and mesentery opened.
All arteries form arcades at different levels of their divisions. This allows for the mobility of the intestinal loops. At the left colic flexure, the middle colic artery forms a functionally important anastomosis (arc of RIOLAN) with the left colic artery from the inferior mesenteric artery. This facilitates the formation of collateral circulations in the case of occlusion of one of the arteries. The venous branches correspond to the arteries.

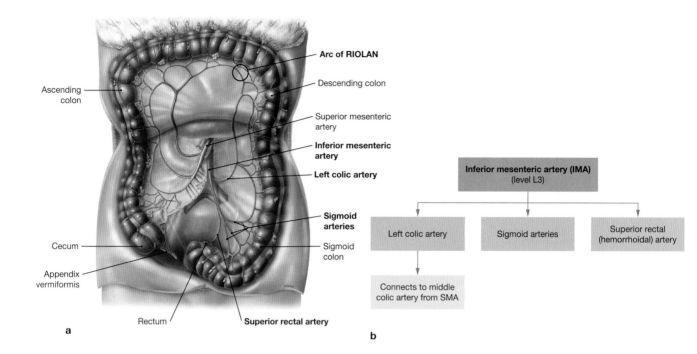

a

b

Fig. 6.75a und b Inferior mesenteric artery (IMA); anterior view **(a);** transverse colon reflected cranially and schematic illustration of IMA branches **(b).** a [L238], b [L231]
The unpaired inferior mesenteric artery branches off the abdominal aorta to the left at the vertebral level L2/L3, approximately 5 cm (2 in) cranial to the aortic bifurcation.

The branches of the IMA:
- **Sigmoid arteries:** several branches within the sigmoid mesocolon to the sigmoid colon,
- **Superior rectal artery:** descends to the upper two-thirds of the rectum and supplies the rectal cavernous bodies in the submucosa (corpus cavernosum recti), clin. term: **superior hemorrhoidal artery,**
- **Left colic artery:** ascends along the descending colon and anastomoses via the left colic artery with the middle colic artery from the SMA (arc of RIOLAN).

Fig. 6.76 Course of the inferior mesenteric artery and vein in the retroperitoneal space; anterior view; transverse colon reflected cranially and small intestinal loops to the right side.
The superior rectal artery **(superior hemorrhoidal artery)** is the most inferior branch of the IMA and descends into the pelvis within the posterior aspect of the mesorectal sleeve (➤ Fig. 7.30).
The inferior mesenteric vein enters the renal vein behind the body of pancreas.

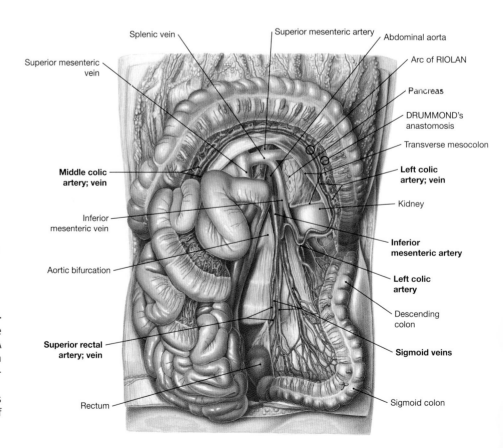

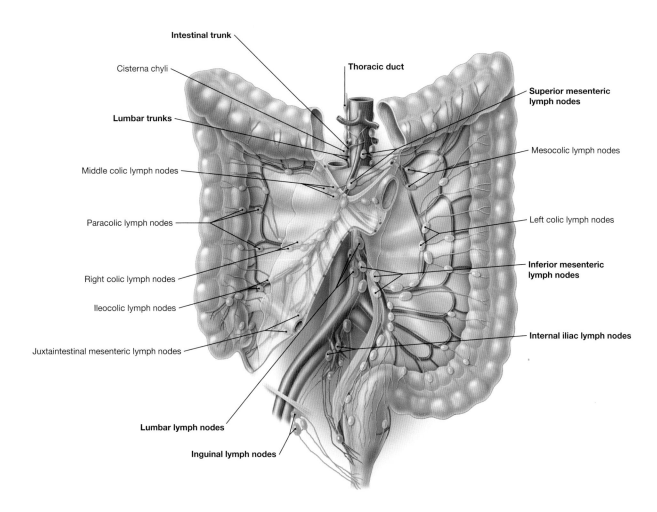

Fig. 6.77 Lymphatic drainage of the intestines; anterior view; transverse colon reflected cranially. [L238]
The left colic (splenic) flexure of the colon is the demarcation between the developmental midgut (green) and the hindgut (yellow).

This is reflected by the associated blood vessels, the lymphatic drainage pathways and the autonomic innervation. The retroperitoneal position of the ascending colon explains that alternative lymphatic drainage is into the lumbar trunks.

Overview of the Blood Supply, Innervation and Lymphatic Drainage of the Intestines			
Origin	**Midgut**	**Hindgut**	**Proctodeum**
		Endoderm	Ectoderm
Intestinal sections	Intestines distal to major duodenal papilla up to left colic flexure	Colon from left colic flexure to pectinate line of the rectum	Rectum and anal canal distal to pectinate line
Arteries	Superior mesenteric artery	Inferior mesenteric artery	Internal iliac artery
Veins	Superior mesenteric vein	Inferior mesenteric vein	Internal iliac vein
Lymphatics (All intestinal lymph finally enters the cisterna chyli and the thoracic duct)	1. Superior mesenteric nodes 2. Intestinal trunks	1. Inferior mesenteric nodes 2. Retroperitoneal para-aortic nodes 3. Lumbar trunks	1. Internal iliac nodes and superficial inguinal nodes 2. Lumbar trunks
Innervation	Parasympathetics from vagus nerve [CN X]	Parasympathetics from S2–S4, intermediolateral column	Somatic innervation via pudendal nerve

Clinical Remarks

The entire intestinal tract is associated with numerous lymph follicles which as a whole are referred to as **gut-associated lymphoid tissue (GALT)** or as a part of all **mucosa-associated lymphoid tissue (MALT)** which includes the lymphatic tissue in the respiratory tract. The lymphatic tissue associated with the mucosal lining is the largest immunological organ in the body.

PEYER's patches in the terminal ileum and the appendix vermiformis show these prominent lymphatic nodules of GALT. The gut associated lymphatic tissue contributes to inflammatory bowel diseases such as CROHN's and colitis ulcerosa.

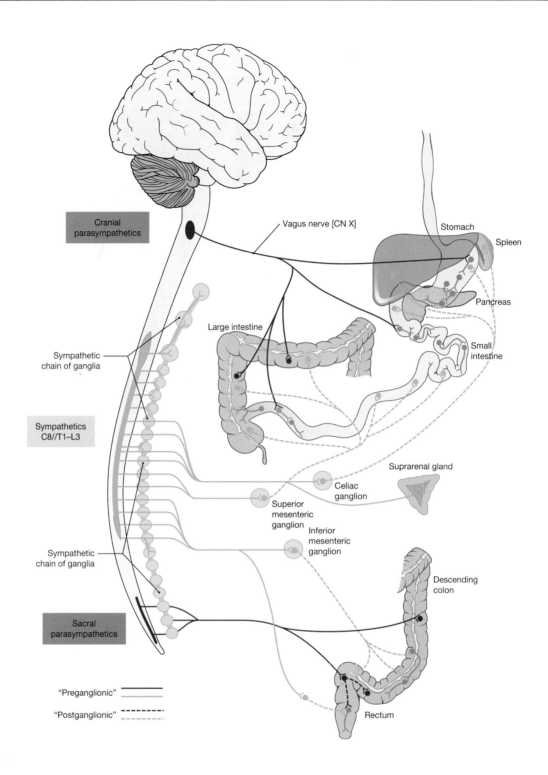

Fig. 6.78 Autonomic innervation of the intestinal tract; schematic illustration. [L126]

Structure/Function

Sympathetic (green) innervation of the abdominal intestinal tract:

Preganglionic sympathetic fibers originate from the thoracic spinal cord and travel as **greater** (T5–T9) or **lesser** (T10–T11) **splanchnic nerves** to the ganglia of the aortic plexus. Aortic plexus also receives contributions from the **lumbar splanchnic nerves.** The aortic plexus is named according to the major arterial branches as celiac, superior and inferior mesenteric plexus. Postsynaptic sympathetics course with the respective arteries to reach their target organs.

Parasympathetic (purple) innervation of the abdominal intestinal tract:

Preganglionic parasympathetics derive from the dorsal nucleus of the vagus nerve [CN X] in the brain stem and reach the abdomen as anterior and posterior vagal trunk. They travel in the celiac and superior mesenteric plexus to reach the target organs and are synapsed in intramural ganglia. Sacral preganglionic parasympathetics ascend through the inferior mesenteric plexus or directly to their target organs.

Thus, periarterial autonomic nerve plexus contain sympathetic and parasympathetic fibers, but the ganglia around aortic branches are exclusively sympathetic.

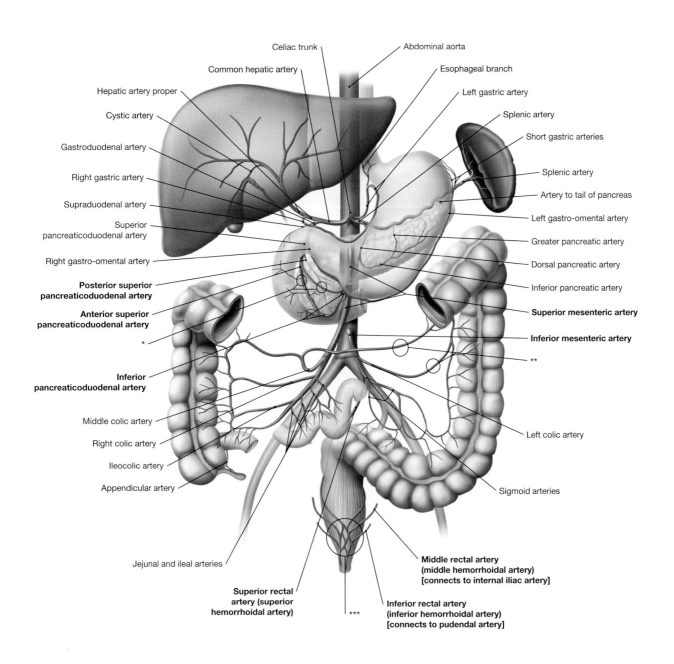

Celiac trunk

Abdominal aorta

Common hepatic artery

Esophageal branch

Hepatic artery proper

Left gastric artery

Cystic artery

Splenic artery

Gastroduodenal artery

Short gastric arteries

Right gastric artery

Splenic artery

Supraduodenal artery

Artery to tail of pancreas

Superior pancreaticoduodenal artery

Left gastro-omental artery

Right gastro-omental artery

Greater pancreatic artery

Posterior superior pancreaticoduodenal artery

Dorsal pancreatic artery

Inferior pancreatic artery

Anterior superior pancreaticoduodenal artery

Superior mesenteric artery

*

Inferior mesenteric artery

**

Inferior pancreaticoduodenal artery

Middle colic artery

Right colic artery

Left colic artery

Ileocolic artery

Appendicular artery

Sigmoid arteries

Jejunal and ileal arteries

Middle rectal artery (middle hemorrhoidal artery) [connects to internal iliac artery]

Superior rectal artery (superior hemorrhoidal artery)

***

Inferior rectal artery (inferior hemorrhoidal artery) [connects to pudendal artery]

Fig. 6.79 Arteries of the abdominal viscera; semi-schematic illustration; anterior view. The most important anastomoses are marked by black circles. [L275]

For *, ** and *** see Structure/Function box below.

Structure/Function

The **three unpaired arteries** to the abdominal viscera derive from the abdominal aorta:
1. **Celiac trunk** at the level of T12/L1,
2. **Superior mesenteric artery** (SMA) at the level of L1/L2,
3. **Inferior mesenteric artery** (IMA) at the level of L3.

The superior mesenteric artery has its origin directly below the celiac trunk. All three arteries anastomose with each other and with branches of the internal iliac artery. This may prevent ischemic infarction in cases of an occlusion of one of these vessels.

The **anastomoses** are:
- Between the celiac trunk and the superior mesenteric artery via pancreaticoduodenal arteries (*),
- Between the superior and inferior mesenteric arteries: RIOLAN's anastomosis between the middle colic artery and left colic artery (**),
- Plexus of rectal arteries: here the superior rectal artery from the inferior mesenteric artery connects to the middle and inferior rectal arteries from the internal iliac artery (***).

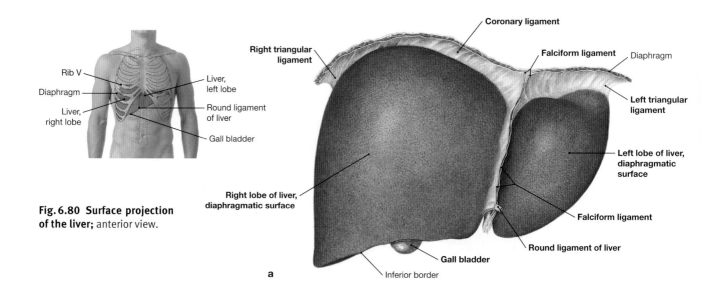

Rib V
Diaphragm
Liver, right lobe
Liver, left lobe
Round ligament of liver
Gall bladder

Coronary ligament
Right triangular ligament
Falciform ligament
Diaphragm
Left triangular ligament
Left lobe of liver, diaphragmatic surface
Falciform ligament
Round ligament of liver
Right lobe of liver, diaphragmatic surface
Gall bladder
Inferior border

Fig. 6.80 Surface projection of the liver; anterior view.

a

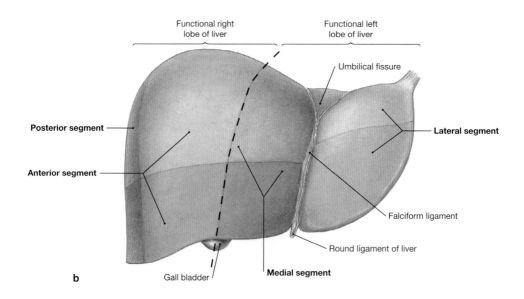

Functional right lobe of liver
Functional left lobe of liver
Umbilical fissure
Posterior segment
Lateral segment
Anterior segment
Medial segment
Falciform ligament
Round ligament of liver
Gall bladder
Medial segment

b

Fig. 6.81a and b Liver (a) and liver segments (b); anterior view.
The liver is divided in a larger right and a smaller left lobe which are separated ventrally by the **falciform ligament**. The latter continues as **coronary ligament** which then becomes the right and left **triangular ligament** connecting to the diaphragm. The left triangular ligament continues into the fibrous appendix of the liver. The free margin of the falciform ligament contains the **round ligament of liver** (ligamentum teres, remnant of the prenatal umbilical vein). Both ligaments connect to the ventral abdominal wall.

The three almost vertically oriented hepatic veins divide the liver into **four adjacent segments.** The lateral segment corresponds to the anatomical left lobe of the liver and is bordered by the falciform ligament, which is adjacent to the left liver vein. The medial segment is located between the falciform ligament and the gall bladder at the level of the middle liver vein. Functionally, the lateral and medial segments belong to the left portal triad system and thus, comprise the **left functional lobe of the liver.**

Clinical Remarks

The liver is attached to the diaphragm and moves inferiorly with inspiration. The liver is normally covered by ribs 7–11 and crosses the midline in the upper epigastrium. The craniocaudal diameter of the normal liver does not exceed 12 cm (4.5 in) in the midclavicular line. The anatomy of the lungs and the position of the diaphragm determine the position of the liver. Palpation of a firm and blunted/rounded or nodular inferior **liver margin** during deep inspiration may suggest a pathology of the liver. Changes in consistency and size may suggest certain pathological conditions such as **fatty liver** or **liver cirrhosis.**
[L126, K340]

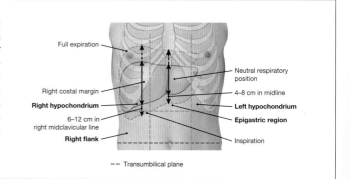

Full expiration
Neutral respiratory position
Right costal margin
4–8 cm in midline
Right hypochondrium
Left hypochondrium
6–12 cm in right midclavicular line
Epigastric region
Right flank
Inspiration
Transumbilical plane

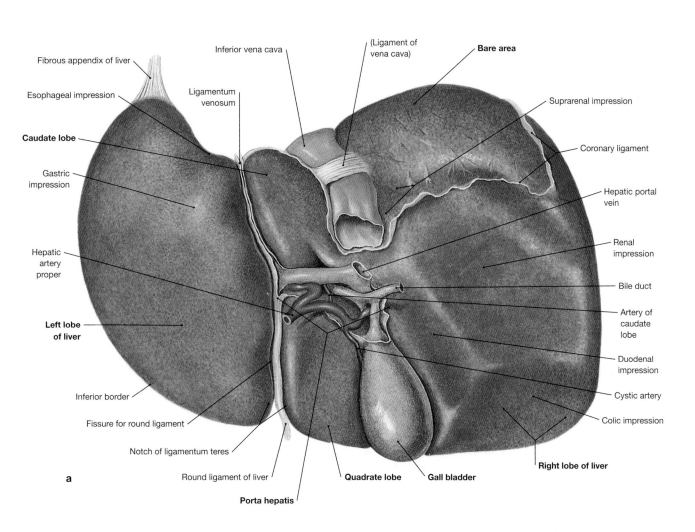

a

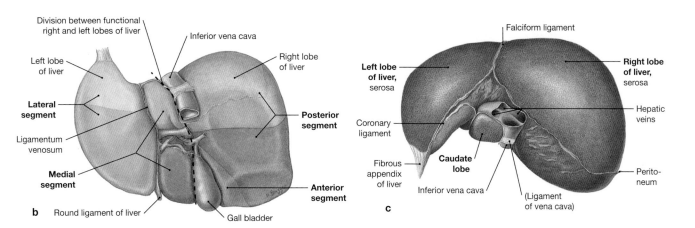

b

c

Fig. 6.82a to c Liver (a) and liver segments (b), visceral surface, inferior views **(a** and **b);** superior view **(c).**
At the **visceral surface (a)** the **porta hepatis** (hilum of the liver) is located which harbors the vascular structures to and from the liver (except for the hepatic veins):
* Hepatic portal vein,
* Hepatic artery proper,
* Common hepatic duct.

The **ligamentum venosum** (remnant of the prenatal ductus venosus) is shown superiorly. The structure on the visceral liver surface resembles the letter 'H' in which the ligamentum teres and ligamentum venosum on the left side and the inferior vena cava and gall bladder on the right side delineate two rectangular areas on both sides of the porta hepatis, the anterior quadrate lobe and the posterior caudate lobe.

The **diaphragmatic surface (c)** is partly adherent to the diaphragm and lacks the peritoneal lining in this area **(bare area).**
The liver is not covered by peritoneum in four larger areas: bare area, porta hepatis, bed of the gall bladder, and groove of the inferior vena cava.

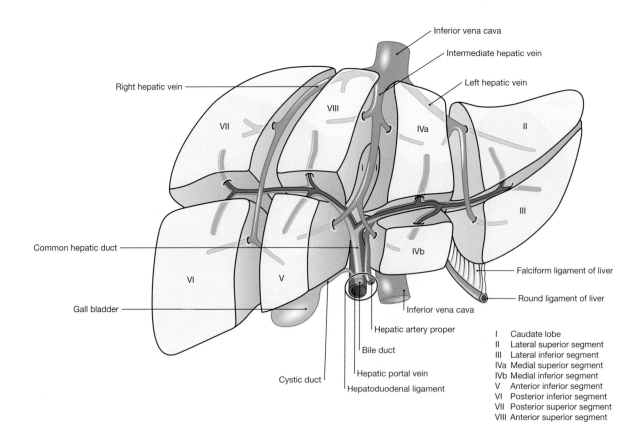

I Caudate lobe
II Lateral superior segment
III Lateral inferior segment
IVa Medial superior segment
IVb Medial inferior segment
V Anterior inferior segment
VI Posterior inferior segment
VII Posterior superior segment
VIII Anterior superior segment

Fig. 6.83 Schematic illustration of the liver segments and their relations to the intrahepatic blood vessels and the bile ducts; anterior view. [L126]
The liver is divided into **eight functional segments** which are supplied by one branch of the **portal triad** each (hepatic portal vein, hepatic artery proper, common hepatic duct) and are therefore functional units of the liver. Two segments each are combined by

the vertically oriented three liver veins to four adjacent liver segments (➤ Fig. 6.84 and ➤ Fig. 6.88). It is of functional importance that segments I to IV are supplied by branches of the left portal triad and can be combined to a functional left liver lobe. **As a result, the border between the functional right and left liver lobes is located in the sagittal plane between the inferior vena cava and gall bladder and not at the level of the falciform ligament of the liver.**

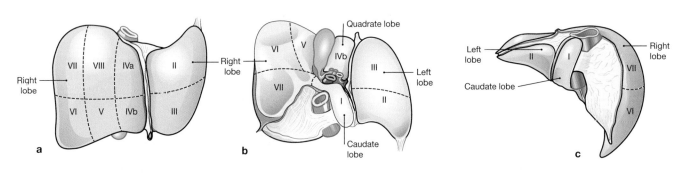

Fig. 6.84a to c Segments of the liver; anterior view **(a)**, posterior-inferior view **(b)** and superior view **(c)**. [L126]

Clinical Remarks

In visceral surgery, the liver segments are of great relevance. The existence of liver segments allows the resection of individual segments and their supporting vessels without extensive blood loss. Localized liver pathologies, such as **solitary liver metastases**, can be treated by the surgical resection of individual segments in different parts of the liver without compromising the liver function as a whole. The ligation of the individual branches of the segmental vessels and the subsequent discoloration of the respective segment due to lack of perfusion enables the surgeon to identify each segment.
[S008-3, P497]

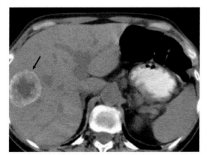

Abdomen CT showing liver with metastasis (arrow)

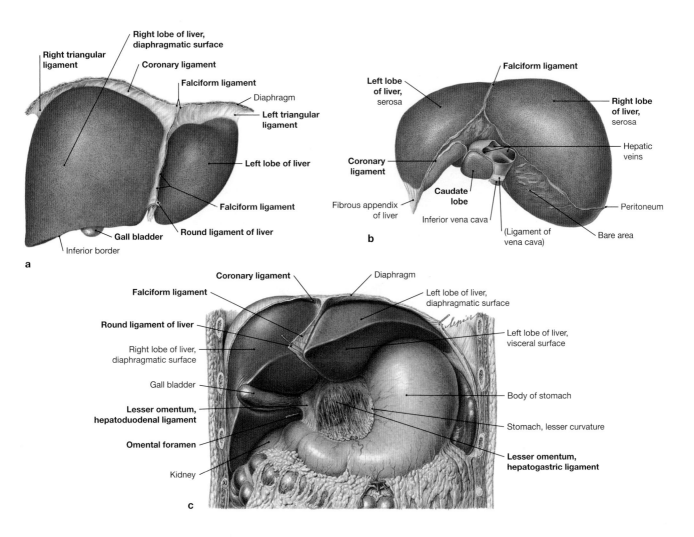

Fig. 6.85a to c Peritoneal attachments of the liver; anterior view **(a),** superior view **(b)** and anterior in situ view **(c).**
The liver develops into the ventral mesogastrium and keeps its attachment to the anterior abdominal wall: the **falciform ligament,** a double-layered peritoneal fold. At its free margin, the **round ligament of liver** represents the obliterated umbilical vein. The falciform ligament splits cranially into the **right and left coronary ligaments** which transition to the **right and left triangular ligaments.**

Coronary and triangular ligaments continue to the parietal peritoneum of the diaphragm and surround the bare area of the liver. The part of the embryological ventral mesogastrium between the liver and the stomach remains as **lesser omentum** (➤ Fig. 6.29). The latter consists of the **hepatoduodenal ligament** which contains the portal triad (hepatic artery proper, hepatic portal vein and bile duct) and the **hepatogastric ligament** to the lesser curvature of the stomach.

Structure/Function

The **superior recess of the omental bursa (a)** behind the caudate lobe of the liver, the **hepatorenal recess (b;** MORRISON's pouch) behind the right lobe of the liver and anterior to the right kidney and adrenal gland and the **subphrenic recess (c)** ventral to the right lobe of the liver are important superior and posterior recesses of the supracolic compartment of the peritoneal abdominal cavity adjacent to the liver. These recesses may accumulate ascites fluid or other pathological content of the peritoneal cavity.

The falciform ligament of the liver separates the right and left subphrenic recess. MORRISON's pouch communicates superiorly and anteriorly with the right subhepatic recess and inferiorly through the right paracolic gutter with the pelvic peritoneal cavity. Thus ascites fluid may shift between these peritoneal locations depending on the position of the patient.
[L126]

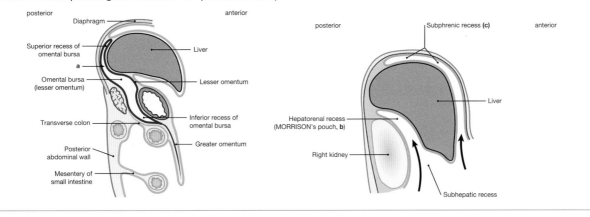

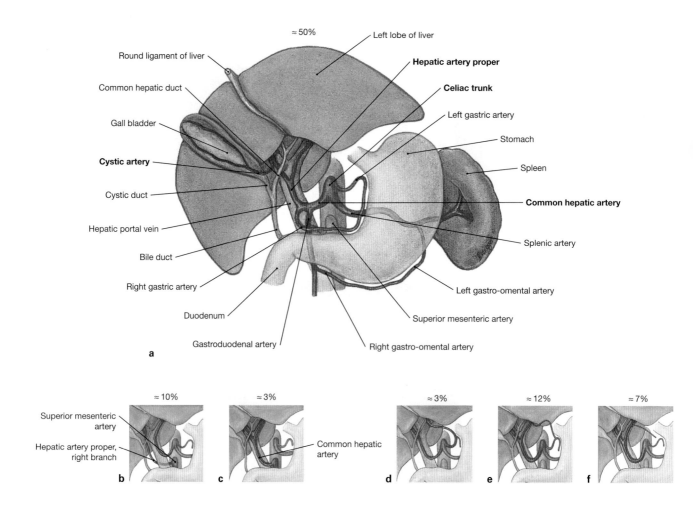

Fig. 6.86a to f Arteries of the liver and the gall bladder.
The liver is supplied by the **hepatic artery proper** which courses within the **hepatoduodenal ligament** together with the hepatic portal vein and the bile duct. At the hilum of the liver this artery divides into the right branch and the left branch to the liver lobes. The right branch gives rise to the cystic artery to the gall bladder. In 10–20% of all cases, the superior mesenteric artery contributes to the blood supply of the right liver lobe, and the left gastric artery contributes to the supply of the left liver lobe.

Variations of the blood supply of the liver, frequencies in the population are indicated in %:
a Textbook case,
b Contribution of the superior mesenteric artery to the blood supply of the right liver lobe,
c Origin of the common hepatic artery by the superior mesenteric artery,
d Blood supply of the left liver lobe by the left gastric artery,
e Contribution of a branch of the left gastric artery to the blood supply of the left liver lobe in addition to the left branch of the hepatic artery proper,
f Blood supply of the lesser curvature of the stomach by an accessory branch of the hepatic artery proper.

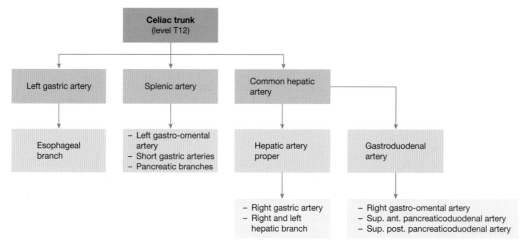

Fig. 6.87 Branches of the celiac trunk; schematic illustration.
[L231]

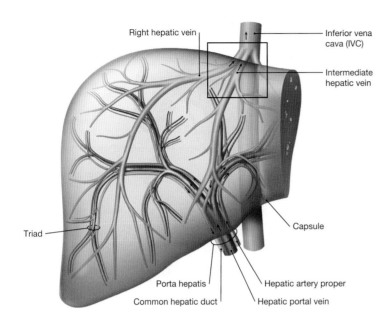

Right hepatic vein

Inferior vena cava (IVC)

Intermediate hepatic vein

Capsule

Triad

Porta hepatis

Common hepatic duct

Hepatic artery proper

Hepatic portal vein

Fig. 6.88 Blood flow through the liver; schematic illustration. [L275]

75–80% of the blood to the liver derives from the **hepatic portal vein**, 20–25% from the **proper hepatic artery** which supports the liver parenchyma. The hepatic portal vein transports nutrient-rich blood from the intestinal tract for metabolic processing in the liver. The right, middle and left **hepatic veins** collect venous blood from the central veins and open into the inferior vena cava just below the diaphragm at the level of **T10**. The boxed insert depicts the region corresponding to the ultrasound image below.

Hepatocytes produce bile continuously and secrete the bile into the bile canaliculi. The bile is eventually collected in the common hepatic bile duct. **Hepatic bile duct, hepatic portal vein** and **hepatic artery proper** emerge at the porta hepatis (hilum of the liver) and course within the hepatoduodenal ligament.

The **hepatic portal vein** is different from a classical vein of the systemic circulation as it connects the capillary system of the intestines and the sinusoid blood vessels of the spleen, respectively, with the sinusoid blood vessels of the liver.

Structure/Function

The hexagonal **classical liver lobule** centers around one central vein and features six portal triads. The **liver acinus** represents a functional segment centered around the most oxygenated (hepatic artery) and nutrient rich (portal vein) blood from the blood vessels of the portal triad. The diamond-shaped liver acinus centers between two liver lobules. The periphery is marked by the central veins of neighboring classical liver lobules. The liver acinus functionally reflects the liver perfusion (oxygen gradient) and metabolite activity and shows the severity of liver toxicity and ischemia. The **portal lobule** centers around the structures of the portal triad and functionally emphasizes the bile secretory function of the liver.

Absorbed lipids bypass the liver as they travel with the lymphatic system of the intestines to reach the systemic circulation via the thoracic duct.
[L126]

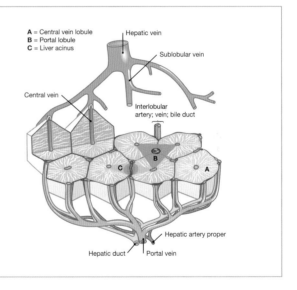

A = Central vein lobule
B = Portal lobule
C = Liver acinus

Hepatic vein

Sublobular vein

Central vein

Interlobular artery; vein; bile duct

Hepatic artery proper

Hepatic duct

Portal vein

Clinical Remarks

Ultrasonographic examination **(sonography)** of the liver enables a noninvasive investigation of the liver parenchyma and allows the detection of structural changes, for example by the local or general increased echogenicity in cases of a fatty liver degeneration in hepatitis or liver cirrhosis. Focal tumors or cysts are also detectable. Subsequently, liver biopsies or a laparoscopic investigation of the liver may be performed to reach a diagnosis. The ultrasound image shows the confluence of the hepatic veins with the inferior vena cava.

* abdominal wall

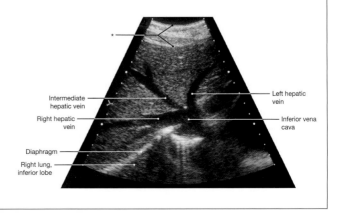

Intermediate hepatic vein

Right hepatic vein

Diaphragm

Right lung, inferior lobe

Left hepatic vein

Inferior vena cava

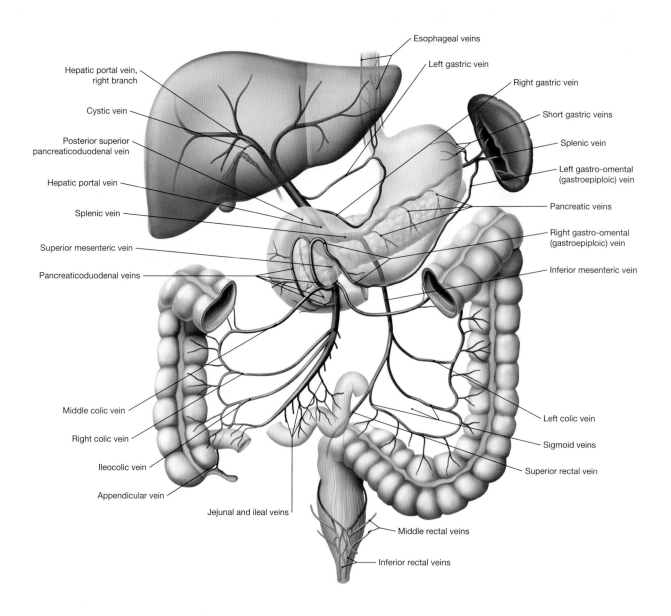

Fig. 6.89 Tributaries of the hepatic portal vein; schematic illustration; anterior view. [L275]

The hepatic portal vein collects the nutrient-rich blood from the unpaired abdominal organs (stomach, intestines, pancreas, spleen) and brings it, together with the arterial blood from the common hepatic artery, into the sinusoids of the liver lobules. **Thus, the portal system connects two capillary systems.**

The portal vein forms at the level of L1. Behind the head of pancreas, the superior mesenteric vein merges with the splenic vein to form the hepatic portal vein. In most cases (70%), the inferior mesenteric vein drains into the splenic vein; in the remaining cases (30%) it drains into the superior mesenteric vein.

Structure/Function

Tributaries of the splenic vein (collecting blood from spleen and parts of the stomach and pancreas):
* Short gastric veins,
* Left gastro-omental vein,
* Pancreatic veins (from the pancreatic tail and body).

Tributaries of the superior mesenteric vein (collecting blood from parts of the stomach and pancreas, from the entire small intestine, the ascending colon, and transverse colon):
* Right gastro-omental vein with pancreaticoduodenal veins,
* Pancreatic veins (from the pancreatic head and body),
* Jejunal and ileal veins,
* Ileocolic veins,
* Right colic vein,
* Middle colic vein.

Tributaries of the inferior mesenteric vein (collecting blood from sigmoid descending colon and upper rectum):
* Left colic vein,
* Sigmoid veins,
* Superior rectal vein: the vein anastomoses with the middle rectal vein and the inferior rectal vein, which drain into the inferior vena cava.

In addition, there are veins which drain **directly into the portal vein** once the main venous branches have merged:
* Cystic vein (from the gall bladder),
* Paraumbilical veins (via veins in the round ligament of liver from the abdominal wall around the umbilicus),
* Right and left gastric veins (from the lesser curvature of the stomach).

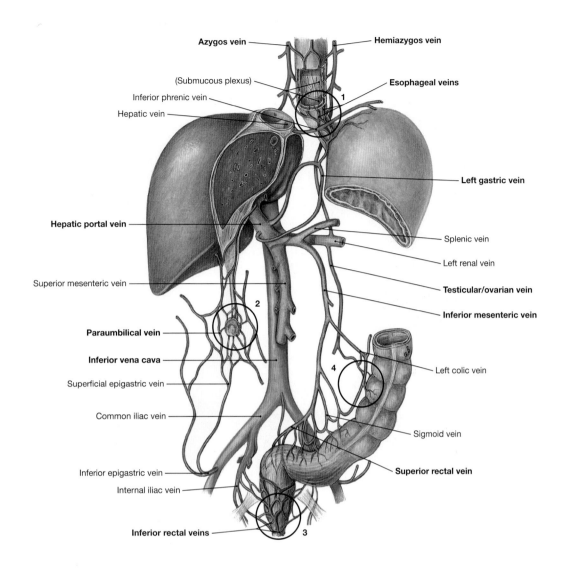

Fig. 6.90 Portocaval anastomoses are portal-systemic collateral pathways connecting between the portal vein and the superior/inferior vena cava. Tributaries to the superior/inferior vena cava (blue), tributaries to the hepatic portal vein (purple).
There are four possible collateral circulations via portocaval anastomoses (marked by black circles):
1. Right and left gastric veins via esophageal veins and veins of the azygos system to the superior vena cava. This may result in the dilation of submucosal veins of the esophagus (esophageal varices).

2. Paraumbilical veins via veins of the ventral abdominal wall (deep: superior and inferior epigastric veins; superficial: thoracoepigastric vein and superficial epigastric vein) to the superior and inferior vena cava. Dilation of the superficial veins may appear as caput medusae.
3. Superior rectal vein via veins of the distal rectum and anal canal and via the internal iliac vein to the inferior vena cava.
4. Retroperitoneal anastomoses via the inferior mesenteric vein to the testicular/ovarian vein with connection to the inferior vena cava.

Clinical Remarks

In cases of high blood pressure in the portal system **(portal hypertension),** such as in liver cirrhosis, collateral pathways (portocaval anastomoses) be-tween the portal and systemic venous systems may develop much stronger. Clinically important are the connections to the esophageal veins because rupture of esophageal varices may result in life threatening hemorrhage, the most common cause of death in patients with liver cirrhosis. The connections to superficial veins of the ventral abdominal wall are only of diagnostic value. Although the caput medusae is rare, the appearance is so characteristic that a liver cirrhosis cannot be overlooked.
[L238]

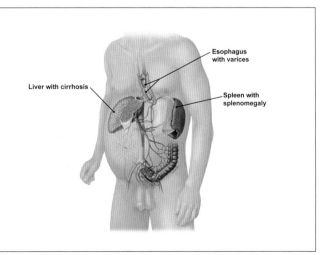

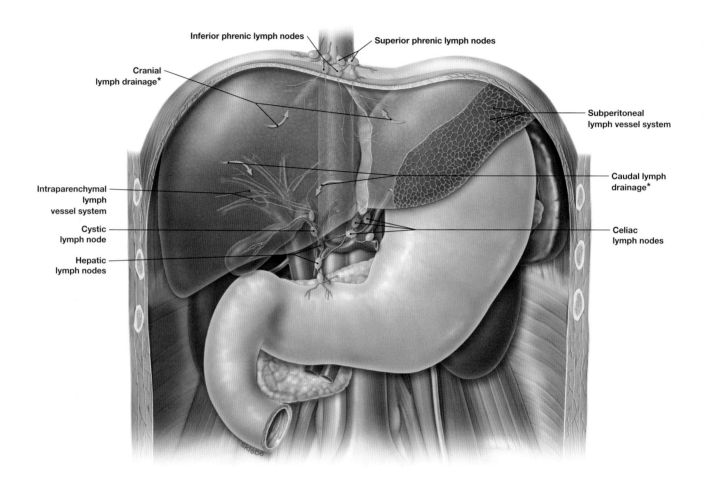

Inferior phrenic lymph nodes

Superior phrenic lymph nodes

Cranial
lymph drainage*

Subperitoneal
lymph vessel system

Intraparenchymal
lymph
vessel system

Caudal lymph
drainage*

Cystic
lymph node

Celiac
lymph nodes

Hepatic
lymph nodes

Fig. 6.91 Lymph vessels and lymph nodes of the liver and bile duct system. [L238]

The liver has two lymph vessel systems:
- The **subperitoneal system** at the surface of the liver,
- The **intraparenchymal system** alongside the structures in the portal triad to the hilum of the liver,

With respect to the regional lymph nodes, there are **two major lymph drainage routes:**
- In **caudal direction to the hilum of the liver** (most important) via the hepatic nodes at the hilum of the liver and from there via the celiac nodes to the intestinal trunk,
- In **cranial direction passing the diaphragm** via the inferior and superior phrenic nodes into the anterior and posterior media-stinal nodes which drain into the bronchomediastinal trunks; using this drainage pathway, carcinomas of the liver may also metastasize into thoracic lymph nodes.

There are **two minor lymph drainage routes:**
- To the anterior abdominal wall via the lymph vessels in the round ligament of liver to the inguinal and axillary lymph nodes,
- To the stomach and pancreas from the left lobe of the liver.

The **gall bladder** usually has its own cystic node in the area of the neck, which drains into the lymph nodes at the hilum of the liver (in the caudal direction).

* The green arrows depict the direction of lymph drainage from the parenchyma via the cranial or caudal route.

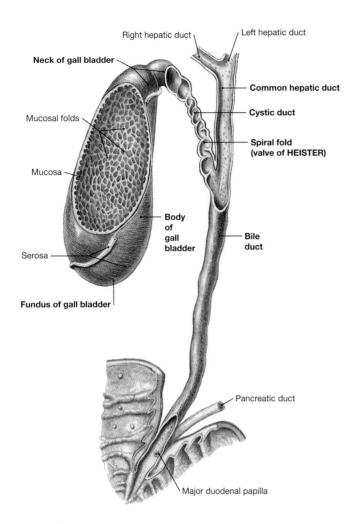

Right hepatic duct

Left hepatic duct

Neck of gall bladder

Common hepatic duct

Mucosal folds

Cystic duct

**Spiral fold
(valve of HEISTER)**

Mucosa

**Body
of
gall
bladder**

**Bile
duct**

Serosa

Fundus of gall bladder

Pancreatic duct

Major duodenal papilla

**Fig. 6.92 Gall bladder and extrahepatic bile
ducts;** anterior view.
The gall bladder consists of a body, fundus and
neck. A spiral fold (valve of HEISTER) at the terminal end of the neck closes the opening of the
excretory **cystic duct**, which then fuses with the
common hepatic duct to form the **bile duct**
(choledochus) which courses within the hepatoduodenal ligament.
In 60% of all cases, the bile duct fuses with the
main pancreatic duct to form the **hepatopancreatic ampulla**, which enters the duodenum
at the major duodenal papilla. At its distal end,
smooth muscles of the common bile duct
create the sphincter of the bile duct, also referred to as **sphincter of ODDI**.

Structure/Function

The fundus of the gall bladder is located in close proximity to the
superior part of the duodenum and the transverse colon. This
close spatial relation is the reason for the potential development
of fistulations **(cholecystocolic fistula; cholecystoduodenal fistula)** between the lumen of the gall bladder and the adjacent intestines in cases of inflammatory reactions (cholecystolithiasis).
The inflammation of the wall and the peritoneal lining leads to
adhesions and transmural inflammation.

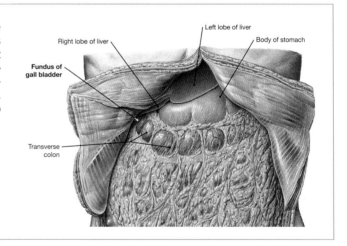

Right lobe of liver

Left lobe of liver

Body of stomach

Fundus of
gall bladder

Transverse
colon

Clinical Remarks

Gallstones are common and may obstruct the neck of the gall
bladder or the bile duct system causing inflammation of the gall
bladder **(cholecystolithiasis).** This ultrasound image shows a solitary gall stone. The calculus appears 'echogenic' within the 'an-
echoic' bile fluid. The 'acoustic shadow' is caused by the reflection of the ultrasound waves.
Pain from cholecystolithiasis travels with the sympathetic fibers
of the splanchnic nerves and is referred to the right epigastric region (dermatome T8–T11).
[E355]

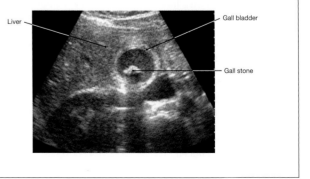

Liver

Gall bladder

Gall stone

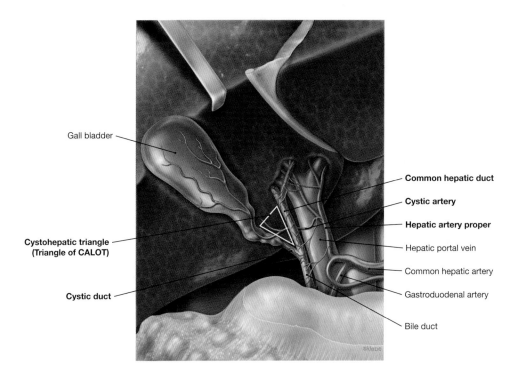

Gall bladder

Cystohepatic triangle
(Triangle of CALOT)

Cystic duct

Common hepatic duct

Cystic artery

Hepatic artery proper

Hepatic portal vein

Common hepatic artery

Gastroduodenal artery

Bile duct

Fig. 6.93 Triangle of CALOT, cystohepatic triangle; inferior view.
[L238]
The cystic duct, the common hepatic duct and the inferior area of
the liver together form the cystohepatic triangle, also referred to as

triangle of CALOT. In 75 % of all cases, the cystic artery originates in
this triangle from the right branch of the hepatic artery proper and
courses posteriorly through this triangle to reach the cystic duct
and the neck of the gall bladder.

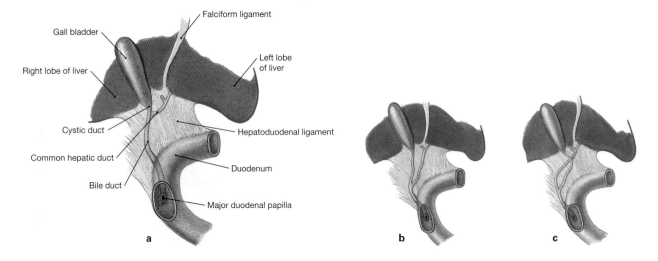

Falciform ligament

Gall bladder

Right lobe of liver

Cystic duct

Common hepatic duct

Bile duct

Left lobe
of liver

Hepatoduodenal ligament

Duodenum

Major duodenal papilla

a

b

c

**Fig. 6.94a to c Variations of the bile ducts regarding the conjunc-
tion of the common hepatic duct and cystic duct.**

a High junction,
b Low junction,
c Low junction with crossing.

Clinical Remarks

Laparoscopy is minimally invasive surgery for which a fiber-optic
instrument is inserted into the peritoneal cavity through the abdominal wall to inspect or perform surgery in the abdomen. Using
a laparoscope and one or two additional entrance ports for light
sources, camera, or biopsy instruments, the entire abdominal
cavity can be inspected and biopsies can be taken under visual
control.
The **triangle of CALOT** is an important landmark during the surgical removal of the gall bladder. Prior to removal of the gall bladder, all structures are identified before the cystic artery and the
cystic duct are ligated. This way, the risk of an accidental ligation
of the common bile duct with subsequent stasis of the bile
(cholestasis) is reduced.

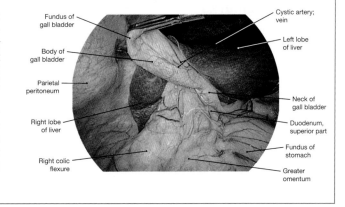

Fundus of
gall bladder

Body of
gall bladder

Parietal
peritoneum

Right lobe
of liver

Right colic
flexure

Cystic artery;
vein

Left lobe
of liver

Neck of
gall bladder

Duodenum,
superior part

Fundus of
stomach

Greater
omentum

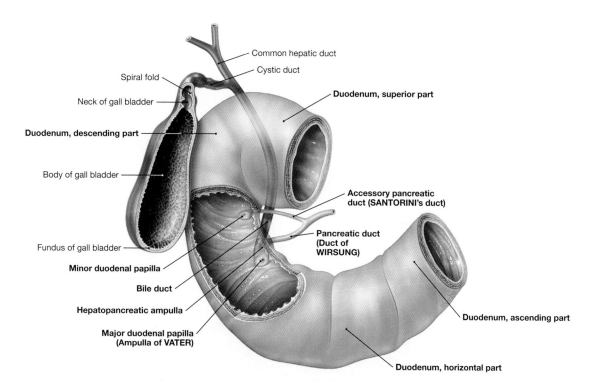

Fig. 6.95 Divisions of the duodenum together with the extrahepatic bile ducts and pancreatic ducts; anterior view. [L238]
The **bile duct** (choledochus) and **major pancreatic duct (duct of WIRSUNG)** frequently unite to form the **hepatopancreatic ampulla** and enter the descending part of the duodenum on the **major duo-**denal papilla (of VATER) which is found 8–10 cm (3–4 in) distal to the pylorus. Commonly, an accessory pancreatic duct **(SANTORINI's duct)** empties into a smaller **minor duodenal papilla** 2 cm (1 in) proximal to the papilla of VATER. Both ducts enter at the posteromedial wall of the descending duodenum.

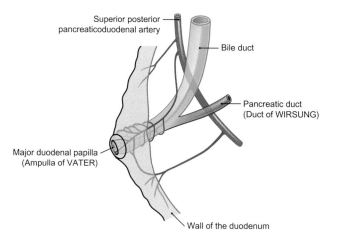

Fig. 6.96 Arteries of the hepatopancreatic ampulla. [L126]

Fig. 6.97 Sphincters of the bile duct and pancreatic duct at the major duodenal papilla. [L238]

Clinical Remarks

Radiography after intravenous administration of contrast medium allows the visualization of the gall bladder and bile ducts, including the detection of noncalcified bile concrements. Malignant tumors of the bile ducts **(cholangiocarcinomas)** or of the pancreas **(pancreatic carcinomas)** may cause cholestasis which appears as dilation of the bile ducts.

This radiograph in anteroposterior (A/P) beam projection shows the normal anatomy of the gall bladder and intrahepatic and extrahepatic bile ducts; after administration of contrast medium; patient in upright position; ventral view.

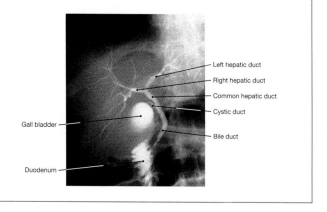

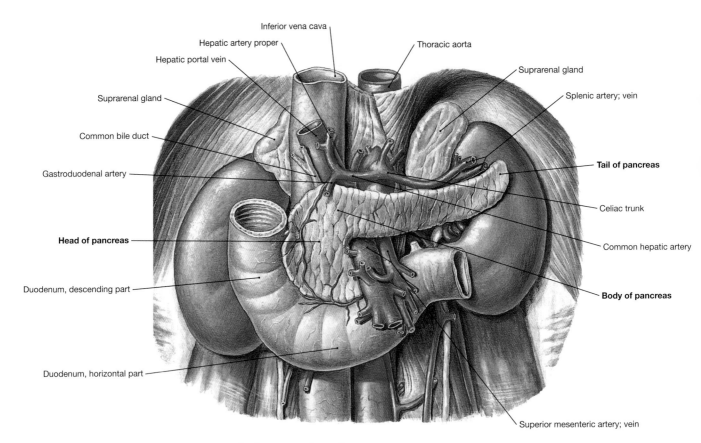

Fig. 6.98 **Spatial relations of the pancreas in the retroperitoneal space;** anterior view.

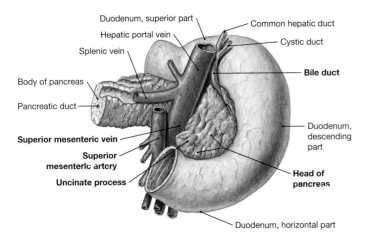

Fig. 6.99 **Pancreas and duodenum;** posterior view.

Structure/Function

- Vertebral level **L1:** body and tail of pancreas. The body creates an anterior hump in the omental bursa behind the stomach, the **omental tuberosity** (➤ Fig. 6.32).
- Vertebral level **L2:** head and uncinate process.
- The pancreas tail extends to the hilum of the spleen.
- The splenic artery courses at the superior border of the body and tail. The splenic vein is posterior to the body and merges with the SMV posterior to the neck of pancreas forming the hepatic portal vein.
- The SMA arises posterior to the body of pancreas and crosses the tip of uncinate process and the horizontal part of the duodenum anteriorly.
- The IVC lies posterior to the head of pancreas.
- The bile duct enters the head of pancreas from posterior.

Clinical Remarks

If the movement of the ventral pancreatic bud towards the dorsal pancreatic bud during development results in circular parenchymal growth around the duodenum **(anular pancreas),** the lumen of the descending part of the duodenum is constricted. Ileus with vomiting may occur which is particularly evident in newborns. In these cases, the duodenum is mobilized, cut, and positioned next to the pancreas or surgically bypassed.
[E247-09]

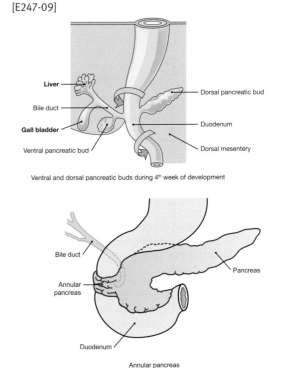

Ventral and dorsal pancreatic buds during 4th week of development

Annular pancreas

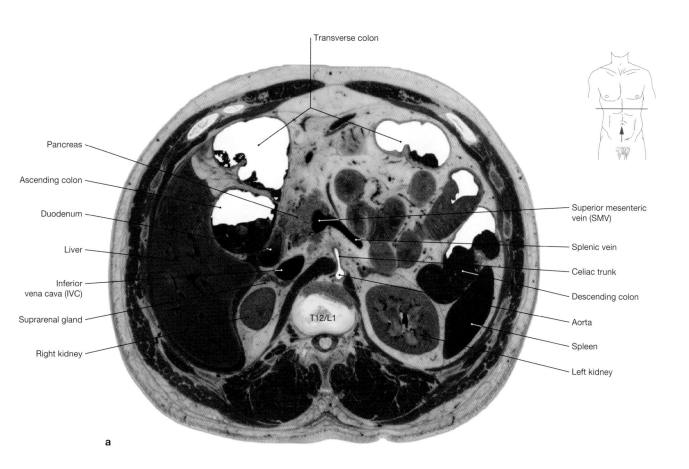

a

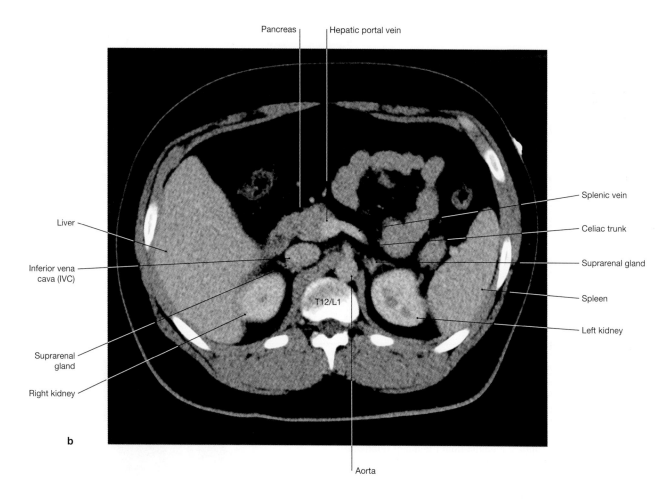

b

Fig. 6.100a and b Cross-sectional anatomy (a) and abdominal CT cross-section (b) at the level of T12/L1. The cross-sections show the spatial relation of the pancreas to the inferior vena cava and the superior mesenteric artery and vein and the splenic vein. [X338]

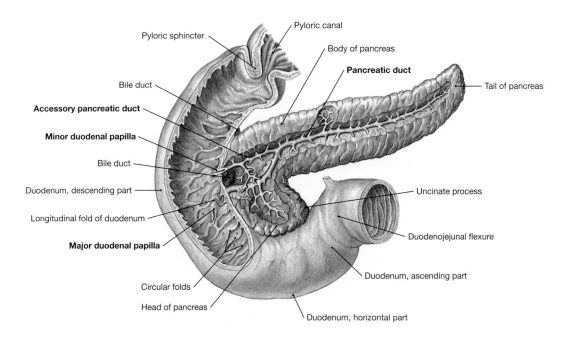

Pyloric sphincter

Pyloric canal

Body of pancreas

Pancreatic duct

Bile duct

Tail of pancreas

Accessory pancreatic duct

Minor duodenal papilla

Bile duct

Duodenum, descending part

Longitudinal fold of duodenum

Major duodenal papilla

Uncinate process

Duodenojejunal flexure

Duodenum, ascending part

Circular folds

Head of pancreas

Duodenum, horizontal part

Fig. 6.101 Excretory duct system of the pancreas; anterior view. The **main pancreatic duct** (duct of WIRSUNG) fuses with the terminal segment of the **bile duct** (ductus choledochus) in 60% of all cases to form the hepatopancreatic ampulla. The latter enters the descending part of the duodenum at the **major duodenal papilla.** In 65% of all cases an **accessory pancreatic duct** (duct of SANTORINI) exists which opens into the duodenum proximally at the **minor duodenal papilla.**

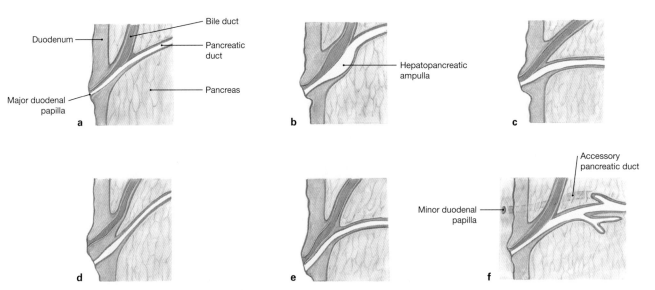

Duodenum

Bile duct

Pancreatic duct

Pancreas

Major duodenal papilla

a

Hepatopancreatic ampulla

b

c

d

e

Accessory pancreatic duct

Minor duodenal papilla

f

Fig. 6.102a to f Variations of the pancreatic and bile duct at the major duodenal papilla.
a Long common portion,
b Ampullary dilation of the terminal part (60% of all cases),
c Short common portion,
d Separate entrance,
e Common entrance with septated common duct,
f Accessory pancreatic duct (65% of all cases).

Clinical Remarks

Sonography and computer tomography are performed for the imaging of the pancreas. **Endoscopic retrograde cholangiopancreatography** (ERCP) is performed to diagnose and treat obstructions of the bile and/or pancreatic ducts.
ERCP image example to the right: to visualize the duct systems in the radiograph, the excretory duct of the pancreas and the bile duct were filled with contrast medium from the major duodenal papilla via an endoscope.

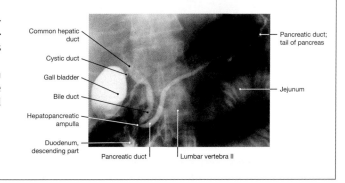

Common hepatic duct

Cystic duct

Gall bladder

Bile duct

Hepatopancreatic ampulla

Duodenum, descending part

Pancreatic duct

Lumbar vertebra II

Pancreatic duct; tail of pancreas

Jejunum

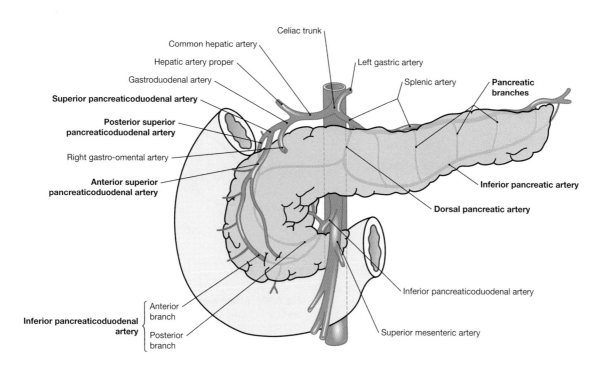

Fig. 6.103 Arteries of the pancreas; schematic illustration. [L126]
The pancreas is supplied by **two separate arterial systems** for the pancreatic head and the pancreatic body and tail, respectively.
- **Head:** double arterial arches from the anterior and posterior superior pancreaticoduodenal arteries (from the gastroduodenal artery) and from the inferior pancreaticoduodenal artery with an anterior and a posterior branch (from the superior mesenteric artery).

- **Body and tail:** pancreatic branches from the splenic artery which give rise to a dorsal pancreatic artery behind the pancreas and an inferior pancreatic artery at the inferior border of the gland.

The **veins** of the pancreas correspond to the arteries and drain via the superior mesenteric vein and the splenic vein into the hepatic portal vein.

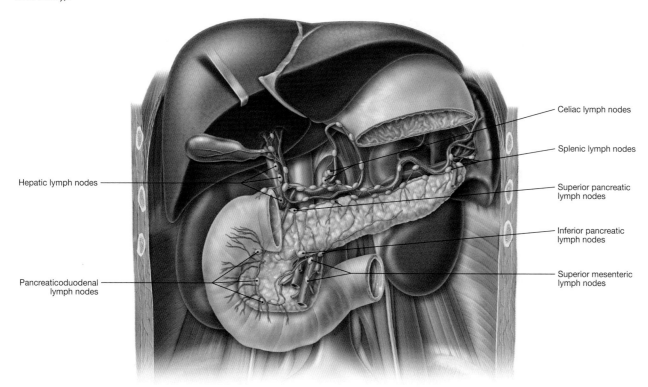

Fig. 6.104 Lymphatic drainage pathways of the pancreas; anterior view. [L238]
- **Head:** anterior and posterior pancreaticoduodenal lymph nodes, then via hepatic lymph nodes to the **celiac lymph nodes** or directly to the **superior mesenteric lymph nodes** and finally to the intestinal trunk.

- **Body:** superior and inferior pancreatic lymph nodes along the splenic artery and vein; from there to the **celiac lymph nodes** and to the **superior mesenteric lymph nodes**. There are also connections to the retroperitoneal **lumbar lymph nodes**.
- **Tail:** splenic lymph nodes.

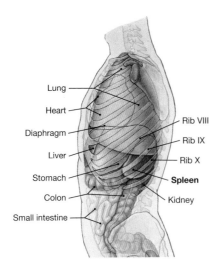

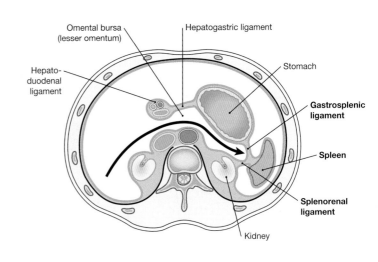

Fig. 6.105 Projection of the viscera onto the body surface; left side.

The spleen is located intraperitoneally in the posterior left epigastrium. Its longitudinal axis projects onto rib X. A normal-sized spleen is not palpable beyond the costal margin. Due to its large contact area with the diaphragm, the position of the spleen is dependent on respiration. The spleen lies in the so-called **splenic niche** which is confined inferiorly by the phrenicocolic ligament between the left colic flexure and diaphragm.

Fig. 6.106 Attachment of the spleen to the posterior abdominal wall; schematic section. [L126]

The spleen develops in the dorsal mesogastrium dividing it into the **gastrosplenic ligament** and the **splenorenal ligament**. The gastrosplenic ligament contains the short gastric and the left gastroepiploic blood vessels.

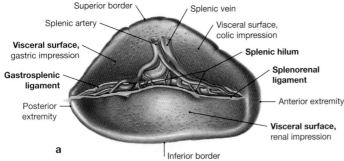

Fig. 6.107a and b Spleen; medial anterior view **(a)** and lateral superior view **(b)**.

The spleen weighs 150 g (5.3 oz), is 11 cm (4.3 in) long, 7 cm (2.8 in) wide and 4 cm (1.6 in) high. The spleen is a secondary lymphatic organ and plays a role in the immune system as well as in filtering of the blood. Its **diaphragmatic surface** is convex, its **visceral surface** is facing the left kidney, the left colic flexure, and the stomach. The blood vessels enter and exit at the splenic hilum. The spleen is anchored to the surroundings by two peritoneal duplicatures, both of which insert at the splenic hilum. The **gastrosplenic ligament** connects the spleen to the stomach and continues as **splenorenal ligament** to the posterior wall of the trunk.

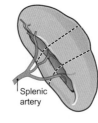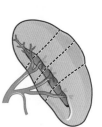

Fig. 6.108 Segments of the spleen. [L126]

The branching pattern of the blood vessels reflects the segmentation of the spleen.

┌─ Clinical Remarks ──────────────

Following abdominal trauma a rupture of the spleen may result in life-threatening hemorrhage. Because of the segmental structure of the spleen, longitudinal lacerations will affect several splenic segments and cause intense bleeding; transverse lacerations bleed weakly since splenic arteries are terminal arteries. This also explains the wedge-shaped area of infarction between the segmental borders – see abdominal CT image to the right. [G169]

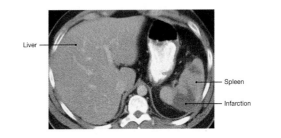

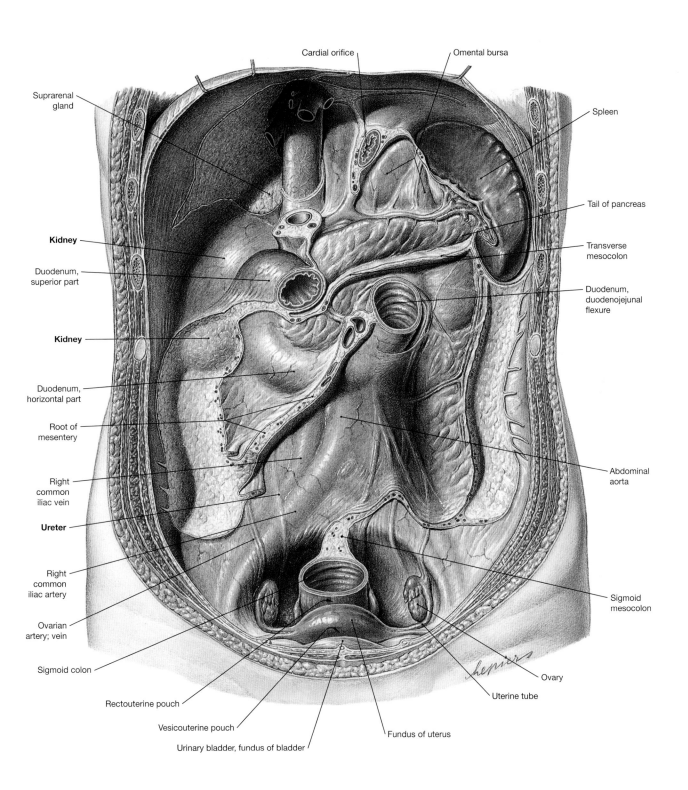

Fig. 6.109 Posterior wall of the peritoneal cavity with spleen (intraperitoneal); anterior view.

The kidneys and ureters are in retroperitoneal position and the parietal peritoneum is shown here covering the retroperitoneal structures.

Structure/Function

Retroperitoneal anatomical structures of the abdomen are located posterior to the parietal peritoneum:
- Kidneys and ureters,
- Suprarenal (adrenal) glands,
- Abdominal aorta and its branches,

- Inferior vena cava and its tributaries,
- Lymph nodes,
- Somatic nerves of the lumbar plexus,
- Psoas, iliacus and quadratus lumborum muscles.

Note: The muscles of the posterior abdominal wall are shown in ➤ chapter 2.

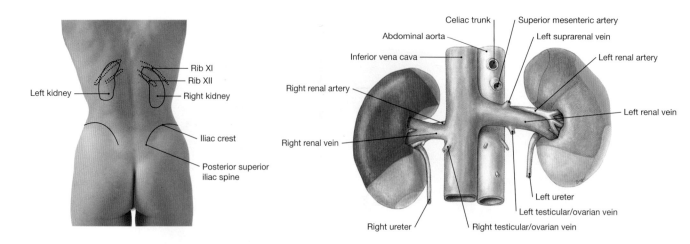

Fig. 6.110 **Projection of the kidneys onto the dorsal body wall.**
Left kidney:
* **Superior pole:** 12th thoracic vertebra, rib XI,
* **Hilum:** 2nd lumbar vertebra,
* **Inferior pole:** 3rd lumbar vertebra.

Due to the size of the liver, the right kidney is located about half a vertebra further inferior. The proximity to the diaphragm causes the downward movement (about 3 cm [1 in]) of both kidneys during inspiration.

Fig. 6.111 **Spatial relation of the kidneys;** anterior view.
The dorsal aspect of the kidney is adjacent to the posterior abdominal wall. The kidneys are embedded within the renal fascia – see ➤ Fig. 6.113.

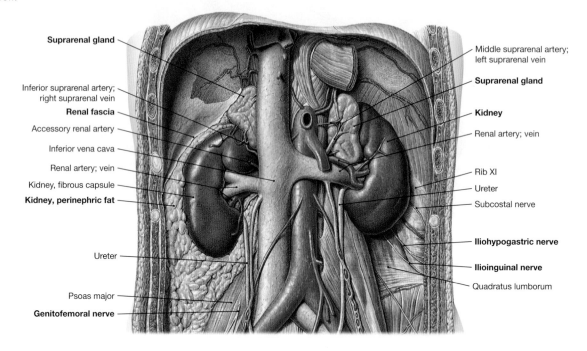

Fig. 6.112 **Position of the kidneys, ureter and adrenal gland in the retroperitoneal space;** anterior view.

Clinical Remarks

The metanephros develops at the level of S1–S4 vertebrae and ascends during embryonal weeks 6–9. This is a relative ascent since the part of the developing body caudal to the inferior pole of the kidney grows faster (**a** and **b**). If the kidneys fail to ascend, a **pelvic kidney (c)** is present. A **horseshoe kidney** develops if both inferior renal poles position in close proximity to each other and fuse **(d).** The horseshoe kidney does not fully ascend because the root of the inferior mesenteric artery presents an obstacle.

Pelvic kidneys and horseshoe kidneys are usually accidental findings and have no clinical relevance if the ureter is not compromised.   [L126]

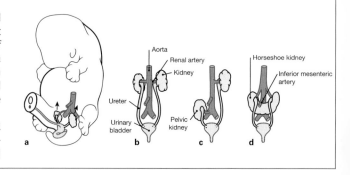

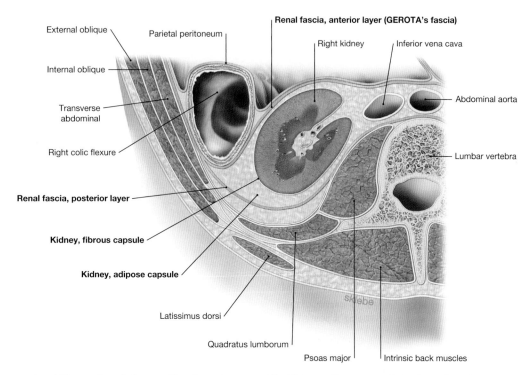

External oblique
Parietal peritoneum
Renal fascia, anterior layer (GEROTA's fascia)
Right kidney
Inferior vena cava
Internal oblique
Transverse abdominal
Abdominal aorta
Right colic flexure
Lumbar vertebra
Renal fascia, posterior layer
Kidney, fibrous capsule
Kidney, adipose capsule
Latissimus dorsi
Quadratus lumborum
Psoas major
Intrinsic back muscles

Fig. 6.113 Cross-sectional illustration of the renal fascia at the level of L3. [L238]

The kidney adipose capsule is also referred to as perirenal adipose capsule.

Structure/Function

The anterior and posterior layers of the renal fascia are fused superiorly and laterally and include the suprarenal gland. The renal fascia is open and connected to the retroperitoneal space medially and caudally for the entrance of the renal blood vessels and the exit of the ureters.

The anterior leaf of the renal fascia is referred to as GEROTA's fascia.

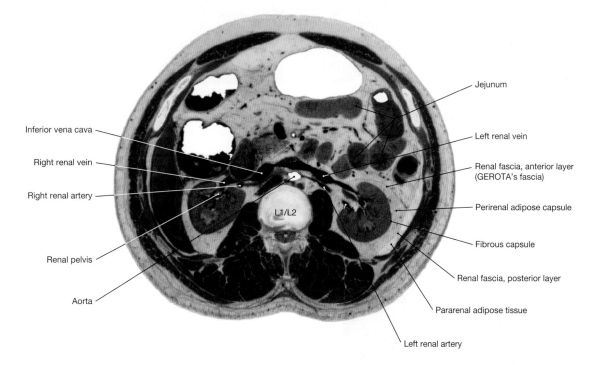

Inferior vena cava
Right renal vein
Right renal artery
Renal pelvis
Aorta
L1/L2
Jejunum
Left renal vein
Renal fascia, anterior layer (GEROTA's fascia)
Perirenal adipose capsule
Fibrous capsule
Renal fascia, posterior layer
Pararenal adipose tissue
Left renal artery

Fig. 6.114 Anatomical cross-section at the level of the L1/L2 intervertebral disc. The hilum of the kidney and the renal capsule and fascia are visible. [X338]

Clinical Remarks

The fascial systems and the topographical relationships of the kidneys are clinically relevant. In cases of **malignant tumors,** the kidney is always removed together with the adrenal gland and including the GEROTA's fascia **(nephrectomy).**

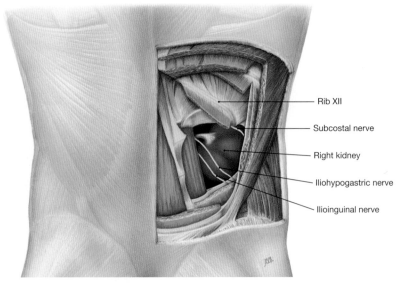

Right kidney

Subcostal nerve

Rib XII

Iliohypogastric nerve

Ilioinguinal nerve

Fig. 6.115 Position of the kidney in relation to the nerves of the lumbar plexus; view from a window through the right posterior body wall. [L285]

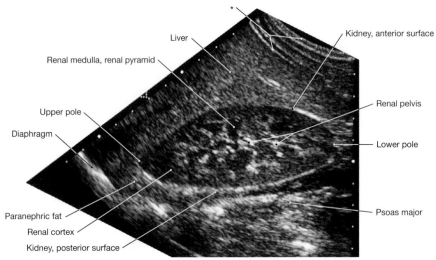

Liver

Renal medulla, renal pyramid

Upper pole

Diaphragm

Paranephric fat

Renal cortex

Kidney, posterior surface

*

Kidney, anterior surface

Renal pelvis

Lower pole

Psoas major

Fig. 6.116 Kidney; right side; ultrasound image; lateral view; transducer positioned almost vertically.

* abdominal wall

Clinical Remarks

Large benign **renal cysts** may be accidental findings but can be symptomatic when adjacent nerves of the lumbar plexus are affected. This causes pain in the groin region (L1 dermatome).
Surgical access to the kidney is preferentially achieved from the posterior wall of the trunk as the kidney is retroperitoneal. Removal of the kidney **(nephrectomy)** for renal malignancies includes the removal of the suprarenal gland, the adipose capsule

(perirenal fat) and GEROTA's fascia. For **renal transplantation** surgery the donor kidney is also accessed from posterior, but the suprarenal gland remains attached to the blood vessels of the donor. The kidney is then usually transplanted into the iliac fossa of the greater pelvis, renal blood vessels are connected to the external iliac artery and vein and the ureter is anastomosed to the urinary bladder.   a [T975], b [L275]

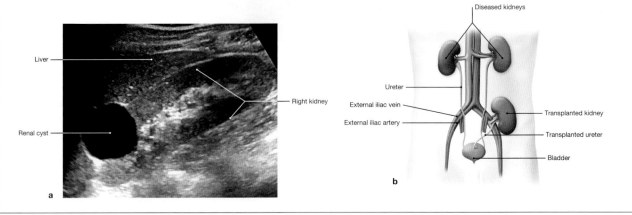

Liver

Renal cyst

Right kidney

Diseased kidneys

Ureter

External iliac vein

External iliac artery

Transplanted kidney

Transplanted ureter

Bladder

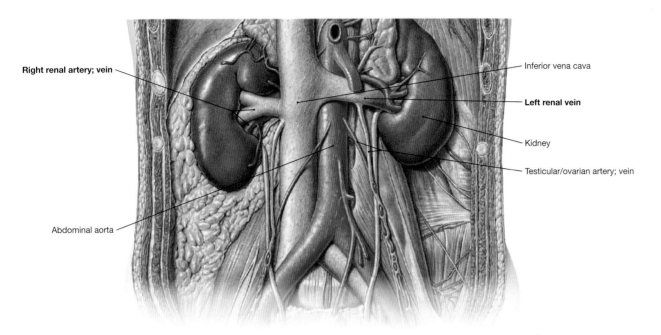

Fig. 6.117 Course of the renal artery and vein; anterior view.
The paired **renal arteries** arise from the abdominal aorta at the level of L2 and course posterior to the veins to the hilum of the kidney. The right renal artery crosses the inferior vena cava posteriorly. **At the hilum, they divide into several branches,** the segmental arteries.

The **renal veins** drain into the inferior vena cava.
The **left renal vein** receives blood from three tributaries, whereas on the right side these veins enter the inferior vena cava directly:
* Left suprarenal vein,
* Left testicular/ovarian vein,
* Left inferior phrenic vein.

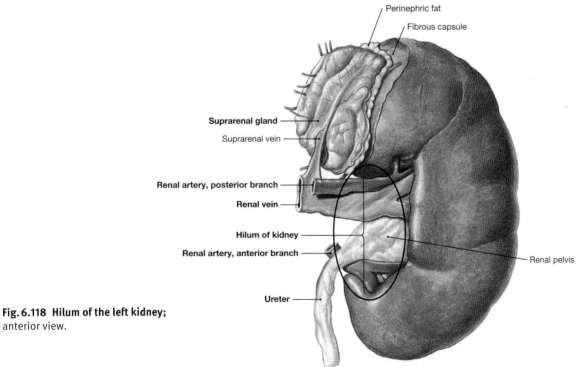

Fig. 6.118 Hilum of the left kidney; anterior view.

Structure/Function

The topography at the hilum of the kidney from ventral to dorsal is: renal vein, renal artery and the ureter as the most inferior and posterior structure. At the hilum the renal artery already branches into the anterior and posterior principal branch which further divide into the **five segmental arteries**: the anterior branch of the renal artery supplies the superior, the two anterior and the inferior renal segments; the posterior branch supplies the posterior segment.

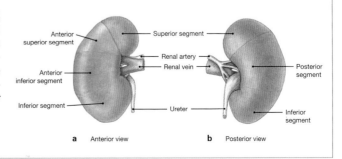

351

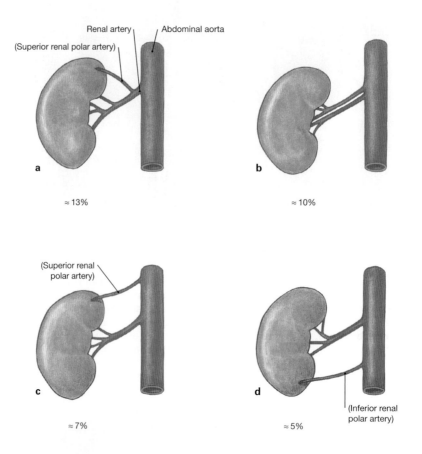

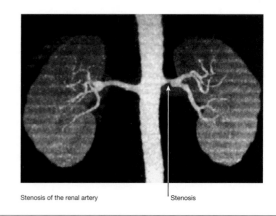

Fig. 6.119a to d Accessory renal arteries originate from the aorta independently.

Polar arteries do not enter the kidney at the hilum, but reach the parenchyma of the upper or lower kidney pole. Accessory renal arteries and their frequencies in the population:

a Renal artery with a branch as superior polar artery,
b Two renal arteries to the hilum of the kidney,
c Accessory superior polar artery,
d Accessory inferior polar artery.

Clinical Remarks

In patients with high blood pressure **(arterial hypertension)** a stenosis of one of the renal arteries needs to be excluded. Reduced blood pressure in the afferent arteriole of the renal glomerulus causes the release of renin and subsequent activation of the **renin-angiotensin pathway** with consecutive increased systemic blood pressure.
[F264-003]

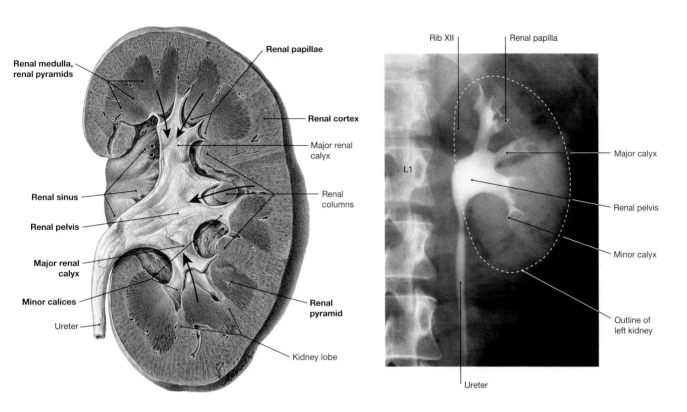

Fig. 6.120

Renal medulla, renal pyramids

Renal papillae

Renal cortex

Major renal calyx

Renal sinus

Renal columns

Renal pelvis

Major renal calyx

Minor calices

Renal pyramid

Ureter

Kidney lobe

Fig. 6.121

Rib XII

Renal papilla

L1

Major calyx

Renal pelvis

Minor calyx

Outline of left kidney

Ureter

Fig. 6.120 Kidney; left side; anterior view.
The cortex of the kidney contains the glomerula (➤ Fig. 6.121). The medulla consists of the renal pyramids which are separated by the renal columns. The renal lobe comprises one pyramid and adjacent cortical area. At the tip of each pyramid, the urine is released into the **minor renal calyx.** Two or three minor calyces merge to a **major renal calyx.** Arrows depict the urine release from the renal pyramids into the calyces. The major calyces merge to the renal pelvis.

Fig. 6.121 Intravenous (IV) pyelogram; anteroposterior view. [G130]
Normal anatomy of minor and major calices, the renal pelvis and the ureter is shown.

Clinical Remarks

Diagnostic imaging of the minor and major renal calyces is performed by intravenous (IV) pyelography using a radiocontrast agent that is exclusively eliminated by the kidney. A normal IV pyelogram is shown in ➤ Fig. 6.121. Urinary outflow (obstructive uropathy) may be caused by concrements in the renal pelvis or the ureters (renal calculi, kidney stones) or as lower urinary tract obstruction with a urethral obstruction e.g. in cases of prostate enlargements. Urinary outflow obstruction may be uni- or bilateral and may cause a dilation of the renal pelvis **(hydronephrosis).** The IV pyelography image to the right shows a hydronephrosis of the right kidney with substantial dilation of the renal calices and renal pelvis and the right ureter suggesting an obstruction of the distal ureter on the right side. The left kidney and renal pelvis is normal.
[H080]

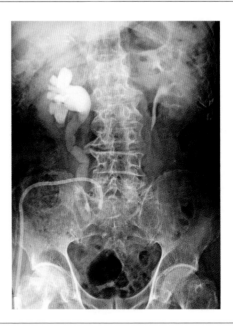

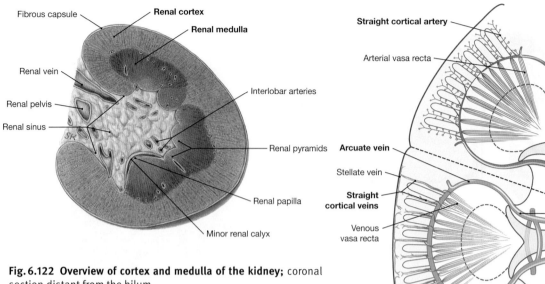

Fig. 6.122 Overview of cortex and medulla of the kidney; coronal section distant from the hilum.

Structure/Function

The function of the kidney is the removal of waste products and excretion or reabsorption of salts.

The kidneys produce and release the protease **renin** for the regulation of arterial blood pressure.

The kidney also produces the hormone erythropoietin **(EPO)** and expresses 1α-hydroxylase, an enzyme contributing to the active form of vitamin D, calcitriol (1,25-dihydroxyvitamin D).

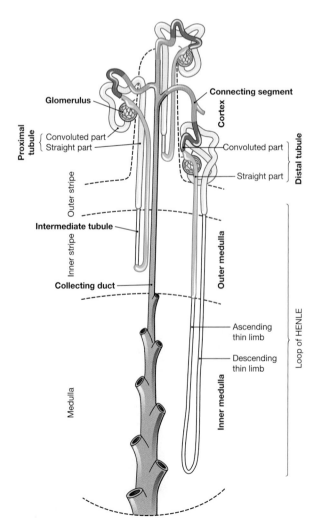

Fig. 6.123 Course of arteries (red), veins (blue), and nephrons (gray) in the renal parenchyma; schematic illustration. [L126]

The **renal artery and vein** divide at the hilum and ascend as **interlobar artery and vein** at the edge of the pyramids. They arch around the base of the pyramids as **arcuate artery and vein** and from there give rise to the **cortical radiate arteries and veins** to reach the capsule. In contrast to the communicating veins, the arteries are terminal arteries. Therefore, the occlusion of an artery, for example by a blood clot (embolism), will cause a **renal infarction.**

Within the lobes of the kidney the nephrons are arranged radially.

Fig. 6.124 Organization of nephron and collecting ducts; schematic illustration. [L126]

The nephron is the functional unit of the kidney and consists of the **renal corpuscle (glomerulus)** and the connected system of tubules. Filtration of blood and primary urine production occurs in the renal corpuscle. The **proximal tubule** begins with a convoluted part and a consecutive straight part. This is continued by the **intermediate tubule** which consists of a descending limb and an ascending limb followed by the **distal tubule** (again with straight part and convoluted part). The **connecting segment (collecting tubule)** is the transition to the **collecting duct** which finally releases the urine into the renal pelvis.

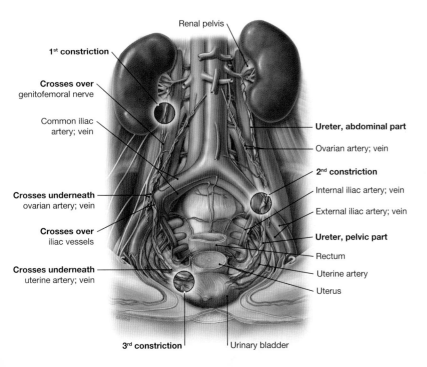

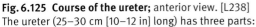

Fig. 6.125 Course of the ureter; anterior view. [L238]

The ureter (25–30 cm [10–12 in] long) has three parts:

- **Abdominal part:** from renal pelvis to pelvic brim,
- **Pelvic part:** from pelvic brim to urinary bladder,
- **Intramural part:** within bladder wall (➤ chapter 7 Pelvis).

Location of the **three ureteric constrictions**:

1. Pelviureteric junction (PU),
2. Crossing over the common iliac artery bifurcation at the pelvic brim,
3. Vesicoureteric junction (VU).

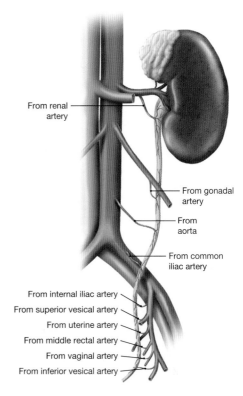

Fig. 6.126 Blood supply of the ureter. [L275]

Structure/Function

The ureter descends in the retroperitoneal space from the renal pelvis to the urinary bladder. It enters the pelvis anterior to the sacroiliac joints at the **level of the pelvic brim** at the bifurcation of the common iliac blood vessels, then courses anterior to the internal iliac artery in the pelvis. The **left ureter** is closely adjacent to the left colic artery, the inferior mesenteric vein and the sigmoid mesentery.

Specific spatial relations: The ureter courses anterior to the genitofemoral nerve, then **posterior to** the gonadal artery and vein, **crosses over** the common iliac artery and vein and **crosses underneath** the uterine artery (women) – 'water under the bridge' – or vas deferens (men) in the pelvis.

Clinical Remarks

Common variations are the **bifid renal pelvis (a),** the **bifid ureter (b)** and the duplicated ureter **(ureter duplex; c).** In all cases two renal pelvices are present. The bifid ureter is often an accidental finding and has no clinical relevance. In contrast, cases of a duplicated ureter are frequently associated with malformations of the ureteric opening into the urinary bladder, a condition potentially causing **reflux of urine which** promotes ascending **urinary tract infections** (UTIs) or incontinence. Frequently, the ureter from the superior renal pelvis crosses the ureter from the lower renal pelvis and may enter the urinary bladder more inferiorly or even directly enters the urethra resulting in urinary incontinence. a–c [L126], [E377]

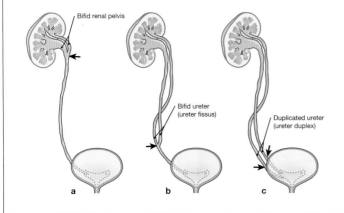

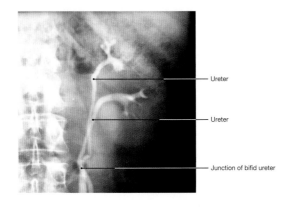

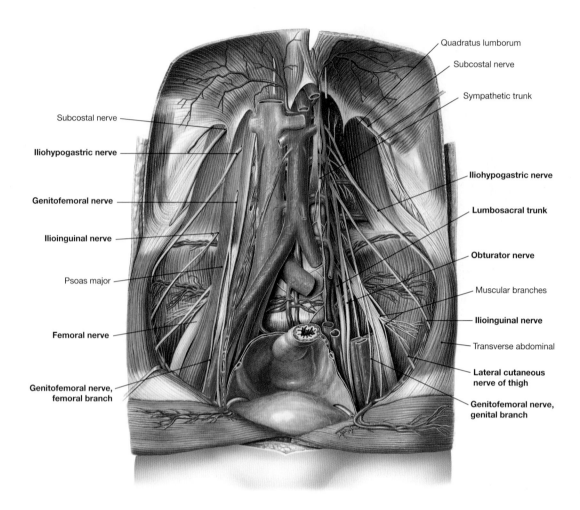

Subcostal nerve

Iliohypogastric nerve

Genitofemoral nerve

Ilioinguinal nerve

Psoas major

Femoral nerve

Genitofemoral nerve, femoral branch

Quadratus lumborum

Subcostal nerve

Sympathetic trunk

Iliohypogastric nerve

Lumbosacral trunk

Obturator nerve

Muscular branches

Ilioinguinal nerve

Transverse abdominal

Lateral cutaneous nerve of thigh

Genitofemoral nerve, genital branch

Fig. 6.127 Somatic nerves of the retroperitoneal space; anterior view.

The nerves of the **lumbar plexus** serve the innervation of the antero-lateral abdominal wall, the inguinal region and the anterior aspect of the thigh. The lumbosacral trunk is the connection to the sacral plexus in the lesser pelvis (➤ chapter 4). Together with the iliohypogastric and ilioinguinal nerves of the lumbar plexus the subcostal nerve (T12) provides motor innervation to the muscles of the anterolateral abdominal wall.

Note: Details to the nerves of the lumbar plexus can be found in ➤ *chapter 4 (Lower Extremity).*

Structure/Function

Nerves of the lumbar plexus (T12–L4):
- Motor branches to iliopsoas and quadratus lumborum (T12–L4),
- Iliohypogastric nerve (T12, L1),
- Ilioinguinal nerve (T12, L1),
- Genitofemoral nerve (L1, L2),
- Lateral femoral cutaneous nerve (L2, L3),
- Femoral nerve (L2–L4),
- Obturator nerve (L2–L4).

Clinical Remarks

The close proximity of the kidney to the iliohypogastric and ilio-inguinal nerves explains why certain diseases of the kidney such as inflammation of the renal pelvis **(pyelonephritis)** or concrements in the renal pelvis **(nephrolithiasis)** may cause **radiating pain into the inguinal region. Renal concrements** may dislodge, descend in the ureter and obstruct the ureter at the site of its constrictions. This causes intense, colic-like pain (ureteral colic) from waves of muscular contraction and distension of the ureter.
a [L126], b [L238]

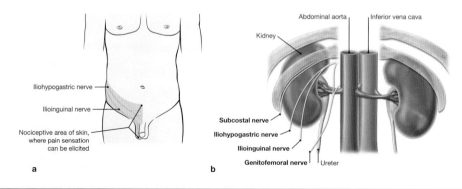

Iliohypogastric nerve

Ilioinguinal nerve

Nociceptive area of skin, where pain sensation can be elicited

Abdominal aorta

Inferior vena cava

Kidney

Subcostal nerve

Iliohypogastric nerve

Ilioinguinal nerve

Genitofemoral nerve

Ureter

a

b

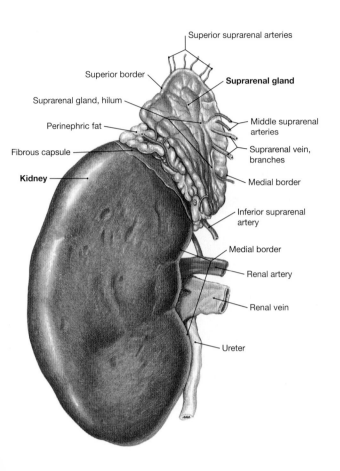

Fig. 6.128 Kidney and suprarenal gland; right side; anterior view.
The suprarenal (adrenal) gland is adjacent to the superior pole of
the kidney and separated from the fibrous capsule of the kidney by
a layer of perirenal fat. The suprarenal gland is located within the
renal fascia.

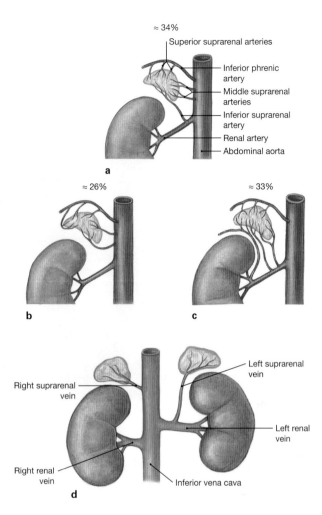

Fig. 6.129a to d Suprarenal arteries and veins; anterior view.
Usually there are three arteries to the adrenal gland:
* **Superior suprarenal artery:** derives from the inferior phrenic
  artery,
* **Middle suprarenal artery:** arises directly from the aorta,
* **Inferior suprarenal artery:** branch of the renal artery.
Variations of the arteries to the suprarenal gland; frequencies in
the population are indicated in %,
a Arterial supply via three arteries,
b Arterial supply without tributary from the renal artery,
c Arterial supply without a direct branch of the aorta,
d In contrast, **only one suprarenal vein** exists for each adrenal
gland. The suprarenal vein drains into the inferior vena cava on the
right side, and into the left renal vein on the left side.

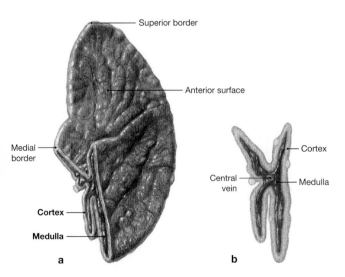

Fig. 6.130a and b Suprarenal gland; right side; anterior view **(a)**;
sagittal section **(b)**.
The paired suprarenal (adrenal) glands are vital organs and consist
of a cortex and a medulla. The right suprarenal gland has a triangular shape, the left gland is more crescent-shaped.

Structure/Function

* The suprarenal **cortex** develops from the mesoderm and
  produces steroid hormones, glucocorticoids, mineralocor-
  ticoids and androgens (dehydroepiandrosterone).
* The suprarenal **medulla** originates from the neural crest as
  a modified sympathetic ganglion. Preganglionic sympathetic neurons traveling with the greater (T5–T9) and lesser splanchnic nerves (T10, T11) directly stimulate the release of (nor)epinephrine into the bloodstream. Thus, the
  suprarenal gland is an important organ for the stress response.
* The suprarenal glands position at the level of T11/T12.
* The right suprarenal gland is adjacent to the IVC and the
  right crus of the lumbar diaphragm.
* The left suprarenal gland is located adjacent to the aorta
  near the celiac trunk and to the left crus of the diaphragm.
  It is posterior to the lesser sac of the abdominal peritoneal
  cavity near the splenic artery and the pancreas.

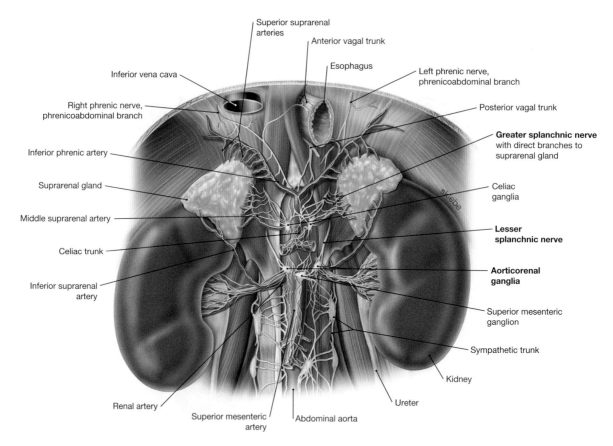

Superior suprarenal
arteries

Anterior vagal trunk

Esophagus

Inferior vena cava

Left phrenic nerve,
phrenicoabdominal branch

Right phrenic nerve,
phrenicoabdominal branch

Posterior vagal trunk

Greater splanchnic nerve
with direct branches to
suprarenal gland

Inferior phrenic artery

Suprarenal gland

Celiac
ganglia

Middle suprarenal artery

**Lesser
splanchnic nerve**

Celiac trunk

**Aorticorenal
ganglia**

Inferior suprarenal
artery

Superior mesenteric
ganglion

Sympathetic trunk

Kidney

Renal artery

Ureter

Superior mesenteric
artery

Abdominal aorta

Fig. 6.131 Innervation of the kidney and suprarenal gland; anterior view. [L238]
The predominantly **sympathetic innervation** of the kidney occurs via postganglionic sympathetic fibers of the aorticorenal ganglion which are mostly synapsed from fibers traveling with the **lesser splanchnic nerve** (T10, T11). Sympathetic innervation leads to vasoconstriction and release of the protease renin.

The **autonomic innervation** of the suprarenal gland is exclusively sympathetic and derives from preganglionic (!) sympathetic nerve fibers traveling with the **greater splanchnic nerve** (T5–T9) to reach the gland directly or via the celiac plexus (the adrenal medulla represents a **sympathetic paraganglion**). Sympathetic stimulation causes the immediate release of (nor)epinephrine into the blood.

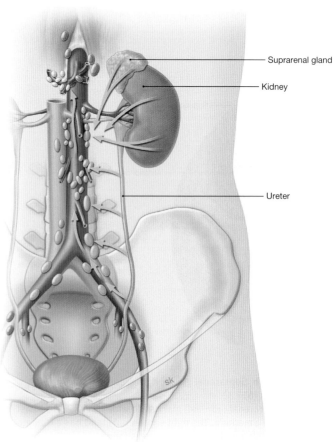

Suprarenal gland

Kidney

Ureter

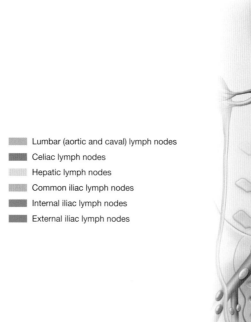

▨ Lumbar (aortic and caval) lymph nodes
▨ Celiac lymph nodes
▨ Hepatic lymph nodes
▨ Common iliac lymph nodes
▨ Internal iliac lymph nodes
▨ External iliac lymph nodes

Fig. 6.132 Lymphatic drainage of the kidney, ureter and suprarenal gland; schematic illustration. [L238]
The lymph of the ureter, kidney and suprarenal gland is drained through the lumbar nodes into the lumbar trunks and the thoracic duct.

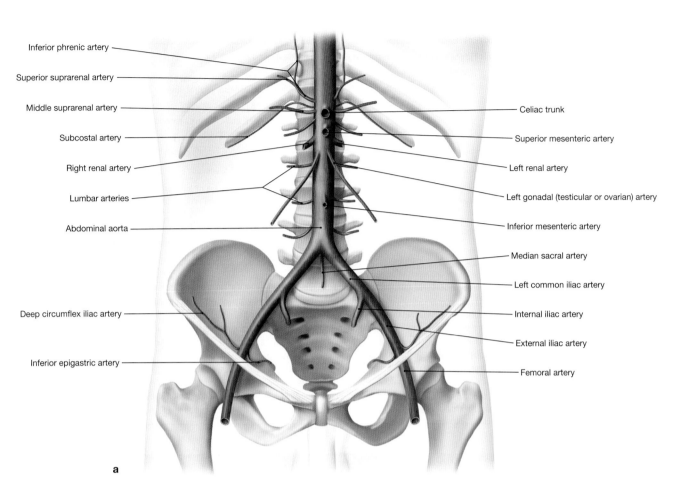

Inferior phrenic artery

Superior suprarenal artery

Middle suprarenal artery

Subcostal artery

Right renal artery

Lumbar arteries

Abdominal aorta

Deep circumflex iliac artery

Inferior epigastric artery

Celiac trunk

Superior mesenteric artery

Left renal artery

Left gonadal (testicular or ovarian) artery

Inferior mesenteric artery

Median sacral artery

Left common iliac artery

Internal iliac artery

External iliac artery

Femoral artery

a

Fig. 6.133a and b Branches of the abdominal aorta; schematic illustration. a [L238], b [L126] **(a)** Paired and unpaired branches of the abdominal aorta; **(b)** cross-sectional schematic of the vascular planes:
1. **Midline:** unpaired branches to viscera,
2. **Lateral:** paired branches to viscera,
3. **Posterolateral:** paired branches to the wall of the trunk.

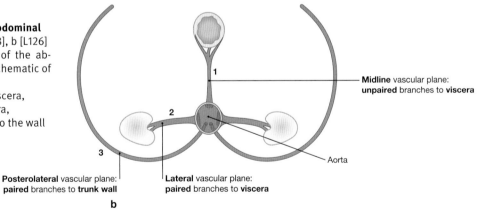

Midline vascular plane: **unpaired** branches to **viscera**

Posterolateral vascular plane: **paired** branches to **trunk wall**

Lateral vascular plane: **paired** branches to **viscera**

Aorta

b

Branches of the Abdominal Aorta	Vertebral Level	Vascular Plane	See ➤ Fig. 6.133b
Celiac trunk	T12	Unpaired, midline, gastrointestinal tract	1
Superior mesenteric artery (SMA)	L1		
Inferior mesenteric artery (IMA)	L3		
Median sacral artery	L4	Unpaired, midline	
Middle suprarenal arteries	L1	Paired, lateral, endocrine and urogenital viscera	2
Renal arteries	L1–L2		
Gonadal arteries (ovarian, testicular)	L2		
Common iliac arteries	L4	Paired terminal branches of the aorta	
Inferior phrenic arteries	T12	Paired, posterolateral, body wall	3
Subcostal artery	T12		
Lumbar arteries	L1–L4		

Sympathetic Innervation of Abdominal Viscera

CNS Origin (Spinal Cord)	Preganglionic Fibers	Prevertebral Ganglia and Plexus	Target Organs
T5–T9	Greater splanchnic nerve	Celiac	Lower esophagus, stomach, spleen, liver, gall bladder, duodenum, pancreas
		Superior mesenteric	Pancreas, duodenum, jejunum, ileum, cecum, colon to left colic flexure: ascending and transverse colon, gonads (ovary, testis)
T10, T11	Lesser splanchnic nerve	Aorticorenal ganglion and renal plexus	Kidneys, upper ureter, suprarenal (adrenal) glands
T12	Lowest splanchnic nerve		Kidneys, ureter
L1, L2	Lumbar splanchnic nerves (from L1–L2 lumbar ganglion)	Inferior mesenteric	Colon distal of left colic flexure: descending and sigmoid colon, upper rectum (associated with peritoneal lining)
L1, L2	Lumbar splanchnic nerves (from L3–L5 lumbar ganglion)	Superior and inferior hypo-gastric	Middle and lower rectum, pelvic viscera

Structure/Function

- **Sympathetics** derive from the intermediolateral column of the thoracolumbar spinal cord (T5–L2).
- Splanchnic nerves contain preganglionic sympathetic fibers that have not been synapsed in the ganglia of the sympathetic chain. These fibers are synapsed in one of the prevertebral sympathetic ganglia (celiac **(A),** aorticorenal, superior **(B)** and inferior **(C)** mesenteric, superior hypogastric; **D).**
- Postganglionic fibers from the prevertebral ganglia course along branches of the aorta to reach their target organs, e.g. along the arterial branches within the mesenteries.

- The organ-specific nerve plexus is named accordingly and con-tains mixed sympathetic and parasympathetic nerves.
- **Function:** sympathetic innervation of the gastrointestinal tract results in vasoconstriction and inhibition of peristalsis and glandular secretion. Afferent **visceral pain** fibers also travel with sympathetics.

Note: postganglionic fibers from the ganglia of the sympathetic chain join the somatic nerves (gray rami communicantes) to reach the skin via their cutaneous branches. A few postganglionic fibers also course with periarte-rial nerves to reach visceral targets.

Parasympathetic Innervation of Abdominal Viscera

CNS Origin	Preganglionic Fibers	Ganglia and Plexus	Target Organs
Dorsal nucleus of vagus nerve in the brain stem	Vagus nerve [CN X]	Organ-specific or intramural	Esophagus, stomach, liver, gallbladder, spleen, duodenum, pancreas, kidney, ureter, small intestines, cecum, colon proximal to left colic flexure
S2–S4 sacral spinal cord	Pelvic splanchnic nerves	Inferior hypogastric or intramural	Colon distal to left colic (splenic) flexure, rectum

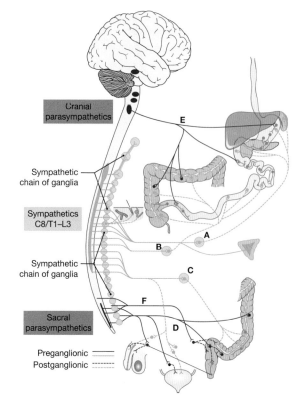

Fig. 6.134 Organization of the autonomic innervation to the abdominopelvic viscera. [L126]

Structure/Function

- **Parasympathetics** derive from the cranial, dorsal nucleus of vagus nerve [CN X] in the brain stem, or from the inter-mediolateral column of the sacral spinal cord (S2–S4 seg-ments).
- Preganglionic parasympathetic fibers travel with the **va-gus nerve (E)** and with the **pelvic splanchnic nerves (F)** to join autonomic nerve plexus around their target organs. They course along branches of the aorta, e.g. along the ar-terial branches within the mesenteries.
- Preganglionic parasympathetic fibers are synapsed in small intramural ganglia of the abdominopelvic viscera or in small ganglia of autonomic organs (e.g. inferior hypo-gastric plexus)
- **Function:** parasympathetic innervation of the gastrointes-tinal tract results in vasodilation and stimulation of peri-stalsis and glandular secretion.

Note: the left colic (splenic) flexure marks the demarcation for the para-sympathetic innervation from the cranial and the sacral origin.

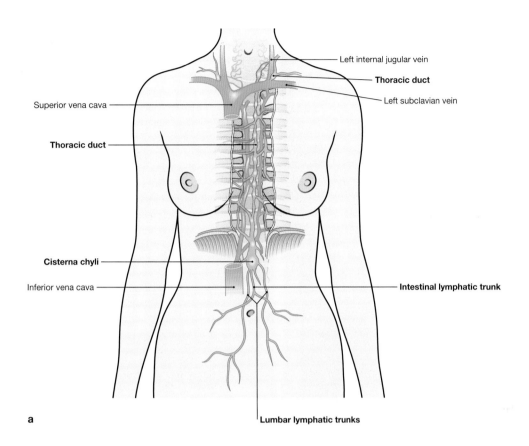

a

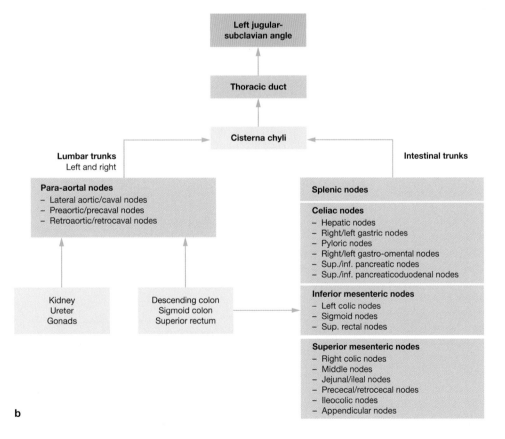

b

Fig. 6.135a and b Lymphatic drainage pathways of the abdomen; schematic illustration. a [L126], b [L231]

Structure/Function

- The cisterna chyli is located just below the diaphragm.
- All lymph nodes listed here to drain into the celiac nodes may also directly drain into the intestinal trunks.

- The lumbar trunks also receive all lymph from the perineum and the lower limbs.

Pelvis

Surface Anatomy 364

Male and Female Pelvis 365

Pelvic Floor 367

Pelvic Viscera – Overview 369

Rectum and Anal Canal 371

Urinary Bladder 376

Male Urethra 378

Female Urethra 379

Male Pelvic Viscera 380

Female Pelvic Viscera 385

Male Genitalia 397

Perineum 405

Female Perineum 406

Male Perineum 413

Ischioanal Fossa 416

Perineal Spaces 417

Pelvic Arteries 419

Pelvic Veins 420

Pelvic Nerves 421

7

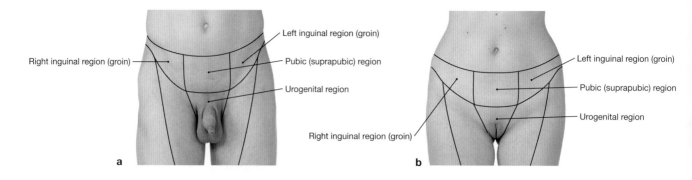

Fig. 7.1a and b Body regions in the male **(a)** and female **(b)**; anterior view. [K340]

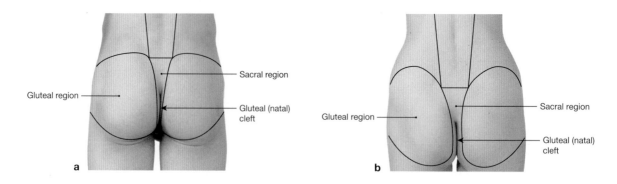

Fig. 7.2a and b Body regions in the male **(a)** and female **(b)**; posterior view. [K340]

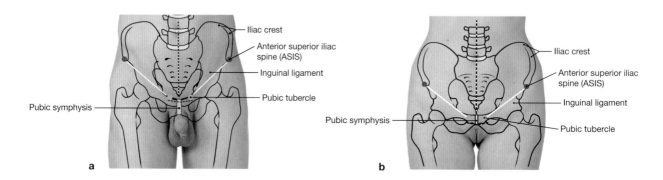

Fig. 7.3a and b Surface projection of the pelvic bones and surface landmarks in the male **(a)** and female **(b)**; anterior view. [K340]

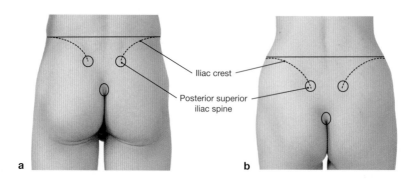

Fig. 7.4a and b Surface projection of the pelvic bones and surface landmarks in the male **(a)** and female **(b)**; posterior view. [K340]

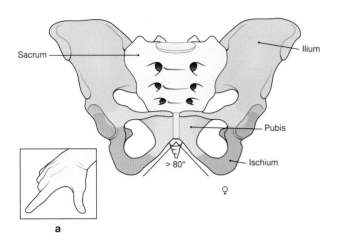

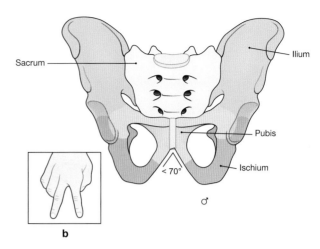

Fig. 7.5a and b Differences between female (a) and male (b) pelvices. [L126]
The parts of the os coxae (innominate bone) are coloured in green (ilium), red (ischium) and yellow (pubis). The position of the fingers demonstrates the infrapubic angle (➤ Fig. 4.6).

	Female Pelvis	Male Pelvis
Greater pelvis	Shallow	Deep
Lesser pelvis	Wide and shallow	Narrow and deep
Pelvic inlet	Oval, rounded	Heart-shaped
Pelvic outlet	Round, spacious	Narrow
Pubic arch and suprapubic angle	Wide > 80°	Narrow < 70°
Sacrum	Short and wide	Long and more convex

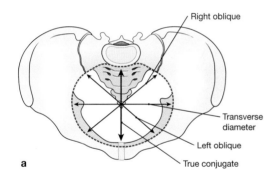

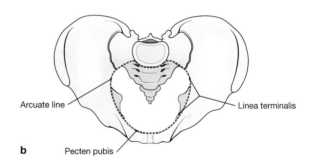

Fig. 7.6a and b Pelvic inlet plane in the female (a) and male (b) pelvices; superior view. [L126]

The pelvic inlet plane is bordered by the promontory and the pelvic brim, a bony ridge formed by the arcuate line of the ilium and the pecten pubis. The pelvic inlet plane separates the greater (false) from the lesser (true) pelvis (➤ Fig. 4.4, ➤ Fig. 4.5)

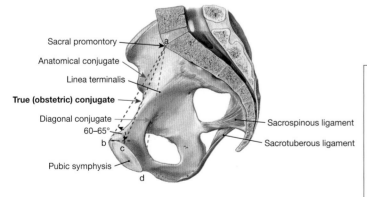

Fig. 7.7 Pelvic diameters; medial view from the left side.
The **true (obstetric) conjugate** is the narrowest anteroposterior pelvic diameter of the birth canal that does not widen. It is usually 11 cm (4.3 in) or greater.
Anatomical conjugate: distance between a and b, true (obstetric) conjugate: distance between a and c, diagonal conjugate: distance between a and d.

Clinical Remarks

The obstetric conjugate can be manually assessed by measuring the distance between the promontory and the inferior margin of the pubic symphysis (diagonal conjugate) using the middle finger minus 1.5 cm (0.6 in). [L126]

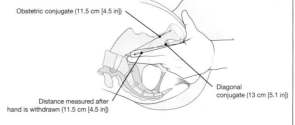

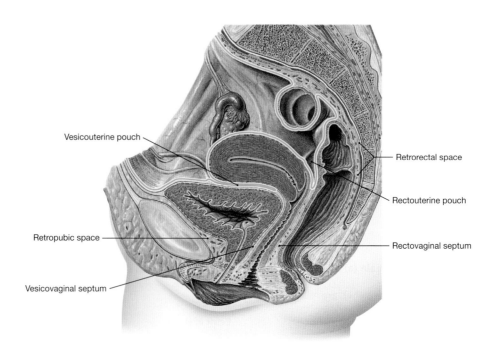

Fig. 7.8 Female pelvis; median section; view from the left side. The peritoneal lining is shown in green color. It separates the peritoneal cavity of pelvis from the extraperitoneal space of the pelvis.

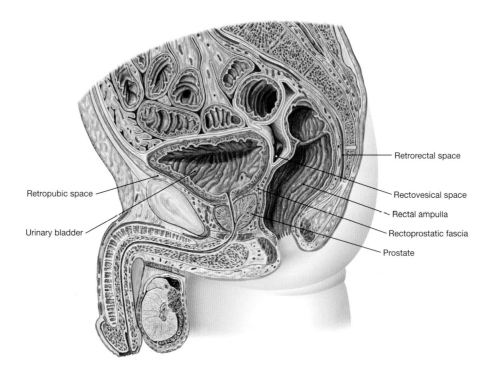

Fig. 7.9 Male pelvis; median section; view from the left side. The peritoneal lining is shown in green color. It separates the peritoneal pelvic cavity from the extraperitoneal space of the pelvis.

Clinical Remarks

In woman, the **rectouterine pouch (pouch of DOUGLAS)** is the most inferior recess of the peritoneal cavity. It can be accessed through the posterior fornix of the vagina. The **pelvic fascia** is the connective tissue between the peritoneal lining and the muscular walls and floor of the pelvis which contains nerves, blood vessels and lymphatics. The **retropubic space (space of RETZIUS)** behind the pubic symphysis and the retrorectal space are regions of the pelvic fascia containing loose connective tissue for the bladder and rectum to expand.

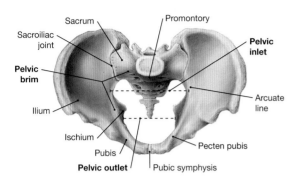

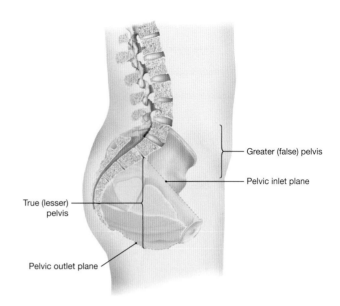

Fig. 7.10 Pelvis; superior view.
Key features of the bony pelvis are shown. The inferior opening of the bony pelvis is closed by the dynamic myofascial pelvic floor (➤ Fig. 7.12 and ➤ Fig. 7.13).

Fig. 7.11 True (lesser) pelvic; view from the right side. [L280]

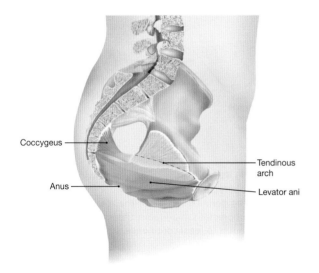

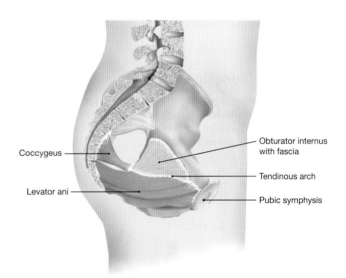

Fig. 7.12 Schematic drawing of the pelvic floor; median section; view from the right side. [L280]
The funnel-shaped pelvic floor, also referred to as pelvic diaphragm, is an essential dynamic myofascial inferior support structure for pelvic viscera and its position is indicated here in green.

Fig. 7.13 Muscles of the pelvic floor; median section; view from the right side. [L280]
The levator ani and coccygeus muscles together form the funnel-shaped pelvic floor (pelvic diaphragm). Its tonic contraction supports the position of the abdominopelvic viscera and is essential for maintaining urinary and fecal continence. The area inferior to the pelvic floor is the perineum.

Clinical Remarks

The muscles of the pelvic floor are actively contracted – together with the diaphragm and the abdominal muscles – to increase abdominal pressure during coughing, sneezing, forced expiration and weight lifting. Women more frequently suffer from **pelvic floor insufficiency** due to the extensive dilation of the levator hiatus during vaginal deliveries.

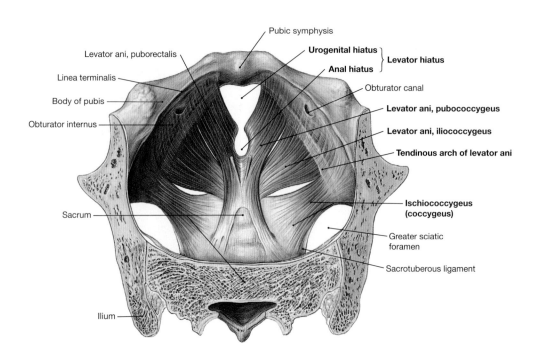

Fig. 7.14 Pelvic floor (female); superior view.
The pelvic floor comprises the following muscles:
- Levator ani: pubococcygeus, iliococcygeus, and puborectalis
- Ischiococcygeus

The muscles of both sides spare the levator hiatus between them (urogenital hiatus) for the passage of urethra, vagina and rectum. Innervation: direct branches of the sacral plexus (S3–S4).

Structure/Function

The puborectalis slings around the anorectal junction and pulls the rectum towards the pubic symphysis. This puborectalis loop is the basis for the **perineal flexure** of the rectum and maintains the **anorectal angle.**

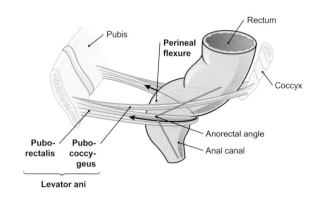

Fig. 7.15 Puborectalis; schematic drawing. [L126]
The puborectalis loop of the levator ani muscle stabilizes the perineal flexure of the rectum. The tonus of the puborectalis maintains the anorectal angle and contributes to fecal continence.

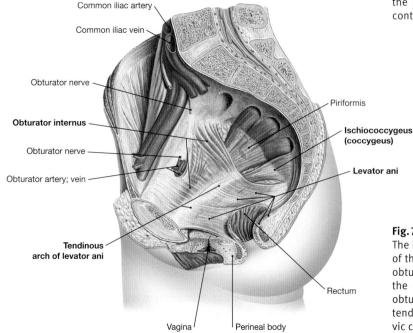

Fig. 7.16 Pelvic floor (female); view from the left side. The levator ani broadly attaches to the tendinous arch of the levator ani, a reinforcement of the fascia of the obturator internus. The obturator internus is pierced by the obturator canal containing the obturator artery, obturator vein and obturator nerve. The levator ani extends to the sacrum and the coccyx and closes the pelvic cavity caudally.

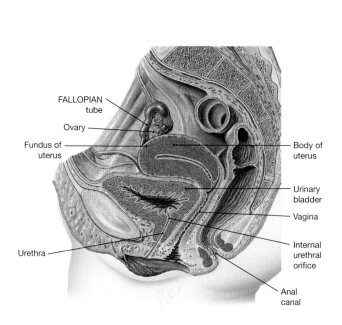

FALLOPIAN tube

Ovary

Fundus of uterus

Urethra

Body of uterus

Urinary bladder

Vagina

Internal urethral orifice

Anal canal

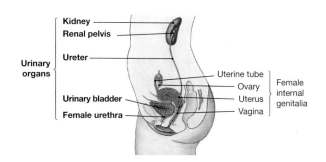

Kidney
Renal pelvis

Urinary organs

Ureter

Uterine tube
Ovary
Uterus
Vagina

Female internal genitalia

Urinary bladder

Female urethra

Fig. 7.17 Genital and urinary organs in the female; schematic drawing.

Fig. 7.18 Female pelvis, median section; view from the left side. The uterus lies above the urinary bladder. Its fundus and body are covered by peritoneum.

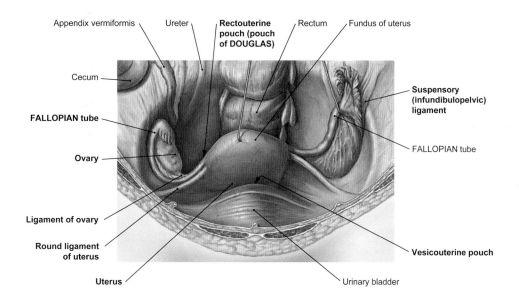

Appendix vermiformis

Ureter

Rectouterine pouch (pouch of DOUGLAS)

Rectum

Fundus of uterus

Cecum

FALLOPIAN tube

Ovary

Ligament of ovary

Round ligament of uterus

Uterus

Urinary bladder

Vesicouterine pouch

FALLOPIAN tube

Suspensory (infundibulopelvic) ligament

Fig. 7.19 Uterus, ovary, and uterine tube, with peritoneal duplicatures; anterior view.
Uterus, uterine tubes, and ovaries have an **intraperitoneal** position. Their peritoneal duplicatures (broad ligament of uterus, mesosalpinx, mesovarium) form a transverse fold in the lesser pelvis. The **round ligament** of uterus extends ventrally from the utero-

tubal junction to the lateral wall of the lesser pelvis and traverses the inguinal canal to merge with the connective tissue of the labia majora. The **ligament of ovary** connects uterus and ovary. The **suspensory** (clin. term: **infundibulopelvic**) **ligament** of the ovary connects the ovary to the lateral pelvic wall and contains the ovarian artery and vein.

Clinical Remarks

The **vesicouterine pouch** is a peritoneal recess between the uterus and the urinary bladder. The **rectouterine pouch** (pouch of DOUGLAS, clin. term: cul-de-sac) posterior to the uterus is the most caudal extension of the peritoneal cavity in women and may collect fluids and pus in cases of inflammatory abdominal processes. The pouch of DOUGLAS can be accessed through the

posterior fornix of the vagina. The close topographical relationship between the adnexa (ovary and uterine tube) and the appendix vermiformis of the colon explain why inflammations of the appendix **(appendicitis)** and of the uterine tube **(salpingitis)** may cause similar pain in the right lower abdominal quadrant.

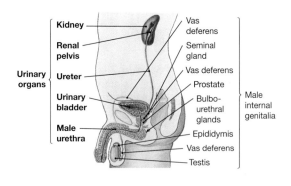

Fig. 7.20 Genital and urinary organs in the male; schematic drawing.

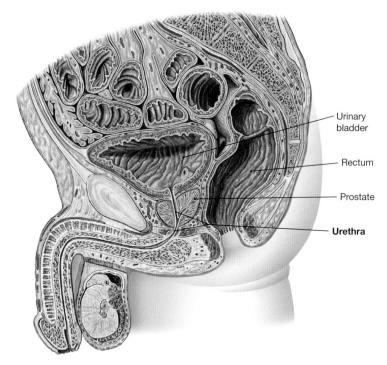

Fig. 7.21 Male pelvis; median section; view from the left side.
The prostate is positioned beneath the urinary bladder and surrounds the proximal male urethra.

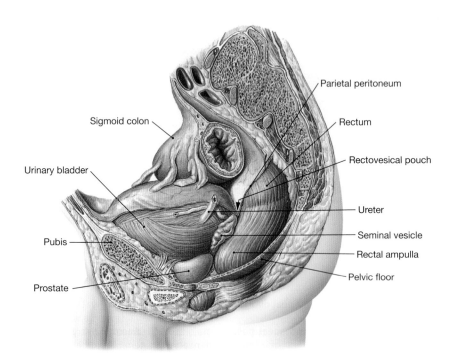

Fig. 7.22 Male pelvis; view from the left side.
The upper rectum and the superior and posterior aspect of the urinary bladder are lined by parietal peritoneum. The peritoneal reflection forms the **rectovesical pouch**, the most inferior peritoneal recess in men. In the extraperitoneal pelvic space beneath the peritoneum (subperitoneal), the anterior aspect of the rectum is adjacent to the posterior wall of the urinary bladder and the seminal vesicles and further caudally to the prostate.

Clinical Remarks

The prostate gland is separated from the rectum only by the thin rectoprostatic fascia (DENONVILLIERS' fascia) and the prostate can be assessed by digital rectal examination (DRE). Due to the high incidence of **benign prostatic hyperplasia** (BPH) and **prostatic carcinoma**, the digital rectal examination is part of a complete physical examination in men over 50 years of age.

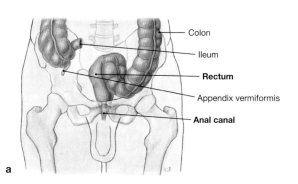

a

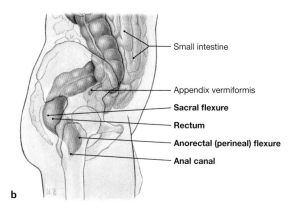

b

Fig. 7.23a and b Projection of the rectum and of the anal canal on-to the body surface; anterior view **(a)** and lateral view **(b).**
The rectum begins at the level of the 2nd or 3rd sacral vertebrae and ends on the pelvic diaphragm which is traversed by the anal canal.

The rectum has two bends: the posteriorly convex **sacral flexure** and the anteriorly convex **perineal** or **anorectal flexure.**

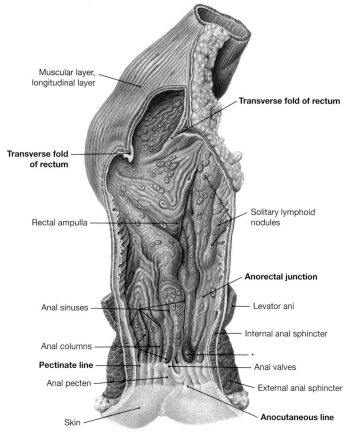

Fig. 7.24 Rectum and anal canal; anterior view.
The inner relief of the rectum shows transverse folds **(HOUSTON's valves).** One of the three folds is palpable regularly at about 6–7 cm (2.3–2.8 in) above the anus (KOHLRAUSCH's fold). Below this fold,

the rectum is dilated to form the **rectal ampulla.** The anorectal line marks the anorectal junction.

* hemorrhoidal knots

Structure/Function

The **anal canal** has three segments:
- **Columnar zone:** contains longitudinal folds (anal columns) formed by the underlying corpus cavernosum of rectum.
- **Anal pecten:** the stratified non-keratinized squamous epithelium creates a white zone in the mucosa; the superior border

of this zone is referred to as **pectinate line** (clinical term: dentate line).
- **Cutaneous zone:** external skin, inconsistently limited by the anocutaneous line).

Clinical Remarks

Inspection of the mucosa of a prolapse allows the visual discrimination between a rectal (transverse folds) versus an anal (longitudinal folds) **prolapse.** Both result in fecal incontinence. Above the anal valves, the anal sinuses are located as depres-

sions in which proctodeal glands (anal glands) enter the anal canal. These glands may traverse the sphincter muscles and cause fistulas when inflamed and, thus, potentially facilitate the spread of the inflammation into the ischioanal fossa.

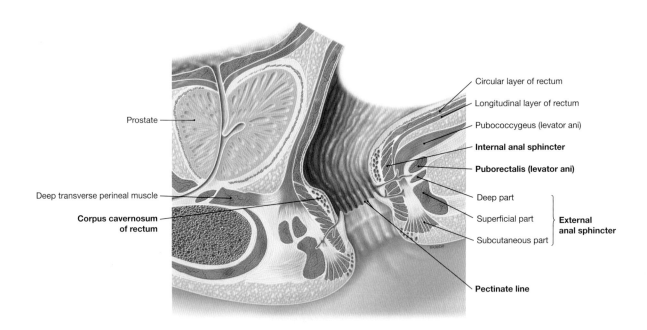

Prostate

Deep transverse perineal muscle

Corpus cavernosum of rectum

Circular layer of rectum

Longitudinal layer of rectum

Pubococcygeus (levator ani)

Internal anal sphincter

Puborectalis (levator ani)

Deep part

Superficial part

Subcutaneous part

External anal sphincter

Pectinate line

Fig. 7.25 Anal sphincter apparatus in men; median section; view from the left side. [L238]

The pectinate line is the developmental border between the hindgut and the proctodeum and marks the border between the columnar zone and the anal pecten in the adult. The pectinate line marks the watershed for neurovascular structures and serves as clinically important landmark in the anal canal. The continence organ of the anal canal comprises the anus, sphincter muscles, and the corpus cavernosum of rectum. In resting condition, the anus is closed by the constant tonus of the internal anal sphincter. The corpus cavernosum of rectum is supplied by the superior rectal (hemorrhoidal) artery and it warrants a gas-tight closure of the anal canal.

Anal Sphincters	Innervation	Function
Puborectalis as part of levator ani (puborectalis sling)	Pudendal nerve (S2–S4); branches of sacral plexus	**Constant tonus** maintains the perineal flexure of the rectum and the anorectal angle
External anal sphincter (deep/superficial/subcutaneous parts)	Pudendal nerve (S2–S4)	Conscious activation for enforced closure of the anal canal
Internal anal sphincter: circular smooth muscle with a longitudinal part (corrugator ani)	Sympathetic lumbar splanchnic nerves (T12–L2) via hypogastric plexus	**Constant high tonus** mediates closure of the anal canal; relaxation enables defecation

Structure/Function

The **anal sphincter muscles** comprise:
- **Internal anal sphincter** (smooth muscle, involuntary sympathetic innervation): continuation of the circular muscular layer
- **Corrugator ani** (smooth muscle): continuation of the longitudinal muscular layer
- **External anal sphincter** (striated muscle, voluntary control via the pudendal nerve): has different segments (subcutaneous, superficial, deep parts)

- **Puborectalis** (striated muscle, voluntary control via direct branches of the sacral plexus and some contribution by the pudendal nerve): part of the levator ani; loops behind the rectum creating the perineal flexure. Essential to maintain the anorectal angle and for the storage of feces in the rectal ampulla.

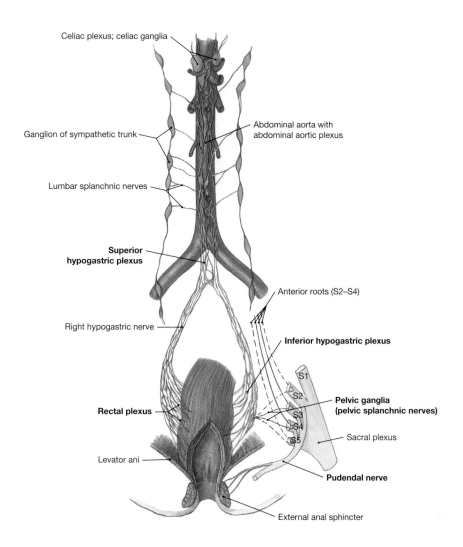

Celiac plexus; celiac ganglia

Ganglion of sympathetic trunk

Abdominal aorta with
abdominal aortic plexus

Lumbar splanchnic nerves

**Superior
hypogastric plexus**

Anterior roots (S2–S4)

Right hypogastric nerve

Inferior hypogastric plexus

S1

S2

**Pelvic ganglia
(pelvic splanchnic nerves)**

Rectal plexus

S3

S4

S5

Sacral plexus

Levator ani

Pudendal nerve

External anal sphincter

Fig. 7.26 Innervation of rectum and anal canal; schematic drawing; anterior view.

The rectal plexus continues from the inferior hypogastric plexus and contains sympathetic (green) and parasympathetic (purple) nerve fibers (➤ Fig. 12.68).

Preganglionic **sympathetic fibers** (T10–L2) descend via the lumbar splanchnic nerves and the superior hypogastric plexus and from the sacral ganglia of the sympathetic trunk via the sacral splanchnic nerves. They are synapsed mostly in the inferior hypogastric plexus. Postganglionic fibers reach the rectum and anal canal via the rectal plexus. Sympathetic fibers activate the internal anal sphincter.

Preganglionic **parasympathetic fibers** derive from the sacral division of the parasympathetic nervous system (S2–S4) and reach the ganglia of the inferior hypogastric plexus via pelvic splanchnic nerves. They are synapsed to postganglionic fibers either here or in the vicinity of the intestines for the stimulation of peristalsis and the relaxation of the internal anal sphincter to facilitate defecation. Visceral afferent fibers travel with the parasympathetic fibers to the sensory ganglia of the sacral spinal cord.

Inferior to the **pectinate line** sensory innervation of the mucosa and skin of the anal canal is conveyed by the somatic **pudendal nerve** (S2–S4). Thus, **anal lesions** inferior to the pectinate line are extremely painful. In addition, the pudendal nerve conveys motor fibers to the external anal sphincter and, in part, to the puborectalis and thus, facilitates voluntary closure of the anus.

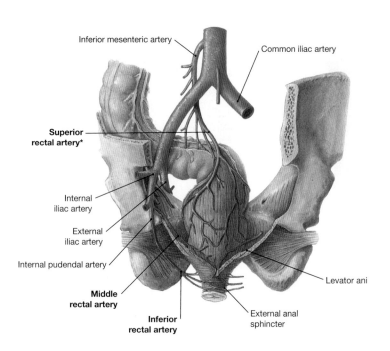

Inferior mesenteric artery

Common iliac artery

Superior rectal artery*

Internal iliac artery

External iliac artery

Internal pudendal artery

Levator ani

Middle rectal artery

Inferior rectal artery

External anal sphincter

Fig. 7.27 Rectal arteries; posterior view.
Rectum and anal canal are supplied by three arteries:

- **Superior rectal (hemorrhoidal) artery** (unpaired): from the inferior mesenteric artery
- **Middle rectal artery** (paired): from the internal iliac artery above the pelvic floor (weak and inconsistent)
- **Inferior rectal artery** (paired): from the internal pudendal artery beneath the pelvic floor

The pectinate line marks the border between the arterial supply from the inferior mesenteric artery and the internal iliac artery. There are numerous anastomoses between these arteries. Distal from its anastomosis with the sigmoid arteries (clinical term: SUDECK's point) the superior rectal artery is considered a terminal artery.

* clin. term: superior hemorrhoidal artery

Fig. 7.28 Venous drainage of rectum and anal canal; anterior view. Tributaries to the hepatic portal vein (purple) and to the inferior vena cava (blue).

- **Superior rectal vein** (unpaired): access to the hepatic portal vein via the inferior mesenteric vein
- **Middle rectal vein** (paired): access to the inferior vena cava via the internal iliac vein
- **Inferior rectal vein** (paired): access to the inferior vena cava via the internal pudendal and the internal iliac veins

The pectinate line marks the watershed between the venous drainage to the hepatic portal vein and the inferior vena cava. This illustration demonstrates the venous anastomoses between the drainage pathways to the portal vein and to the inferior vena cava. With increased blood pressure in the portal system (portal hypertension) these **portocaval anastomoses** are utilized for the drainage of blood to the inferior vena cava.

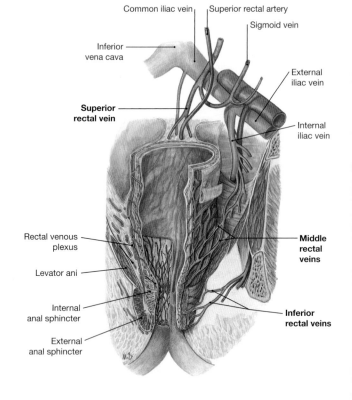

Common iliac vein

Superior rectal artery

Sigmoid vein

Inferior vena cava

External iliac vein

Superior rectal vein

Internal iliac vein

Rectal venous plexus

Levator ani

Internal anal sphincter

External anal sphincter

Middle rectal veins

Inferior rectal veins

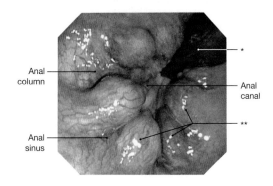

Anal column

Anal canal

Anal sinus

*

**

Fig. 7.29 Anal canal, rectoscopy; superior view. [T901]
Dilations of the corpus cavernosum of rectum are referred to as superior (or internal) **hemorrhoids.** Six substantially enlarged knots are visible.

*   coloscope
** three hemorrhoidal knots

Clinical Remarks

The corpus cavernosum of rectum is primarily supplied by the superior rectal artery. Therefore, bleedings of hemorrhoids, which represent dilated rectal cavernous bodies, are arterial bleedings as shown by the bright red color.

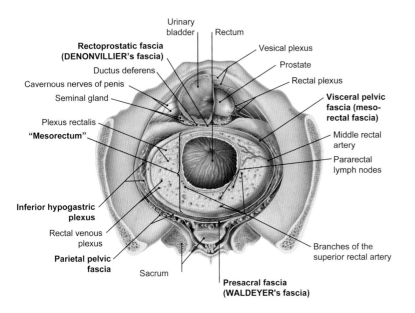

Urinary bladder

Rectum

Rectoprostatic fascia (DENONVILLIER's fascia)

Vesical plexus

Ductus deferens

Prostate

Cavernous nerves of penis

Rectal plexus

Seminal gland

Visceral pelvic fascia (meso-rectal fascia)

Plexus rectalis

"**Mesorectum**"

Middle rectal artery

Pararectal lymph nodes

Inferior hypogastric plexus

Rectal venous plexus

Parietal pelvic fascia

Sacrum

Branches of the superior rectal artery

Presacral fascia (WALDEYER's fascia)

Fig. 7.30 Mesorectum, transverse section; schematic drawing; superior view. [L238]
The **mesorectal fascia** forms a sleeve around the rectum below the peritoneal reflection. It separates the rectum from the seminal vesicles and prostate gland (men) or from the uterine cervix and posterior vaginal fornix (women). The **mesorectum** comprises the rectal wall, the perirectal adipose tissue with pararectal lymph nodes and the mesorectal fascia.

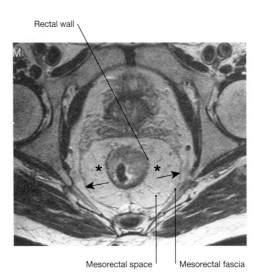

Rectal wall

Mesorectal space

Mesorectal fascia

Fig. 7.31 T2 weighted turbo-spin echo MRI. [E393]
The mesorectal fascia is shown with black arrows. Asterisks mark the mesorectal space between the rectal wall and the mesorectal fascia.

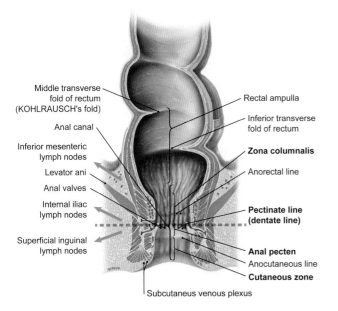

Middle transverse fold of rectum (KOHLRAUSCH's fold)

Rectal ampulla

Inferior transverse fold of rectum

Anal canal

Zona columnalis

Inferior mesenteric lymph nodes

Anorectal line

Levator ani

Anal valves

Pectinate line (dentate line)

Internal iliac lymph nodes

Superficial inguinal lymph nodes

Anal pecten

Anocutaneous line

Cutaneous zone

Subcutaneus venous plexus

Fig. 7.32 Rectum and anal canal; schematic coronal section of the rectum and anal canal. [L238]
Lymphatic and venous drainage of the rectum and anal canal.

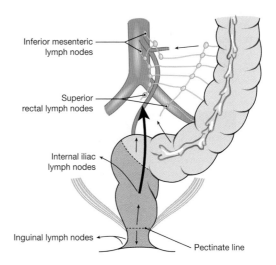

Inferior mesenteric lymph nodes

Superior rectal lymph nodes

Internal iliac lymph nodes

Inguinal lymph nodes

Pectinate line

Fig. 7.33 Lymphatic drainage of the rectum; schematic drawing. [L126]
The main lymphatic drainage of the supralevator part of the rectum is to the inferior mesenteric lymph nodes.

Clinical Remarks

Knowledge of lymphatic drainage pathways in the anorectal region is essential in cases of cancer in the anorectal region. **Total mesorectal excision** (TME) for rectal cancer removes pararectal lymph nodes within the mesorectum and spares the inferior hypogastric plexus and the presacral venous plexus located outside of the mesorectal fascia. The **pectinate line** inferior to the anal sinuses marks the border between the embryological hindgut (superior part of the anal canal) and the proctodeum (inferior part of the anal canal). Anal carcinoma proximal to the pectinate line metastasise to the pelvic nodes, distal carcinomas spread first to the inguinal nodes. Anal malignancies are staged according to their proximity to the anocutaneous line.

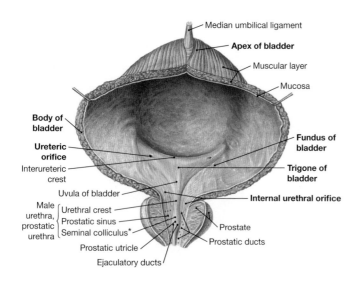

Fig. 7.34 Urinary bladder and opening into the male urethra.

The urinary bladder is located below the peritoneum and comprises a body with apex and fundus. At the fundus, the internal urethral orifice and the two ureteric openings form the **trigone** of bladder. The urinary bladder holds about 500–1,500 ml (17–51 fl oz) of urine. The wall consists of the internal mucosal layer (Tunica mucosa) followed by three layers of smooth muscle fibres (Tunica muscularis = detrusor muscle), and the outer adventitial layer (Tunica adventitia) or the cranial serosa (peritoneum), respectively. The median umbilical ligament connects the apex to the umbilicus. In women the bilateral pubovesical ligaments and in men the bilateral puboprostatic ligaments anchor the bladder to the bony pelvis.

* clin. term: verumontanum

Fig. 7.35 Sphincter mechanisms of the male urinary bladder and urethra; median section; view from the left side.
Sphincter mechanisms for urinary bladder and urethra:

- **Internal urethral sphincter:** smooth muscle fibers of the circular muscle layer of the urethra; sympathetic innervation; prevents retrograde ejaculation in men.
- **External urethral sphincter:** in men a separation of the deep transverse perineal muscle, in woman single striated muscle fibers surrounding the urethra; innervated by the pudendal nerve. (➤ Fig. 7.43)

In addition, the **pelvic floor** (pelvic diaphragm) is important in supporting the urinary bladder, maintaining the vesicourethral angle and thus ensuring urinary continence. During micturition the smooth muscles of the wall of the bladder (detrusor) contract following parasympathetic activation. At the same time, the striated muscles of the pelvic floor relax allowing the bladder to descend, the urethral sphincters to relax, and urination to occur.

* smooth muscles of the urethra

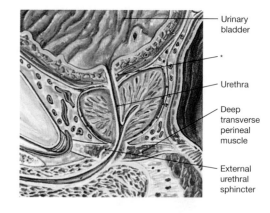

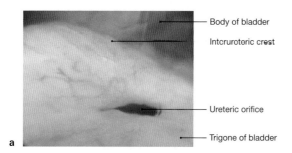

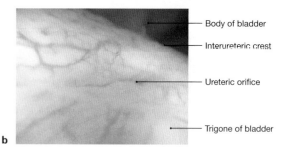

Fig. 7.36a and b Ureteric orifice; cystoscopy. [T898]
a Opened ureteric orifice, a peristaltic wave has released urine into the bladder;
b Closed ureteric orifice.

The valve-like ureteric orifice contributes substantially to the prevention of urine reflux which may endanger the kidneys via ascending urinary tract infections.

Clinical Remarks

The internal openings of the ureters are usually closed. Contraction of the detrusor muscle for micturition firmly closes the ureteric openings to prevent reflux of urine into the ureters. Extreme dilation of the bladder wall compromises the ureteric closure mechanisms frequently causing a reflux of urine.

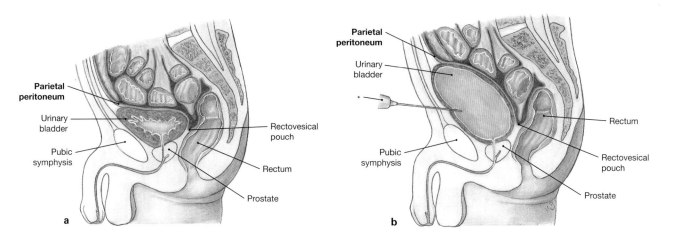

a

b

Fig. 7.37a and b Urinary bladder, empty (a) and filled (b); schematic median section; view from the left side.
The urinary bladder is located subperitoneal, surrounded by paravesical adipose tissue including the anterior **space of RETZIUS** (ret-

ropubic space) and is covered by parietal peritoneum on its upper surface. When filled with urine, the bladder rises above the pubic symphysis **(b)**.
* puncture needle for suprapubic transcutaneous access

Clinical Remarks

Suprapubic cystostomy: The empty bladder is positioned behind the pubic symphysis. Filled with urine, the bladder rises up to 10 cm (3.9 in) above the pubic symphysis pushing its peritoneal lining cranially towards the umbilicus. The bladder is then

adjacent to the abdominal wall and can be accessed without opening the peritoneal cavity (suprapubic cystostomy) for cystoscopy or insertion of a suprapubic catheter.

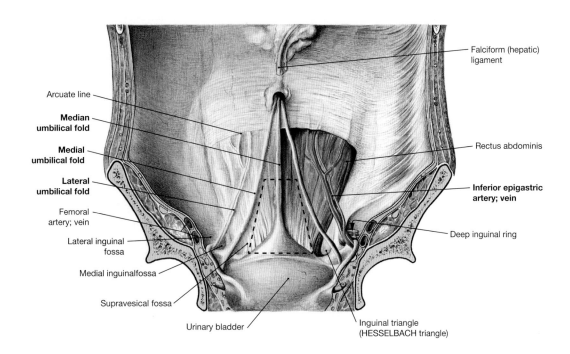

Fig. 7.38 Ventral abdominal wall; inside view.
The dotted line marks the area of the ventral abdominal wall through which the bladder can be accessed. This area above the pubic symphysis along the median umbilical ligament is devoid of

major vessels (note the distance to the inferior epigastric artery and vein) or nerves. It can be penetrated for suprapubic access to the urinary bladder when the bladder is filled.

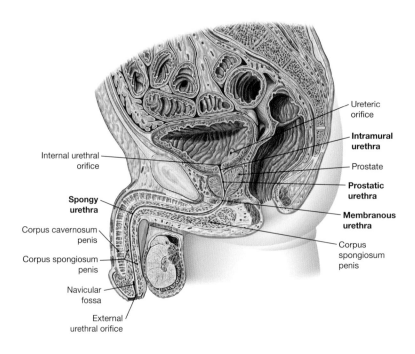

Fig. 7.39 Male pelvis, median section; view from the left side.
The illustration shows the course and the parts of the male urethra:
intramural, prostatic, membranous and **spongy urethra.**

The urethra has two bends:
*   at the transition from the membranous to the spongy urethra
*   in the middle part of the spongy urethra

Fig. 7.40 Urinary bladder and male urethra; anterior view; urinary bladder and urethra opened ventrally.
Parts of the urethra:
*   **Intramural urethra** (1 cm, 0.4 in): within the wall of the urinary bladder
*   **Prostatic urethra** (3.5 cm, 1.4 in): traverses the prostate. Here the following ducts enter the urethra: ejaculatory ducts (common duct of vas deferens and seminal vesicle) on the seminal colliculus and the prostatic ducts on both sides.
*   **Membranous urethra** (1–2 cm, 0.4–0.8 in): traverses the pelvic floor.
*   **Spongy urethra** (15 cm, 5.9 in): embedded in the corpus spongiosum penis, continues to the external urethral orifice. COWPER's glands (bulbourethral glands) and LITTRÉ's glands (urethral glands) enter here. The terminal part is dilated to form the navicular fossa.
The urethra has the following constrictions:
*   Internal urethral orifice
*   Membranous urethra
*   External urethral orifice

* clin. term: verumontanum

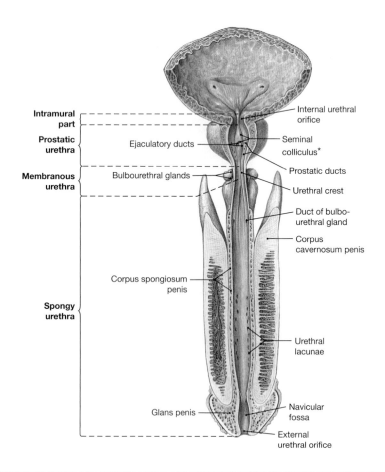

Clinical Remarks

The most common injury of the male urethra during transurethral catheterization occurs in the membranous part. The bends of the urethra have to be straight prior to inserting a catheter to avoid painful perforations of the membranous urethra or the prostatic urethra with consecutive profuse bleedings or extravasation of urine. The seminal colliculus (verumontanum) serves as anatomical landmark for the urinary sphincter during **transurethral resection of the prostate** (TURP) in cases of benign prostatic hypertrophy.

Fig. 7.41 Female pelvis and female urethra; median section; view from the left side.
The illustration shows the course and the external orifice of the female urethra. The female urethra is 3–5 cm (1.2–2.0 in) long and enters the vestibule of vagina directly in front of the vagina. Urethrovaginal connective tissue, a part of the endopelvic fascia, adheres the anterior wall of the vagina to the posterior wall of the female urethra.

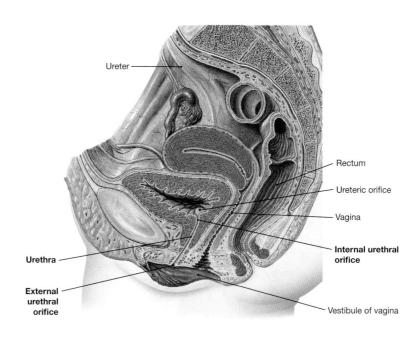

Ureter

Rectum

Ureteric orifice

Vagina

Internal urethral orifice

Urethra

External urethral orifice

Vestibule of vagina

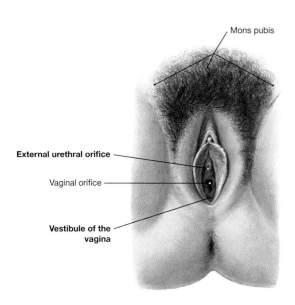

Mons pubis

External urethral orifice

Vaginal orifice

Vestibule of the vagina

Fig. 7.42 Female urethra, external orifice; inferior view.
The illustration shows the external orifice of the female urethra located anterior to the vaginal orifice within the vestibule of vagina. The vestibule is bordered by the labia minora.

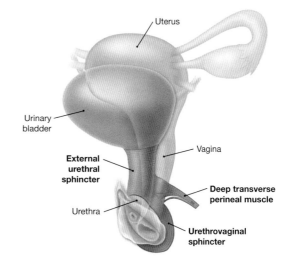

Uterus

Urinary bladder

Vagina

External urethral sphincter

Deep transverse perineal muscle

Urethra

Urethrovaginal sphincter

Fig. 7.43 Voluntary sphincter muscles of the urinary bladder (female). [L238]
The deep transverse perineal muscle in women does not form a continuous muscular plate. Instead, individual striated muscle fibers around the urethra form the **external urethral sphincter** which constitutes the voluntary sphincter of the urinary bladder. Some muscle fibers continue to surround the distal vagina and are referred to as **urethrovaginal sphincter.** These external urethral sphincters are innervated by the **pudendal nerve.**

Clinical Remarks

Because of the shorter length of the female urethra, ascending infections of the urinary bladder **(cystitis)** are more common in women than in men. Positioning of a **transurethral catheter** is easier in women due to the straight course of the shorter urethra. The urethral orifice in the vestibule is located **ventral** to the vagina.

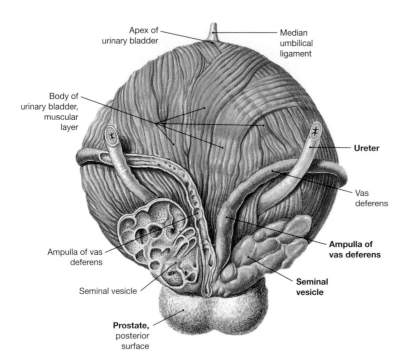

Fig. 7.44 Urinary bladder, vas deferens, seminal vesicle, and prostate; posterior view.
In men, the following paired anatomical structures are positioned posterior and adjacent to the bladder, from medial to lateral:
- dilated part (ampulla) of the vas deferens
- seminal vesicle
- ureter

The urinary bladder is positioned directly superior to the prostate. The terminal part of the vas deferens combines with the excretory duct of the seminal vesicle to form the ejaculatory duct, which enters the prostatic urethra of the male.

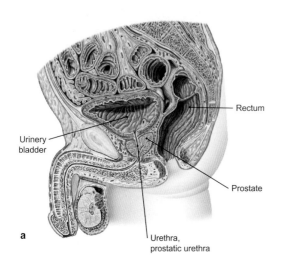

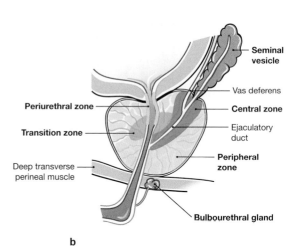

Fig. 7.45a and b   Position of prostata gland (a) and schematic drawing of male accessory sex glands (b); median section; view from the left side. b [L126]
The accessory sex glands consist of:
- **Prostate:** unpaired gland beneath the base of the bladder. The prostate measures 4 × 3 × 2 cm / 1.6 × 1.2 × 0.8 in (20 g) and has a superior base and an inferior apex. The prostate discharges its secretions into the centrally traversing prostatic urethra.
- **Seminal vesicle** (seminal gland): paired gland at the dorsal aspect of the urinary bladder (➤ Fig. 7.44). The seminal vesicles are elongated oval glands (5 × 1 × 1 cm / 2.0 × 0.4 × 0.4 in). Their excretory ducts combine with the vas deferens to form the ejaculatory duct and enter the prostatic urethra.
- **COWPER's gland** (bulbourethral gland): paired gland located within the perineal muscles (➤ Fig. 7.40). The excretory ducts of the lentil-sized COWPER's glands enter the spongy urethra.

The prostate has three clinically important zones:
- **Peripheral zone:** 70% of the gland, mostly the posterior aspect of the gland
- **Central zone:** 20% of the gland adjacent to the transition zone, between the ejaculatory ducts
- **Transition zone:** 10% of the gland; surrounding the prostatic urethra

The **periurethral zone** contains submucosal glands to the urethra. Seminal vesicles and prostate produce the liquid component of the ejaculate which nurtures the spermatozoa. The viscous alkaline secretions of the COWPER's glands enter the urethra prior to ejaculation and function in lubrication and neutralization of the acidic urine in the urethra.

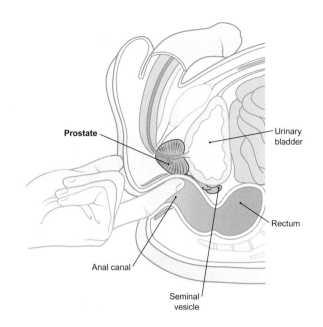

Prostate

Urinary bladder

Rectum

Anal canal

Seminal vesicle

Fig. 7.46 Palpation of the prostate: digital rectal examination (DRE); schematic sagittal section. [L126]
The prostate is separated from the rectum only by the thin rectoprostatic fascia (DENONVILLIERS' fascia) and can be palpated from the rectal ampulla.

Clinical Remarks

Prostate carcinoma is one of the three most common malignant tumors in men. It usually develops from the histologically distinct peripheral zone of the gland and may be palpated through the rectal wall. Therefore, symptoms related to micturition are only found with advanced stages. Due to the fact that the prostate is separated from the rectum only by the thin rectoprostatic fascia (DENONVILLIERS' fascia; ➤ Fig. 7.46) prostate carcinomas may be palpable through the rectum. The digital rectal ex-

amination (DRE) is therefore part of a complete physical examination in men over 50 years of age.
The **benign prostatic hyperplasia (BPH)** is a benign tumor of the prostate. BPH is a condition usually present in various degrees in all men over 70 years of age. Since BPH develops from the transition zone of the gland, constriction of the urethra and resulting micturition difficulties are early signs of this condition.

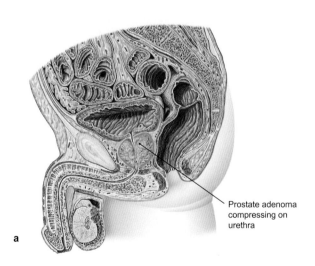

a

Prostate adenoma compressing on urethra

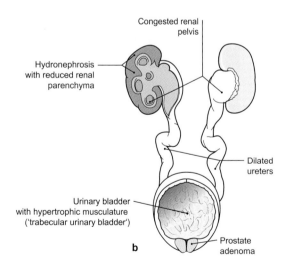

Congested renal pelvis

Hydronephrosis with reduced renal parenchyma

Dilated ureters

Urinary bladder with hypertrophic musculature ('trabecular urinary bladder')

Prostate adenoma

b

Fig. 7.47a and b Prostate enlargement and clinical consequences; schematic sagittal section. b [L126]
Benign prostatic hyperplasia **(a)** and clinical scenario with dilated urinary bladder, bilaterally dilated ureters and bilateral hydronephrosis **(b)**. The benign prostatic hyperplasia originates in the transition zone of the prostate (➤ Fig. 7.45) and causes a compression of the prostatic urethra and a functional constriction of the internal

urethral orifice upon detrusor contraction. Long-term, this condition leads to hypertrophy of the detrusor muscle with a trabeculated bladder wall and to increasing amounts of residual urine in the bladder which causes insufficient closure of the ureteric orifices and reflux of urine into the ureters and renal pelvis (hydronephrosis).

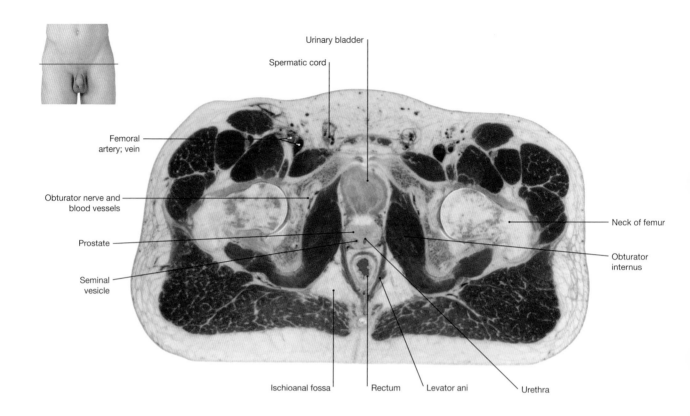

Fig. 7.48 **Cross-sectional anatomy of the male pelvis;** transverse section at the level of the head of femur. [X338]

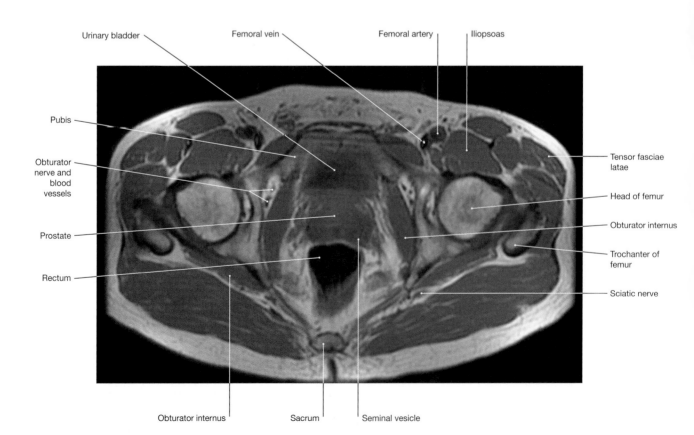

Fig. 7.49 **T2w MRI of the male pelvis;** transverse section at the level of the head of the femur. [G744]

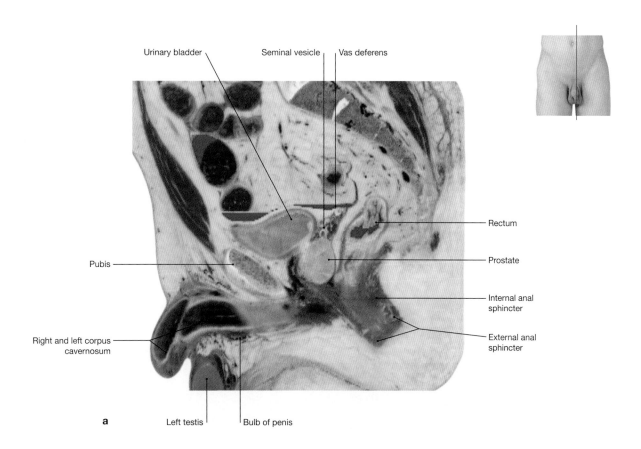

Urinary bladder   Seminal vesicle   Vas deferens

Pubis

Right and left corpus
cavernosum

Rectum

Prostate

Internal anal
sphincter

External anal
sphincter

a   Left testis   Bulb of penis

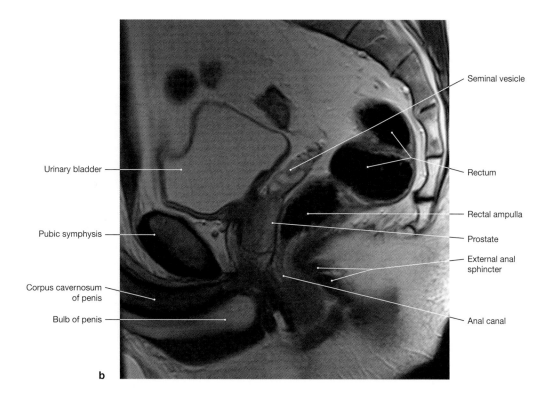

Urinary bladder

Pubic symphysis

Corpus cavernosum
of penis

Bulb of penis

Seminal vesicle

Rectum

Rectal ampulla

Prostate

External anal
sphincter

Anal canal

b

Fig. 7.50a and b Male pelvis; parasagittal section. a [X338], b [T975]
a Cross-sectional anatomy of the male pelvis; left parasagittal
plane through the seminal vesicle.

b Parasagittal T2w MRI of the male pelvis. The seminal vesicle is
shown behind the urinary bladder.

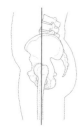

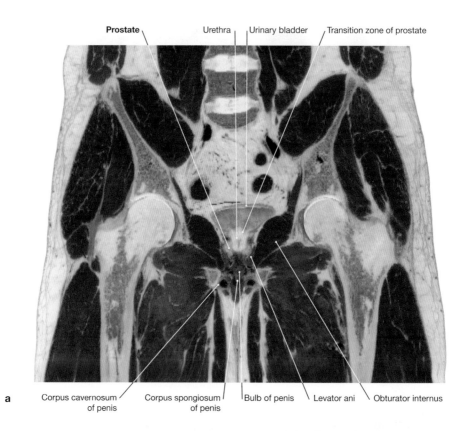

Prostate | Urethra | Urinary bladder | Transition zone of prostate

a

Corpus cavernosum of penis | Corpus spongiosum of penis | Bulb of penis | Levator ani | Obturator internus

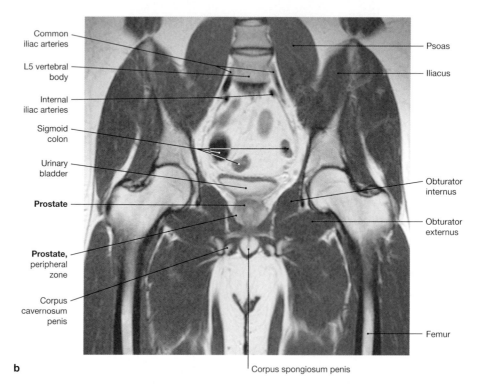

Common iliac arteries

L5 vertebral body

Internal iliac arteries

Sigmoid colon

Urinary bladder

Prostate

Prostate, peripheral zone

Corpus cavernosum penis

Psoas

Iliacus

Obturator internus

Obturator externus

Femur

b

Corpus spongiosum penis

Fig. 7.51a and b Male plevis, coronal plane. a [X338], b [G745]
a Cross-sectional anatomy; coronal section through the anterior prostate.

b Coronal T2w MRI of the male pelvis. The position of the prostate inferior to the neck of the bladder is shown.

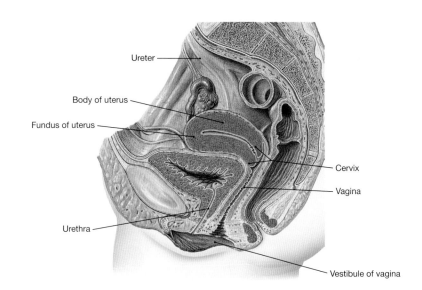

Fig. 7.52 Position of the uterus in the female pelvis; median section.
The uterus is positioned above the empty urinary bladder and its fundus points anteriorly towards the abdominal wall. Fundus and corpus are lined with peritoneum (intraperitoneal), the cervix is located below the peritoneal lining (infraperitoneal). The axes of urethra and vagina are parallel and the anterior wall of the vagina is adherent to the posterior wall of the urethra.

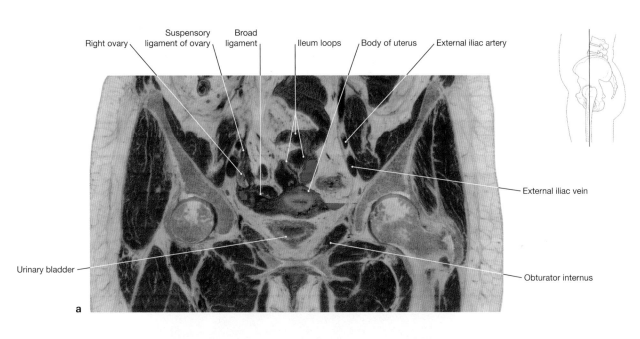

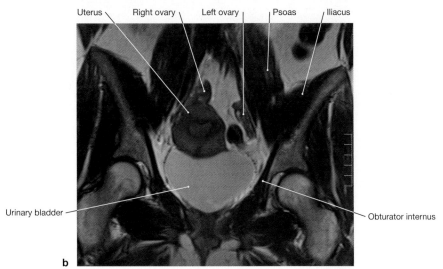

Fig. 7.53a and b Female pelvis, coronal plane at the level of the hip joint. **a** Cross-sectional anatomy; **b** coronal T2w MRI. a [X338], b [T975]

The body of uterus is positioned above the urinary bladder and the ovaries are visible.

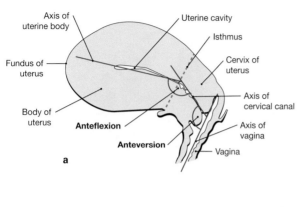

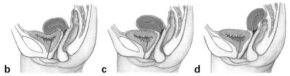

Fig. 7.54a to d Position of uterus and vagina; view from the right side.
a Normally, the uterus has an anteverted and anteflexed position. Anteversion: angle between the axis of the vagina and the axis of the cervix. Anteflexion: angle between the axis of the cervix and the axis of the body of uterus. This position prevents a prolapse of the uterus through the vagina during increased intra-abdominal pressure (coughing, sneezing).
b Anteversion, anteflexion = normal position
c Anteversion, lack of anteflexion
d Retroversion, retroflexion

Clinical Remarks

In cases of retroflexion and/or retroversion of the uterus, the weight of the body of uterus is pushing down towards the vagina with increased intra-abdominal pressure. A retroverted uterus is therefore more likely to **prolapse** through the vagina, especially in cases with **pelvic floor insufficiency.** As a consequence, a lowering (**descensus**) or prolapse of uterus and vagina may occur. The level of uterine decent determines the staging of the prolapse: first **(a),** second **(b)** or third **(c)** degree prolapse. This condition is often combined with a prolapse of the bladder (**cystocele**) and the rectum **(rectocele)** resulting in urinary and fecal incontinence.
[G302]

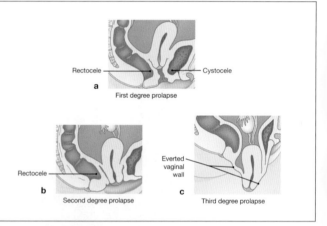

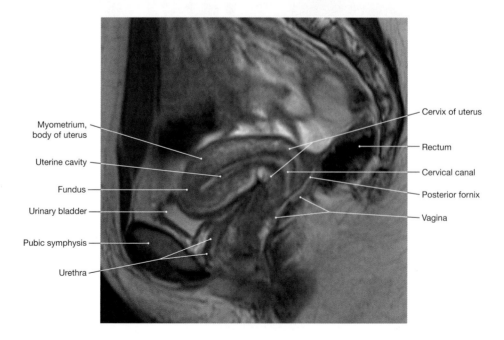

Fig. 7.55 T2w MRI of female pelvis; sagittal section; view from the right side. [T975]
Note the anteversion and anteflexion of the uterus. The fundus and body of uterus rest on the empty urinary bladder. The posterior for-nix of the vagina reaches behind the cervix and is adjacent to the anterior wall of the rectum.

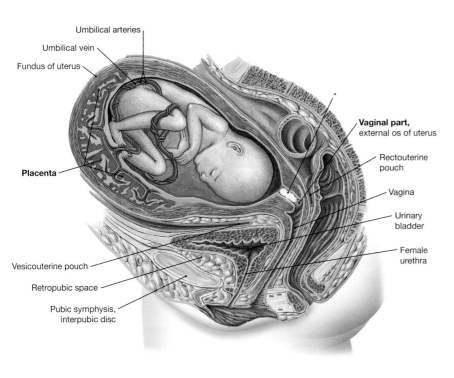

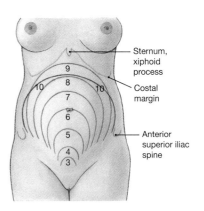

Fig. 7.57 Level of the fundus of uterus during pregnancy; anterior view.

The numbers represent the end of the respective month of pregnancy. In the 6th month (week 24) the fundus of uterus is at the level of the umbilical region, in the 9th month (week 36) at the costal margin. Up to parturition, the volume of uterus increases 800–1,200 times and its weight increases from 30–120 g (1–4.2 oz) to 1,000–1,500 g (35–53 oz).

Fig. 7.56 Uterus with placenta and fetus; median section of the pelvis except for the fetus; view from the left side.

The developing child in the uterus is nourished via the placenta which develops from maternal and fetal tissues after implantation. The cervix of uterus is closed during pregnancy by the mucous plug of KRISTELLER (*).

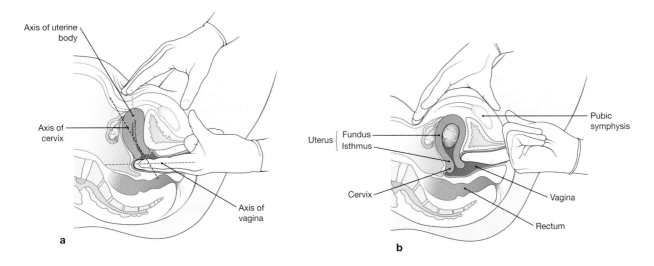

Fig. 7.58a and b Manual palpation of the uterus; schematic sagittal section. [L126]

a Bimanual palpation to assess the size and position of the uterus;

b Palpation to assess the softening of the isthmus of the uterus during pregnancy.

Clinical Remarks

Bimanual palpation allows to assess the size and position of the uterus. The examiner inserts two fingers of one hand into the posterior fornix of vagina to push the cervix anteriorly. The other hand (> Fig. 7.58a) presses on the pubic region to palpate the fundus of uterus. Palpation of the cervix from the anterior fornix of vagina may reveal softening of the isthmus of uterus during early pregnancy (**HEGAR's sign;** > Fig. 7.58b).

The vagina is remarkably distensible. This allows the manual palpation of bony landmarks such as the promontory of sacrum for the assessment of the diagonal conjugate (> Fig. 7.58) and the ischial spine for a pudendal nerve block (> Fig. 7.108). Substantial **vaginal distension** occurs during parturition.

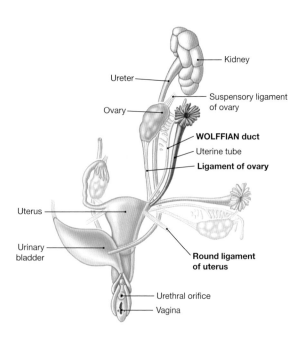

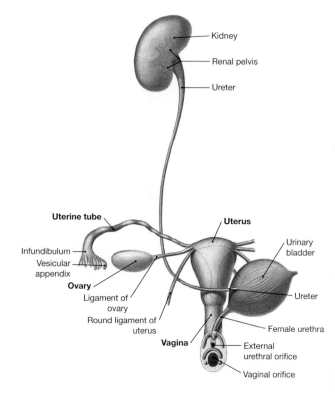

Fig. 7.59 Development of the internal female genitalia. [L126]
The internal genitalia develop identically in both sexes up to week 7 (sexual indifferent stage). In the female, the primordial gonad then develops into the ovary in the lumbar region at the level of the mesonephros. The ovary is then relocated caudally to the lesser pelvis without leaving the peritoneal cavity. Thus, ovary and uterine tube have an **intraperitoneal** position.

Without the suppressing effects of the anti-MÜLLERIAN hormone from the testis, the MÜLLERIAN **(paramesonephric)** ducts differentiate into female genitalia. Beginning in week 12, the **MÜLLERIAN ducts** form the uterine tube. Their distal portions merge to form the uterus and the upper vagina. The lower vagina develops from the urogenital sinus. The **ligament of ovary** and **round ligament** of uterus are remnants of the gubernaculum, a fibromuscular cord which in males guides the testis into the scrotum.

Fig. 7.60 Female urinary and genital organs; ventral view.
The internal genitalia comprise:
• Vagina
• Uterus
• Uterine tube
• Ovary
Uterine tube and ovary are paired organs and are collectively referred to as uterine adnexa.

Structure/Function

The internal genitalia in women are reproductive and sex organs. Functionally, the ovary serves as a maturation site for follicles (and ova) and as a production site of female sex hormones (estrogens and progesterone). The uterine tube provides the place for fertilization of ova and transports the zygote to the uterus where the embryo/fetus develops and grows during pregnancy. The vagina serves the sexual intercourse and is part of the birth canal.

Clinical Remarks

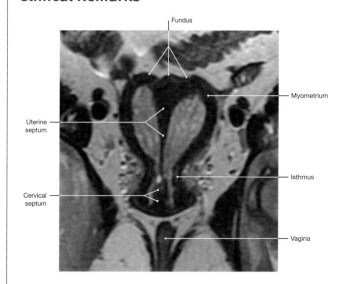

Coronal T2 weighted MRI; ventral view.
The image demonstrates a completely septate uterus with a relatively flat fundus; the septum divides the uterine cavity and cervix. If the MÜLLERIAN ducts fail to fuse, a septate (uterus septus or subseptus) or a double uterus (uterus duplex, uterus didelphys) may result.
[T975]

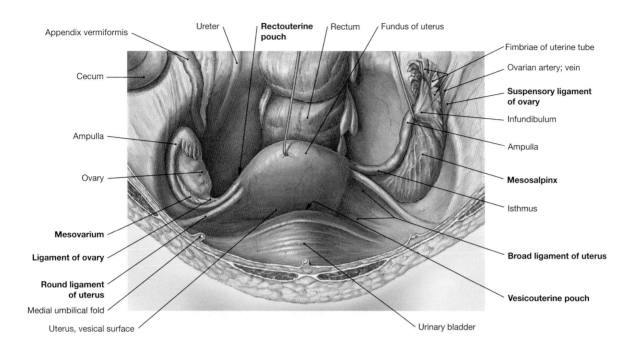

Fig. 7.61 Uterus, ovary, and uterine tube, with peritoneal duplicatures; anterior view.
Uterus, uterine tubes, and ovaries have an intraperitoneal position. Their peritoneal ligaments are duplicatures of peritoneum (broad ligament of uterus, mesosalpinx, mesovarium) which form a transverse fold in the lesser pelvis. The round ligament of uterus

reaches ventral from the uterotubal junction to the lateral wall of the lesser pelvis and traverses the inguinal canal to merge with the connective tissue of the labia majora. The ligament of ovary connects uterus and ovary. The suspensory ligament of ovary (clin. **infundibulopelvic ligament**) connects ovary and lateral pelvic wall and contains the ovarian artery and vein and lymphatics.

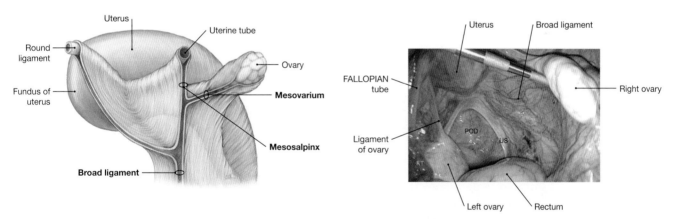

Fig. 7.62 Mesovarium and mesosalpinx; schematic parasagittal section through the broad ligament of uterus. [L285]
Mesovarium and mesosalpinx are peritoneal duplicatures that are continuous with the broad ligament and envelope the neurovascular structures to the uterine tube (FALLOPIAN tube) and the ovary.

Fig. 7.63 Laparoscopic view of the female peritoneal pelvic cavity in a woman of reproductive age. [G746]
The probe pushes the uterus anteriorly; the rectouterine pouch (pouch of DOUGLAS, POD) and the posterior aspect of the body of uterus are visible. The attachment of the ovaries to the posterolateral abdominal wall by the suspensory (infundibulopelvic) ligament causes the posterior orientation of the FALLOPIAN tubes and ovaries. The uterosacral peritoneal folds (US) result from the uterosacral ligament of the pelvic fascia.

Clinical Remarks

The close topographical relationship between the adnexa (ovary and uterine tube) and the appendix vermiformis of the colon explains why inflammations of the appendix **(appendicitis)** as well as those of the uterine tube **(salpingitis)** may cause similar pain in the right lower abdominal quadrant. The adnexa are always

oriented posteriorly due to their peritoneal attachment (infundibulopelvic ligament) to the posterior abdominal wall. This posterior attachment serves as orientation for laparoscopic images (➤ Fig. 7.63).

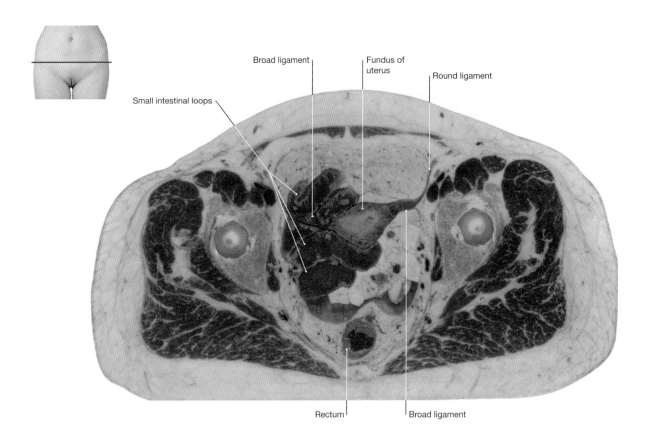

Fig. 7.64 Cross-sectional anatomy of the female pelvis; just above the hip joint. [X338]

The fundus of uterus and the broad ligament are visible. Small intestinal loops are positioned anterior and posterior to the uterus demonstrating its intraperitoneal position.

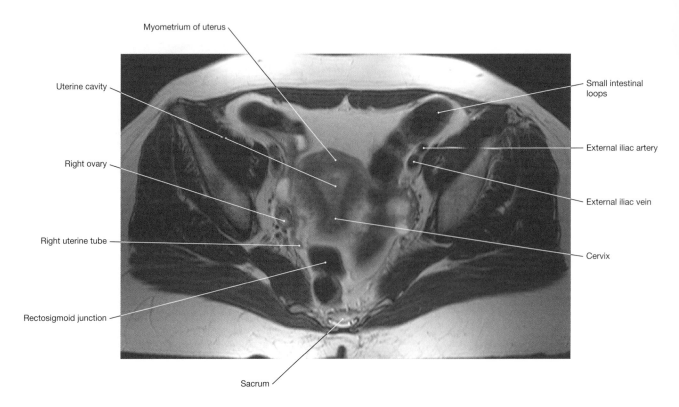

Fig. 7.65 T2w MRI of the female pelvis; transverse section (just above the hip joint). [G744]

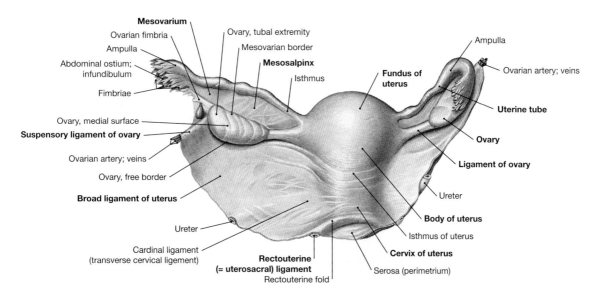

Mesovarium
Ovarian fimbria
Ampulla
Abdominal ostium;
infundibulum
Fimbriae
Ovary, medial surface
Suspensory ligament of ovary
Ovarian artery; veins
Ovary, free border
Broad ligament of uterus
Ureter
Cardinal ligament
(transverse cervical ligement)

Ovary, tubal extremity
Mesovarian border
Mesosalpinx
Isthmus

**Rectouterine
(= uterosacral) ligament**
Rectouterine fold

Ampulla
Ovarian artery; veins
**Fundus of
uterus**
Uterine tube
Ovary
Ligament of ovary
Ureter
Body of uterus
Isthmus of uterus
Cervix of uterus
Serosa (perimetrium)

Fig. 7.66 Uterus, ovary, and uterine tube, with peritoneal duplicatures; posterior view.

Structure/Function

Peritoneal ligaments and attachments relevant for surgical procedures:
- **Broad ligament of uterus:** frontal peritoneal fold
- **Mesovarium** and **mesosalpinx:** peritoneal duplicatures of ovary and uterine tube, respectively, connected to the broad ligament
- **Round ligament of uterus:** coursing within the broad ligament from the uterotubal junction through the inguinal canal to the labia majora; not visible in the posterior view of ➤ Fig. 7.66

- **Ligament of ovary** (ovarian ligament): the ovarian ligament connects ovary and uterus
- **Suspensory ligament of ovary** (clinical term: infundibulopelvic ligament): connects the ovary to the posterolateral pelvic wall, carries the ovarian artery and vein.

The transverse cervical ligament (cardinal ligament) and the uterosacral (rectonerine) ligament are attachments of the cervix below the peritoneal lining (➤ Fig. 7.66).

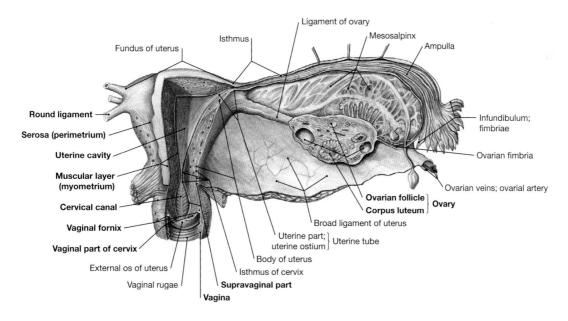

Fundus of uterus
Isthmus
Ligament of ovary
Mesosalpinx
Ampulla

Round ligament
Serosa (perimetrium)
Uterine cavity
**Muscular layer
(myometrium)**
Cervical canal
Vaginal fornix
Vaginal part of cervix
External os of uterus
Vaginal rugae
Vagina

Infundibulum;
fimbriae
Ovarian fimbria
Ovarian veins; ovarial artery
Ovarian follicle } Ovary
Corpus luteum
Broad ligament of uterus
Uterine part;
uterine ostium } Uterine tube
Body of uterus
Isthmus of cervix
Supravaginal part

Fig. 7.67 Uterus, vagina, ovary, and uterine tube, frontal section; posterior view.
The lumen of the uterus is divided into the uterine cavity in the body and the cervical canal in the cervix of uterus. The lower portion of the cervix is referred to as vaginal part of cervix, its upper portion as the supravaginal part. The vagina is a muscular hollow organ of about 10 cm (4 in) in length in a subperitoneal location. The vaginal fornix surrounds the vaginal part of cervix.

Clinical Remarks

The female genital tract communicates with the peritoneal cavity. Thus, inflammation of the FALLOPIAN tube **(salpingitis)** may occur with infections of the peritoneal cavity and vice versa.

80 % of **extrauterine (ectopic) pregnancies** occur in the ampulla of the FALLOPIAN tube and may result in rupture of the uterine tube and severe hemorrhage into the abdominopelvic cavity.

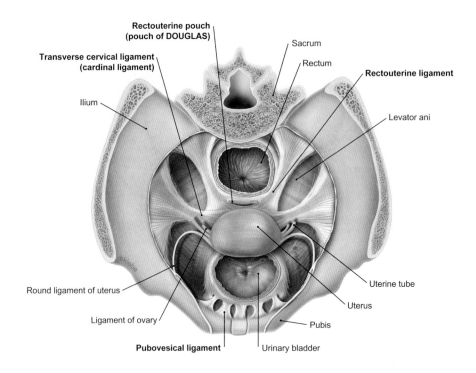

Fig. 7.68 Extraperitoneal pelvic attachments of the uterus; superior view. [L238]
Connective tissue attachments in the subperitoneal pelvic fascia stabilize the cervix and support the uterus in the pelvis:

- the cardinal (MACKENRODT) ligament (transverse cervical ligament): in lateral direction and
- the uterosacral (rectouterine) and pubovesical ligaments in anteroposterior direction.

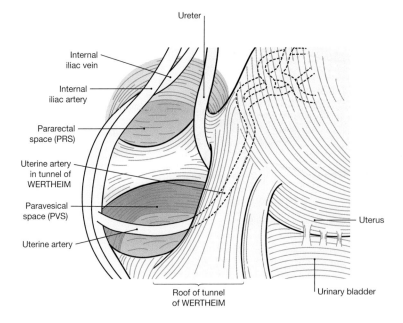

Fig. 7.69 Schematic drawing of the ureter and uterine artery in the pelvic fascia; superior view, right side. The drawing shows the ureter and the uterine artery entering the 'tunnel of WERTHEIM'. [L231]
Loose connective tissue of the pelvic fascia defines the pararectal space posterior to the cardinal ligament and the paravesical space anterior to the cardinal ligament.

Structure/Function

The tunnel of WERTHEIM presents a surgical landmark in the pelvic fascia to locate the uterine artery and the ureter in their close spatial relationship to the cervix. The tunnel of WERTHEIM is confined by the broad ligament superiorly and the cardinal ligament inferolaterally. The ureter descends over the cardinal ligament and crosses inferior to the uterine artery ('water under the bridge') at the base of the broad ligament (roof of the tunnel) to reach the urinary bladder.

Clinical Remarks

Surgical removal of the uterus **(hysterectomy)** requires its separation from peritoneal and subperitoneal attachments and ligation of the uterine artery. The uterine artery crosses the ureter anteriorly and superiorly: 'water under the bridge'. The identification of the pulsating artery and the peristaltic waves of the ureter and a careful separation of both structures in the tunnel of WERTHEIM are essential.

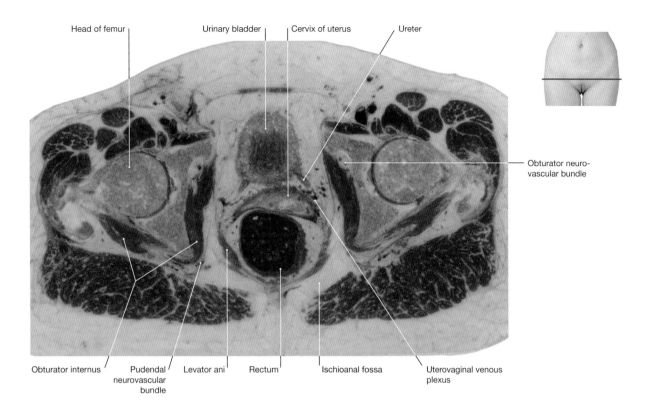

Head of femur | Urinary bladder | Cervix of uterus | Ureter

Obturator neuro-vascular bundle

Obturator internus | Pudendal neurovascular bundle | Levator ani | Rectum | Ischioanal fossa | Uterovaginal venous plexus

Fig. 7.70 Cross-section of the subperitoneal female pelvic viscera; level of the hip joint. [X338]
The subperitoneal cervix of uterus and the uterovaginal venous plexus are shown. The ureters entering the bladder from posterior are visible.

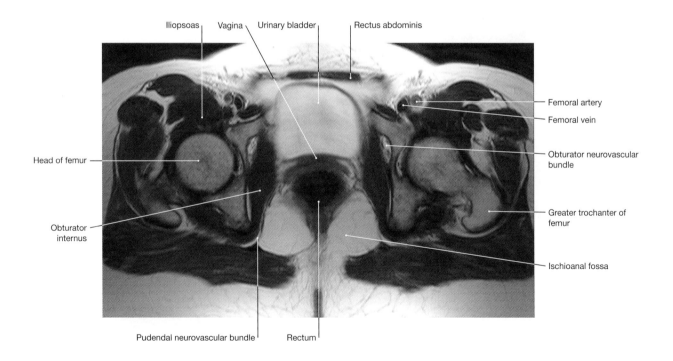

Iliopsoas | Vagina | Urinary bladder | Rectus abdominis

Femoral artery
Femoral vein

Head of femur

Obturator neurovascular bundle

Obturator internus

Greater trochanter of femur

Ischioanal fossa

Pudendal neurovascular bundle | Rectum

Fig. 7.71 T2w MRI of the female pelvis; transverse section at the level of the head of femur. [G744]

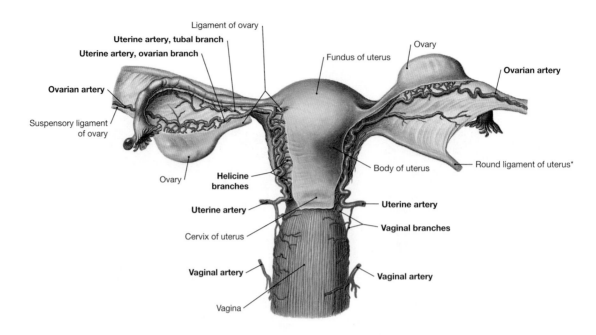

Fig. 7.72 Arteries of the internal female genitalia; posterior view.
The internal female genitalia are supplied by three paired arteries:
1. **Uterine artery** (from the internal iliac artery) with vaginal, ovarian and tubal branches,
2. **Ovarian artery** (from the abdominal aorta), and

3. **Vaginal artery** (from the internal iliac artery).
There are substantial variations in the anastomoses between these arteries.

* clin. term: round ligament

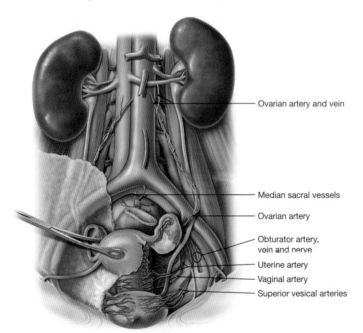

Fig. 7.73 Course of the ovarian arteries; anterior view. [L238]
The paired ovarian artery arises from the abdominal aorta at the level of L2. It descends in the retroperitoneal space and crosses the ureter anteriorly. At the pelvic brim it crosses over the common iliac blood vessels and travels in the suspensory (clin. term: **infundibulopelvic**) ligament of ovary to reach the intraperitoneal ovary.

Fig. 7.74 Course of the uterine artery;
right side; anterior view. [L285]
The uterine artery originates either directly from the anterior division of the internal iliac artery or from the umbilical artery. It travels at the base of the broad ligament to reach the uterus at the body to cervix transition. It ascends to the fundus along the lateral side of the body of uterus and gives rise to the tubal and ovarian branches. In the pelvic fascia the uterine artery crosses over the distal ureter.

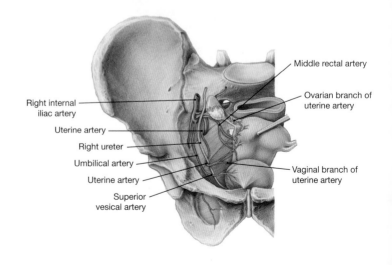

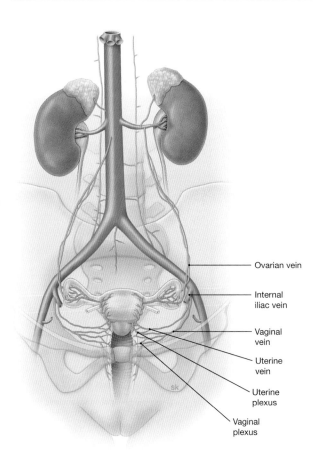

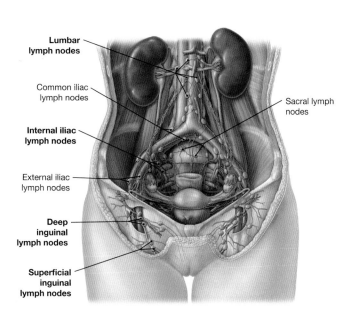

Fig. 7.76 Lymphatic vessels and lymph nodes of the external and internal female genitalia; anterior view. [L238]

Fig. 7.75 Veins of the internal female genitalia; schematic drawing. [L238]
The uterine and vaginal venous plexus drain into the internal iliac vein. The right ovarian vein drains into the inferior vena cava and the left ovarian vein into the left renal vein.

Fig. 7.77 Lymphatic drainage of the female genitalia; anterior view. [L127]
Pelvic (internal iliac; sacral) lymph nodes:
- Upper ⅔ of vagina
- Part of the uterine fundus, body and cervix

Lumbar (preaortic) lymph nodes:
- Ovary
- Uterine tube (FALLOPIAN tube)
- Part of the uterine fundus

Superficial inguinal lymph nodes:
- Lower ⅓ of vagina
- Fundus and body of uterus (via round ligament of uterus)
- Superficial and deep inguinal nodes drain into the external iliac nodes. External and internal inguinal nodes drain via the common iliac nodes into the lateral aortic nodes, also known as preaortic or lumbar nodes.

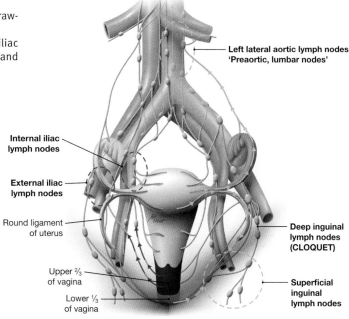

┌ Clinical Remarks

Carcinoma of the vulva **metastasizes** to the superficial inguinal lymph nodes. A metastatic spread to deep inguinal lymph nodes **(CLOQUET's node)** raises concern of further spreading of cancer cells into the pelvis. Endometrial carcinoma in the corpus area spreads within the broad ligament to the iliac lymph nodes, but when located near the uterine tubes (FALLOPIAN tubes) in the fundus it may also metastasize along the round ligament to inguinal lymph nodes or along the uterine tubes (FALLOPIAN tubes) to lumbar lymph nodes.

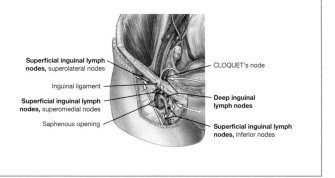

Fig. 7.78 Innervation of the female genitalia, schematic drawing; ventral view. Inferior hypogastric plexus and uterovaginal plexus contain sympathetic (green) and parasympathetic (purple) nerve fibers.

Preganglionic **sympathetic** nerve fibers (T10–L2) descend

- from the abdominal aortic plexus via the **hypogastric nerves** or
- via the pelvic sympathetic trunk and the **sacral splanchnic nerves** to the **inferior hypogastric plexus.**

From the inferior hypogastric plexus, postsynaptic sympathetic fibers reach the uterus, uterine tube and vagina via the **regional uterovaginal plexus.**

The mostly postganglionic sympathetic nerves to the ovary descend from the aorticorenal ganglia alongside the ovarian artery.

Preganglionic **parasympathetic** nerve fibers (S2–S4) reach the **inferior hypogastric plexus** via the **pelvic splanchnic nerves.** They synapse in ganglia of the inferior hypogastric or the **uterovaginal plexus** to reach the corpora cavernosa of clitoris and the greater vestibular (BARTHOLIN's) glands.

Somatic innervation by the **pudendal nerve** (S2–S4) conveys sensory innervation to the lower part of the vagina and the labia minora and majora via the posterior labial nerves and to the clitoris via the dorsal nerve of clitoris.

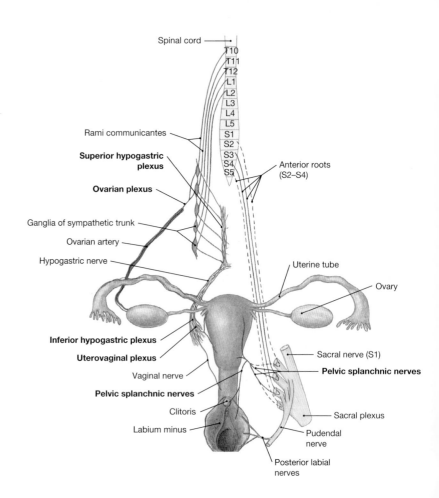

Clinical Remarks

Common options for anesthesia during childbirth:

1. **Spinal anesthesia:** catheter is advanced between L4/L5 spinous processes; anesthetic administered in the lumbar cistern abrogates all pain from the female genitalia; anesthesia of the lower limbs.

2. **Epidural anesthesia:** most commonly used anesthetic method during childbirth: catheter dwells in the epidural space and affects spinal nerve roots with a more local effect. With **caudal epidural anesthesia** the catheter is advanced through the sacral canal and dwells in the sacral canal; abrogates all pain from the lower birth canal (S2-S4; visceral and somatic); mother is aware of and feels pain from uterine contractions ['pelvic pain line']; limbs not affected. In contrast, the **lumbar epidural anesthesia** at the level of L4/L5 leads to a greater level of pain relief but some sensory and motor deficits in the lower extremity may occur.

3. **Pudendal nerve block:** this peripheral nerve block only abrogates somatic pain from the lower third of the vagina and the perineum; useful also for repair of perineal tears after vaginal delivery.

The line connecting the superior palpable iliac crests crosses the vertebral column at the level of L4. This is an important surface landmark for the lumbar puncture for spinal anesthesia (L3/L4) or placement of the catheter for a lumbar epidural anesthesia.

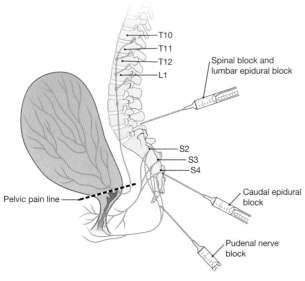

Fig. 7.79 Pain afferents with afferent visceral pain fibers from female genitalia; schematic drawing. [L126]

The imaginary **pelvic pain line** roughly marks the separation between female genitalia above and below the peritoneal lining. **Visceral pain** fibers from the intraperitoneal fundus and corpus of uterus travel with sympathetic branches to the T10–L2 spinal segments, but from the subperitoneal cervix and upper two-thirds of the vagina travel with parasympathetic branches to the S2–S4 spinal segments. **Somatic pain fibers** from the lower third of the vagina and the perineum course with the **pudendal nerve** (S2–S4).

Internal male genitalia comprise the testis, epididymis, vas deferens, seminal vesicle and prostate.
External male genitalia are defined as the penis, scrotum and urethra.

Internal and external male genitalia associated with the perineum are shown on the following pages. The prostate, seminal vesicles and ejaculatory ducts are shown as male pelvic viscera in ➤ Fig. 7.21, ➤ Fig. 7.44, ➤ Fig. 7.45, ➤ Fig. 7.48, ➤ Fig. 7.49 ➤ Fig. 7.50 and ➤ Fig. 7.51.

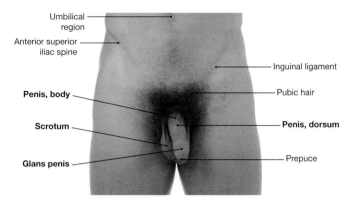

Fig. 7.80 Surface anatomy of the external male genitalia; anterior view.

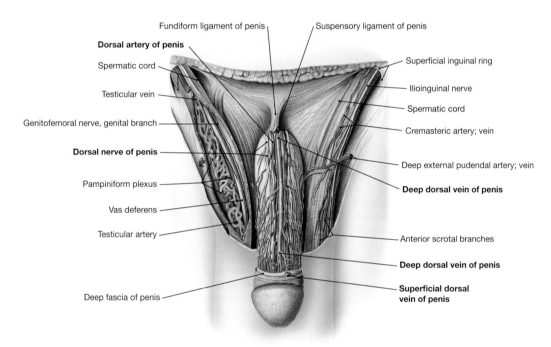

Fig. 7.81 External male genitalia with neurovascular structures; anterior view; after removal of the fascia of penis.
The paired dorsal arteries (from internal pudendal arteries) and sensory dorsal nerves of penis (from pudendal nerves) course together with the unpaired deep dorsal vein of penis beneath the deep fascia of penis.

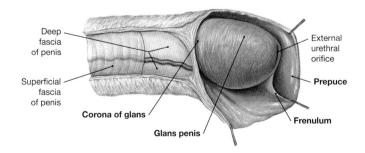

Fig. 7.82 Penis with glans and prepuce; view from the right side.
The distal end of the penis is enlarged to form the glans penis and shows a ridge (corona of glans) at its base. In the flaccid state, the glans is covered by the prepuce. At its underside, the prepuce is connected by a small ligament (frenulum).

Clinical Remarks

If the prepuce is very narrow **(phimosis)** and cannot be retracted, problems in micturition and infections may occur.

In this case, the removal of the prepuce by circumcision is required.

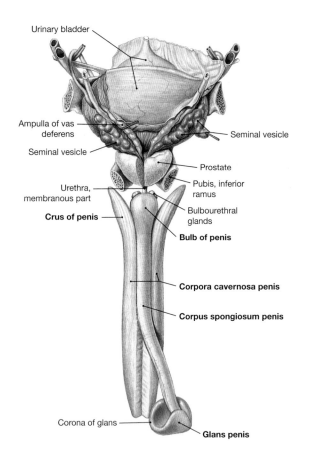

Urinary bladder

Ampulla of vas
deferens

Seminal vesicle

Urethra,
membranous part

Crus of penis

Seminal vesicle

Prostate

Pubis, inferior
ramus

Bulbourethral
glands

Bulb of penis

Corpora cavernosa penis

Corpus spongiosum penis

Corona of glans

Glans penis

Fig. 7.83 Urinary bladder, prostate and penis with exposed corpora cavernosa; posterior view.

In a flaccid state, the penis is usually about 10 cm (4 in) long and divided into the body, glans, and base or root of penis. It consists of the paired corpora cavernosa which are enclosed in a dense fibrous covering (tunica albuginea) and separated by a septum. The other component is the corpus spongiosum surrounding the urethra. The proximal parts (crura of penis) of the corpora cavernosa are fixed to the inferior pubic rami. The proximal and distal parts of each corpus spongiosum are dilated to form the bulb of penis and the glans of penis, respectively. All cavernous bodies together are ensheathed by the fascia of penis, which was removed in this illustration.

For the different parts of the male urethra ➤ Fig. 7.40.

Structure/Function

The penis receives its **arterial blood supply** from three paired arteries arising from the internal pudendal artery:
- **Dorsal artery of penis:** paired; courses deep to the deep fascia of penis, supplies skin and glans of penis;
- **Deep artery of penis:** located within the corpora cavernosa; regulates the filling of the corpora cavernosa;
- **Artery of bulb of penis:** supplies the urethra and the corpus spongiosum.

The **venous blood** is collected by three venous systems:
- **Superficial dorsal vein of penis:** paired or unpaired, courses superficial to the deep fascia of penis, drains blood from the skin of penis to the external pudendal vein;

- **Deep dorsal vein of penis:** unpaired, covered by the deep fascia of penis, drains blood from the corpora cavernosa to the prostatic venous plexus;
- **Vein of bulb of penis:** paired, drains blood from the bulb of penis to the deep dorsal vein of penis.

Innervation
- **sensory:** dorsal nerve of penis (from the pudendal nerve);
- **autonomic:** cavernous nerves of penis (from the inferior hypogastric plexus) penetrate the pelvic floor and course adjacent to the dorsal nerve of penis (sympathetic stimulation causes vasoconstriction, parasympathetic stimulation causes vasodilation, arterial blood flow to the erectile tissues of the corpora cavernosa and consecutive erection).

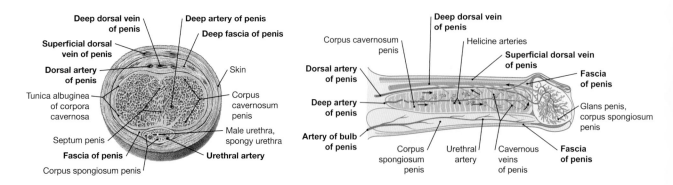

Fig. 7.84 Penis, cross-section at the midlevel of the body of penis; anterior view.

Following parasympathetic innervation, dilation of the deep artery of penis causes the filling of the corpora cavernosa. These compress the deep dorsal vein of penis beneath the tough fascia of penis and prevent venous drainage.

Fig. 7.85 Arteries and veins of the penis; parasagittal view. [L126]

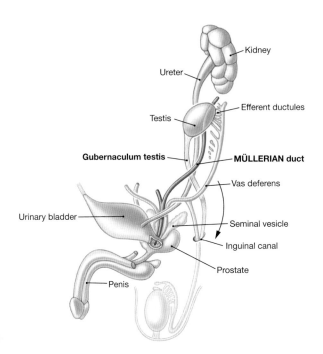

Fig. 7.86 Development of the internal male genitalia. [L126]
Up to week 7, development of the internal genitalia is identical in both sexes (sexual indifferent stage). The testis develops in the lumbar region at the level of the mesonephros which contributes several canaliculi as a connection between the testis and the epididymis. The testis is then relocated caudally **(testicular descent)** but remains connected to its vascular structures. Along the inferior mesenchymal **gubernaculum testis** a peritoneal pouch is formed **(processus vaginalis)** which reaches down to the future scrotum and serves in guiding the descent of the testis, a process normally completed at birth. Postnatally, the processus vaginalis obliterates in the area of the spermatic cord, but its distal part remains and forms a part of the testicular coverings (tunica vaginalis testis).

The sex hormones of the testis (mainly testosterone) induce the final differentiation of the WOLFFIAN duct to the internal male genitalia (epididymis, vas deferens), the seminal vesicles, and other accessory sex glands (prostate, COWPER's glands) from the urogenital sinus. The anti-MÜLLERIAN hormone suppresses the differentiation of the MÜLLERIAN ducts into female genitalia.

Clinical Remarks

Persistent incomplete testicular descent within the first years of life **(cryptorchidism)** may result in infertility and increases the risk of testicular cancer.

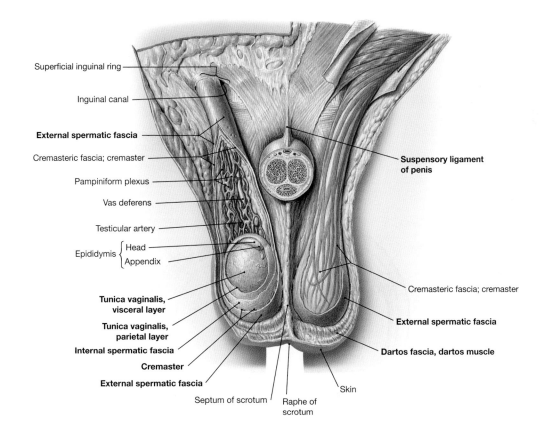

Fig. 7.87 Scrotum; ventral view; the scrotum is opened and the penis sectioned in the front.
The scrotum is divided internally by a septum which at the skin surface corresponds to the scrotal raphe (raphe of scrotum).
For fascial coverings of the spermatic cord ➤ Fig. 6.12 (abdominal wall):

The testis is covered with the **tunica vaginalis** which consists of an external parietal layer **(periorchium)** and an internal visceral layer **(epiorchium)**. Both are connected by the mesorchium and create between them the serosal cavity of the scrotum.

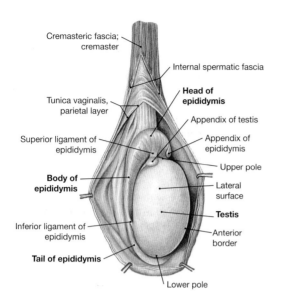

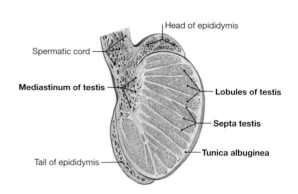

Fig. 7.89 Testis and epididymis, sagittal section; view from the right side.

At the mediastinum of testis neurovascular structures enter and exit the testis, and here the seminiferous tubules are connected to the head of epididymis.

Fig. 7.88 Testis and epididymis (➤ Fig. 6.16, ➤ Fig 6.20); view from the right side.

The testis is 4 × 3 cm (1.6 × 1.2 in) in size (20–30 g [0.7–1.1 oz]). The epididymis is attached to it by a superior and an inferior ligament. The epididymis has the following parts: head, body and tail of epididymis which continues as vas deferens.

Clinical Remarks

If the processus vaginalis fails to obliterate, accumulation of fluids may occur (even in adulthood) in the tunica vaginalis **(hydrocele testis)** which presents as scrotal swelling (➤ Fig. 7.90). Also, abdominal organs may prolapse into the scrotum **(congenital inguinal hernia;** ➤ Fig. 6.21). When blood enters the serosal cavity around the testis a **hematocele testis** forms.

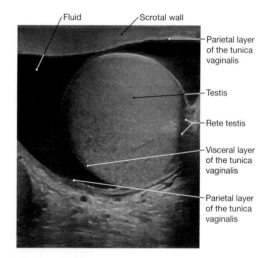

Fig. 7.90 Ultrasound image of a hydrocele testis. [T975]
Fluid accumulation within the serosal cavity (tunica vaginalis) of the testis.

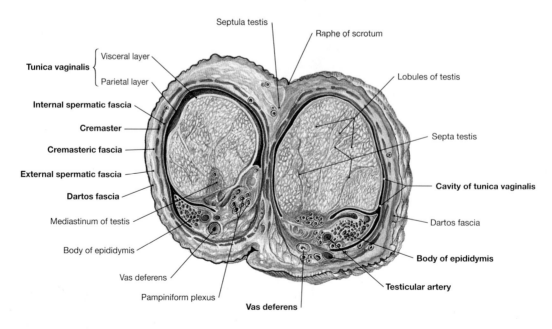

Fig. 7.91 Testis and epididymis, transverse section; superior view.

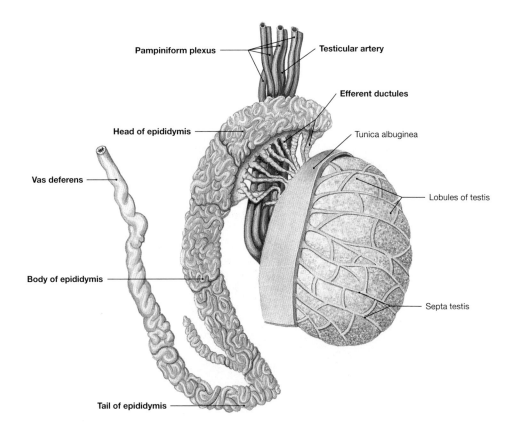

Fig. 7.92 Testis and epididymis, with blood vessels; view from the right side.

The testis is connected to the head of epididymis via efferent ductules. The epididymis itself consists of a 6 m (236 in) long convoluted duct which continues as vas deferens. The vas deferens (35–40 cm/ 14–16 in long, 3 mm/0.1 in thick) courses within the spermatic cord and through the inguinal canal to the dorsal aspect of the urinary bladder.

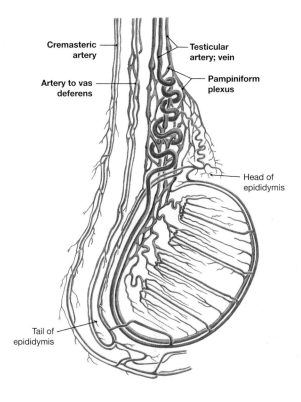

Fig. 7.93 Blood vessels of the internal male genitalia; view from the right side.

Clinical Remarks

The descent of the testis explains why the testicular blood vessels arise at the level of the kidneys and why the regional lymph nodes of the testis are positioned at this level in the retroperitoneal space. Lymph node metastases from **testicular cancer** are to be expected in the lumbar periaortic region, not in the inguinal region. Twisting of the spermatic cord presents as **testicular torsion,** an urologic emergency from ischemia of the testis. Doppler ultrasound is used to detect a loss of perfusion of the testis as shown in the example below. An abnormal enlargement of the pampiniform veins is referred to as **varicocele testis** and more commonly occurs on the left side.
[G724]

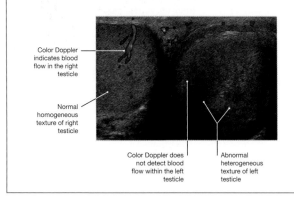

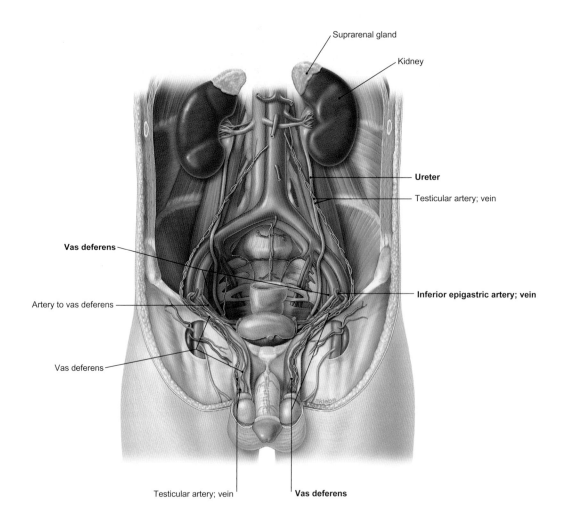

Fig. 7.94 Course of the vas deferens; ventral view. [L238]
The vas deferens crosses the ureter anteriorly in the pelvis. It enters the inguinal canal through the deep inguinal ring lateral to the inferior epigastric blood vessels.

Blood Vessels of the Internal Genitalia		
	Organ	**Blood Vessel**
Arteries	Testis and epididymis	Testicular artery (from the abdominal aorta)
	Vas deferens	Artery to vas deferens (usually from the umbilical artery)
	Spermatic cord (cremaster)	Cremasteric artery (from the inferior epigastric artery)
	Accessory sex glands	Inferior vesical artery and middle rectal artery (from the internal iliac artery)

Blood Vessels of the Internal Genitalia		
	Organ	**Blood Vessel**
Veins	Testis, epididymis, vas deferens, spermatic cord	Pampiniform plexus: plexus of veins that merge to form the testicular vein which drains into the inferior vena cava on the right side and into the left renal vein on the left side
	Accessory sex glands	Vesical and prostatic venous plexus with outflow into the internal iliac vein

Structure/Function

Innervation of male genitalia

Sympathetic innervation (green)

- Preganglionic sympathetic fibers (T10–L2) descend via the **superior hypogastric plexus** and **hypogastric nerves** some derive from the sacral ganglia of the sympathetic trunk via the sacral splanchnic nerves to the ganglia of the **inferior hypogastric plexus (IHP).** Postganglionic fibers reach the pelvic viscera, including the accessory sex glands and the smooth muscles of the vas deferens. Sympathetic stimulation facilitates emission through contraction of the smooth muscles in the vas deferens and the seminal vesicles.
- Autonomic fibers to the testis descent along the testicular blood vessels. The (mostly) postganglionic sympathetic fibers to the testis and epididymis are synapsed in the aorticorenal ganglia or the superior hypogastric plexus and course in the testicular plexus alongside the testicular artery.

Parasympathetic innervation (purple)

- Preganglionic parasympathetic fibers derive from the sacral division of the parasympathetic nervous system (S2–S4) via the **pelvic splanchnic nerves** and reach the ganglia of the **inferior hypogastric plexus (IHP).** They are synapsed either here or in the vicinity of the pelvic viscera to postganglionic neurons for the accessory sex glands and the vas deferens.
- The **cavernous nerves** penetrate the pelvic floor to reach the corpora cavernosa (partly adjacent to the dorsal nerve of penis). Parasympathetic stimulation facilitates **penile erection** through smooth muscle relaxation in the helicine arteries within the corpora cavernosa.

Somatic innervation

- The **pudendal nerve** (S2–S4) conveys sensory innervation to the penis and posterior scrotum via the dorsal nerve of penis and the posterior scrotal nerves.
- Motor innervation to the bulbospongiosus and ischiocavernosus via the perineal branches of the pudendal nerve initiates their contraction during ejaculation.

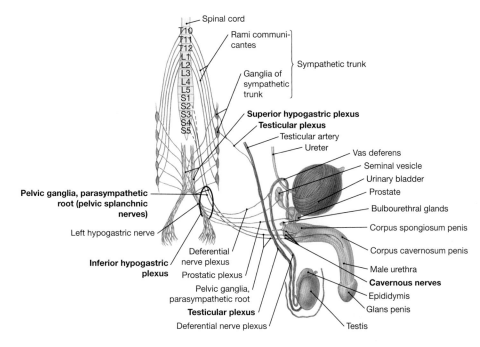

Fig. 7.95 Innervation of the male genitalia; schematic drawing; ventral and lateral view.
Note: Autonomic innervation to the testis and epididymis travels with the testicular plexus around the testicular artery. Parasympathetics derive from the vagus nerve and sympathetic fibers from the lumbar ganglia of the sympathetic trunk.

Preganglionic Autonomic Nerves	Postganglionic Autonomic Nerves	Function
Preganglionic **sympathetic** fibers (T10–L2) descend in the superior hypogastric plexus	Reach the sympathetic ganglia of the **inferior hypogastric plexus;** postganglionic fibers travel within pelvic organ plexus	Stimulate peristalsis of the vas deferens and contraction of the seminal vesicles during **emission**
Preganglionic **sympathetic** fibers (T10–L2) synapse in the aorticorenal ganglia	Postganglionic sympathetic fibers descend in the testicular plexus along the testicular artery	Vasomotor function for testis and epididymis
Preganglionic **parasympathetic** fibers (S2–S4) travel as **pelvic splanchnic nerves**	Reach the parasympathetic ganglia of the **inferior hypogastric plexus** and **pelvic organ plexus;** postganglionic fibers travel within pelvic organ plexus	The cavernous nerves penetrate the pelvic floor to reach the corpora cavernosa of the penis. Parasympathetic stimulation facilitates penile **erection**

Somatic innervation via the pudendal nerve (S2–S4) conveys sensory innervation to the penis and posterior scrotum via the dorsal nerve of penis and motor innervation to the bulbospongiosus and ischiocavernosus via the perineal nerves.

Clinical Remarks

Surgical procedures on the prostate or the rectum may injure the parasympathetic nerve fibers to the penis causing **erectile dysfunction.** Surgical procedures involving the abdominal aorta or the larger pelvic arteries have a risk for injury to the sympathetic fibers potentially compromising emission as well as subsequent ejaculation with resulting impotence.

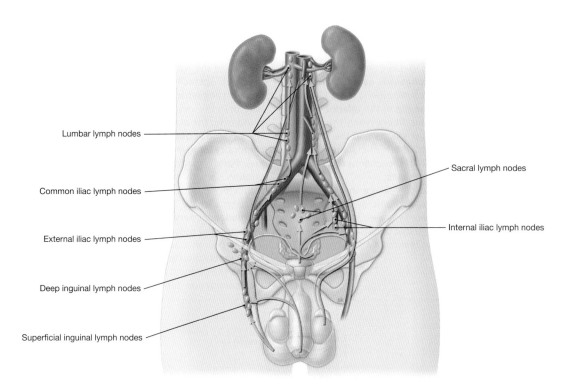

Fig. 7.96 Lymphatic drainage of the external and internal male genitalia; anterior view. [L238]
In men, the lymphatic drainage of external and internal genitalia do not communicate.

External genitalia:
* Penis and scrotum drain via the perineal lymphatic pathways to reach the inguinal lymph nodes: the scrotum via the superficial inguinal nodes and the penis directly into the deep inguinal nodes;

Internal genitalia:
* Testis and epididymis drain via lymphatics within the spermatic cord through the inguinal canal to reach the lumbar lymph nodes at the level of the kidneys;
* Vas deferens, spermatic cord, and accessory sex glands drain to the internal/external iliac and sacral lymph nodes.

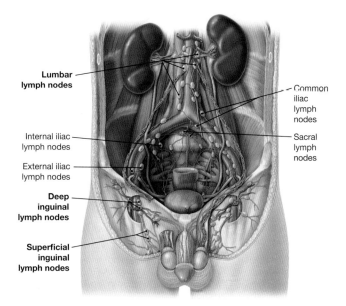

Fig. 7.97 Lymphatic vessels and lymph nodes of the external and internal male genitalia; anterior view. [L238]
The regional lymph nodes for the external genitalia are the inguinal lymph nodes. In contrast, the first regional lymph nodes for testis and epididymis are located in the retroperitoneal space at the level of the kidneys (**lumbar [para-aortic] lymph nodes**).

Clinical Remarks

Lymphatic metastases of **testicular cancer** metastasize to the retroperitoneal space, but those of **penile carcinoma** appear in the inguinal region. Transscrotal testicular biopsy must be avoided when suspecting testicular carcinoma since this may cause the dissemination of malignant cells into the inguinal nodes. In these cases, biopsies must be taken from the inguinal canal.

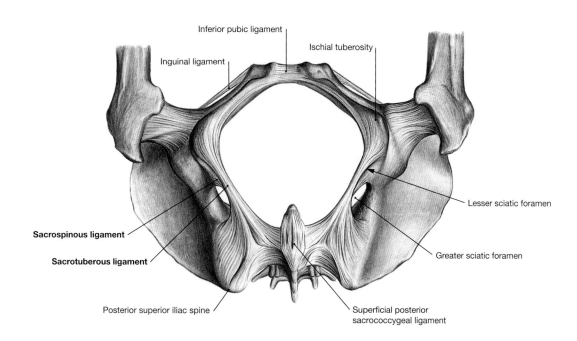

Fig. 7.98 Bones and ligaments of the female pelvic outlet; lithotomy position; caudal view.
The bony and ligamentous confinements of the pelvic outlet are shown: (1) the coccyx and the superficial posterior sacrococcygeal ligament; (2) the ischial tuberosities and the sacrotuberous ligaments; (3) the pubic symphysis with inferior pubic ligament and the ischiopubic rami.

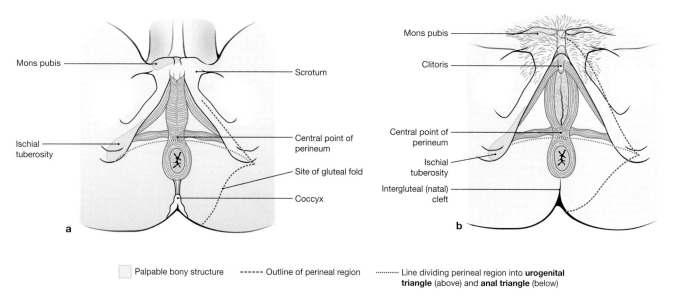

Fig. 7.99a and b Surface projection of perineal structures in the male (a) and female (b); lithotomy position. [L126]
The anterior **urogenital triangle** is separated from the posterior **anal triangle** by an imaginary line connecting the ischial tuberosities through the perineal body. The urogenital triangle contains the external genitalia in both sexes.

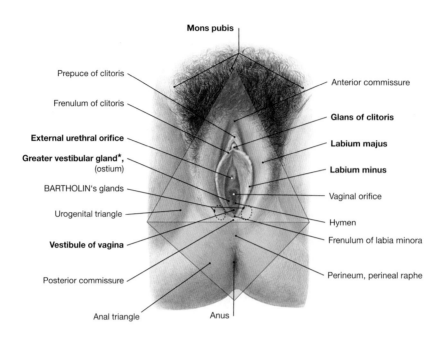

Fig. 7.100 **External female genitalia,** lithotomy position; inferior view.
The perineal region is divided into the anterior **urogenital triangle** and the posterior **anal triangle.** The external genitalia are located in the urogenital triangle and referred to as vulva. They comprise: mons pubis, labia majora, labia minora, clitoris, vestibule, greater vestibular glands (*BARTHOLIN's glands; position indicated with black circles). The vestibule extends to the hymen at the vaginal orifice.

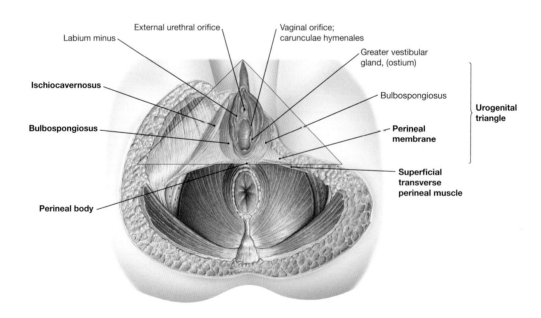

Fig. 7.101 **Perineal region in woman: urogenital triangle shaded;** lithotomy position; inferior view; all neurovascular structures removed.
The diamond-shaped perineal region reaches from the inferior margin of the pubic symphysis to the ischial tuberosities and the tip of the coccyx. The term perineal body (clin. term: perineum) describes exclusively the connective tissue bridge between the labia majora and the anus. The perineal membrane spans between the ischiopubic rami and separates the **deep** from the **superficial perineal pouch (space).** The bulbospongiosus, ischiocavernosus and superficial transverse perineal muscles are attached to and located inferior to the perineal membrane.

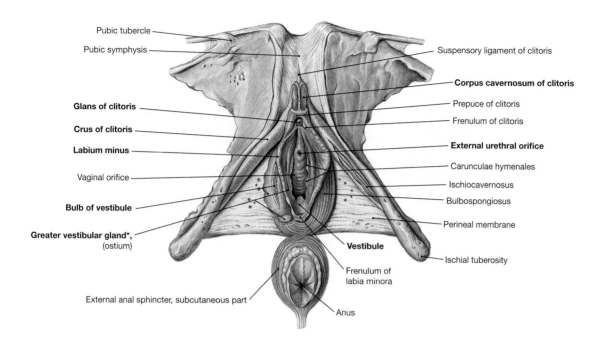

Pubic tubercle
Pubic symphysis
Glans of clitoris
Crus of clitoris
Labium minus
Vaginal orifice
Bulb of vestibule
Greater vestibular gland*,
(ostium)
External anal sphincter, subcutaneous part

Suspensory ligament of clitoris
Corpus cavernosum of clitoris
Prepuce of clitoris
Frenulum of clitoris
External urethral orifice
Carunculae hymenales
Ischiocavernosus
Bulbospongiosus
Perineal membrane
Vestibule
Ischial tuberosity
Frenulum of labia minora
Anus

Fig. 7.102 External female genitalia; inferior view; body fascia and neurovascular structures removed.
The labia majora are removed in this illustration. They cover the corpus cavernosum of clitoris (bulb of vestibule). The labia minora surround the vestibule and continue anteriorly as frenulum of clitoris to the glans of clitoris. The vestibular glands (greater vestibular glands [* BARTHOLIN's glands] and lesser vestibular glands) enter the vestibule from lateral. The clitoris is the sensory organ for sexual arousal. The corpora cavernosa form a short body of clitoris with the glans at the inferior end. The crura of clitoris are attached inferiorly to the ischiopubic rami and covered by the ischiocavernosus on both sides. The bulbospongiosus stabilizes the bulb of vestibule.

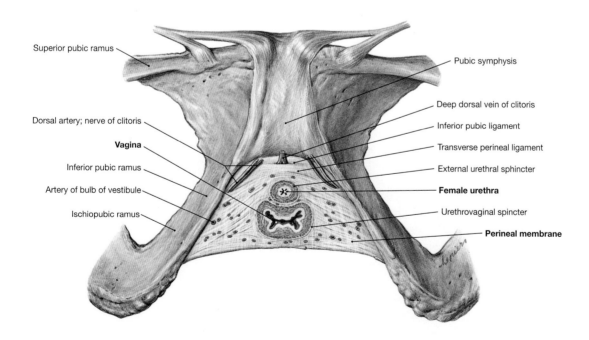

Superior pubic ramus
Dorsal artery; nerve of clitoris
Vagina
Inferior pubic ramus
Artery of bulb of vestibule
Ischiopubic ramus

Pubic symphysis
Deep dorsal vein of clitoris
Inferior pubic ligament
Transverse perineal ligament
External urethral sphincter
Female urethra
Urethrovaginal spincter
Perineal membrane

Fig. 7.103 Deep perineal muscles in women; inferior view; all other muscles removed.
In women, the deep transverse perineal muscle, which only consists of single muscle fibers embedded in connective tissue, is weak and does not form a muscular plate. Therefore, the term 'urogenital diaphragm' is not used anymore. The **perineal membrane** connects the ischiopubic rami and serves as attachment for the external genitalia. The deep perineal space superior to the perineal membrane contains the vagina and the urethra and the external urethral sphincter and is traversed by deep branches of the pudendal nerve and internal pudendal artery and vein before they reach the vulva.

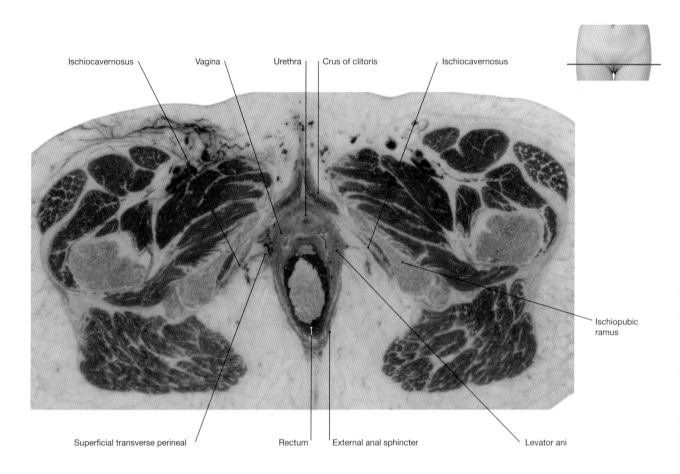

Fig. 7.104 Cross-sectional anatomy of the female perineum; at the
level just below the pubic symphysis. [X338]
The collapsed vagina is posteriorly adjacent to the urethra. The
ischiocavernosus is marked on both sides and the superficial
transverse perineal muscle is visible on the right side.

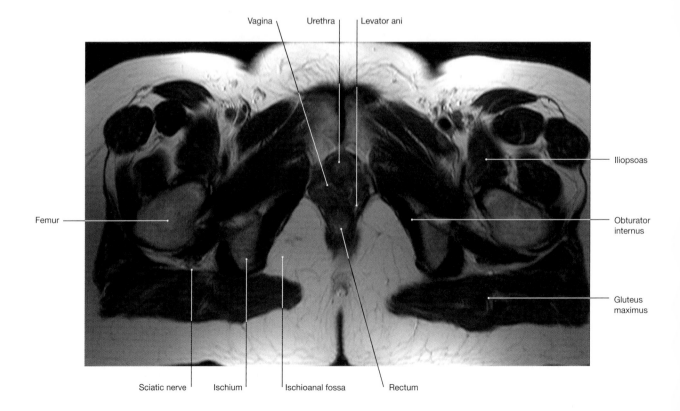

Fig. 7.105 T2w MRI of the female pelvis; transverse section. [G744]

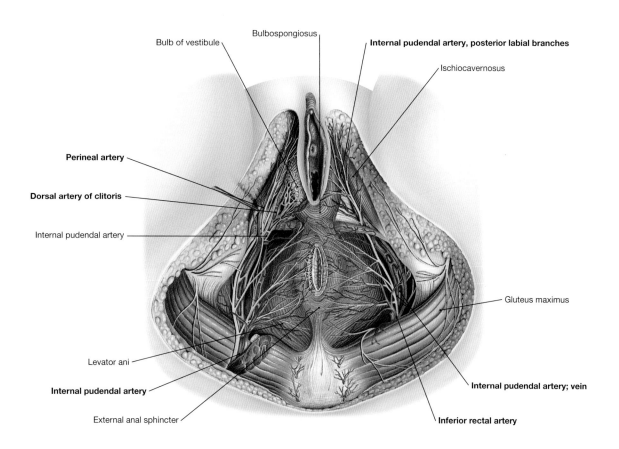

Fig. 7.106 Branches of the internal pudendal artery, female perineum; inferior view.
The inferior rectal artery branches off from the internal pudendal artery, leaves the pudendal canal (ALCOCK's canal) and crosses together with the inferior rectal vein and nerve the ischioanal fossa to reach the anal region. The remaining perineal branches of the internal pudendal artery are shown.

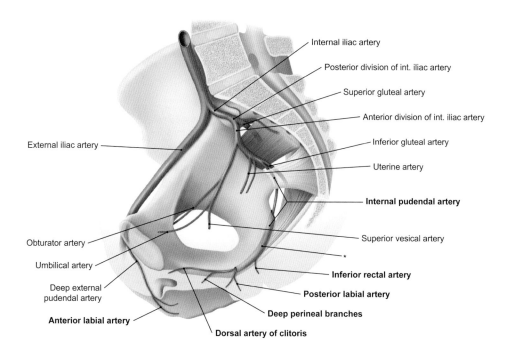

Fig. 7.107 Blood supply of the female perineum; schematic drawing; lateral view. [L275]
Arterial supply to the perineum derives from the internal and external pudendal arteries. The internal pudendal artery is a branch of the anterior division of the internal iliac artery. It leaves the pelvis below the piriformis through the greater sciatic foramen, winds around the ischial spine and courses through the lesser sciatic foramen and then within the pudendal canal (* ALCOCK's canal), a duplicature of the internal obturator fascia, to reach the perineum. It supplies perineal structures in the deep and superficial perineal pouches. Its terminal branch is the dorsal artery of clitoris. The labia majora are supplied from the **anterior labial artery** of the external pudendal artery, a branch of the external iliac artery, and the **posterior labial artery,** a branch of the internal pudendal artery.

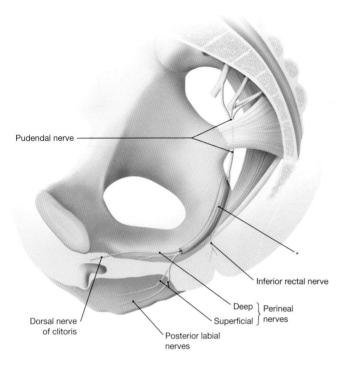

Pudendal nerve

Dorsal nerve
of clitoris

Posterior labial
nerves

Deep ⎱ Perineal
Superficial ⎰ nerves

Inferior rectal nerve

Fig. 7.108 Course of the pudendal nerve in the female; schematic drawing; view from the left side. [L275]
The pudendal nerve derives from the sacral plexus and has contributions from S2–S4 spinal segments. It leaves the pelvis (➤ Fig. 4.10) through the greater sciatic foramen inferior to the piriformis, loops around the ischial spine and passes through the lesser sciatic foramen to enter the pudendal canal (*, shaded in brown), a duplicature of the obturator internus fascia. After branching off the inferior rectal nerve, the perineal branches of the pudendal nerve course in the deep and superficial perineal pouches.

Pudendal Nerve	Innervated Structures	Functional Aspects
Inferior rectal nerve	**Motor** fibers to external anal sphincter and puborectalis **Sensory** fibers to perianal skin and anus inferior to the pectinate line	• Voluntary closure of anus • Facilitating the perineal flexure of the rectum (puborectalis muscle) • Anal reflex
Deep perineal nerves Terminal branch: dorsal nerve of clitoris	Deep perineal pouch: **Motor** fibers to deep transverse perineal muscles, to external urethral and urethrovaginal sphincters **Sensory** fibers to clitoris	• Voluntary closure of the urethra • Sexual arousal
Superficial perineal nerves including the posterior labial nerve	Superficial perineal pouch: **Motor** fibers to ischiocavernosus, bulbospongiosus, and superficial transverse perineal muscles **Sensory** fibers to posterior labia majora, vestibule of vagina, labia minora, lower third of vagina and lower urethra, greater vestibular (BARTHOLIN's) glands.	• Supports orgasm • Sexual arousal • Pain sensation from perineum

Clinical Remarks

To achieve a **pudendal nerve block** the ischial spine is palpated from the vagina. The anesthetic is then administered around the ischial spine on both sides. This peripheral nerve block relaxes the perineal muscles and abrogates somatic pain from the perineal skin, the posterior vulva and the mucosa of the lower third of vagina and lower urethra. It is not effective for uterus, cervix and upper vagina. Sensory fibers to the anterior vulva, the anterior labial nerves, derive from the lumbar plexus (L1: ilioinguinal and genitofemoral nerves) and are not anesthesized with a pudendal nerve block. Application of a local anesthetic may be required to reach analgesia.
[R388]

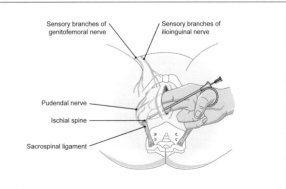

Sensory branches of
genitofemoral nerve

Sensory branches of
ilioinguinal nerve

Pudendal nerve

Ischial spine

Sacrospinal ligament

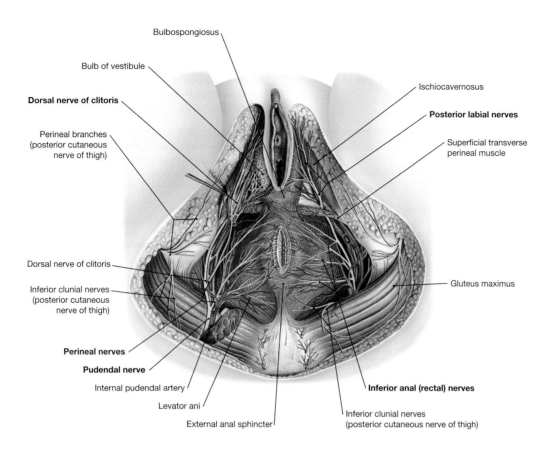

Bulbospongiosus

Bulb of vestibule

Dorsal nerve of clitoris

Perineal branches
(posterior cutaneous
nerve of thigh)

Dorsal nerve of clitoris

Inferior clunial nerves
(posterior cutaneous
nerve of thigh)

Perineal nerves

Pudendal nerve

Internal pudendal artery

Levator ani

External anal sphincter

Ischiocavernosus

Posterior labial nerves

Superficial transverse
perineal muscle

Gluteus maximus

Inferior anal (rectal) nerves

Inferior clunial nerves
(posterior cutaneous nerve of thigh)

Fig. 7.109 Branches of the pudendal nerve, female perineum; inferior view.
The inferior rectal nerve branches off the pudendal nerve, leaves the pudendal canal (ALCOCK's canal) and crosses together with the inferior rectal artery and vein the ischioanal fossa (➤ Fig. 4.10) to reach the anal region. The remaining perineal branches of the pudendal nerve are shown.

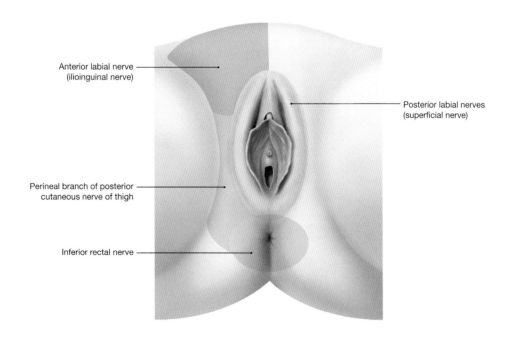

Anterior labial nerve
(ilioinguinal nerve)

Posterior labial nerves
(superficial nerve)

Perineal branch of posterior
cutaneous nerve of thigh

Inferior rectal nerve

Fig. 7.110 Sensory innervation of the perineum, female perineum; inferior view. [L275]
The pudendal nerve conveys most of the sensory innervation of the perineum through the superficial perineal nerves and the inferior rectal nerves. But branches of the ilioinguinal nerve (L1, lumbar plexus) and the posterior cutaneous nerve of thigh (S1–S3, sacral plexus) provide sensory innervation to most of the anterior and lateral perineal region.

Clinical Remarks

An episiotomy is a surgical incision in the perineum to enlarge the vaginal opening and reduce resistance during second stage labor and to avoid extensive perineal lacerations of the mother during the transition of the baby's head.
[E754]

Both procedures, the median (midline) and the mediolateral episiotomy, require that the perineal skin, the vaginal mucosa, the urethrovaginal sphincter (➤ Fig. 7.43) are transsected.
The specific anatomical structures to be transsected distinctly for each procedure are listed below:

Median Episiotomy	Mediolateral Episiotomy
Specific anatomical structures incised are: • junction of superficial transverse perineal and bulbospongiosus muscles with perineal body • perineal body Offers the advantage of **less pain and blood** loss, easier and better cosmetic repair; Disadvantages include higher incidence of lacerations of the anal sphincter and rectum.	Specific anatomical structures incised are: • superficial transverse perineal and bulbospongiosus muscles • greater vestibular (BARTHOLIN's) gland and duct • bulb of vestibule • perineal membrane Offers advantage of protecting **maternal anal sphincter and rectum** from injury when extended; Disadvantages are greater blood loss, longer time for surgical repair and more often faulty healing.
Midline incision	Mediolateral incision

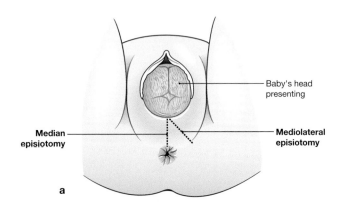

Fig. 7.111a and b Median versus mediolateral episiotomy; lithotomy position; caudal view. [L126]
For a median (midline) episiotomy the vaginal mucosa and vaginal wall are cut and the incision is continued along the perineal raphe without injuring the anal sphincter. For a mediolateral episiotomy the incision is directed away from the anus either on the right or the left side **(a)**. The muscles of the perineum and the pelvic floor are shown **(b)**.

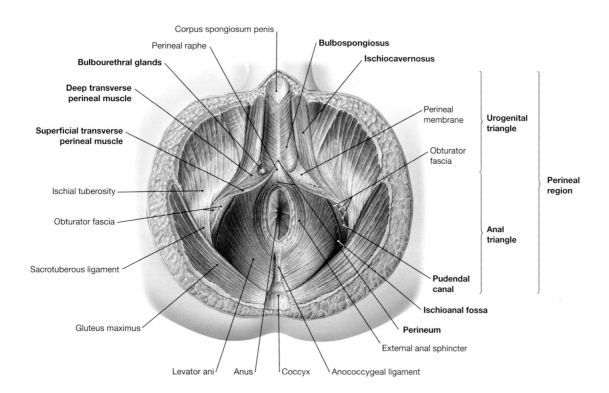

Fig. 7.112 Muscles of the perineal region in the male; inferior view; all neurovascular structures removed.

The perineal region extends from the inferior margin of the pubic symphysis to the tip of the coccyx (coccygeal bone). The term perineal body, however, exclusively describes the small bridge of con-nective tissue between the root of penis and the anus. The perineal body serves as attachment for the muscles of the anterior urogenital region (bulbospongiosus, ischiocavernosus, superficial and deep perineal muscles) and the posterior anal region (external anal sphincter muscles).

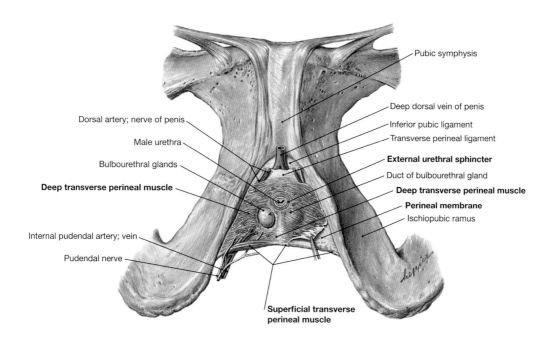

Fig. 7.113 Deep perineal muscles in the male; inferior view; all other muscles removed.

The perineal muscles in the male comprise the strong deep transverse perineal muscle and the thin superficial transverse perineal muscle located at its posterior margin. The voluntary sphincter of the urinary bladder, the **external urethral sphincter,** is a part of the deep transverse perineal muscle. The deep transverse perineal muscle is covered inferiorly by the **perineal membrane.** The deep perineal space (pouch) above this membrane contains: urethra, COWPER's glands (bulbourethral glands), deep branches of the pudendal nerve and the internal pudendal artery and vein. The superficial perineal space (pouch) lies inferior to the perineal membrane.

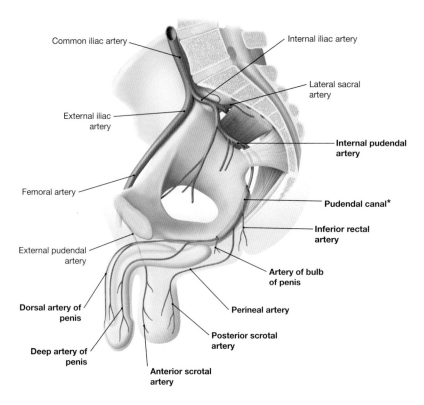

Fig. 7.114 Blood supply of the perineum in the male; schematic drawing; lateral view. [L275]
Arterial supply of the perineum derives from the internal and external pudendal arteries. The internal pudendal artery is a branch of the anterior division of the internal iliac artery. It leaves the pelvis below the piriformis through the greater sciatic foramen, winds around the ischial spine and courses through the lesser sciatic foramen and then within the pudendal canal to reach the perineum. The **pudendal canal (* ALCOCK's canal;** shaded in brown) contains the internal pudendal artery and vein, and the pudendal nerve after their passage from the gluteal region through the lesser sciatic foramen. The internal pudendal artery supplies perineal structures in the deep and superficial perineal pouch. Its terminal branch is the dorsal artery of penis. The scrotum is supplied from the anterior scrotal artery of the external pudendal artery, a branch of the external iliac artery, and the posterior scrotal artery, a branch of the internal pudendal artery.

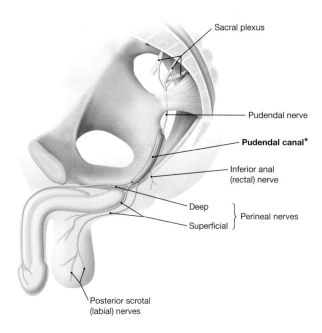

Fig. 7.115 Course of the pudendal nerve in the male; schematic drawing; view from the left side. [L275]
The pudendal nerve derives from the sacral plexus and has contributions of the S2–S4 spinal segments. It leaves the pelvis (➤ Fig. 4.10) through the greater sciatic foramen inferior to the piriformis, loops around the ischial spine and passes through the lesser sciatic foramen to enter the **pudendal canal (* ALCOCK's canal;** shaded in brown), a duplicature of the obturator internus fascia. When entering the pelvis below the ischial spine the pudendal nerve courses below the pelvic diaphragm to reach the perineum. After branching off the inferior rectal nerve, the perineal branches of the pudendal nerve course in the deep and superficial perineal pouches.

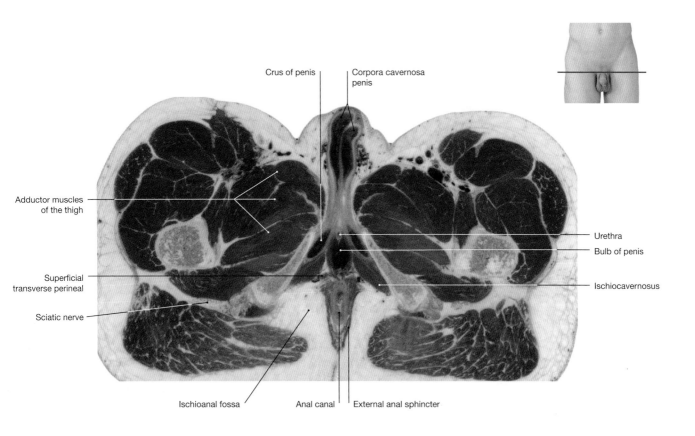

Crus of penis

Corpora cavernosa penis

Adductor muscles of the thigh

Superficial transverse perineal

Sciatic nerve

Urethra

Bulb of penis

Ischiocavernosus

Ischioanal fossa

Anal canal

External anal sphincter

Fig. 7.116 Cross-sectional anatomy of the male perineum and ischioanal fossa (➤ Fig. 4.10, ➤ Fig. 4.85). [X338]

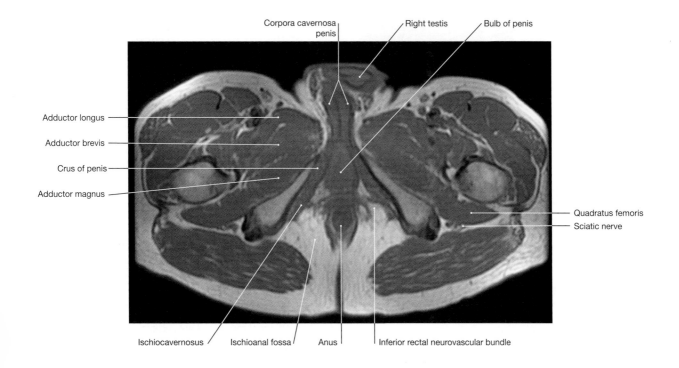

Corpora cavernosa penis

Right testis

Bulb of penis

Adductor longus

Adductor brevis

Crus of penis

Adductor magnus

Quadratus femoris

Sciatic nerve

Ischiocavernosus

Ischioanal fossa

Anus

Inferior rectal neurovascular bundle

Fig. 7.117 T2w MRI of the male perineum. [G744]

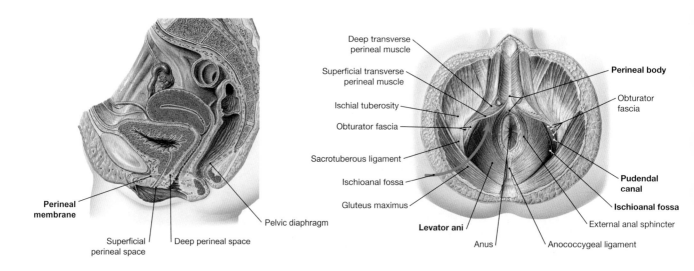

Fig. 7.118 Deep and superficial perineal spaces in the female; sagittal section; view from the left.

The position of the pelvic diaphragm and of the perineal membrane are indicated with dotted lines. The **perineal membrane** separates the deep from the superficial perineal space. The anterior recess of the ischioanal fossa is a part of the deep perineal space.

Fig. 7.119 Ischioanal fossa in the male; inferior view.

The pyramid-shaped ischioanal fossa has a very similar anatomy in men and women. The fossa is filled with adipose tissue (removed here). The **anterior recess of the ischioanal fossa** extends anteriorly above the perineal membrane towards the pubic symphysis. The anterior recess is continuous with the **deep perineal pouch.**

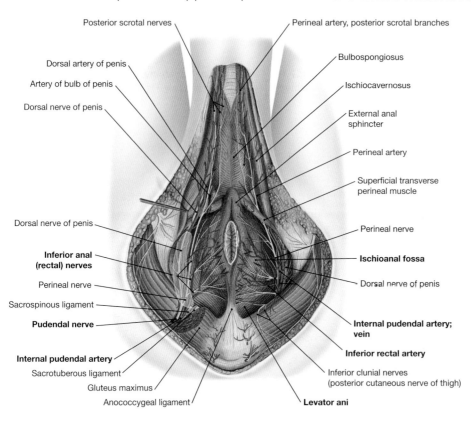

Fig. 7.120 Neurovascular structures in the ischioanal fossa, male; inferior view. The pudendal canal (ALCOCK's canal), a fascial duplicature of the obturator internus muscle, is highlighted in yellow. It covers the pudendal vessels and nerve. The neurovascular structures then continue ventrally to the penis and the two perineal spaces. Inferior rectal artery, vein and nerve leave the pudendal canal and cross the fossa to the anus.

Borders of the Ischioanal Fossa	
Medial and cranial	External anal sphincter and levator ani
Lateral	Obturator externus
Dorsal	Gluteus maximus and sacrotuberous ligament
Ventral	Posterior margin of the superficial and the deep perineal spaces; anterior recess reaches to the pubic symphysis
Caudal	Skin of the perineum

Clinical Remarks

The ischioanal fossa is of great clinical relevance because of its expansion to both sides of the anus. Collections of pus (abscesses) may expand within the entire ischioanal fossa, including its anterior recesses, and even extend to the pubic symphysis. Perianal abcesses can occur with inflammatory bowel disease (IBD), are extremely painful and may cause anal fistulations. Scarring from recurrent transsphincteric fistulation may compromise fecal continence.

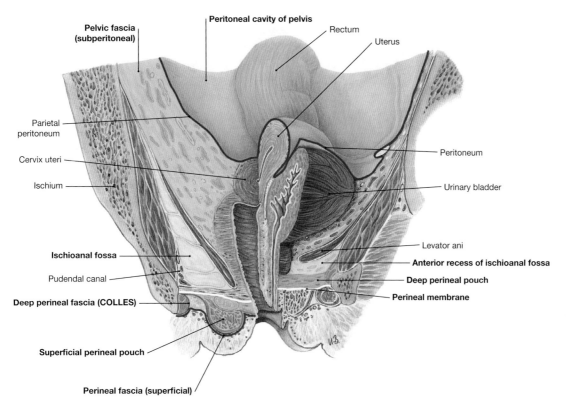

Fig. 7.121 Pelvic spaces in the female; median section, and frontal section on the right side; anterior view.
The frontal section shows three levels of the female pelvis:
• **Peritoneal cavity** of the pelvis caudally bordered by the parietal peritoneum;
• **Subperitoneal pelvic space,** caudally bordered by the levator ani of the pelvic floor;

• **Perineal region** inferior to the pelvic floor. The anterior portion contains two perineal spaces which are separated by the perineal membrane. The deep perineal space includes the variably expanded anterior recess of ischioanal fossa.
The ischioanal fossa is illustrated here at two different frontal planes for the right and left sides.

Structure/Function

The **deep perineal space (deep perineal pouch)** comprises connective tissue, single muscle fibers of the deep transverse perineal muscle. The anterior recess of the ischioanal fossa is continuous with the deep perineal pouch.
The **deep perineal space (deep perineal pouch) in the female** is traversed by:
• Branches of the pudendal nerve (dorsal nerve of clitoris)
• Branches of the internal pudendal artery and vein (dorsal artery of clitoris, deep artery of clitoris)
• Vagina
• Urethra

The **superficial perineal space (superficial perineal pouch)** is located between the perineal membrane and the membranous layer of the perineal fascia (COLLES fascia).
The superficial perineal space contains:
• Superficial transverse perineal muscle
• Proximal parts of the corpora cavernosa of clitoris (crura of clitoris), covered by ischiocavernosus
• **Greater vestibular glands (BARTHOLIN's glands)**
• Bulb of the vestibule, covered by bulbospongiosus
• Branches of the pudendal nerve (perineal nerves with branch to the bulb of vestibule)
• Branches of the internal pudendal artery and vein (perineal artery with artery to the bulb of vestibule)

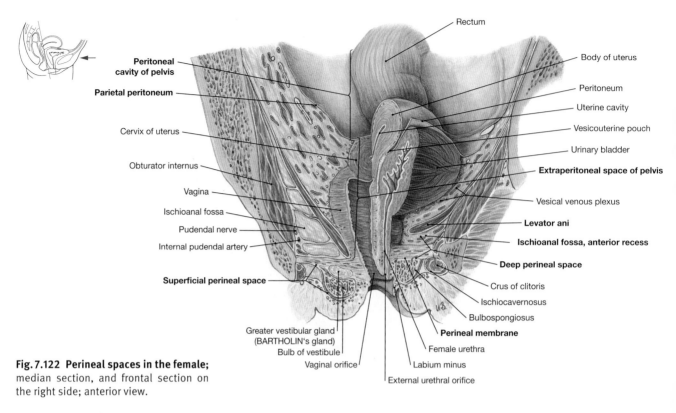

Fig. 7.122 Perineal spaces in the female; median section, and frontal section on the right side; anterior view.

Structure/Function

The **deep perineal space (deep perineal pouch) in the male** contains:
- Deep transverse perineal muscle
- External urethral sphincter muscle
- Anterior recess of the ischioanal fossa
- **Bulbourethral glands (COWPER's glands)**
- Branches of the pudendal nerve (dorsal nerve of penis)
- Branches of the internal pudendal artery and vein (dorsal artery of penis, deep artery of penis)
- Urethra, membranous part

The **superficial perineal space (superficial perineal pouch) in the male** contains:
- Superficial transverse perineal muscle
- Proximal parts of the corpora cavernosa of the penis (crura of penis), covered by ischiocavernosus muscle
- Spongy urethra, proximal part
- Bulb of the penis, covered by bulbospongiosus muscle
- Branches of the pudendal nerve (perineal nerves to erectile bodies and surrounding muscles)
- Branches of the internal pudendal artery and vein (perineal branches to erectile bodies and surrounding muscles)

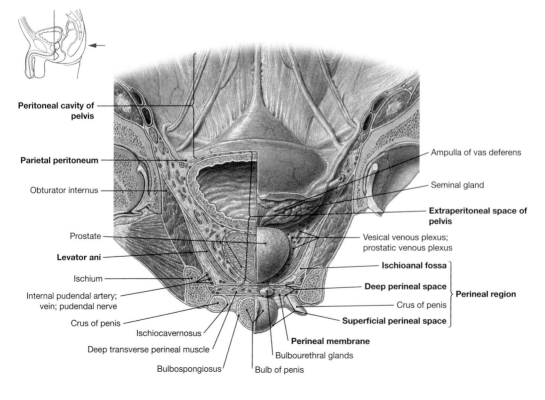

Fig. 7.123 Perineal spaces in the male; left side; frontal section at the level of the femoral head; posterior view.
The frontal section shows three levels of the male pelvis:
- Peritoneal cavity of the pelvis,
- Subperitoneal space,
- Perineal region, below the pelvic floor.

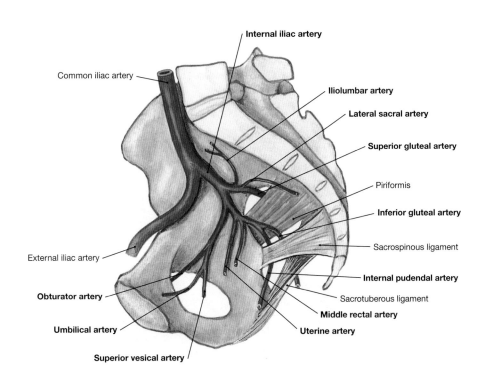

Fig. 7.124 Branches of the internal iliac artery in the female pelvis; view from the left side.
In most cases (60%), the internal iliac artery divides into an anterior and a posterior division. The sequence for the consecutive branching is highly variable. The arterial branches are categorized according to their perfusion area in parietal branches for the pelvic wall and the external genitalia and in visceral branches for the pelvic viscera.

Posterior Division		
Arterial Branch	**Anatomical Remarks**	**Structures Supplied**
Iliolumbar artery		Iliacus, psoas, and quadratus lumborum
Lateral sacral arteries	Enter the anterior sacral foramina	Sacral canal
Superior gluteal artery	Exits through greater sciatic foramen, between lumbosacral trunk and S1 anterior ramus	Gluteal region, gluteus medius and gluteus minimus

Anterior Division		
Arterial Branch	**Anatomical Remarks**	**Structures Supplied**
Obturator artery	Exits through obturator canal	Obturator muscles
Internal pudendal artery	Exits through greater sciatic foramen	Perineum (skin, muscles, erectile tissues, anus)
Inferior gluteal artery	Separates S1 from S2 anterior rami; exits through greater sciatic foramen	Levator ani (in part), gluteus maximus, hamstrings, quadratus femoris
Umbilical artery*	Distally obliterated to medial umbilical ligament	Gives rise to superior vesical arteries
Superior vesical artery*		Bladder and distal ureter
Middle rectal artery*		Inferior rectum
Inferior vesical artery (men)*		Neck of bladder, seminal vesicle and prostate
Uterine artery (women)*	May arise from umbilical artery or directly from anterior division	Uterus, uterine tubes (FALLOPIAN tubes), upper vagina Vaginal artery may branch off directly from umbilical or internal iliac arteries.

* Visceral branches

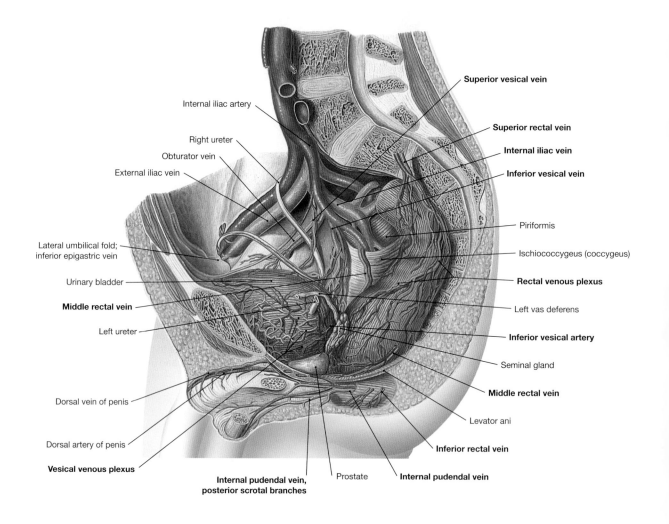

Fig. 7.125 Blood drainage from the pelvic viscera in the male (➤ Fig. 4.88); view from the left side.

The venous blood drains into the internal iliac vein. Its tributaries form communicating venous plexuses around the pelvic viscera. These are in close proximity to autonomic nerve plexuses in the pelvic fascia.

- **Rectal venous plexus:** connected via the superior rectal vein to the portal venous system and via the middle and inferior rectal veins to the drainage system of the inferior vena cava (porto-caval anastomosis).

- **Vesical venous plexus:** at the base of the urinary bladder, also collects the venous blood from the accessory sex glands.
- **Prostatic venous plexus:** drains not only the venous blood from the prostate, but also from the corpora cavernosa of penis (deep dorsal vein of penis). Connections to the venous plexuses around the vertebral column explain the frequently occurring vertebral metastases in patients with prostatic carcinoma.

In **the female,** the **uterovaginal venous plexus** drains blood from the uterus and vagina.

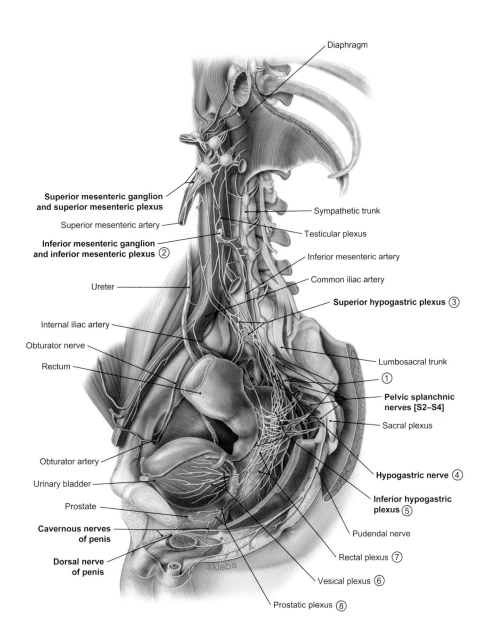

Fig. 7.126 **Autonomic and somatic nerves in the male pelvis;** view from the left side. [L238]

Note: Circled numbers in this figure correspond to the numbers in the table on the next page.

Structure/Function

Sympathetic Nerves of the Pelvis

Sacral Sympathetic Chain ①	Superior Rectal Plexus (Periarterial)	Hypogastric Plexus (Presacral)

• Continuation of lumbar splanchnic trunks
• Descend behind the common iliac vessels medial to the sacral foramina
• Connect to sacral spinal nerves by gray rami communicantes only [comprise postsynaptic sympathetic fibers from T12–L2]
• Provide sympathetic innervation to the **lower limbs**
1. **Sudomotor**
2. **Pilomotor**
3. **Vasomotor**
	• Continuation of periarterial inferior mesenteric plexus ②
	• Accompany the superior rectal (hemorrhoidal) artery to reach the superior rectal (hemorrhoidal) plexus
	• Course *within the mesorectum!*
	• Provides sympathetic innervation to lower sigmoid colon and rectum
	  – **vasomotor**
	  – **inhibition of peristalsis**
	[the inferior mesenteric plexus also contains parasympathetic fibers which ascend from the pelvis to sigmoid and descending colon]
		• Continuation of aortic plexus
		• **Lumbar splanchnic nerves synapse** in ganglia of the **superior hypogastric plexus (SHP)** ③
		• Located in front of L5/sacral promontory
		• Main continuation of sympathetic fibers into the pelvis
		• Also contain afferent fibers which convey reflex information and pain from pelvic viscera (superior to pelvic pain line)
		• Divides in two trunks at the level of the sacral promontory: **Hypogastric nerves** ④ which descend along the lateral pelvic wall to the **inferior hypogastric plexus (IHP)** ⑤
		  – **Inhibition of peristalsis**
		  – **Stimulation of sphincters and pelvic genital organs**
		  – **Vasomotor**

Parasympathetic Nerves of the Pelvis (T12–L2)

- Exit the anterior sacral foramina as preganglionic **pelvic splanchnic nerves**
- Provide parasympathetic innervation to the pelvic viscera, including descending and sigmoid colon (craniosacral distribution of the parasympathetic nervous system; vagus nerve conveys parasympathetics until the left/splenic colic flexure)
- Convey afferent fibers concerned with reflexive activity (micturition, defecation, erection and pelvic pain)
- Parasympathetic innervation is more important for pelvic reflexes and for the conduction of pain from pelvic viscera than sympathetic afferents in the hypogastric plexus
- **Inferior hypogastric plexus (IHP)** ⑤
  - Presents a mix of sympathetic and parasympathetic pre- and postsynaptic fibers, small autonomic ganglia and afferent fibers and continues as the pelvic plexus in the connective tissue of the lateral pelvic wall
  - Organ-specific subplexuess (such as vesical ⑥, rectal ⑦, prostatic ⑧, utero-vaginal) derive from the IHP/pelvic plexus
- Parasympathetics fibers have no connections to the somatic nerves of the sacral plexus (no contribution to the lower limbs)

Note: Circled numbers in the table correspond to the numbers in ➤ Fig. 7.126.

Head

Surface Anatomy 425

Skull 426

Facial Muscles 439

Neurovascular Supply 442

Nose and Nasal Cavity 448

Paranal Sinuses 452

Neurovascular Supply
to the Nasal Cavity 454

Oral Cavity 455

Bones of the Oral Cavity 456

Temporomandibular Joint 458

Muscles of Mastication 460

Dentition and Gingiva 461

Dentition 462

Hard Palate 464

Neurovascular Supply
to the Teeth 465

Mucosa and Innervation
of the Tongue 467

Muscles of the Tongue 468

Neurovascular Supply
of the Tongue 470

Tonsils 471

Soft Palate 472

Hyoid Bone and Floor
of Oral Cavity 473

Floor of Mouth 474

Salivary Glands 475

Innervation of Glands of the Head .. 479

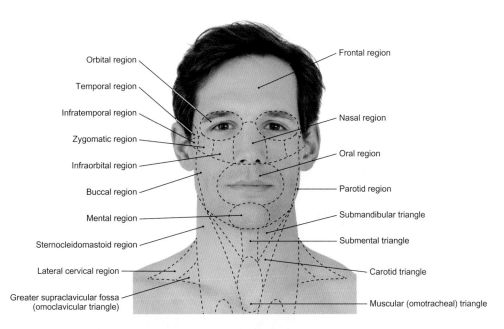

Orbital region
Temporal region
Infratemporal region
Zygomatic region
Infraorbital region
Buccal region
Mental region
Sternocleidomastoid region
Lateral cervical region
Greater supraclavicular fossa (omoclavicular triangle)

Frontal region
Nasal region
Oral region
Parotid region
Submandibular triangle
Submental triangle
Carotid triangle
Muscular (omotracheal) triangle

Fig. 8.1 Regions of the head and neck; frontal view. [K340]

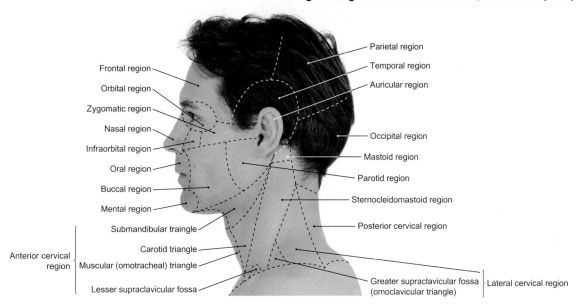

Frontal region
Orbital region
Zygomatic region
Nasal region
Infraorbital region
Oral region
Buccal region
Mental region

Parietal region
Temporal region
Auricular region
Occipital region
Mastoid region
Parotid region
Sternocleidomastoid region
Posterior cervical region

Anterior cervical region
Submandibular traingle
Carotid triangle
Muscular (omotracheal) triangle
Lesser supraclavicular fossa

Greater supraclavicular fossa (omoclavicular triangle)
Lateral cervical region

Fig. 8.2 Regions of the head and neck; lateral view. [K340]

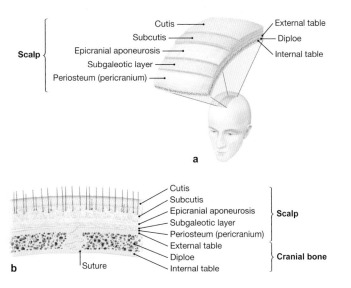

Scalp
Cutis
Subcutis
Epicranial aponeurosis
Subgaleotic layer
Periosteum (pericranium)

External table
Diploe
Internal table

a

Cutis
Subcutis
Epicranial aponeurosis
Subgaleotic layer
Periosteum (pericranium)
External table
Diploe
Internal table

Scalp

Cranial bone

b
Suture

Fig. 8.3a and b Scalp layers; the scalp consists of five distinct soft tissue layers that cover the cranial vault. [L127]

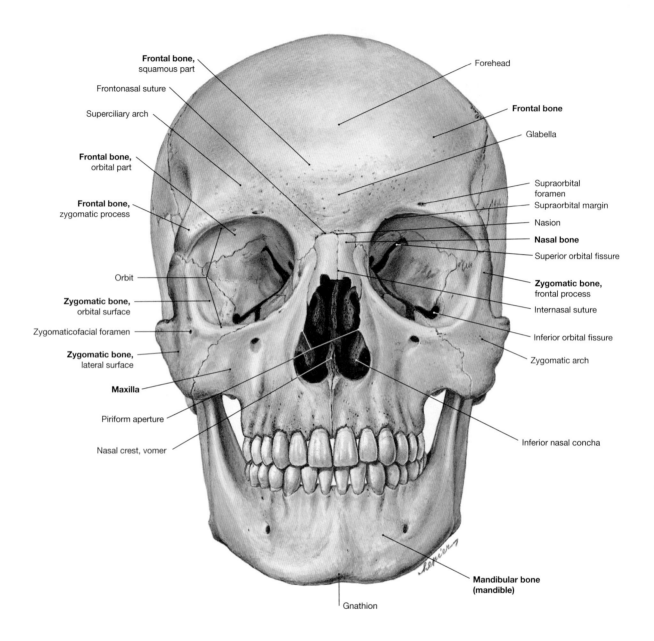

Fig. 8.4 Cranial bones; frontal view.

Frontal bone,
squamous part

Frontonasal suture

Superciliary arch

Frontal bone,
orbital part

Frontal bone,
zygomatic process

Orbit

Zygomatic bone,
orbital surface

Zygomaticofacial foramen

Zygomatic bone,
lateral surface

Maxilla

Piriform aperture

Nasal crest, vomer

Gnathion

Forehead

Frontal bone

Glabella

Supraorbital
foramen

Supraorbital margin

Nasion

Nasal bone

Superior orbital fissure

Zygomatic bone,
frontal process

Internasal suture

Inferior orbital fissure

Zygomatic arch

Inferior nasal concha

Mandibular bone
(mandible)

Structure/Function

The **neurocranium** (blue) is composed of eight bones: the paired parietal and temporal bones, and the unpaired frontal, ethmoid, sphenoidal, and occipital bones.

The **viscerocranium** (also named splanchnocranium, orange) is composed of the paired nasal, zygomatic and lacrimal bones and inferior nasal conchae, as well as four unpaired bones: the vomer, maxillary (maxilla), mandibular (mandible), and palatine bones.

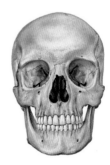

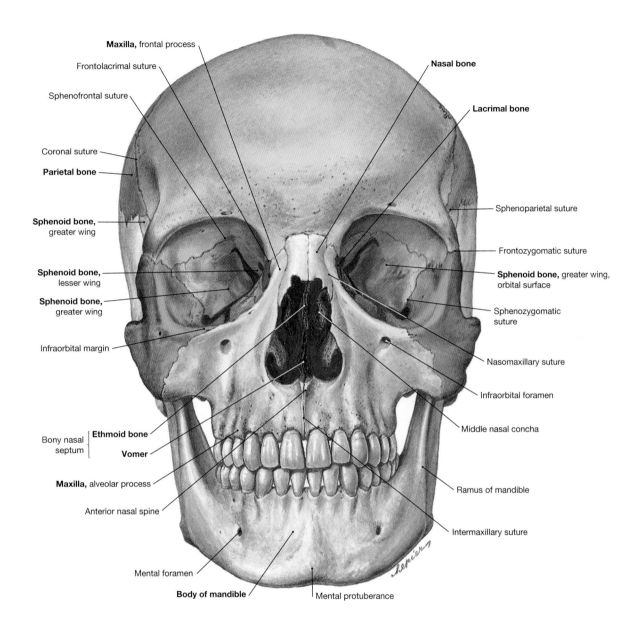

Maxilla, frontal process

Frontolacrimal suture

Sphenofrontal suture

Coronal suture

Parietal bone

Sphenoid bone, greater wing

Sphenoid bone, lesser wing

Sphenoid bone, greater wing

Infraorbital margin

Bony nasal septum · **Ethmoid bone** · **Vomer**

Maxilla, alveolar process

Anterior nasal spine

Mental foramen

Body of mandible

Nasal bone

Lacrimal bone

Sphenoparietal suture

Frontozygomatic suture

Sphenoid bone, greater wing, orbital surface

Sphenozygomatic suture

Nasomaxillary suture

Infraorbital foramen

Middle nasal concha

Ramus of mandible

Intermaxillary suture

Mental protuberance

Fig. 8.5 Cranial sutures and bones in color; frontal view; for color chart see p. VIII.

Clinical Remarks

Central fractures (red lines) of the midface are frequently caused by car accidents and are classified according to LE FORT:
- LE FORT I: *horizontal fracture line* with isolated detachment of the maxillary alveolar rim ('floating palate')
- LE FORT II: *pyramidal facture line* involving the maxilla in the floor of orbit; affected are the ethmoid bones, anterior skull base, and sometimes nasal bones as well
- LE FORT III: *transverse fracture line* with craniofacial dissociation

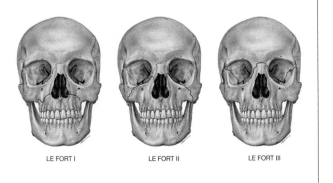

LE FORT I   LE FORT II   LE FORT III

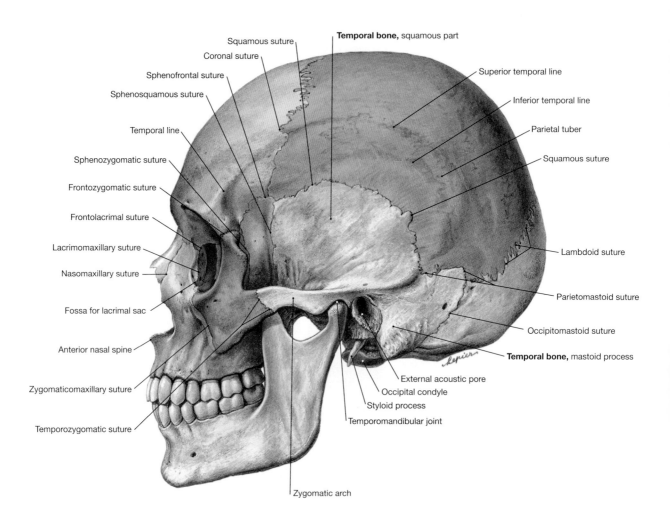

Squamous suture

Coronal suture

Sphenofrontal suture

Sphenosquamous suture

Temporal line

Sphenozygomatic suture

Frontozygomatic suture

Frontolacrimal suture

Lacrimomaxillary suture

Nasomaxillary suture

Fossa for lacrimal sac

Anterior nasal spine

Zygomaticomaxillary suture

Temporozygomatic suture

Temporal bone, squamous part

Superior temporal line

Inferior temporal line

Parietal tuber

Squamous suture

Lambdoid suture

Parietomastoid suture

Occipitomastoid suture

Temporal bone, mastoid process

External acoustic pore

Occipital condyle

Styloid process

Temporomandibular joint

Zygomatic arch

Fig. 8.6 Cranial sutures and bones in color; lateral view; for color chart see p. VIII.

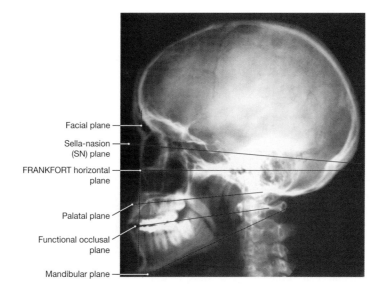

Facial plane

Sella-nasion (SN) plane

FRANKFORT horizontal plane

Palatal plane

Functional occlusal plane

Mandibular plane

Fig. 8.7 Reference lines of the skull. [E460]

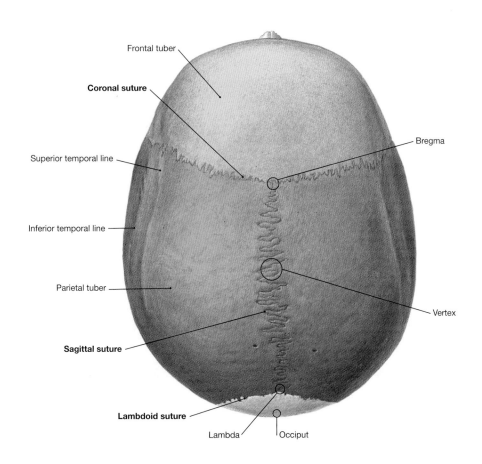

Fig. 8.8 Cranial sutures and bones in color; superior view; for color chart see p. VIII.

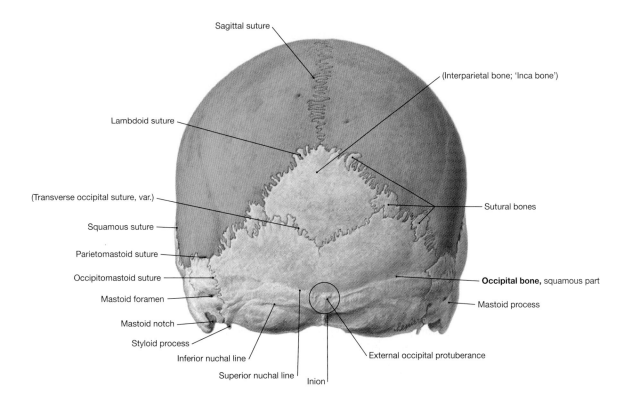

Fig. 8.9 Cranial bones in color; posterior view; for color chart see p. VIII.

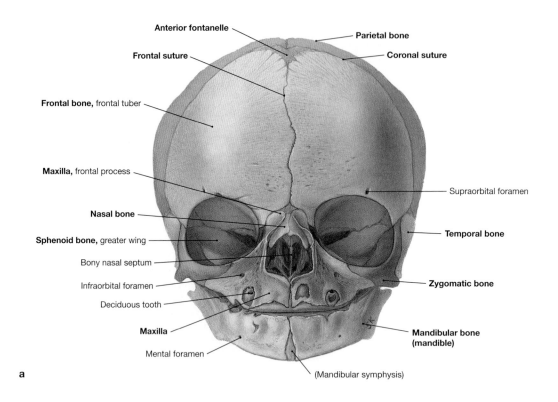

a

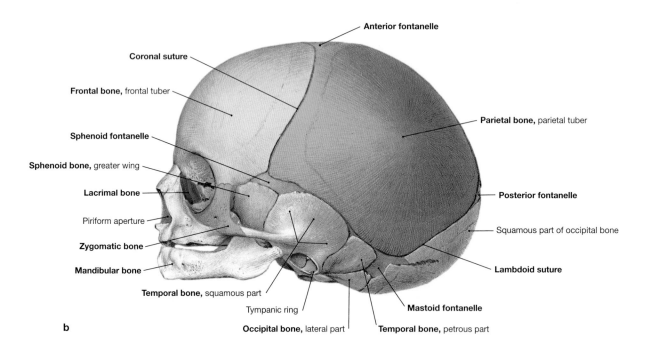

b

Fig. 8.10a and b Skull, cranium, of a newborn; frontal view **(a)** and lateral view **(b);** for color chart see p. VIII.

At birth, the newborn has six fontanelles (fonticuli), two unpaired (anterior and posterior fontanelles) and two paired (sphenoid and mastoid fontanelles). During delivery, sutures and fontanelles serve as reference structures to assess the location and position of the fetal head. Shortly before birth, the posterior fontanelle be- comes the leading part of the head during normal cephalic pre- sentation. In concert with the sutures, the fontanelles allow limited deformation of the fetal skull during delivery. The remarkable post- natal growth results in the fontanelles becoming rapidly smaller. Complete closure normally occurs by the end of the third year of life.

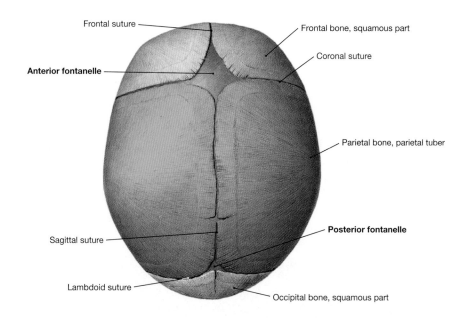

Frontal suture
Frontal bone, squamous part
Coronal suture
Anterior fontanelle
Parietal bone, parietal tuber
Posterior fontanelle
Sagittal suture
Lambdoid suture
Occipital bone, squamous part

Fig. 8.11 Skull, cranium, of a newborn; superior view; for color chart see p. VIII.

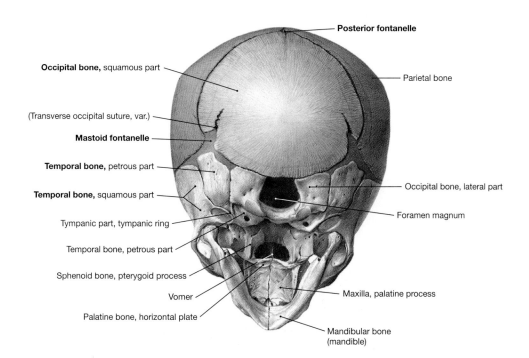

Posterior fontanelle
Occipital bone, squamous part
Parietal bone
(Transverse occipital suture, var.)
Mastoid fontanelle
Temporal bone, petrous part
Occipital bone, lateral part
Temporal bone, squamous part
Foramen magnum
Tympanic part, tympanic ring
Temporal bone, petrous part
Sphenoid bone, pterygoid process
Vomer
Maxilla, palatine process
Palatine bone, horizontal plate
Mandibular bone (mandible)

Fig. 8.12 Skull, cranium, of a newborn; posterior view; for color chart see p. VIII.
At birth, the cranial sutures that separate the bony plates of the skull cap (calvaria) are filled with interstitial tissue. Sutures are widened to fontanelles in regions where more than two bones meet. Important sutures include the lambdoid suture, frontal suture, sagittal suture, and coronal suture which gradually fuse at about 50 years of age. The frontal suture closes already between the first and second year of life.

Fontanelle	Number	Closure (Months of Life)
Anterior fontanelle (large fontanelle)	Unpaired	Approx. 36
Posterior fontanelle (small fontanelle)	Unpaired	Approx. 3
Sphenoid fontanelle (anterior lateral fontanelle)	Paired	Approx. 6
Mastoid fontanelle (posterior lateral fontanelle)	Paired	Approx. 18

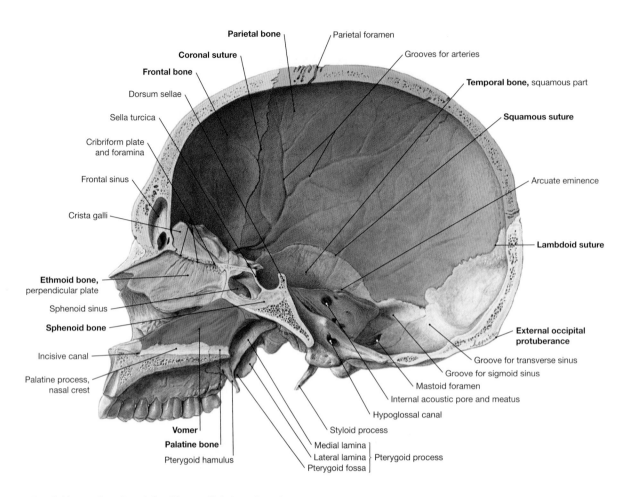

Fig. 8.13 Cranial bones in color, right side; medial view; for color chart see p. VIII.

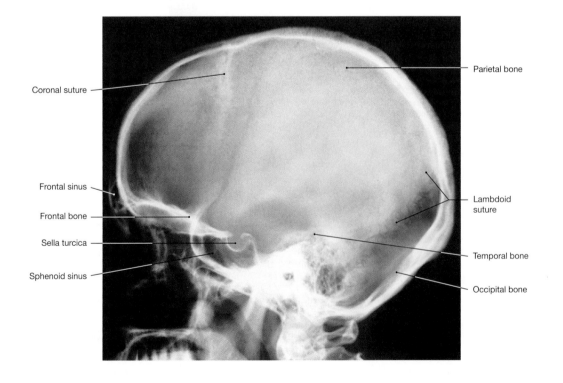

Fig. 8.14 X-ray image of a normal human skull, right side; medial view. [G198]

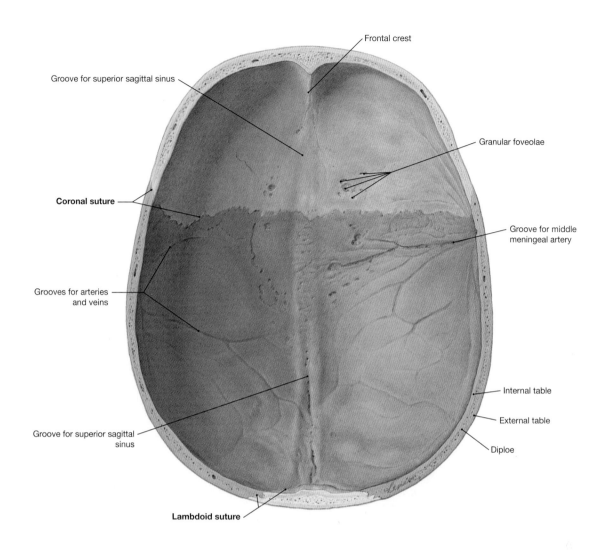

Frontal crest

Groove for superior sagittal sinus

Granular foveolae

Coronal suture

Groove for middle meningeal artery

Grooves for arteries and veins

Internal table

External table

Groove for superior sagittal sinus

Diploe

Lambdoid suture

Fig. 8.15 **Roof of the cranium, calvaria;** view from inside; for color chart see p. VIII.

Clinical Remarks

External physical forces can result in **skull fractures.**

1. **Linear fractures** present with clear fracture lines that traverse the full thickness of the skull and usually do not involve displacement of bones.
2. **Depressed skull fractures** contain multiple bony fragments (impression fracture) with inward pointing parts which can lead to compression or tear of dura mater and lesions of brain tissue.
3. **Compound fractures** result in an exposure of the cranial cavity and include tear of epidermis and meninges or affect the sinuses and/or middle ear. Fractures involving the paranasal sinuses or the middle ear are considered open fractures with the associated risk of infection and require surgical intervention.
4. **Diastatic fractures,** also referred to as 'growing fractures', occur along and across sutures in babies and infants and can result in a widening of the suture.
5. **Basal skull fractures** (not shown).

1, 4 [G305], 2 [G198], 3 [G211]

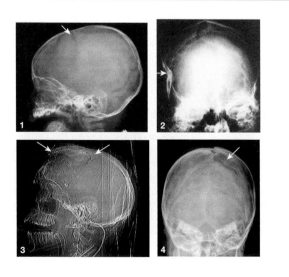

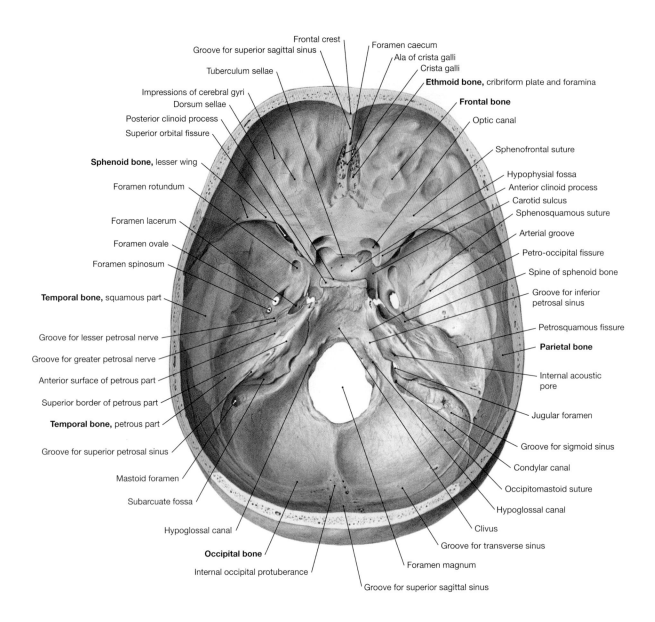

Frontal crest
Groove for superior sagittal sinus
Tuberculum sellae
Impressions of cerebral gyri
Dorsum sellae
Posterior clinoid process
Superior orbital fissure
Sphenoid bone, lesser wing
Foramen rotundum
Foramen lacerum
Foramen ovale
Foramen spinosum
Temporal bone, squamous part
Groove for lesser petrosal nerve
Groove for greater petrosal nerve
Anterior surface of petrous part
Superior border of petrous part
Temporal bone, petrous part
Groove for superior petrosal sinus
Mastoid foramen
Subarcuate fossa
Hypoglossal canal
Occipital bone
Internal occipital protuberance

Foramen caecum
Ala of crista galli
Crista galli
Ethmoid bone, cribriform plate and foramina
Frontal bone
Optic canal
Sphenofrontal suture
Hypophysial fossa
Anterior clinoid process
Carotid sulcus
Sphenosquamous suture
Arterial groove
Petro-occipital fissure
Spine of sphenoid bone
Groove for inferior petrosal sinus
Petrosquamous fissure
Parietal bone
Internal acoustic pore
Jugular foramen
Groove for sigmoid sinus
Condylar canal
Occipitomastoid suture
Hypoglossal canal
Clivus
Groove for transverse sinus
Foramen magnum
Groove for superior sagittal sinus

Fig. 8.16 Inner aspect of the base of the skull; superior view; for color chart see p. VIII.

Structure/Function

The base of skull (from above **(a)**; medial view **(b)**) can be divided into the anterior (light green), middle (orange), and posterior (green) cranial fossae, which form the upper, middle, and lower levels of the skull base, respectively. Bones that form the anterior cranial fossa are: frontal, ethmoid and sphenoid bones; for the middle cranial fossa: sphenoid and temporal bones; and for the posterior cranial fossa: sphenoid, temporal, and occipital bones.

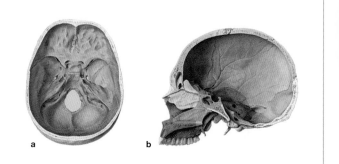

a   b

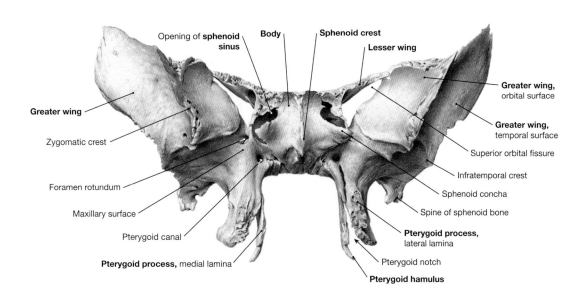

Fig. 8.17 Sphenoid bone; anterior view.
The unpaired sphenoid bone connects the viscerocranium with the neurocranium. The center of the sphenoid bone contains the sphe-noid **sinus.** The sphenoid crest separates the anterior part of the body of sphenoid into two halves.

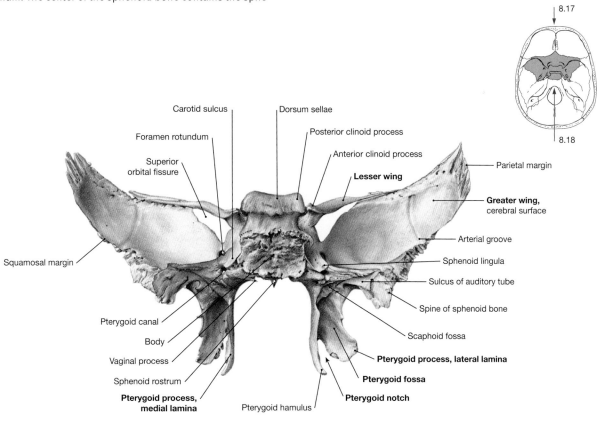

Fig. 8.18 Sphenoid bone; posterior view.
Lesser wing (ala minor) and greater wing (ala major) of the sphe-noid bone participate in the formation of the superior orbital fis-sure. On both sides, the pterygoid process divides into a smaller medial plate (medial lamina) and a larger lateral plate (lateral lam-ina), which create the **pterygoid notch** and enclose the **pterygoid fossa.**

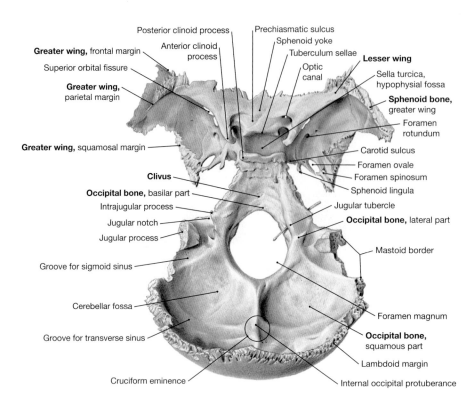

Fig. 8.19 Sphenoid bone and occipital bone; superior view; for color chart see p. VIII.

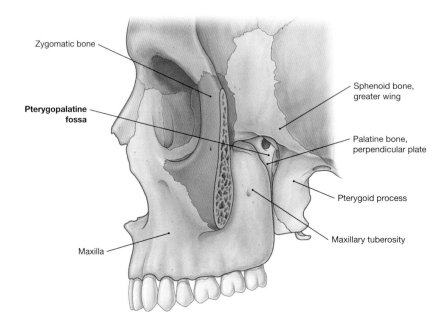

Fig. 8.20 Bony demarcations of the pterygopalatine fossa; lateral view; for color chart see p. VIII. [E402]
Cranial: sphenoid bone, greater wing (ala major); **medial:** perpendicular plate of palatine bone; **rostral:** maxillary tuberosity (tuber maxillae) and orbital process of palatine bone; **lateral:** infratemporal fossa ; **occipital:** pterygoid process; **caudal:** mouth cavity.

Structure/Function

The **pterygopalatine fossa** connects with the
1. Nasal cavity (sphenopalatine foramen)
2. Orbit (inferior orbital fissure)
3. Maxillary tuberosity (posterior alveolar foramina)
4. Medial cranial fossa (foramen rotundum)
5. Outer skull base (pterygoid canal)
6. Oral cavity (greater and lesser palatine canals)

Foramina of the Outer Base of Skull and their Content

Foramina	Content
Incisive foramen	Nasopalatine nerve (maxillary nerve [CN V/2])
Greater palatine foramen	Greater palatine nerve (maxillary nerve [CN V/2]) Greater palatine artery (descending palatine artery)
Lesser palatine foramen	Lesser palatine nerves (maxillary nerve [CN V/2]) Lesser palatine arteries (descending palatine artery)
Inferior orbital fissure	Infraorbital artery (maxillary artery) Inferior ophthalmic vein Infraorbital nerve (maxillary nerve [CN V/2]) Zygomatic nerve (maxillary nerve [CN V/2])
Foramen rotundum (round foramen) (➤ Fig. 8.17, ➤ Fig. 8.18)	Maxillary nerve [CN V/2]
Foramen ovale (oval foramen)	Mandibular nerve [CN V/3] Venous plexus of foramen ovale
Foramen spinosum	Meningeal branch (mandibular nerve [CN V/3]) Medial meningeal artery (maxillary artery)
Sphenopetrosal fissure and foramen lacerum	Lesser petrosal nerve (glossopharyngeal nerve [CN IX]) Greater petrosal nerve (facial nerve [CN VII]) Deep petrosal nerve (internal carotid plexus)
External opening of carotid canal and carotid canal	Internal carotid artery, petrosal part Internal carotid venous plexus Internal carotid plexus (sympathetic trunk, superior cervical ganglion)
Stylomastoid foramen	Facial nerve [CN VII]
Jugular foramen	**Anterior part:** Inferior petrosal sinus Glossopharyngeal nerve [CN IX] **Posterior part:** Posterior meningeal artery (ascending pharyngeal artery) Sigmoid sinus (superior bulb of jugular vein) Vagus nerve [CN X] Meningeal nerve (vagus nerve [CN XI]) Spinal accessory nerve [CN XI]
Mastoid canaliculus	Auricular branch of vagus nerve [CN X]
Hypoglossal canal	Hypoglossal nerve [CN XII] Venous plexus of hypoglossal canal
Condylar canal	Condylar emissary vein
Foramen magnum	Meninges Internal vertebral venous plexus (marginal sinus) Vertebral arteries (subclavian and anterior spinal arteries) Medulla oblongata/spinal cord Spinal roots (spinal accessory nerve [CN XI])

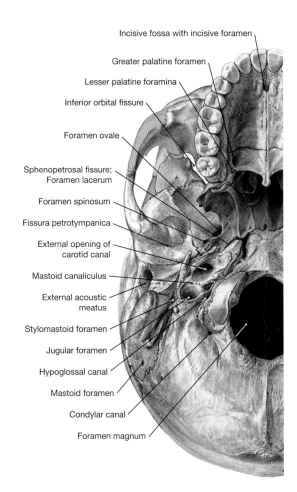

Fig. 8.21 Base of skull, outer aspect, with foramina; inferior view; for color chart see p. VIII.

Incisive fossa with incisive foramen
Greater palatine foramen
Lesser palatine foramina
Inferior orbital fissure
Foramen ovale
Sphenopetrosal fissure; Foramen lacerum
Foramen spinosum
Fissura petrotympanica
External opening of carotid canal
Mastoid canaliculus
External acoustic meatus
Stylomastoid foramen
Jugular foramen
Hypoglossal canal
Mastoid foramen
Condylar canal
Foramen magnum

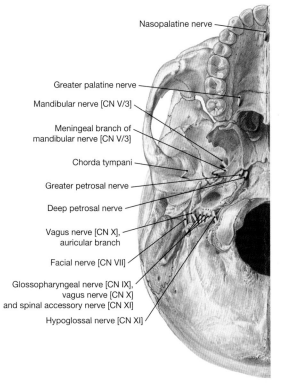

Nasopalatine nerve
Greater palatine nerve
Mandibular nerve [CN V/3]
Meningeal branch of mandibular nerve [CN V/3]
Chorda tympani
Greater petrosal nerve
Deep petrosal nerve
Vagus nerve [CN X], auricular branch
Facial nerve [CN VII]
Glossopharyngeal nerve [CN IX], vagus nerve [CN X] and spinal accessory nerve [CN XI]
Hypoglossal nerve [CN XI]

Fig. 8.22 Nerve exit sites (foramina) of the outer aspect of base of skull; inferior view.

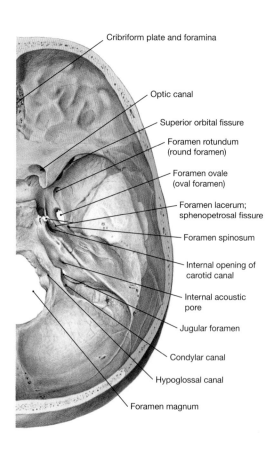

Fig. 8.23 Cranial base, 'inner' aspect, with foramina; superior view; for color chart see p. VIII.

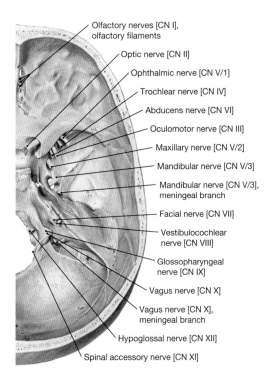

Fig. 8.24 Nerve exit sites at the 'inner' aspect of the cranial base; superior view.

Foramina of the Inner Aspect of the Base of Skull and their Content	
Foramina	**Content**
Cribriform plate	Olfactory nerves [CN I]
	Anterior ethmoid artery (ophthalmic artery)
Optic canal	Optic nerve [CN II]
	Ophthalmic artery (internal carotid artery)
	Meninges; sheath of optic nerve
Superior orbital fissure	**Middle part:**
	Nasociliary nerve (ophthalmic nerve [CN V/1])
	Oculomotor nerve [CN III]
	Abducens nerve [CN VI]
	Lateral part:
	Trochlear nerve [CN IV]
	Frontal nerve (ophthalmic nerve [CN V/1])
	Lacrimal nerve (ophthalmic nerve [CN V/1])
	Orbital branch (medial meningeal artery)
	Superior ophthalmic artery
Foramen rotundum (round foramen)	Maxillary nerve [CN V/2]
Foramen ovale (oval foramen)	Mandibular nerve [CN V/3]
	Plexus venosus of foramen ovale
Foramen spinosum	Meningeal branch (mandibular nerve [CN V/3])
	Medial meningeal artery (maxillary artery)
Sphenopetrosal fissure and foramen lacerum	Lesser petrosal nerve (glossopharyngeal nerve [CN IX])
	Greater petrosal nerve (facial nerve [CN VII])
	Deep petrosal nerve (internal carotid plexus)
Internal opening of carotid canal and carotid canal	Internal carotid artery, petrosal part
	Internal carotid venous plexus
	Internal carotid plexus (sympathetic trunk, superior cervical ganglion)
Internal acoustic meatus and opening (pore)	Facial nerve [CN VII]
	Vestibulocochlear nerve [CN VIII]
	Labyrinthine artery (basilar artery)
	Labyrinthine veins
Jugular foramen	**Anterior part:**
	Inferior petrosal sinus
	Glossopharyngeal nerve [CN IX]
	Posterior part:
	Posterior meningeal artery (ascending pharyngeal artery)
	Sigmoid sinus (superior bulb of jugular vein)
	Vagus nerve [CN X]
	Spinal accessory nerve [CN XI]
	Meningeal branch (vagus nerve [CN X])
Hypoglossal canal	Hypoglossal nerve [CN XII]
	Venous plexus of hypoglossal canal
Condylar canal	Condylar emissary vein
Foramen magnum	Meninges
	Internal vertebral venous plexus (marginal sinus)
	Vertebral arteries (subclavian and anterior spinal arteries)
	Medulla oblongata/spinal cord
	Spinal roots (spinal accessory nerve [CN XI])

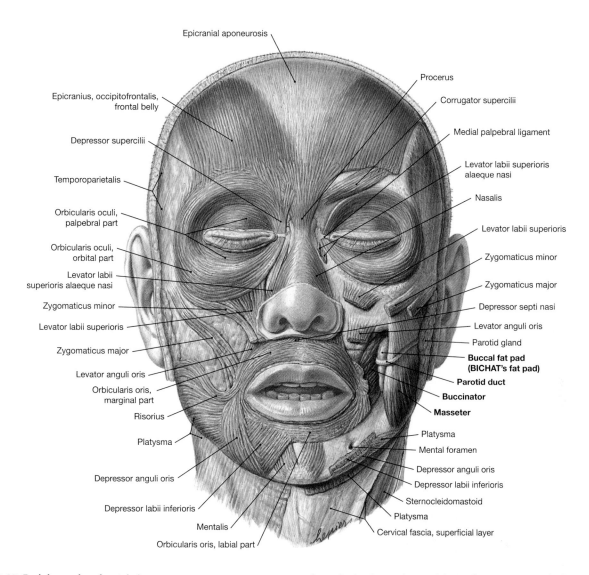

Epicranial aponeurosis

Epicranius, occipitofrontalis, frontal belly

Depressor supercilii

Temporoparietalis

Orbicularis oculi, palpebral part

Orbicularis oculi, orbital part

Levator labii superioris alaeque nasi

Zygomaticus minor

Levator labii superioris

Zygomaticus major

Levator anguli oris

Orbicularis oris, marginal part

Risorius

Platysma

Depressor anguli oris

Depressor labii inferioris

Mentalis

Orbicularis oris, labial part

Procerus

Corrugator supercilii

Medial palpebral ligament

Levator labii superioris alaeque nasi

Nasalis

Levator labii superioris

Zygomaticus minor

Zygomaticus major

Depressor septi nasi

Levator anguli oris

Parotid gland

Buccal fat pad (BICHAT's fat pad)

Parotid duct

Buccinator

Masseter

Platysma

Mental foramen

Depressor anguli oris

Depressor labii inferioris

Sternocleidomastoid

Platysma

Cervical fascia, superficial layer

Fig. 8.25 Facial muscles; frontal view.
With the exception of the buccinator, the facial muscles do not contain a fascia. The parotid duct (STENSON's duct) of the parotid gland passes across the masseter and bends around the muscle's frontal edge in an almost right angle to penetrate the buccinator. A buccal fat pad (BICHAT's fat pad) is located between the masseter and buccinator and contributes to the contour of the region of the cheek.

Clinical Remarks

A **peripheral facial nerve palsy** involves a lesion of the 2nd motor neuron, which can be located anywhere between the nucleus of the facial nerve [CN VII] and its peripheral branches. Most frequent causes are viral infections or nerve injuries during surgery on the parotid gland.

A central (supranuclear) lesion of the facial nerve **(central facial nerve palsy)** results from damage to the 1st motor neuron, mainly caused by bleedings or infarctions in the area of the corticonuclearis tract of the inner capsule on the contralateral side. Contrary to peripheral facial nerve palsy, muscles of the forehead and the orbicularis oculi in the upper eyelid region can still contract on both sides because the temporal branches of the facial nerve contain fibers derived from its contra- and ipsilateral nuclei. However, on the contralateral side the muscles innervated by the zygomatic, buccal, marginal mandibular, and cervical branches are paralysed (so-called lower facial nerve palsy) (➤ Fig. 12.53).

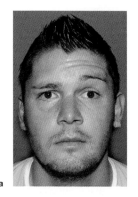
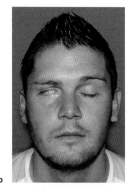

a   **b**

Peripheral facial nerve palsy [CN VII] on the right side. [T620]
a The patient can only raise the eyebrow and wrinkle the forehead on the left side but has lost function of the right occipitofrontalis muscle.
b The eyelid on the injured right side fails to close properly (lagophthalmos). White sclera becomes visible (BELL's phenomenon) because the eyeball automatically turns upwards when the eyelid closes.

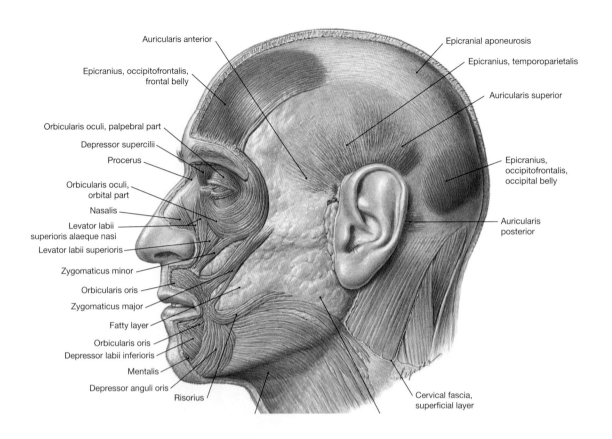

Fig. 8.26 Facial muscles, left side; lateral view.

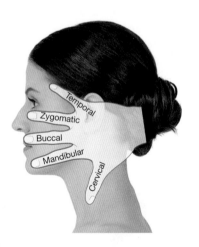

Fig. 8.27 Terminal branches of the facial nerve [CN VII], left side; lateral view. [L126, K340]
The facial nerve [CN VII] creates a nerve plexus within the parotid gland which is divided into a temporofacial and a cervicofacial branch. They generate the terminal branches of the facial nerve: the temporal, zygomatic, buccal, marginal mandibular, and cervical branches. The posterior auricular nerve is another terminal branch of the facial nerve [CN VII] and projects behind the auricle.

Clinical Remarks

The facial nerve [CN VII] forms a nervous plexus within the parotid gland. This plexus is composed of a main superior (temporofacial) and inferior (cervicofacial) branch which project terminal branches (➤ Fig. 8.27). These branches can be damaged by parotid gland tumors and during parotid gland surgery. Surgical incisions at the side of the face should be done along the trajectory of the facial nerve branches to avoid facial nerve paralysis. [E402]

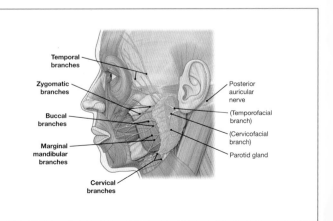

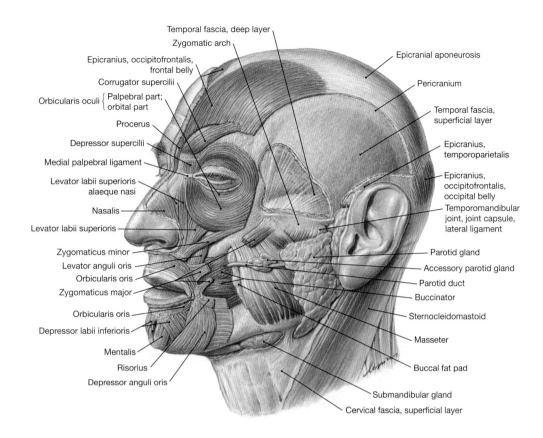

Fig. 8.28 Superficial facial muscles and masticatory muscles; lateral view from an oblique angle.

Temporal fascia, deep layer
Zygomatic arch
Epicranius, occipitofrontalis, frontal belly
Corrugator supercilii
Orbicularis oculi { Palpebral part; orbital part
Procerus
Depressor supercilii
Medial palpebral ligament
Levator labii superioris alaeque nasi
Nasalis
Levator labii superioris
Zygomaticus minor
Levator anguli oris
Orbicularis oris
Zygomaticus major
Orbicularis oris
Depressor labii inferioris
Mentalis
Risorius
Depressor anguli oris

Epicranial aponeurosis
Pericranium
Temporal fascia, superficial layer
Epicranius, temporoparietalis
Epicranius, occipitofrontalis, occipital belly
Temporomandibular joint, joint capsule, lateral ligament
Parotid gland
Accessory parotid gland
Parotid duct
Buccinator
Sternocleidomastoid
Masseter
Buccal fat pad
Submandibular gland
Cervical fascia, superficial layer

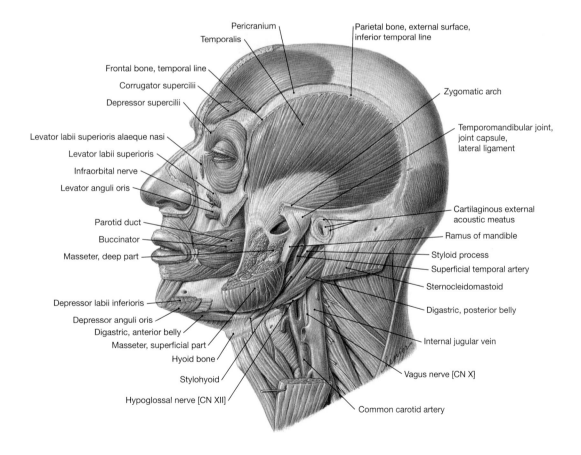

Fig. 8.29 Deep facial muscles and masticatory muscles, left side; lateral view.

Pericranium
Temporalis
Frontal bone, temporal line
Corrugator supercilii
Depressor supercilii
Levator labii superioris alaeque nasi
Levator labii superioris
Infraorbital nerve
Levator anguli oris
Parotid duct
Buccinator
Masseter, deep part
Depressor labii inferioris
Depressor anguli oris
Digastric, anterior belly
Masseter, superficial part
Hyoid bone
Stylohyoid
Hypoglossal nerve [CN XII]

Parietal bone, external surface, inferior temporal line
Zygomatic arch
Temporomandibular joint, joint capsule, lateral ligament
Cartilaginous external acoustic meatus
Ramus of mandible
Styloid process
Superficial temporal artery
Sternocleidomastoid
Digastric, posterior belly
Internal jugular vein
Vagus nerve [CN X]
Common carotid artery

441

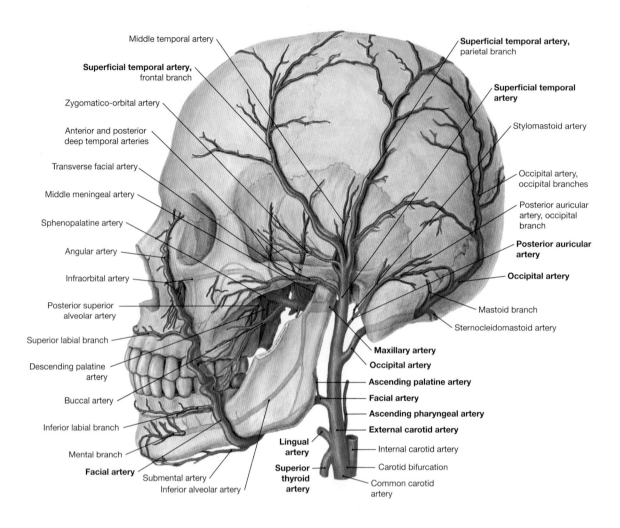

Fig. 8.30 External carotid artery and branches.

Branches of the External Carotid Artery		
1. Superior thyroid artery	*4. Facial artery* • Ascending palatine artery • Submental artery • Inferior labial artery • Superior labial artery • Angular artery	*7. Superficial temporal artery* • Transverse facial artery • Zygomatico-orbital artery • Middle temporal artery • Frontal branch • Parietal branch
2. Ascending pharyngeal artery	*5. Occipital artery* • Mastoid branch • Sternocleidomastoid branches • Occipital branches	*8. Maxillary artery* • Inferior alveolar artery } Mandibular part – Mental branch • Middle meningeal artery • Masseteric artery } Pterygoid part • Deep posterior and anterior temporal arteries • Buccal artery • Posterior superior alveolar artery • Infraorbital artery • Anterior superior alveolar arteries* } Pterygopalatine part • Descending palatine artery • Sphenopalatine artery
3. Lingual artery	*6. Posterior auricular artery* • Stylomastoid artery • Occipital branch	The terminal branches of the maxillary artery are the infraorbital artery, sphenopalatine artery, posterior superior alveolar artery and descending palatine artery.
*not shown		

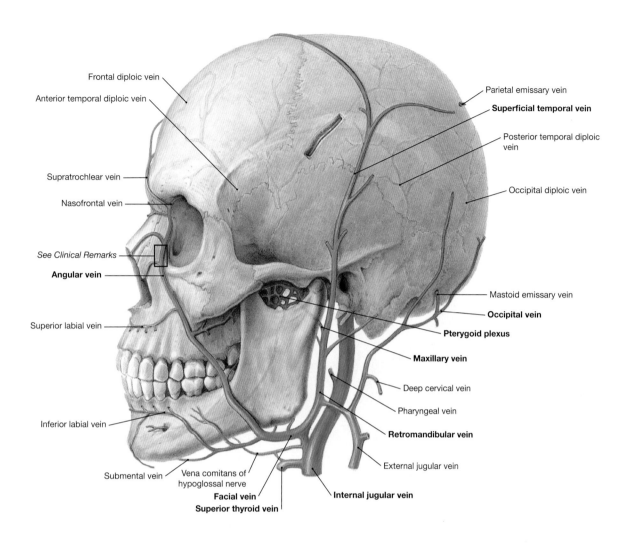

Frontal diploic vein
Anterior temporal diploic vein
Supratrochlear vein
Nasofrontal vein
See Clinical Remarks
Angular vein
Superior labial vein
Inferior labial vein
Submental vein
Vena comitans of hypoglossal nerve
Facial vein
Superior thyroid vein

Parietal emissary vein
Superficial temporal vein
Posterior temporal diploic vein
Occipital diploic vein
Mastoid emissary vein
Occipital vein
Pterygoid plexus
Maxillary vein
Deep cervical vein
Pharyngeal vein
Retromandibular vein
External jugular vein
Internal jugular vein

Fig. 8.31 Internal jugular vein, left side; lateral view.
The internal jugular vein (IJV) starts as a dilated extension of the sigmoid sinus at the cranial base. This biggest vein of the head/neck region drains blood from the skull, brain, face, and parts of the neck. The facial, lingual, pharyngeal, occipital, superior thy-roid, middle thyroid, and emissary veins drain blood from the su-perficial head region into the IJV. From there, the left and right IJV drain into the corresponding brachiocephalic veins which connect to the superior vena cava and right atrium.

Clinical Remarks

Superior ophthalmic vein
Vorticose veins
Cavernous sinus
Pterygoid venous plexus
Inferior rectus
Inferior ophthalmic vein

Supratrochlear vein
Supraorbital vein
Nasofrontal vein
Angular vein
Lateral rectus
Facial vein
(Infraorbital vein)

a   b

The pulse of the jugular vein (jugular pulse) provides useful in-formation on the venous blood pressure. The wave-like charac-teristic of the jugular pulse reflects the function of the right heart.
In rare cases, inflammations of the facial area can spread via the valve-free angular vein to intraorbital veins (superior oph-thalmic vein) and from there to the intracranial cavernous sinus. This can result in a life-threatening phlebitis or venous sinus thrombosis.
a The angular vein locates within the danger triangle of the face.
b The angular vein connects to the cavernosus sinus via orbital veins. a [K340], b [E460]

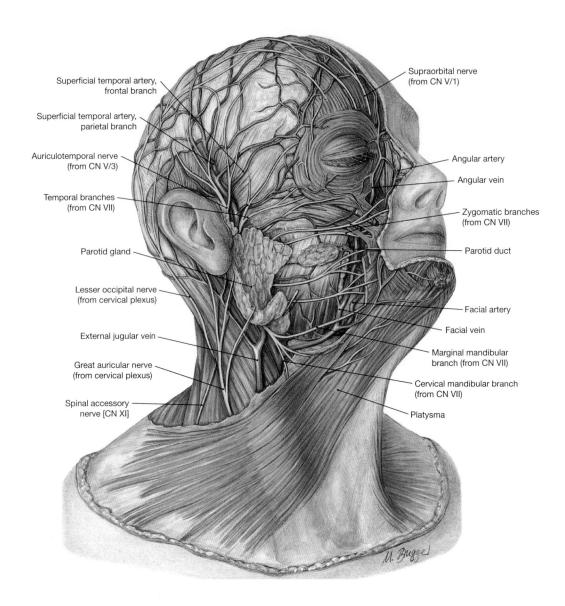

Superficial temporal artery, frontal branch

Superficial temporal artery, parietal branch

Auriculotemporal nerve (from CN V/3)

Temporal branches (from CN VII)

Parotid gland

Lesser occipital nerve (from cervical plexus)

External jugular vein

Great auricular nerve (from cervical plexus)

Spinal accessory nerve [CN XI]

Supraorbital nerve (from CN V/1)

Angular artery

Angular vein

Zygomatic branches (from CN VII)

Parotid duct

Facial artery

Facial vein

Marginal mandibular branch (from CN VII)

Cervical mandibular branch (from CN VII)

Platysma

Fig. 8.32 Vessels and nerves of the head, lateral superficial regions, right side; lateral view.
The branches of the facial artery and the parietal and frontal branches of the superficial temporal artery are the superficial arteries of the face and originate from the external carotid artery. Identically named veins drain the blood into the external jugular vein. The terminal superficial motor branches of the facial nerve [CN VII]

radiate from the intraparotid plexus located within the parotid gland (see also ➤ Fig. 8.27, ➤ Fig. 8.108). The supraorbital and auriculotemporal nerves are branches of the trigeminal nerve (ophtalmic [CN V/1] and mandibular [CN V/3], respectively) and provide sensory innervation to the head. Neck and occipital region receive sensory innervation from the cervical plexus.

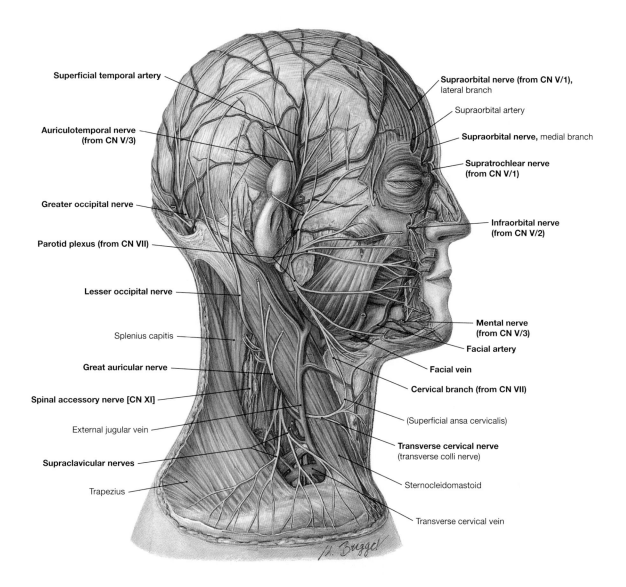

Superficial temporal artery

Auriculotemporal nerve (from CN V/3)

Greater occipital nerve

Parotid plexus (from CN VII)

Lesser occipital nerve

Splenius capitis

Great auricular nerve

Spinal accessory nerve [CN XI]

External jugular vein

Supraclavicular nerves

Trapezius

Supraorbital nerve (from CN V/1), lateral branch

Supraorbital artery

Supraorbital nerve, medial branch

Supratrochlear nerve (from CN V/1)

Infraorbital nerve (from CN V/2)

Mental nerve (from CN V/3)

Facial artery

Facial vein

Cervical branch (from CN VII)

(Superficial ansa cervicalis)

Transverse cervical nerve (transverse colli nerve)

Sternocleidomastoid

Transverse cervical vein

Fig. 8.33 Vessels and nerves of the head, lateral deep regions, right side; lateral view.
Facial muscles and the superficial part of the parotid gland were removed to expose the facial artery, the origin of the terminal branches of the facial nerve [CN VII] derived from the infraparotid plexus, and the terminal sensory branches of the trigeminal nerve [CN V] which originate from its three parts:
- Supraorbital and supratrochlear nerves – ophthalmic nerve [CN V/1]
- Infraorbital nerve – maxillary nerve [CN V/2]
- Mental nerve – mandibular nerve [CN V/3]

On the posterior side of the sternocleidomastoid muscle, four sensory cervical branches exit at the ERB's point. These are the
- transverse cervical,
- great auricular,
- lesser occipital, and
- supraclavicular nerves.

The transverse cervical nerve receives motor fibers via the cervical branches of the facial nerve [CN VII] for the innervation of more distal parts of the platysma. The spinal accessory nerve [CN XI] courses from the posterior border of the sternocleidomastoid to the anterior border of the trapezius.

Clinical Remarks

The four major types of headache include vascular, tension, traction, and inflammatory. Migraine represents the most common type of vascular headache. Tension headache involves the tightening or tensing of facial and neck muscles. Traction and inflammatory headaches are usually warning signs indicating other underlying disorders. This concerns headaches caused by ruptured blood vessels (aneurysms), infection (infectious meningitis), or headaches resulting from diseases of the teeth, ear, sinuses, neck or spine.

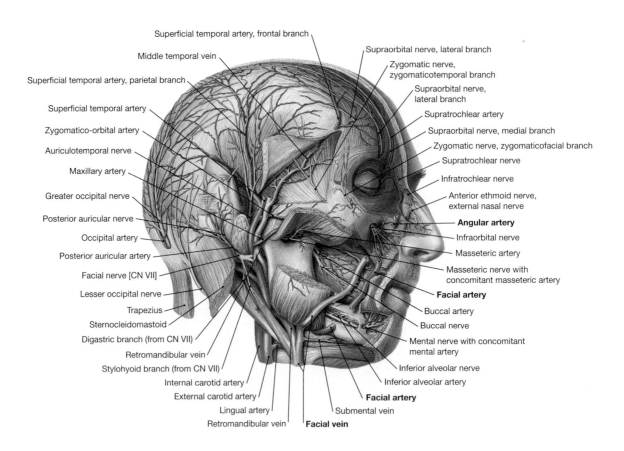

Fig. 8.34 Vessels and nerves of the head, lateral deep regions, right side; lateral view.

The masseter was cut and folded backwards to demonstrate its neurovascular bundle located on the back of this muscle (masseteric nerve – branch of the mandibular nerve [CN V/3]; masseteric artery – branch of the maxillary artery). These supplying structures reach the masseter through the mandibular notch. The facial artery continues as angular artery below the eye and into the orbit where it forms anastomoses with branches of the ophthalmic artery.

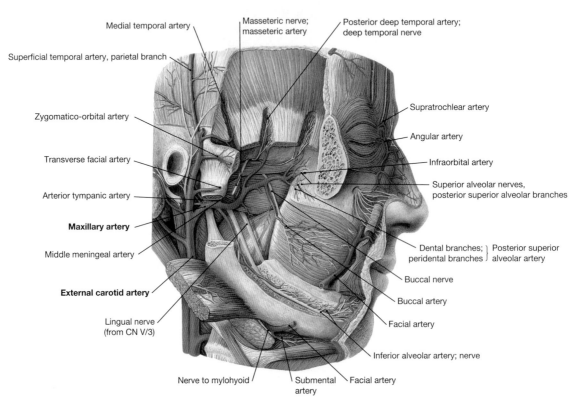

Fig. 8.35 Arteries and nerves of the head, lateral deep regions, right side; lateral view.

In most cases, the maxillary artery courses behind the ramus of mandible. Only rarely does the artery run laterally to the ramus. The maxillary artery continues through the masticatory muscles, supplies these muscles with blood, and provides branches to the buccinator and the mandible. Its terminal branches reach the orbit, nose, maxilla, and palate.

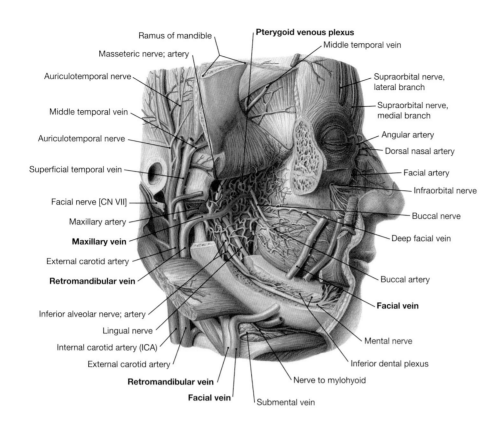

Ramus of mandible
Masseteric nerve; artery
Auriculotemporal nerve
Middle temporal vein
Auriculotemporal nerve
Superficial temporal vein
Facial nerve [CN VII]
Maxillary artery
Maxillary vein
External carotid artery
Retromandibular vein
Inferior alveolar nerve; artery
Lingual nerve
Internal carotid artery (ICA)
External carotid artery
Retromandibular vein
Facial vein
Submental vein
Nerve to mylohyoid
Inferior dental plexus
Mental nerve
Facial vein
Buccal artery
Deep facial vein
Buccal nerve
Infraorbital nerve
Facial artery
Dorsal nasal artery
Angular artery
Supraorbital nerve, medial branch
Supraorbital nerve, lateral branch
Middle temporal vein
Pterygoid venous plexus

Fig. 8.36 Vessels and nerves of the head, lateral deep regions, right side; lateral view.
The pterygoid venous plexus collects blood in the region of the masticatory muscles and drains mainly into the maxillary vein. The pterygoid venous plexus also connects with the facial vein and the cavernous sinus via the deep facial vein and the inferior ophthalmic vein, respectively.

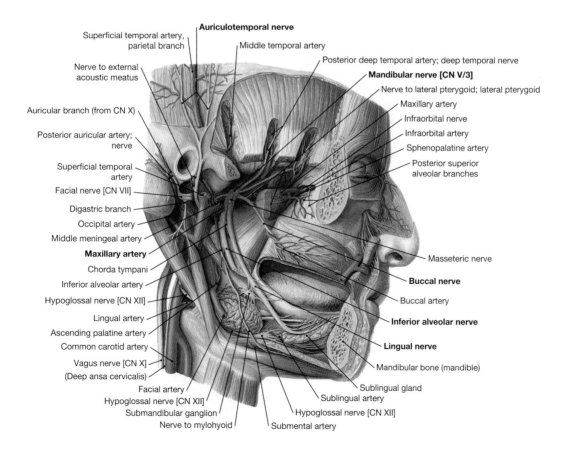

Superficial temporal artery, parietal branch
Nerve to external acoustic meatus
Auricular branch (from CN X)
Posterior auricular artery; nerve
Superficial temporal artery
Facial nerve [CN VII]
Digastric branch
Occipital artery
Middle meningeal artery
Maxillary artery
Chorda tympani
Inferior alveolar artery
Hypoglossal nerve [CN XII]
Lingual artery
Ascending palatine artery
Common carotid artery
Vagus nerve [CN X]
(Deep ansa cervicalis)
Facial artery
Hypoglossal nerve [CN XII]
Submandibular ganglion
Nerve to mylohyoid
Auriculotemporal nerve
Middle temporal artery
Posterior deep temporal artery; deep temporal nerve
Mandibular nerve [CN V/3]
Nerve to lateral pterygoid; lateral pterygoid
Maxillary artery
Infraorbital nerve
Infraorbital artery
Sphenopalatine artery
Posterior superior alveolar branches
Masseteric nerve
Buccal nerve
Buccal artery
Inferior alveolar nerve
Lingual nerve
Mandibular bone (mandible)
Sublingual gland
Sublingual artery
Hypoglossal nerve [CN XII]
Submental artery

Fig. 8.37 Arteries and nerves of the head, lateral deepest regions, right side; lateral view.

Upon exiting the oval foramen, the mandibular nerve [CN V/3] divides into the lingual, inferior alveolar, buccal, and auriculotemporal nerves and sends branches to the masticatory muscles.

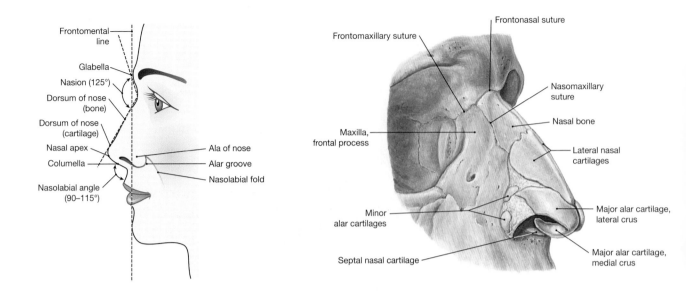

Fig. 8.38 Shape of the nose; angles and reference points. [L126]

Fig. 8.39 Nasal skeleton; frontal view from the right side. Connective tissue attaches the cartilaginous nasal skeleton to the piriform aperture which is formed by the nasal and maxillary bones.

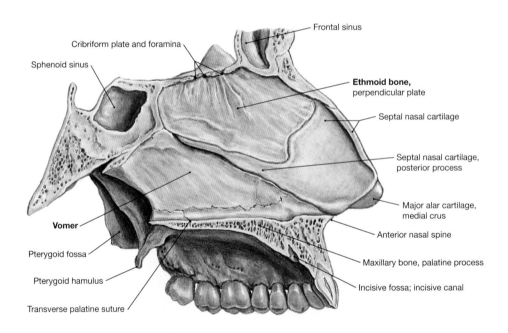

Fig. 8.40 Nasal septum; view from the right side.
The septal nasal cartilage forms the frontal part of the nasal septum and extends as a long cartilaginous posterior process between the bony parts of the nasal septum (top), composed of the perpendicular plate of the ethmoid, and the vomer (bottom).

Clinical Remarks

Fractures or cracks of the nasal bone (arrow in the X-ray) and of the supporting cartilaginous nasal framework are among the most frequent fractures of the facial region and can present as closed or open fractures. Open fractures involve bony parts piercing through the skin and soft tissue. The nasal septum and nasal conchae can also be affected. Fractures of the nose typically occur as a result of violent physical impacts, car accidents, martial arts, boxing, and a variety of team sports.
a [E467], b [G741]

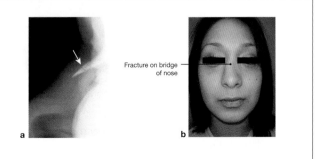

Fracture on bridge of nose

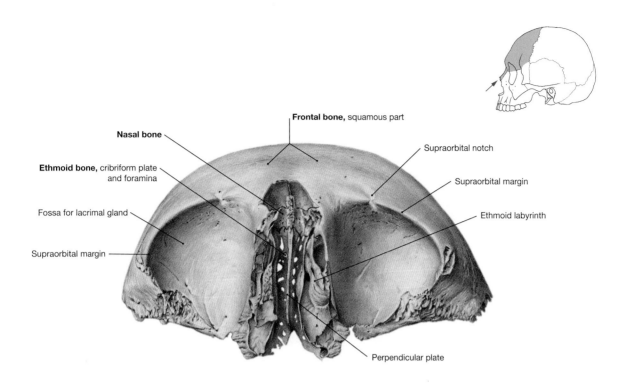

Frontal bone, squamous part

Nasal bone

Supraorbital notch

Ethmoid bone, cribriform plate and foramina

Supraorbital margin

Fossa for lacrimal gland

Ethmoid labyrinth

Supraorbital margin

Perpendicular plate

Fig. 8.41 Ethmoid bone, frontal bone, and nasal bones; inferior view; for color chart see p. VIII.

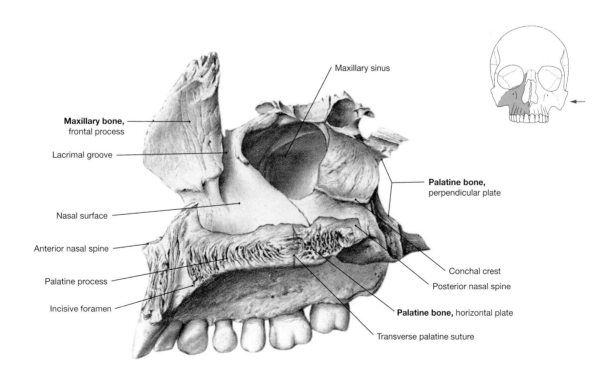

Maxillary sinus

Maxillary bone, frontal process

Lacrimal groove

Palatine bone, perpendicular plate

Nasal surface

Anterior nasal spine

Palatine process

Conchal crest

Posterior nasal spine

Incisive foramen

Palatine bone, horizontal plate

Transverse palatine suture

Fig. 8.42 Anterolateral bony demarcation of the nasal cavity; upper jaw, maxilla, and palatine bone, right side; medial view into the maxillary sinus; for color chart see p. VIII.

449

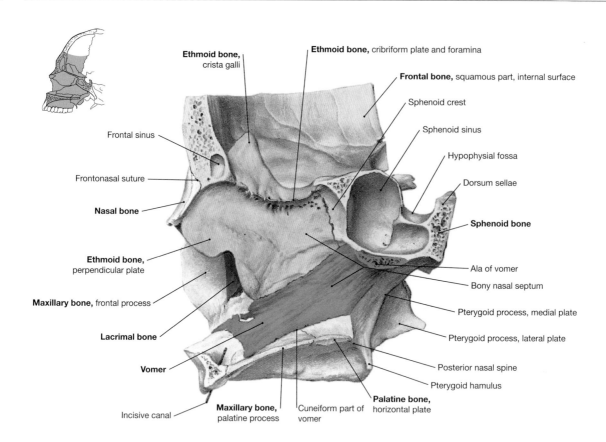

Fig. 8.43 Bony nasal septum; lateral view; for color chart see p. VIII. The perpendicular plate of the ethmoid bone and the vomer create the bony septum of the nose. The perforated cribriform plate is the roof of the nasal cavity and part of the floor of the anterior cranial fossa. The perpendicular plate of the ethmoid bone divides the bony labyrinth of the ethmoid bone into a right part and a left part. The flat and trapezoid vomer forms the largest part of the bony nasal septum.

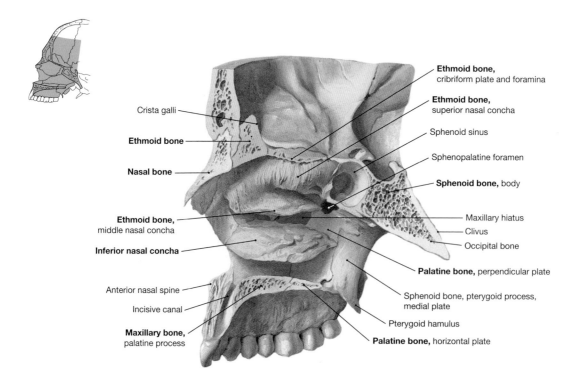

Fig. 8.44 Lateral wall of the nasal cavity, right side; view from the left side; for color chart see p. VIII.
The view onto the lateral wall of the nasal cavity reveals the roof created by the cribriform plate of the ethmoid bone which also forms the upper (superior) and middle nasal conchae. The upper nasal passage (superior nasal meatus) is located between these two nasal conchae. Located below is the inferior nasal concha which is a separate bone.

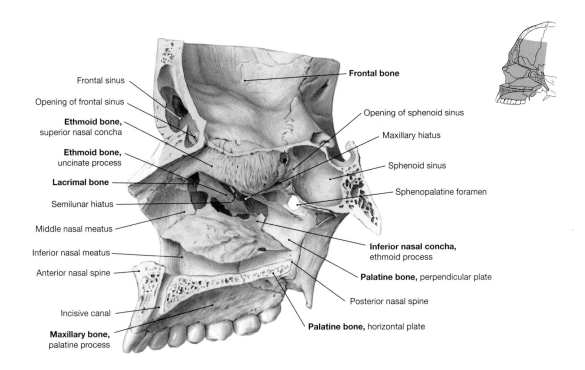

Frontal sinus
Opening of frontal sinus
Ethmoid bone, superior nasal concha
Ethmoid bone, uncinate process
Lacrimal bone
Semilunar hiatus
Middle nasal meatus
Inferior nasal meatus
Anterior nasal spine
Incisive canal
Maxillary bone, palatine process

Frontal bone
Opening of sphenoid sinus
Maxillary hiatus
Sphenoid sinus
Sphenopalatine foramen
Inferior nasal concha, ethmoid process
Palatine bone, perpendicular plate
Posterior nasal spine
Palatine bone, horizontal plate

Fig. 8.45 Lateral wall of the nasal cavity, right side; medial view; after removal of the middle nasal concha; for color chart see p. VIII. Beneath the middle nasal concha the uncinate process of the ethmoid bone incompletely closes the medial wall of the maxillary sinus, with many openings remaining above and below the unci- nate process. One forms the maxillary hiatus. The inferior nasal concha is anchored to the maxilla, the palatine and lacrimal bones and divides the wall of the nasal cavity in a middle nasal meatus and an inferior nasal passage (inferior nasal meatus) located above and below the inferior nasal concha, respectively.

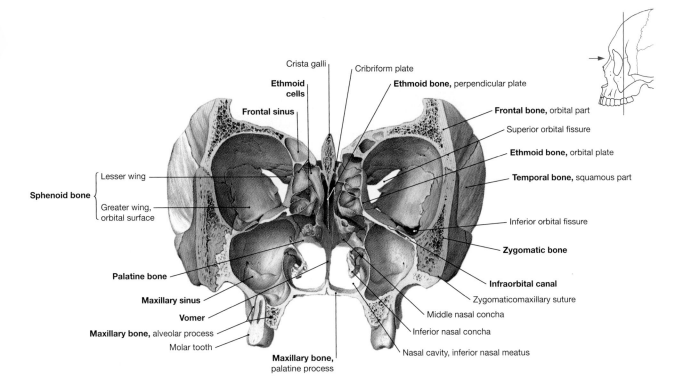

Crista galli
Ethmoid cells
Frontal sinus
Cribriform plate
Ethmoid bone, perpendicular plate
Frontal bone, orbital part
Superior orbital fissure
Ethmoid bone, orbital plate
Temporal bone, squamous part
Inferior orbital fissure
Zygomatic bone
Infraorbital canal
Zygomaticomaxillary suture
Middle nasal concha
Inferior nasal concha
Nasal cavity, inferior nasal meatus

Sphenoid bone { Lesser wing / Greater wing, orbital surface
Palatine bone
Maxillary sinus
Vomer
Maxillary bone, alveolar process
Molar tooth
Maxillary bone, palatine process

Fig. 8.46 Viscerocranium; frontal section at the level of the two orbits; frontal view; for color chart see p. VIII.
The ethmoid bone contains the anterior and posterior ethmoid cells. The perpendicular plate separates the bony labyrinth of the ethmoid bone into a right and a left half and forms the upper part of the bony nasal septum. The lateral walls of the ethmoid cells consist of a thin orbital plate, known as *lamina papyracea,* constitu- ing the major part of the thin medial wall of the orbit. The maxillary sinus is located directly below the orbit. The infraorbital canal is located in its roof which constitutes the floor of the orbit. The cribri- form plate is located below the roof of the orbit.

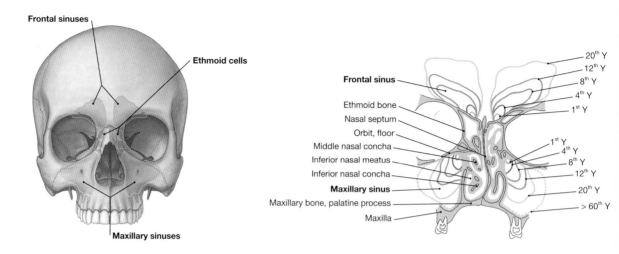

Fig. 8.47 Projection of the paranasal sinuses onto the skull; frontal view. [E402]
The sphenoid sinuses is located deeper within the skull posterior to the ethmoid cells and is not depicted here.

Fig. 8.48 Development of the maxillary and frontal sinuses. Y: year of life.
At about five years of age, the developing frontal sinus reaches the upper margin of the orbit.

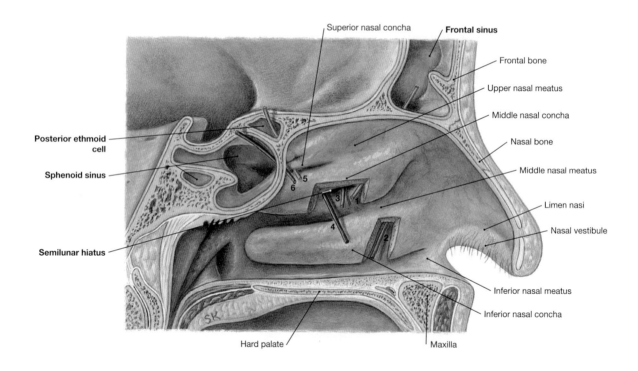

Fig. 8.49 Lateral nasal wall, right side; view from the left side; nasal conchae separated from the wall at the base.
Beneath the middle nasal concha, the frontal (1), anterior ethmoid (3) and maxillary sinuses (4) drain through the hiatus semilunaris

into the middle nasal passage. The nasolacrimal duct opens into the lower nasal passage via the lacrimal fold (HASNER's valve; 2). The posterior ethmoid (5) and sphenoid sinuses (6) drain posterior to the superior nasal concha.

Clinical Remarks

During neurosurgical operations, the nasal access route to the brain involves penetrating the sphenoid sinus. Extensive pneumatization of the sphenoid sinus into the sphenoid bone increases the risk of injury to the internal carotid artery (internal carotid tubercle) and the optic nerve [CN II] (optic nerve tuber-

cle) because of their close proximity to the lateral wall of the sinus. A unilateral inflammation of the maxillary sinus can have an odontogenic origin (odontogenic maxillary sinusitis). This commonly involves an inflammation of the second premolar or the first molar (➤ Fig. 8.51, ➤ Fig. 8.72a).

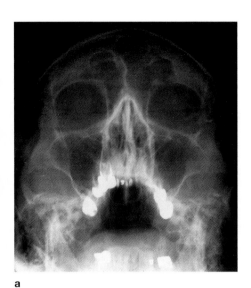

a

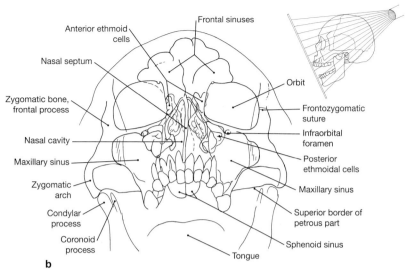

b

Fig. 8.50a and b Paranasal sinuses; radiograph of the skull with opened mouth in posteroanterior (P/A) beam projection.

Anterior ethmoid cells

Frontal sinuses

Nasal septum

Zygomatic bone, frontal process

Nasal cavity

Maxillary sinus

Zygomatic arch

Condylar process

Coronoid process

Tongue

Orbit

Frontozygomatic suture

Infraorbital foramen

Posterior ethmoidal cells

Maxillary sinus

Superior border of petrous part

Sphenoid sinus

Clinical Remarks

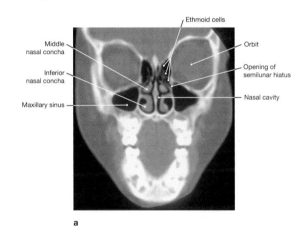

a

Middle nasal concha

Inferior nasal concha

Maxillary sinus

Ethmoid cells

Orbit

Opening of semilunar hiatus

Nasal cavity

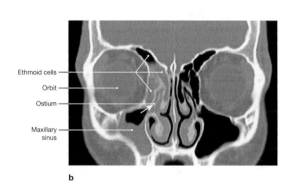

b

Ethmoid cells

Orbit

Ostium

Maxillary sinus

Computed tomography (CT), coronal section of the paranasal sinuses. a [E528], b [E871]
a Normal condition shows air-filled (black) ethmoid maxillary and nasal cavity

b Chronic sinusitis (grey shaded) on the right side, involving the right ethmoid cells, right maxillary sinus, and (swollen) nasal mucosa on the right side. The white arrow points at the congested opening (ostium) between the maxillary sinus and nasal cavity.

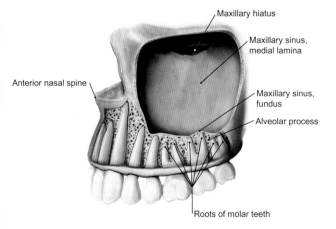

Maxillary hiatus

Maxillary sinus, medial lamina

Anterior nasal spine

Maxillary sinus, fundus

Alveolar process

Roots of molar teeth

Fig. 8.51 Close topographical relationship between the roots of molar teeth and the maxillary sinus. [L266]

Clinical Remarks

The roots of the upper molar teeth may be separated from the maxillary sinus by only a thin bony layer. This can be the reason for toothache during sinus infection. Accidental opening of the maxillary sinus can occur during tooth extractions. Blowing of the nose results in air escaping through the extraction hole. Once the hole is closed, patients should not blow their nose for a week, keep their mouth open if sneezing, avoid vigorous mouth rinsing, and be on a soft diet for several days.

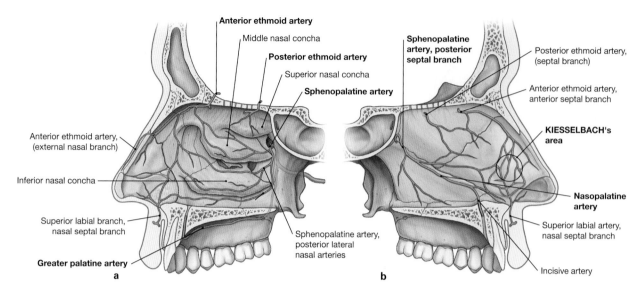

Fig. 8.52a and b Arteries of the nasal cavity, views onto lateral wall of the right nasal cavity **(a)**; and the nasal septum of the right nasal cavity **(b)**. [E402]
Anterior and posterior ethmoid arteries from the ophthalmic artery reach the lateral wall of the nose and the nasal septum by penetrating through the anterior and posterior segments of the ethmoid bone. The sphenopalatine artery, a terminal branch of the maxillary artery, reaches the nasal cavity through the sphenopalatine foramen. There are anastomoses to the facial artery with arterial vessels of the lip. At the nasal septum, the sphenopalatine artery becomes the nasopalatine artery and passes through the incisive canal to reach the oral cavity. Here, it forms anastomoses with the greater palatine artery. The KIESSELBACH's area is an arteriovenous plexus supplied by the nasopalatine artery and the anterior and posterior ethmoid arteries.

Clinical Remarks

- Nosebleed (*epistaxis*) most frequently originates from the KIESSELBACH's area at the nasal septum which has the highest density of subepithelial arteriovenous plexus.
- Basilar skull fractures involving the cribriform plate can lead to the rupture of the anterior and/or posterior ethmoid arteries, resulting in arterial nosebleeds.

- Posterior nasal bleeds originate from the sphenopalatine artery and can cause substantial bleeding that requires posterior packing to stop the bleeding. When a nasal balloon tamponade is unsuccessful in stopping severe bleedings, the sphenopalatine artery has to be ligated.

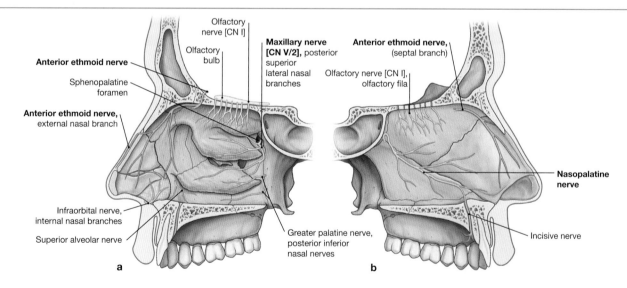

Fig. 8.53a and b Innervation of the nasal cavity; views onto the lateral wall of the right nasal cavity **(a)**; and the nasal septum of the right nasal cavity **(b)**. [E402]
Sensory innervation of the nasal mucosa is provided by branches of the trigeminal nerve [CN V]: ophthalmic nerve [CN V/1] → anterior ethmoid nerve; and maxillary nerve [CN V/2] → nasal branches, nasopalatine nerve. The olfactory nerve [CN I] innervates the olfactory area only.

Clinical Remarks

A fracture of the nasal roof (cribriform plate of ethmoid bone) frequently results in the rupture of the dura mater. This can cause cerebrospinal fluid (CSF) to leak from the nose as clear transparent fluid (rhinorrhea). The diagnosis of CSF is confirmed by the detection of high glucose using glucose test strips. A surgical intervention is mandatory to prevent an ascending infection to the brain.

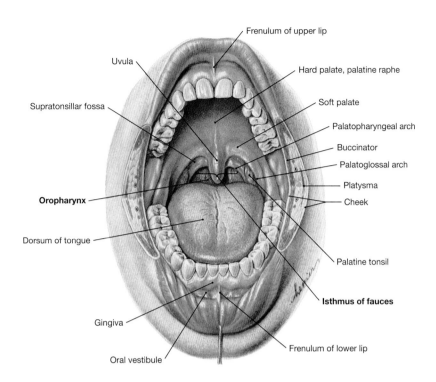

Fig. 8.54 Oral cavity; anterior view; mouth open.
The oral opening represents the entrance to the digestive tract and the oral cavity. With the occlusion of teeth, a space behind the last molar tooth on each side (retromolar space) allows access to the oral cavity by using the flexible tube. In the region of the oropharyngeal isthmus (isthmus of fauces or isthmus faucium) the oral cavity becomes the oral part of the pharynx (oropharynx).

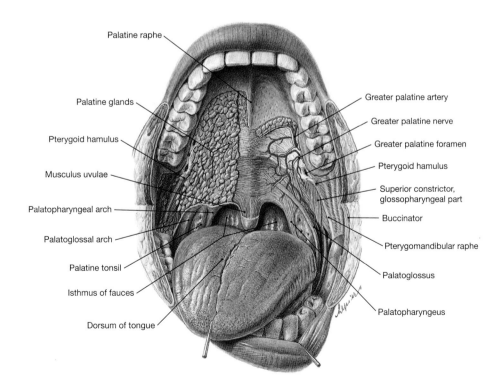

Fig. 8.55 Oral cavity; anterior view; mouth open.
The excretory ducts of numerous smaller salivary glands and those of the three paired large salivary glands all drain into the oral vestibule and the cavity proper. The body of the tongue fills large parts of the oral cavity.

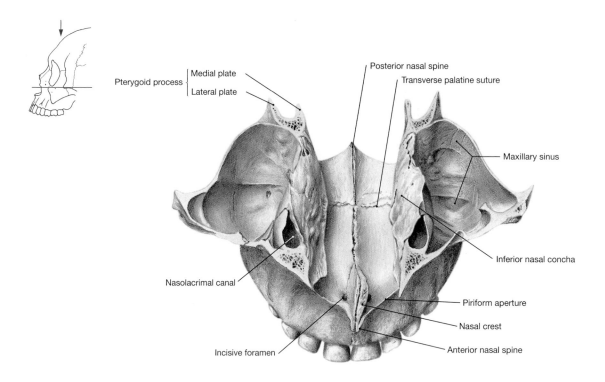

Fig. 8.56 Hard palate; maxillary sinus, and inferior nasal concha; superior view; for color chart see p. VIII.
The hard palate represents a horizontal bony plate created by the maxilla and the palatine bone. It separates the oral front from the nasal cavity. The incisive foramen creates a connection between the oral and the nasal cavity.

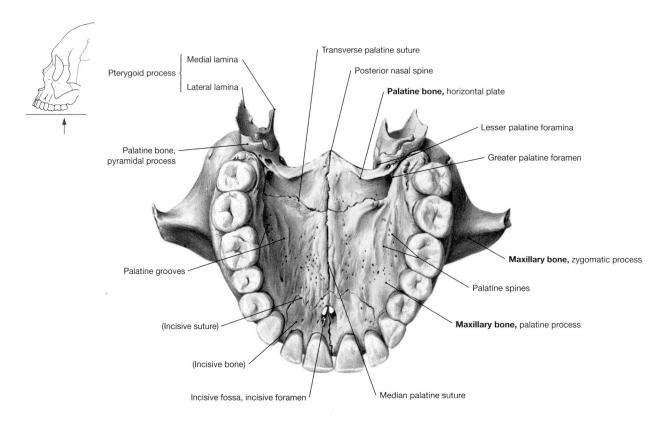

Fig. 8.57 Hard palate; inferior view; for color chart see p. VIII.
The hard palate forms the roof of the mouth and the floor of the nasal cavity. The teeth are attached to the two maxillary alveolar arches. In the midline, the palatine processes are connected by the median palatine suture and dorsally they are connected with the palatine bones through the transverse palatine suture. Located behind the incisors is the incisive canal. Near the posterior margin to both sides of the hard palate are the greater and lesser palatine foramina.

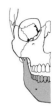

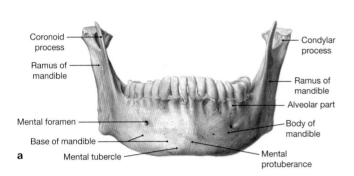

Coronoid process

Ramus of mandible

Mental foramen

Base of mandible

Mental tubercle

Condylar process

Ramus of mandible

Alveolar part

Body of mandible

Mental protuberance

a

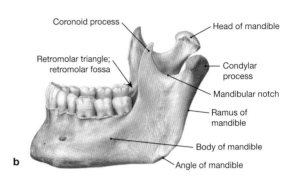

Coronoid process

Retromolar triangle; retromolar fossa

Head of mandible

Condylar process

Mandibular notch

Ramus of mandible

Body of mandible

Angle of mandible

b

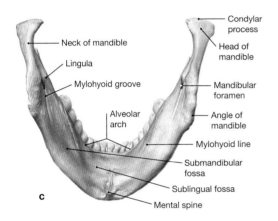

Neck of mandible

Lingula

Mylohyoid groove

Alveolar arch

Condylar process

Head of mandible

Mandibular foramen

Angle of mandible

Mylohyoid line

Submandibular fossa

Sublingual fossa

Mental spine

c

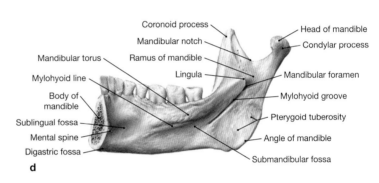

Coronoid process

Mandibular notch

Mandibular torus

Mylohyoid line

Body of mandible

Sublingual fossa

Mental spine

Digastric fossa

Ramus of mandible

Lingula

Head of mandible

Condylar process

Mandibular foramen

Mylohyoid groove

Pterygoid tuberosity

Angle of mandible

Submandibular fossa

d

Fig. 8.58a to d Lower jaw, mandible; frontal view (a), lateral view **(b)**, inferior view **(c)**, inner aspect of the mandibular arch **(d)**.
The mandible consists of a body and two rami. Each ramus divides into a coronoid process and a condylar process. The body of mandible is composed of the base and the alveolar part. The head of mandible sits on top of the condylar process. On the inside of the angle of mandible there are the pterygoid tuberosity and imprints of glands and muscles of the oral cavity. The mandibular foramen is located at the inside of the ramus of mandible. In front thereof, the linea mylohyoidea creates a bony crest which serves as an attachment for the mylohyoid muscle and demarcates the level of the floor of the mouth.

Clinical Remarks

Fractures of the mandible are common. As shown in the panoramic radiograph, the U-shaped structure of the mandible explains the various types of mandibular fractures, in particular at the level of the canines and the third molar teeth (arrows). Extravasated blood at the fracture site collects in the loose tissue of the floor of the mouth and causes small spotted bleeding under the skin (ecchymoses), a typical sign of mandibular fractures.
[E393]

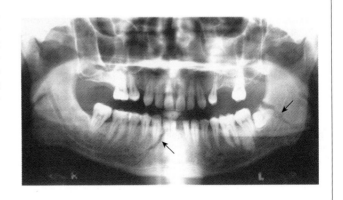

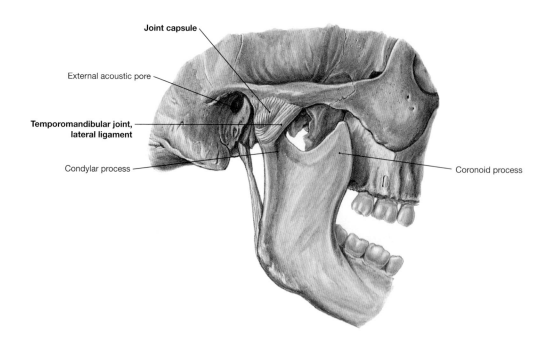

Fig. 8.59 Temporomandibular joint, right side; lateral view.
A wide cone-shaped joint capsule stretching from the temporal bone to the condylar process surrounds the mandibular joint. Extending from the zygomatic arch, the frontal and lateral parts of the lateral ligament reinforce the joint capsule. The lateral ligament assists in guiding joint movements and inhibits posterior movements of the mandibular head. When bite force is applied, the lateral ligament also stabilizes the condyle.

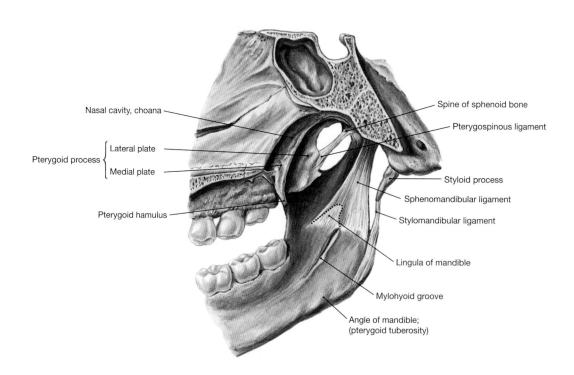

Fig. 8.60 Stylomandibular ligament and sphenomandibular ligament, right side; medial view.
Both ligaments act on the movement of the temporomandibular joint but are not associated with the joint capsule. The pterygo- spinous ligament has no relationship to the temporomandibular joint but has a stabilizing function.

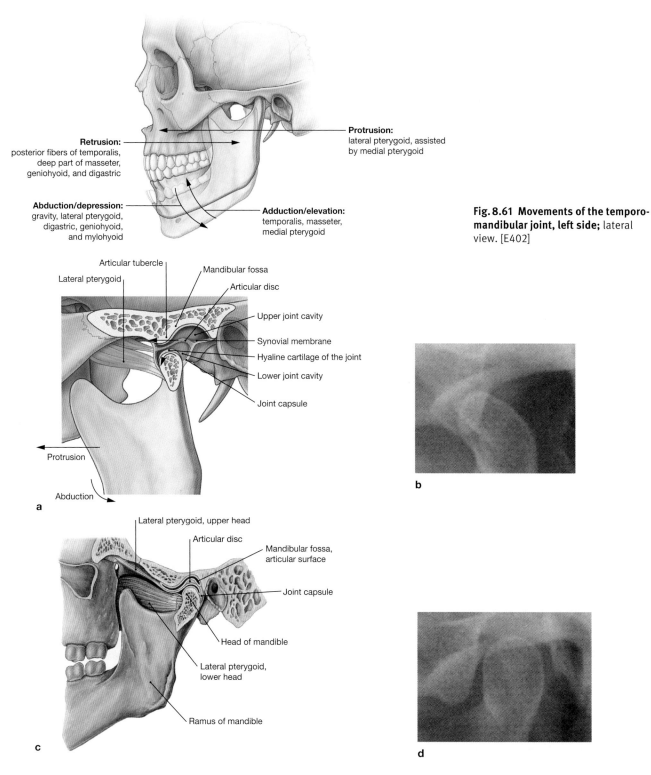

Retrusion:
posterior fibers of temporalis,
deep part of masseter,
geniohyoid, and digastric

Protrusion:
lateral pterygoid, assisted
by medial pterygoid

Abduction/depression:
gravity, lateral pterygoid,
digastric, geniohyoid,
and mylohyoid

Adduction/elevation:
temporalis, masseter,
medial pterygoid

Fig. 8.61 Movements of the temporomandibular joint, left side; lateral view. [E402]

Articular tubercle

Mandibular fossa

Lateral pterygoid

Articular disc

Upper joint cavity

Synovial membrane

Hyaline cartilage of the joint

Lower joint cavity

Joint capsule

Protrusion

Abduction

a

b

Lateral pterygoid, upper head

Articular disc

Mandibular fossa,
articular surface

Joint capsule

Head of mandible

Lateral pterygoid,
lower head

Ramus of mandible

c

d

Fig. 8.62a to d Temporomandibular joint, left side; sagittal section; lateral view; mouth open (**a** and **b**), mouth closed (**c** and **d**).
a, c [E402], b, d [G742]

b and **d** Radiographs of the temporomandibular joint.
An articular disc completely divides the temporomandibular joint into two separate chambers (*dithalamic joint*).

Clinical Remarks

The anterior jaw dislocation is the most frequent type of dislocation, but posterior lateral or superior dislocations of the lower jaw also occur unilaterally or bilaterally. External force to the lower jaw commonly contributes to mandibular dislocations. [L127]

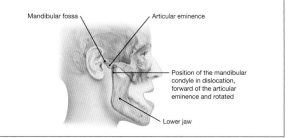

Mandibular fossa

Articular eminence

Position of the mandibular
condyle in dislocation,
forward of the articular
eminence and rotated

Lower jaw

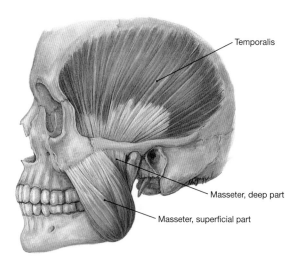

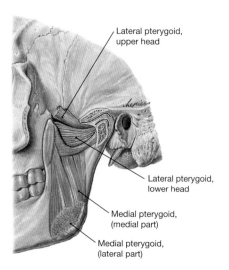

Fig. 8.63 Masseter and temporalis muscles, left side; lateral view.

Fig. 8.64 Temporomandibular joint, medial and lateral pterygoid muscles, left side; lateral view.

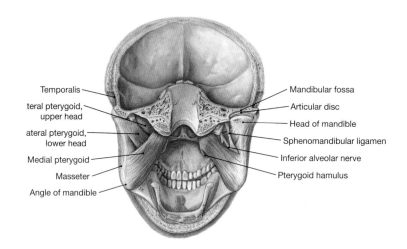

Fig. 8.65 Masticatory muscles; frontal section at the level of the temporomandibular joint; posterior view.

The bilateral insertions of the masseter and medial pterygoid muscles at the angle of mandible suspend the lower jaw like a swing.

Muscle	Attachments (P = proximal, D = distal)	Action/Function	Innervation
Mastication Muscles			
Masseter	**P:** Zygomatic arch of temporal bone **D:** Ramus of mandible	Jaw closure	
Temporalis	**P:** Temporal fossa **D:** Coronoid process of mandible		
Medial pterygoid	**P:** Superficial head: maxillary bone; deep head: lateral pterygoid plate of sphenoid bone **D:** Both parts converge at ramus of mandible near the angle of mandible		
Lateral pterygoid	**P:** Superior head: greater wing of sphenoid bone; inferior head: lateral pterygoid plate of sphenoid bone **D:** Both parts converge at neck of mandible	Jaw opener	Motor branches of mandibular nerve [CN V/3]
Other Muscles			
Mylohyoid	**P:** Mylohyoid line of mandible **D:** Raphe and body of hyoid bone	Elevates hyoid bone, floor of oral cavity, and tongue	
Tensor veli palatini	**P:** Scaphoid fossa, spine of sphenoid bone, cartilage of auditory tube **D:** Tendon loops around hamulus of medial pterygoid plate and inserts into aponeurosis of soft palate	Tenses soft palate	
Tensor tympani	**P:** Auditory tube, greater wing of sphenoid bone, osseus canal of auditory tube **D:** Neck of malleus	Tenses tympanic membrane	

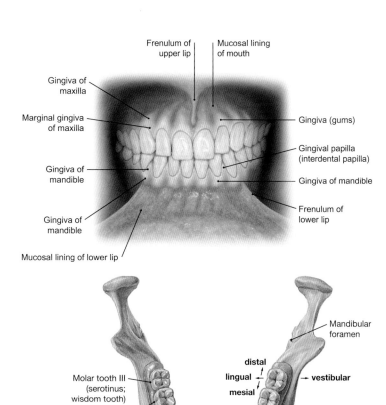

Frenulum of upper lip

Mucosal lining of mouth

Gingiva of maxilla

Marginal gingiva of maxilla

Gingiva (gums)

Gingival papilla (interdental papilla)

Gingiva of mandible

Gingiva of mandible

Gingiva of mandible

Frenulum of lower lip

Mucosal lining of lower lip

Fig. 8.66 Gingiva and oral mucosa. [L127]

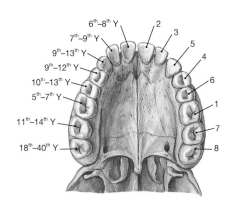

6th–8th Y
7th–9th Y
9th–13th Y
9th–12th Y
10th–13th Y
5th–7th Y
11th–14th Y
18th–40th Y

2
3
5
4
6
1
7
8

Fig. 8.67 Upper dental arch with permanent teeth; left side: average time of tooth eruption in years (Y); right side: sequence of tooth eruption.

Mandibular foramen

Molar tooth III (serotinus; wisdom tooth)

distal
lingual
mesial
→ vestibular

Molar tooth II

Molar tooth I

Mucosal lining of mouth, gingiva

Premolar tooth II

Premolar tooth I

Mental foramen

Canine tooth

Lateral incisor tooth

Medial incisor tooth

Fig. 8.68 Lower dental arch.

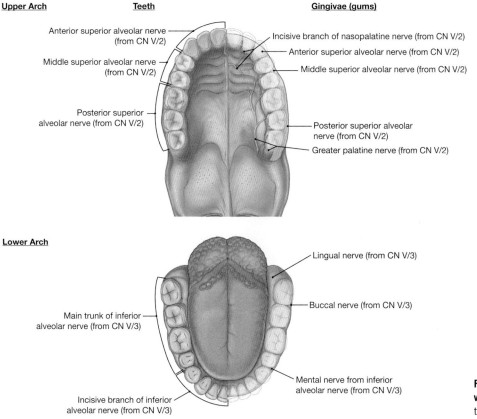

Upper Arch

Teeth

Gingivae (gums)

Anterior superior alveolar nerve (from CN V/2)

Incisive branch of nasopalatine nerve (from CN V/2)

Anterior superior alveolar nerve (from CN V/2)

Middle superior alveolar nerve (from CN V/2)

Middle superior alveolar nerve (from CN V/2)

Posterior superior alveolar nerve (from CN V/2)

Posterior superior alveolar nerve (from CN V/2)

Greater palatine nerve (from CN V/2)

Lower Arch

Lingual nerve (from CN V/3)

Buccal nerve (from CN V/3)

Main trunk of inferior alveolar nerve (from CN V/3)

Mental nerve from inferior alveolar nerve (from CN V/3)

Incisive branch of inferior alveolar nerve (from CN V/3)

Fig. 8.69 Upper and lower arch, with permanent teeth; innervation of teeth and gingiva. [E460]

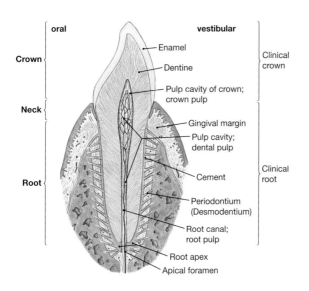

Fig. 8.70 **Structure of a tooth and support system;** incisor.
Each tooth consists of a crown, a cervical part, and a root. The crown of a tooth is covered with enamel.
At the root of a tooth, blood vessels and nerves access the pulp cavity through the apical foramen and the root canal. Collectively, the cementum, desmodontium, alveolar bone, and parts of the gingiva are referred to as the parodontium.

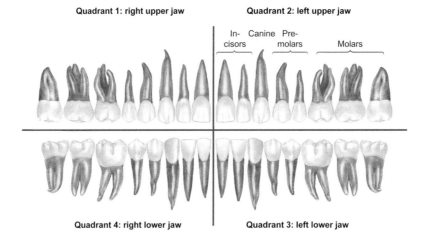

Fig. 8.71 **Permanent teeth;** vestibular view. Human dentition is *heterodont;* the teeth have characteristic shapes as incisors, canines, premolars, and molars.

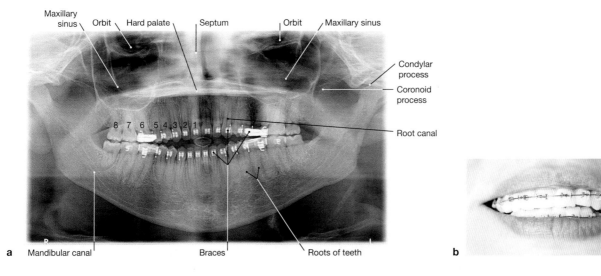

Fig. 8.72a and b **Upper jaw, maxilla, and lower jaw, mandible, of an adult;** panoramic radiography **(a)** and photography **(b).** Orthodontists use dental braces as a temporary aid to align and straighten teeth for a correct bite and improved dental health.
a [P497], b [J787]

1: incisor I; 2: incisor II; 3: canine; 4: premolar I; 5: premolar II; 6: molar I; 7: molar II; 8: molar III (wisdom tooth)

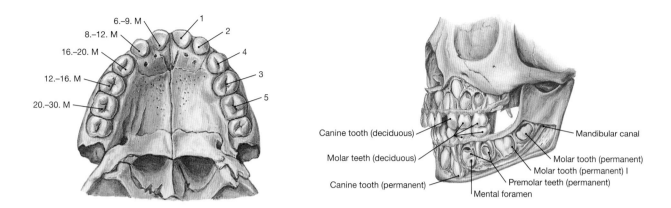

Fig. 8.73 Upper jaw, maxilla, with deciduous teeth (milk teeth) and the first permanent tooth; left side: average time of tooth eruption in months (M); right side: sequence of tooth eruption.

Fig. 8.74 Upper jaw, maxilla, and lower jaw, mandible, of a five year old child; deciduous teeth and primordium of the later permanent teeth.

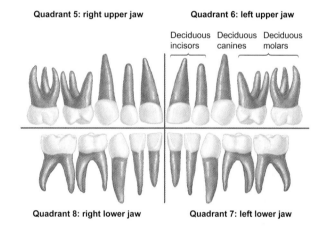

Fig. 8.75 Deciduous (milk) teeth; vestibular view. Human dentition is *diphyodont;* there are two consecutive dentitions, known as deciduous and permanent teeth (dentition).

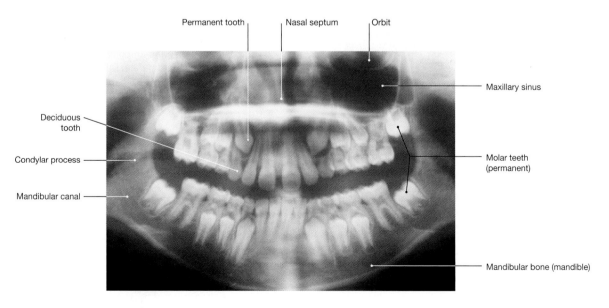

Fig. 8.76 Upper jaw, maxilla, and lower jaw, mandible, of a child; panoramic radiograph. [G743-001]

Permanent teeth develop beneath the deciduous teeth and eventually dislodge and replace the milk teeth.

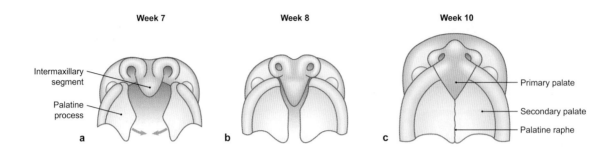

Week 7   Week 8   Week 10

a   **b**   **c**

- Intermaxillary segment
- Palatine process
- Primary palate
- Secondary palate
- Palatine raphe

Fig. 8.77a to c Development of the palate, separation of the nasal and oral cavities. [E838]
The merging of the two medial nasal prominences creates the median palatine process (intermaxillary segment) which is the structural basis for the future philtrum of the upper lip, a part of the maxilla with the four incisors, and the future primary palate. The primary palate extends into the anterior part of the oronasal cavity.

The two opposing palatine processes of maxilla form the major part of the definitive bony (hard) palate. By week 7, the tongue moves into a caudal position, the opposing palatine processes assume a horizontal position, start closing the gap between nose and mouth, and finally merge in the midline as secondary palate. In the anterior part, these palatine processes fuse with the primary palate.

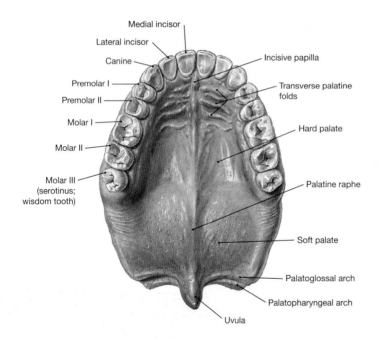

Labels:
- Medial incisor
- Lateral incisor
- Canine
- Premolar I
- Premolar II
- Molar I
- Molar II
- Molar III (serotinus; wisdom tooth)
- Incisive papilla
- Transverse palatine folds
- Hard palate
- Palatine raphe
- Soft palate
- Palatoglossal arch
- Palatopharyngeal arch
- Uvula

Fig. 8.78 Hard palate and soft palate; inferior view.
The hard palate contributes to the phonation of consonants and serves as an abutment for the tongue. Flat transverse palatine mucosal folds (palatine rugae) to both sides of the midline help grind and pin down pieces of food against the hard palate. During swallowing, the flexible soft palate folds back onto the posterior pharyngeal wall blocking off the nasopharynx.

Clinical Remarks

Cleft palate is the result of developmental defects in palate formation. Cleft palate presents as a unilateral (**b** to **e**) or bilateral (**f** to **i**) defect that affects the upper lip, hard and/or soft palate and uvula. Purple line(s)/area show the extent of the cleft palate. Normal condition is shown in **a.**
[L231]

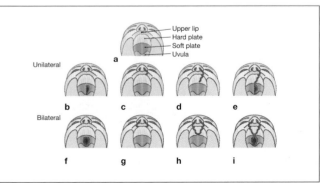

Unilateral   Bilateral

- Upper lip
- Hard plate
- Soft plate
- Uvula

a
b   **c**   **d**   **e**
f   **g**   **h**   **i**

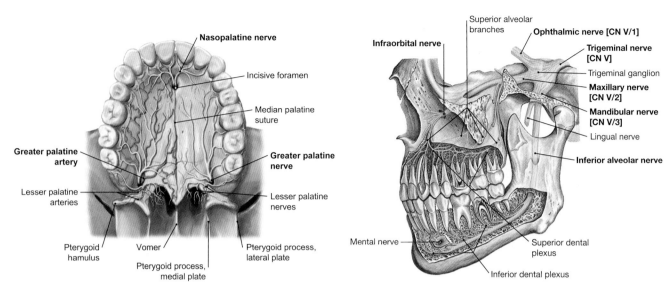

Fig. 8.79 Neurovascular supply to the hard palate. [L266]
The incisive foraminal branches of the nasopalatine nerve [CN V/1] and the branches of the greater and lesser palatine nerves innervate the gingiva of the hard palate.

Fig. 8.80 Innervation of the teeth by branches of the infraorbital and inferior alveolar nerves which originate from the maxillary [CN V/2] and mandibular [CN V/3] branches of the trigeminal nerve [CN V], respectively.

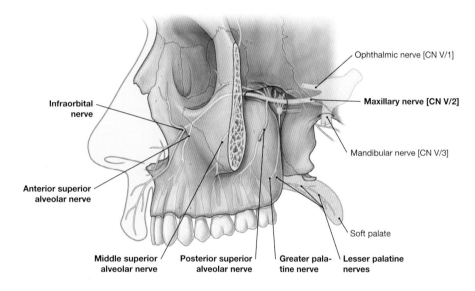

Fig. 8.81 Maxillary nerve [CN V/2], left side; lateral view. [E402]
The maxillary nerve [CN V/2] supplies sensory innervation for the teeth of the upper jaw, gingiva, and upper lips. The greater palatine nerve [from CN V/2] innervates the posterior hard palate and posterior lingual gingiva.

Clinical Remarks

Different sites of local infiltrative anesthesia target different branches of the infraorbital nerve [from CN V/2] and the inferior alveolar nerve [from CN V/3]. Numbness of parts of the gingiva, lips, chin, and tongue occurs since all terminal branches of the infraorbital nerve and inferior alveolar nerve are also anesthetized. Block of the inferior alveolar nerve also anesthetizes the lingual nerve. This sensory block extends to the ipsilateral half of the tongue, with the exception of the tip of tongue.
Abbrevations (in alphabetical order):
c = Canine
i = Incisor
m = Molar
p = Premolar
ASA = Anterior superior alveolar block
B = Buccal block
GP = Greater palatine block
IA = Inferior alveolar block
IN = Incisive block
IO = Infraorbital block
MSA = Middle superior alveolar block
NP = Nasopalatine block
PSA = Posterior superior alveolar block

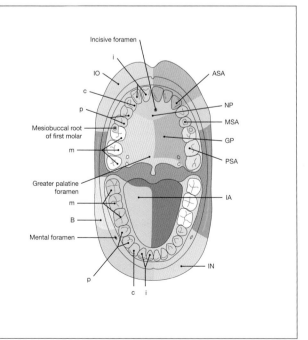

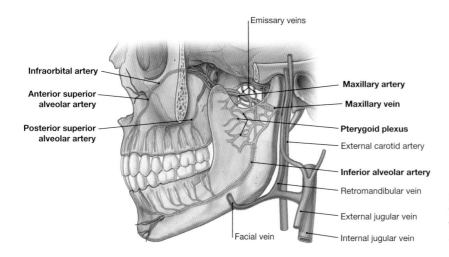

Fig. 8.82 **Blood supply to the teeth** through the superior and inferior alveolar arteries and veins. They originate from the maxillary artery and vein, respectively. [E402]

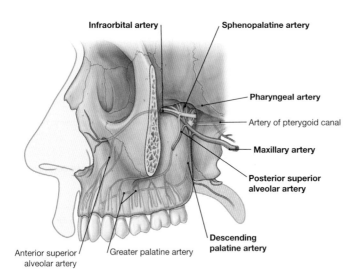

Fig. 8.83 **Maxillary artery in the pterygopalatine fossa, left side;** lateral view. [E402]
Within the pterygopalatine fossa, the maxillary artery divides into its five terminal branches:
- Infraorbital
- Sphenopalatine
- Posterior superior alveolar
- Descending palatine and
- Pharyngeal arteries

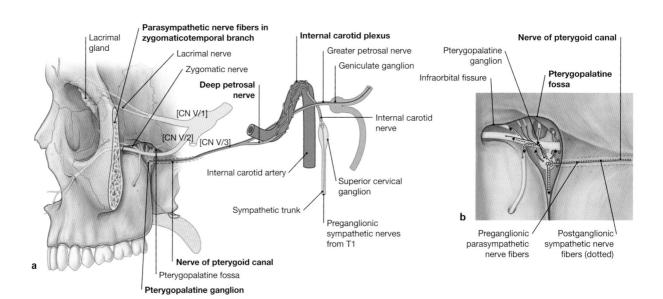

Fig. 8.84a and b **Nerve of pterygoid canal, left side;** lateral view; overview **(a)**; and topography in the pterygopalatine fossa **(b)**. [E402]
Parasympathetic fibers of the facial nerve [CN VII] form the greater petrosal nerve and synapse in the pterygopalatine ganglion. Postganglionic neurons innervate the lacrimal, nasal, and oropharyn-geal glands. Postganglionic sympathetic fibers from the internal carotid plexus enter the pterygopalatine ganglion as the deep petrosal nerve but pass through the parasympathetic ganglion without synapsing to provide sympathetic innervation to the lacri-mal, nasal, and oropharyngeal glands.

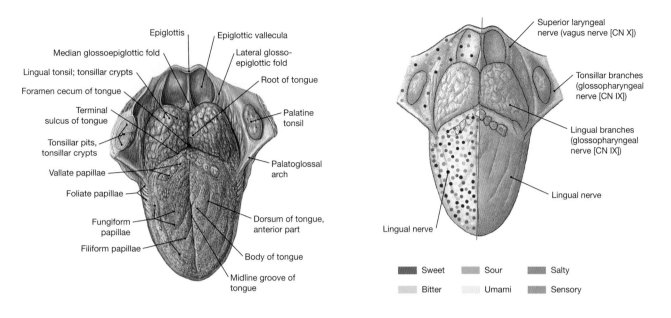

Fig. 8.85 **Tongue;** superior view.

Fig. 8.86 **Innervation and taste qualities of the dorsum of tongue.**

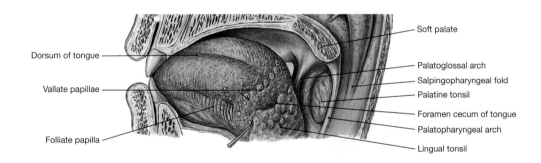

Fig. 8.87 **Tongue;** lateroposterior view.

The lingual tonsil is part of the WALDEYER's ring, as is the palatine tonsil located between the two palatine arches (palatoglossal arch and palatopharyngeal arch).

Taste sensations in the anterior two-thirds of the tongue are conveyed by branches of the facial nerve [CN VII] through the chorda tympani to the upper part of the solitary tract in the brainstem. The perikarya of these sensory nerve fibers are located within the geniculate ganglion. Taste sensations by the posterior third of the tongue are projected to the lower part of the solitary tract by sensory nerve fibers from the glossopharyngeal [CN IX] and vagus nerves [CN X]. The perikarya of these nerve fibers reside in the inferior ganglion of both cranial nerves (CN IX and CN X).

Innervation of the Tongue		
Nerve	**Quality**	**Innervation**
Lingual nerve (branch of CN V/3)	Sensory	Anterior two-thirds of tongue
Glossopharyngeal nerve [CN IX]	Sensory, taste	• Posterior third of tongue • Vallate and foliate papillae of the tongue
Vagus nerve [CN X] Superior laryngeal nerve (branch of CN X)	Sensory, taste	Transition to epiglottis
Chorda tympani (intermedius nerve, as branch of facial nerve [CN VII])	Taste, parasympathetic	• Fungiform papillae • Submandibular gland, sublingual gland, small salivary glands of the oral mucosa
Hypoglossal nerve [CN XII]	Motor	All muscles of the tongue, except palatoglossus muscle
Pharyngeal plexus (branches of CN IX and CN X)	Motor	Palatoglossus muscle

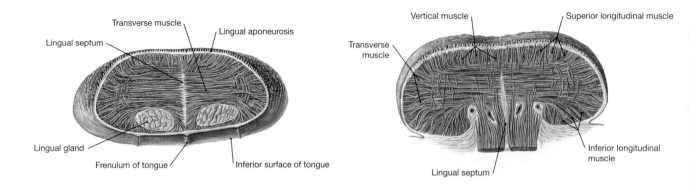

Fig. 8.88 Intrinsic muscles of the tongue; cross-section at the level of the tip of tongue.

Fig. 8.89 Intrinsic muscles of the tongue; cross-section at the level of the middle part.

Intrinsic Muscles of the Tongue *Innervation: [CN XII]*			
Muscles	**Proximal**	**Distal**	**Function**
Superior longitudinal	Lingual aponeurosis	Lingual aponeurosis	Downward vaulting
Transverse	Lingual aponeurosis	Lingual septum	Stretching
Vertical	Lingual aponeurosis, superior site of the tongue	Lingual aponeurosis, inferior site of the tongue	Flattening and furrowing

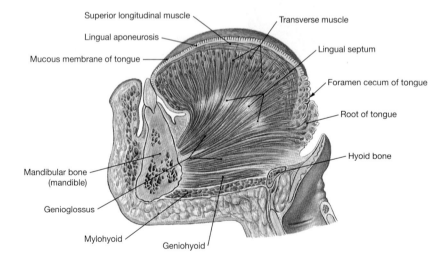

Fig. 8.90 Muscles of the tongue; median section.
Extrinsic muscles of the tongue alter its position, while the intrinsic muscles change the shape of the tongue. Most muscles of the tongue insert at the lingual aponeurosis.

Clinical Remarks

Lesions of the hypoglossal nerve [CN XII] on the right side (see image) cause the protruding tongue to deviate to the affected side. Muscular atrophy occurs on the ipsilateral side of the hypoglossal nerve palsy, sometimes accompanied with wrinkling of the mucosal surface on the paralyzed side.
[G435]

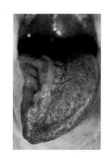

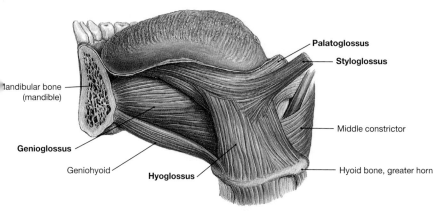

Fig. 8.91 Extrinsic muscles of the tongue, left side; lateral view.
The extrinsic muscles of the tongue are the genioglossus, hyoglossus, styloglossus, and palatoglossus.

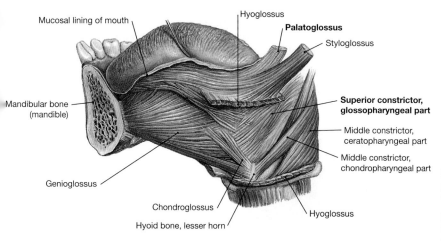

Fig. 8.92 Extrinsic muscles of the tongue, left side; lateral view.
The palatoglossus muscle and the glosso-pharyngeal part of the superior constrictor muscle project into the posterior aspect of the tongue.

Extrinsic Muscles of the Tongue			
Muscle	**Attachments (P = proximal, D = distal)**	**Action/Function**	**Innervation**
Genioglossus	**P:** Mental spine **D:** Body of tongue	Anterior movement, sticking out of tongue	[CN XII]
Styloglossus	**P:** Styloid process **D:** Margin of tongue to apex of tongue	Retraction of tongue	[CN XII]
Hyoglossus	**P:** • Greater horn of hyoid bone (ceratoglossus) • Lesser horn of hyoid bone (chondroglossus) **D:** Body of tongue	Rotation of tongue and flattening of posterior tongue region	[CN XII]
Palatoglossus	**P:** Posterior part of transverse muscle **D:** Palatine aponeurosis	Closure of isthmus of fauces, lowering the soft palate	[CN IX and CN X]; pharyngeal branch

Clinical Remarks

The protrusion of the tongue is facilitated by the genioglossus muscle. In a deep coma, the genioglossus becomes flaccid. In the supine position, the tongue slides back into the pharynx and can suffocate a patient. Unconscious patients should always be placed in the lateral recovery position.

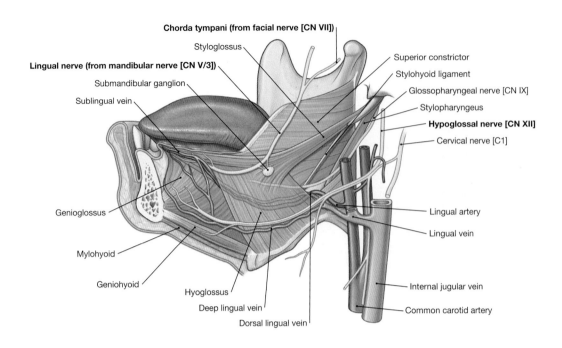

Fig. 8.93 Blood vessels and nerves of the tongue; lateral view; mandibular arch removed. [E460]

The lingual artery from the external carotid artery provides the arterial blood supply of the tongue. The lingual vein runs adjacent to the hyoglossus and drains into the internal jugular vein. The hypo-

glossal nerve [CN XII] provides motor innervation to the tongue (for sensory innervation of the tongue ➤ Fig. 8.86 and ➤ table 'Innervation of the Tongue', p. 467). The submandibular ganglion provides postganglionic parasympathetic nerve fibers for the submandibular, sublingual and small anterior lingual glands (➤ Fig. 8.109).

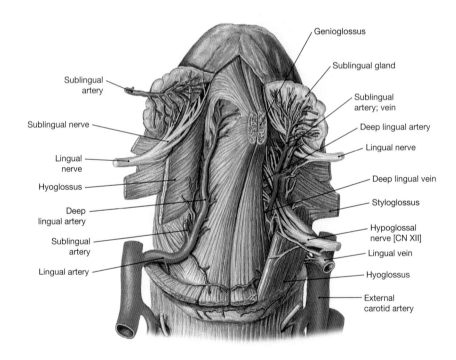

Fig. 8.94 Blood vessels and nerves of the tongue; inferior view.

The deep lingual artery mainly supplies the muscles of the middle and anterior parts of the tongue. The sublingual artery supplies the sublingual gland and the floor of mouth.

Clinical Remarks

A subepithelial venous plexus is located in the mucous membrane lining the underside of the tongue. This facilitates quick resorption of medication when placed underneath the tongue.

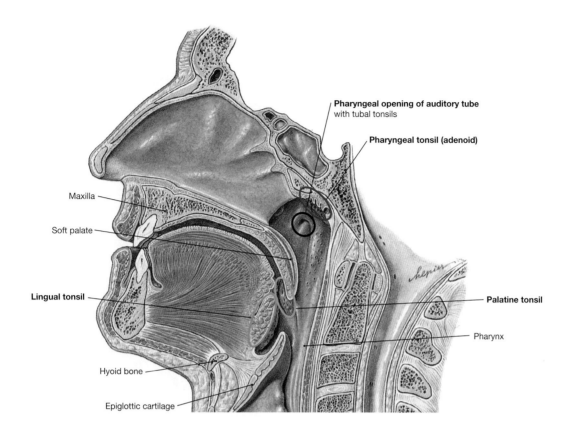

Pharyngeal opening of auditory tube
with tubal tonsils

Pharyngeal tonsil (adenoid)

Maxilla

Soft palate

Lingual tonsil

Palatine tonsil

Pharynx

Hyoid bone

Epiglottic cartilage

Fig. 8.95 Oral cavity and pharynx; midsagittal section.
Location of the tonsils that constitute the lymphatic WALDEYER's ring as part of the mucosa-associated lymphatic tissue (MALT). The pharyngeal tonsil (red circle) is located at the roof of the nasopharynx and is also referred to as adenoid. The lymph of this unpaired tonsil drains into deep cervical and retropharyngeal lymph nodes. The paired tubal tonsils (black circle) are located around the pha-

ryngeal opening of the auditory tube. When enlarged, they can impair middle ear function. The paired palatine tonsil (blue circle) and the unpaired lingual tonsil (green circle) at the oropharyngeal junction complete the lymphatic WALDEYER's ring. Lymph from these tonsils drains into deep cervical and jugulodigastric lymph nodes. All tonsils release lymphocytes into the pharynx.

Clinical Remarks

Recurrent infection of the palatine tonsils is an indication for their surgical removal (tonsillectomy), one of the most frequently conducted surgical interventions concerning ear, nose and throat (ENT). Postoperative bleedings can occur up to three weeks after surgical interventions (in rare cases even later) and can be a serious complication.

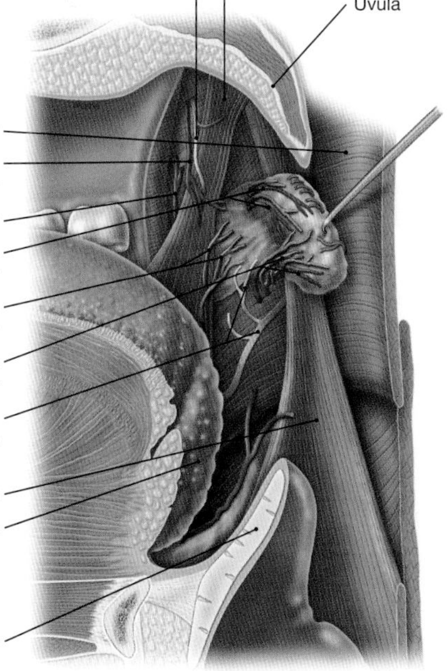

Tonsillar branches
from lesser palatine nerves

Palatoglossus

Uvula

Superior constrictor

Pharyngeal branch
from ascending palatine artery

Ascending pharyngeal artery

Tonsillar branches
from ascending pharyngeal artery

Dorsal lingual branches
from lingual artery

Tonsillar branches
from ascending pharyngeal artery

Glossopharyngeal nerve [CN IX];
tonsillar branches

Palatopharyngeus

Dorsum of tongue

Epiglottis

**Fig. 8.96 Blood and nerve supply of the palatine tonsil,
right side;** medial view. [L238]

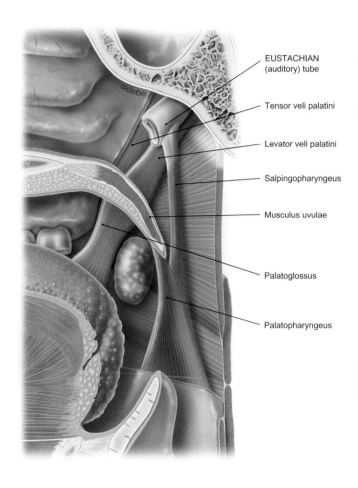

EUSTACHIAN (auditory) tube

Tensor veli palatini

Levator veli palatini

Salpingopharyngeus

Musculus uvulae

Palatoglossus

Palatopharyngeus

Fig. 8.97 Muscles of the soft palate and oropharyngeal region, right side; medial view. [L238]

Muscles and Functions of the Soft Palate			
Muscle	**Attachments (P = proximal, D = distal)**	**Action/Function**	**Innervation**
Levator veli palatini	**P:** Inferior surface of petrosal part of temporal bone and cartilage of auditory tube **D:** Palatine aponeurosis	Tenses and elevates soft palate; opens auditory tube; closes nasopharyngeal space together with superior constrictor muscle; bulges out lateral wall of the nasopharynx	Pharyngeal plexus (branches of CN IX and X; sometimes also CN VII)
Tensor veli palatini	**P:** Medial plate of pterygoid process, greater wing of sphenoid bone, membranous part of auditory tube; bends around the pterygoid hamulus **D:** Palatine aponeurosis	Tenses soft palate, opens auditory tube, changes shape of soft palate to assist in vocalization	Nerve to tensor veli palatini [CN V/3]
Salpingopharyngeus	**P:** Medial cartilage of the auditory tube **D:** Projects into the palatopharyngeus muscle	Elevates pharynx and larynx during deglutition (swallowing); pulls up lateral pharyngeal wall; opens the pharyngeal opening of the auditory tube when swallowing	Pharyngeal plexus [CN X]
Palatopharyngeus	**P:** Palatine aponeurosis, pterygoid hamulus and medial plate of pterygoid process **D:** Lateral wall of pharynx and posterior site of thyroid cartilage	Elevates pharynx; part of palatopharyngeal arch	Pharyngeal plexus (branches of CN IX)
Palatoglossus	**P:** Dorsal secession of transverse muscle of tongue **D:** Palatine aponeurosis	Closes the isthmus of fauces, depresses soft palate; part of palatopharyngeal arch	Pharyngeal plexus (branches of CN IX and X)
Uvular	**P:** Palatine aponeurosis **D:** Mucosa of uvula	Shortens and broadens the uvula	Pharyngeal plexus (branches of CN IX and X)

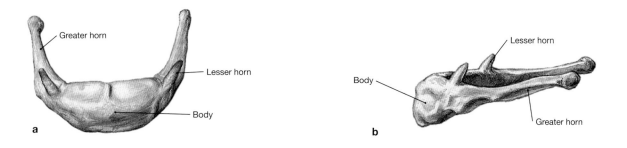

Fig. 8.98a and b Hyoid bone; anterior superior view **(a)** and lateral view **(b)**.

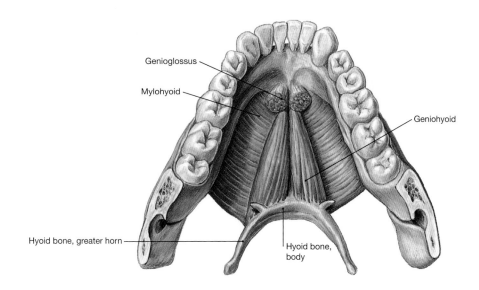

Fig. 8.99 Lower jaw, mandible, muscles of the floor of mouth and hyoid bone; superior view.

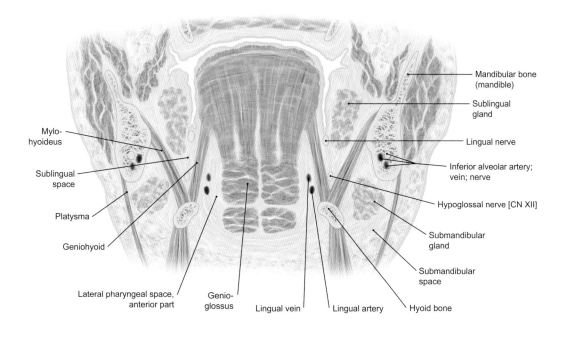

Fig. 8.100 Lower jaw, floor of oral cavity; cross-section at the level of the hyoid bone. [L127]
Topographic representation of anatomical structures and spaces at the floor of mouth. Inflammatory processes or cancer located at the floor of mouth can extend into the spaces (lateral pharyngeal space, sublingual fossa, submandibular fossa) and spread from there to distant parts of the body.

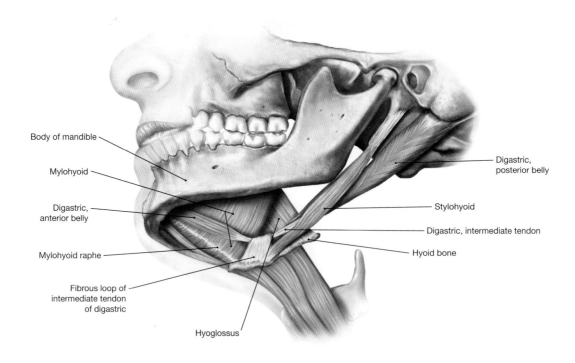

Fig. 8.101 Floor of mouth; lateral inferior view. [L266]

The muscles of the floor of mouth and suprahyoid muscles are attached to the hyoid bone. Functionally, the floor of mouth represents an adjustable abutment for the tongue.

Suprahyoid Muscles and Functions			
Muscle and Innervation	**Proximal**	**Distal**	**Function**
Mylohyoid Nerve to mylohyoid (branch of CN V/3)	Mylohyoid line of mandibular arches (lateral) to central raphe of mylohyoid	Hyoid bone and raphe of mylohyoid	Moves floor of mouth upward during swallowing
Geniohyoid Hypoglossal nerve [CN XII], cervical plexus (C1, C2)	Mental spine	Hyoid bone	Arrests position of hyoid bone (together with posterior belly of digastric muscle and stylohyoid muscle), opens mouth when masticatory muscles arrest position of mandible, moves larynx upward
Digastric, anterior belly Nerve to mylohyoid (branch of CN V/3)	Digastric fossa	Intermediate tendon of digastric muscle at hyoid bone	Moves floor of mouth upward during swallowing
Digastric, posterior belly (not a muscle of the floor of mouth) Digastric branch of facial nerve [CN VII]	Mastoid notch medial of mastoid process	Intermediate tendon of digastric muscle at hyoid bone	Fixes hyoid bone, moves larynx upward
Stylohyoid (not a muscle of the floor of mouth) Stylohyoid branch of facial nerve [CN VII]	Stylohyoid process	Body and greater horn of hyoid bone	Pulls hyoid bone upwards and posterior during swallowing

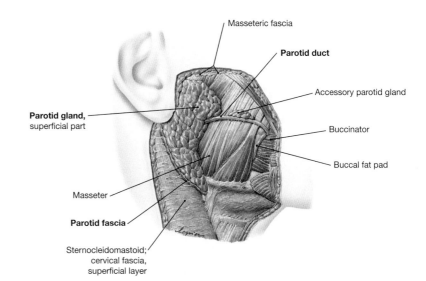

Fig. 8.102 Parotid gland, right side; lateral view.

The exclusively serous parotid gland is the largest salivary gland. The superficial layer of the gland is covered by a tough parotid fascia (cut margins shown). At the anterior margin of the gland, the parotid duct exits, pierces the buccinator muscle and ends in the papilla of parotid duct which opens into the oral vestibule opposite to the second upper molar tooth.

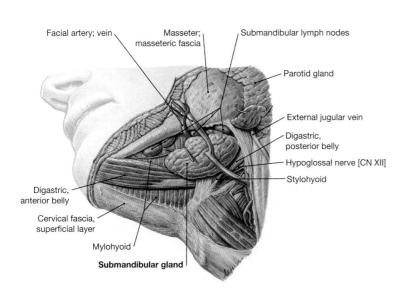

Fig. 8.103 Submandibular gland, left side; inferior view from an oblique lateral angle.

The submandibular gland is located in the submandibular triangle and is surrounded by its own fascia.

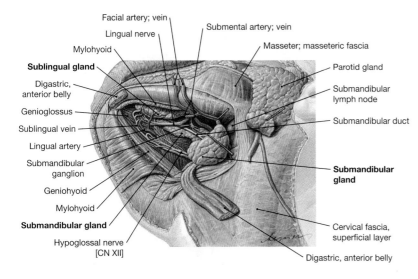

Fig. 8.104 Submandibular gland and sublingual gland, left side; lateral inferior view.

Clinical Remarks

Within the parotid gland, the facial nerve [CN VII] divides into five major branches (➤ Fig. 8.27) which radiate into the face and neck region. A parotid tumor and the surgical removal of the parotid gland can result in lesions of these facial nerve branches and of sympathetic and parasympathetic nerve fibers inner- vating the gland. Incisions should be made along the trajectory of the facial nerve branches to reduce the risk of nerve damage. Epidemic parotitis (mumps) is very painful because the swollen glandular tissue exerts tension on the parotid fascia.

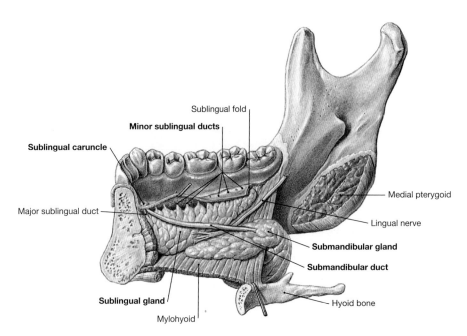

Sublingual fold

Minor sublingual ducts

Sublingual caruncle

Major sublingual duct

Medial pterygoid

Lingual nerve

Submandibular gland

Submandibular duct

Sublingual gland

Mylohyoid

Hyoid bone

Fig. 8.105 Sublingual gland and submandibular gland, right side; medial view.

The sublingual gland creates the sublingual fold at the floor of mouth which contains multiple openings of small excretory ducts (minor sublingual ducts). Bending around the posterior margin of the mylohyoid muscle, the posterior part of the submandibular gland drains its mucous secretions into the submandibular duct (WHARTON's duct) which opens at the sublingual caruncle below the tongue.

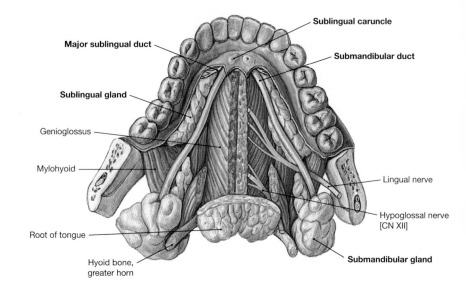

Sublingual caruncle

Major sublingual duct

Submandibular duct

Sublingual gland

Genioglossus

Mylohyoid

Lingual nerve

Hypoglossal nerve [CN XII]

Root of tongue

Hyoid bone, greater horn

Submandibular gland

Fig. 8.106 Sublingual gland and submandibular gland; superior view.

The anterior portion of the sublingual gland contains a single larger excretory duct (major sublingual duct) which merges with the submandibular duct at the sublingual caruncle.

Clinical Remarks

Anomalies of the excretory duct system, in particular of the submandibular duct, can result in a ranula (retention cyst filled with saliva). Salivary stones (sialoliths) can form within the excretory ducts of salivary glands. This can obstruct the duct resulting in episodes of salivary 'colics' and swelling of the gland. Radiation therapy of head and neck tumors can lead to the dry mouth syndrome with difficulties in swallowing and speaking. Inflammations of the salivary glands can present acutely or as chronic progression.

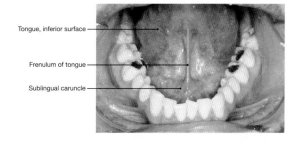

Tongue, inferior surface

Frenulum of tongue

Sublingual caruncle

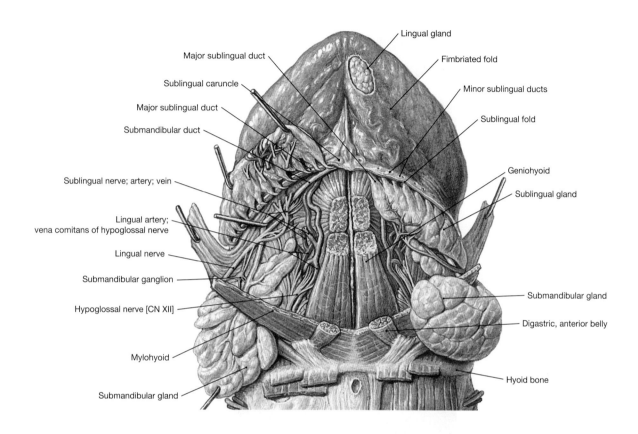

Fig. 8.107 Blood vessels and nerves of the tongue, and large salivary glands; frontal inferior view.

Major Salivary Glands and their Parasympathetic Innervation						
Parasympathetic Nucleus	Preganglionic	Ganglion	Postganglionic	Salivary Gland	Duct	Secretory Fluid
Superior salivatory nucleus (facial nerve [CN VII])	Chorda tympani	Submandibular ganglion	Fibers reach target gland directly	Sublingual gand	Multiple sperate ducts	Sticky mucous fluid
				Submandibular gland	One duct opening at sublingual caruncle	Slightly mucous watery fluid
Inferior salivatory nucleus (glossopharyngeal nerve [CN IX])	Lesser petrosal nerve	Otic ganglion	Auriculotemporal nerve (JACOBSON's nerve)	Parotoid gland	Parotoid duct	Watery fluid

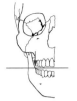

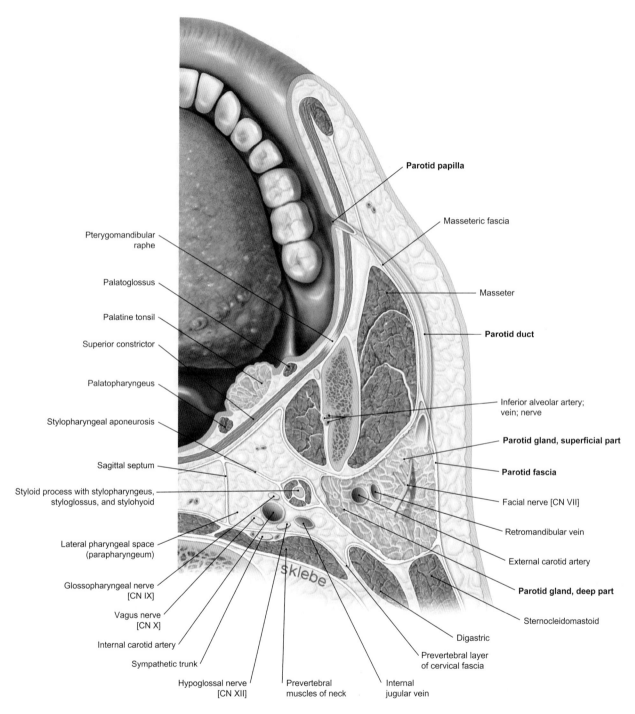

Parotid papilla

Masseteric fascia

Pterygomandibular
raphe

Masseter

Palatoglossus

Palatine tonsil

Parotid duct

Superior constrictor

Palatopharyngeus

Inferior alveolar artery;
vein; nerve

Stylopharyngeal aponeurosis

Parotid gland, superficial part

Sagittal septum

Parotid fascia

Styloid process with stylopharyngeus,
styloglossus, and stylohyoid

Facial nerve [CN VII]

Retromandibular vein

Lateral pharyngeal space
(parapharyngeum)

External carotid artery

Parotid gland, deep part

Glossopharyngeal nerve
[CN IX]

Sternocleidomastoid

Vagus nerve
[CN X]

Digastric

Internal carotid artery

Prevertebral layer
of cervical fascia

Sympathetic trunk

Hypoglossal nerve
[CN XII]

Prevertebral
muscles of neck

Internal
jugular vein

**Fig. 8.108 Topography of anatomical structures and spaces at the
level of the parotid duct;** transverse section. [L238]

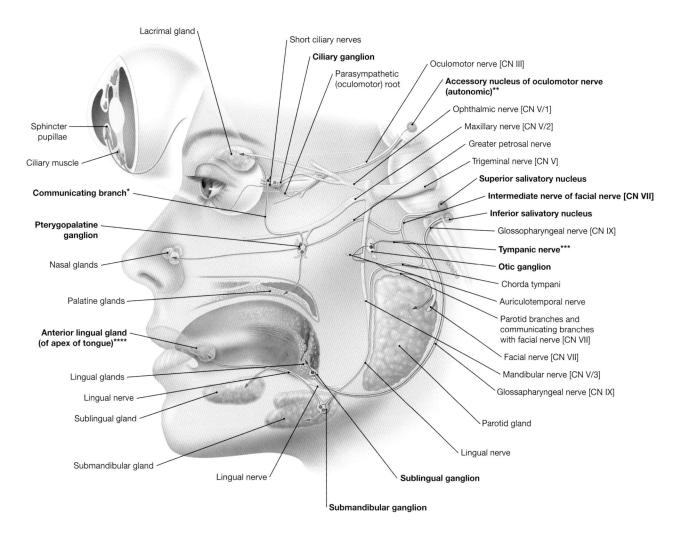

Lacrimal gland

Short ciliary nerves

Ciliary ganglion

Oculomotor nerve [CN III]

Parasympathetic (oculomotor) root

Accessory nucleus of oculomotor nerve (autonomic)**

Ophthalmic nerve [CN V/1]

Maxillary nerve [CN V/2]

Greater petrosal nerve

Trigeminal nerve [CN V]

Sphincter pupillae

Superior salivatory nucleus

Ciliary muscle

Intermediate nerve of facial nerve [CN VII]

Communicating branch*

Inferior salivatory nucleus

Pterygopalatine ganglion

Glossopharyngeal nerve [CN IX]

Tympanic nerve***

Nasal glands

Otic ganglion

Chorda tympani

Palatine glands

Auriculotemporal nerve

Anterior lingual gland (of apex of tongue)****

Parotid branches and communicating branches with facial nerve [CN VII]

Lingual glands

Facial nerve [CN VII]

Lingual nerve

Mandibular nerve [CN V/3]

Sublingual gland

Glossapharyngeal nerve [CN IX]

Parotid gland

Submandibular gland

Lingual nerve

Lingual nerve

Sublingual ganglion

Submandibular ganglion

Fig. 8.109 Parasympathetic innervation of the glands of the head by autonomic ganglia of the head; schematic drawing. [L238] Parasympathetic fibers originate from the upper and lower salivatory nuclei (superior salivatory nucleus and inferior salivatory nucleus). Preganglionic parasympathetic fibers associate with various nerves to reach the **parasympathetic ganglia of the head** (*otic, submandibular, sublingual, pterygopalatine, and ciliary ganglion*). Here, these fibers synapse and short postganglionic fibers reach their glandular targets.
Preganglionic sympathetic fibers for the head originate from the lateral horn of the spinal cord and synapse in the **superior cervical ganglion** (upper ganglion of the sympathetic chain).

Postganglionic fibers create sympathetic plexuses around arteries (e. g. internal carotid artery) and reach their destinations via blood vessels or local nerves.

*   Lacrimal gland anastomosis of parasympathetic secretory fibres from the intermediate nerve (facial nerve [CN VII]) with the lacrimal branch of the ophthalmic nerve [CN V/1] to the lacrimal gland
**   EDINGER-WESTPHAL nucleus
***   JACOBSON's nerve
**** BLANDIN's gland

Eye

Surface Anatomy 482

Eyelids 483

Bones of the Orbit 484

Anterior Orbit 486

Periorbital Blood Supply 487

Lacrimal Gland and Innervation 488

Lacrimal Apparatus 489

Extraocular Muscles 490

Innervation of
Extraocular Muscles 491

Neurovascular Structures
in the Orbit 492

Orbital Levels and Content 493

Eyeball and Blood Supply 495

Iris and Ciliary Body 496

Pupillary Reflexes 497

Ocular Fundus 498

Retina and Central Visual Pathway .. 499

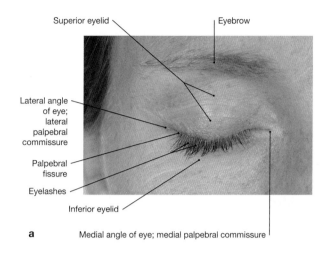

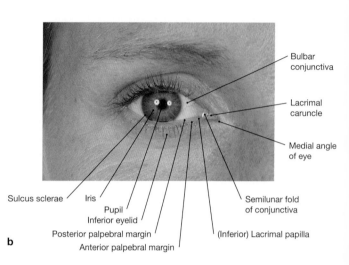

Fig. 9.1a and b Eye, right side; with eyelids closed **(a)** and open **(b).**
On average, a human eye blinks 20 to 30 times per minute. Each eyelid movement distributes a tear film across the surface of the eye. In an adult with eyelids open, the width between the upper and lower eyelid ranges from 6 to 10 mm (0.2 to 0.4 in) and the distance between the lateral and medial angles of eye is 28–30 mm (1–1.2 in).

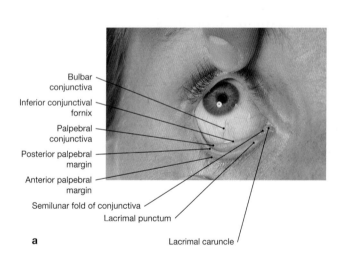

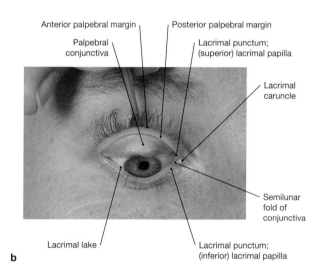

Fig. 9.2a and b Eye, right side; upper and lower eyelids everted **(a)**; with assisted ectropionized upper eyelid **(b).**
The conjunctiva is a translucent thin layer of mucosa with blood vessels. It covers the eyeball (bulbar conjunctiva) and the underside of the eyelids (palpebral conjunctiva) which is in contact with the eye surface. The cornea is free of conjunctiva. The palpebral and bulbar conjunctivae merge at the superior (upper) and inferior (lower) conjunctival fornix. The latter forms the conjunctival sac into which eye drop medication is administered and resorbed through the conjunctival blood vessels.

Clinical Remarks

A *conjunctivitis* is an inflammation of the conjunctiva and causes red eye. It frequently occurs in individuals wearing contact lenses but can have multiple other causes, including viral or bacterial infections and allergies. Anemic patients display a whitish pale conjunctiva because of a low erythrocyte count. Eversion of the lower eyelid and inspection of the conjunctival sac is a simple diagnostic test for this condition.
[G739]

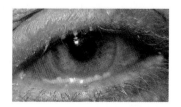

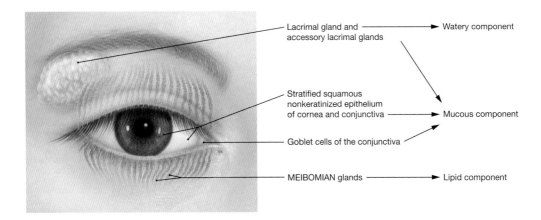

Fig. 9.3 Structures of the eye surface producing the three components of the tear film; schematic drawing. [L238]

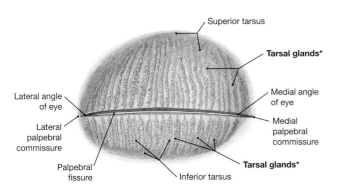

Fig. 9.4 Eyelids, right side; posterior view.
Translucent specimen illustrating the small excretory ducts (ductules) of the tarsal glands (MEIBOMIAN glands). Each eyelid contains approximately 25 to 30 individual glands with their excretory ductules opening at the palpebral fissure.

* MEIBOMIAN glands

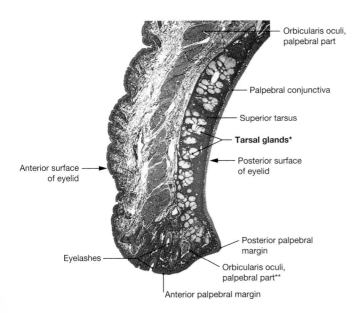

Fig. 9.5 Upper eyelid, histological specimen; azan stain; sagittal section, magnified.
The inner layer of the eyelid consists of conjunctiva, tarsus with integrated MEIBOMIAN glands (tarsal glands, modified sebaceous glands) and, close to the rim of the eyelid, muscle fibers (muscle of RIOLAN) derived from the orbital part of the orbicularis oculi projecting into the tarsus.

*   MEIBOMIAN glands
**   muscle of RIOLAN

Clinical Remarks

a A *stye (hordeolum)* is a painful and frequently putrid inflammation of MEIBOMIAN glands on the inside of the eyelid or sebaceous glands at the outer rim of the eyelid (gland of ZEIS) usually caused by bacteria. A *chalazion* is usually the result of an occluded opening of the excretory duct of a MEIBOMIAN gland. Chalazia are painless.
b An inflammation of the rim of the eyelid can result in *blepharitis* with typical signs of a dry eye, including burning sensation. Blepharitis and generalized eyelid inflammation can cause hordeola and chalazia.
a [G460, E964], b [E282]

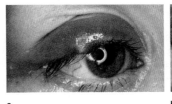
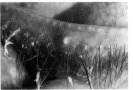

a   b

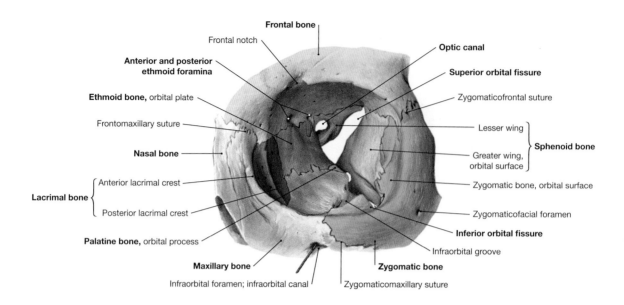

Fig. 9.6 Orbit, left side; frontal view; probe in the infraorbital canal; for color chart see p. VIII.

The ethmoid, lacrimal, palatine, sphenoid, zygomatic, frontal, and maxillary bones create the margins of the orbital cavity. Passages to and from the orbit are the superior and inferior orbital fissures, the optic canal, and the anterior and posterior ethmoid foramina.

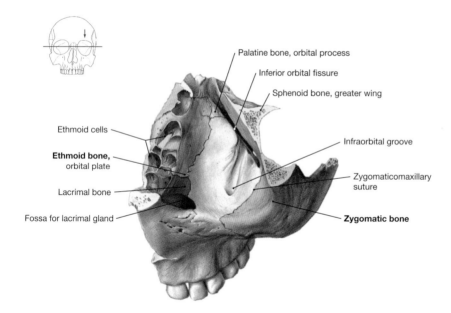

Fig. 9.7 Floor of the orbital cavity, left side; superior view; for color chart see p. VIII.

The floor of the orbit is the roof of the maxillary sinus. On it lies the infraorbital groove, which becomes a bony canal below the floor of the orbit and ends in the infraorbital foramen. It contains the infraorbital nerve and the corresponding blood vessels. The zygomatic bone forms the lateral part of the floor of the orbit. The medial part is composed of the orbital plate of the ethmoid and lacrimal bone.

Fig. 9.8 Roof of the orbit; inferior view; for color chart see p. VIII.

The roof of the orbit is also the floor of the anterior cranial fossa and the floor of parts of the frontal sinus as well. All bones of the ethmoid labyrinth are extremely thin and can be fractured during surgical procedures or external force to the head.

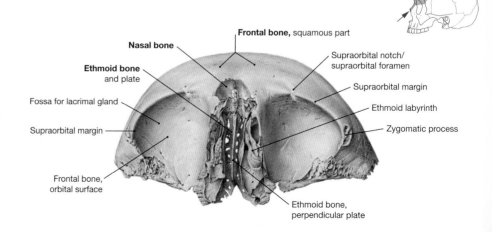

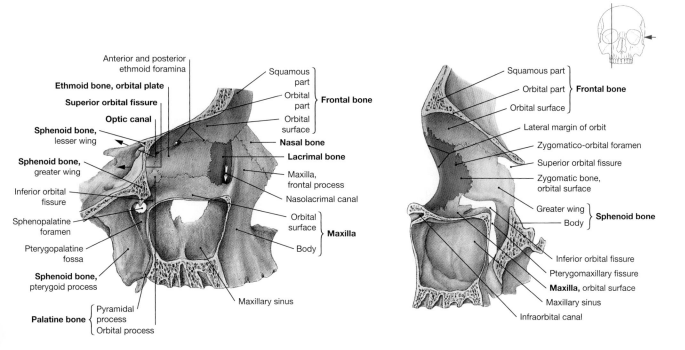

Fig. 9.9 Medial wall of the orbit, right side; lateral view; for color chart see p. VIII.

Fig. 9.10 Lateral wall of the orbit, right side; medial view; for color chart see p. VIII.

Structure/Function

Topographical relationships of the orbit with neighboring regions (red).

Infections in these paraorbital regions can spread to the orbit and vice versa. Bony separations are often thin and pose no real barrier to the spread of aggressive germs.
[L126]

I.   Anterior cranial fossa
II. Frontal sinus
III. Ethmoid cells
IV. Nasal cavity
V.   Maxillary sinus
VI. Temporal fossa

Orbital Connections	Passageways
Anterior cranial fossa	Anterior ethmoid foramen
Middle cranial fossa	Superior orbital fissure and optic canal
Infratemporal fossa	Inferior orbital fissure
Pterygopalatine fossa	Inferior orbital fissure
Ethmoid cells	Posterior ethmoid foramen
Face	Infraorbital and zygomatico-orbital foramina
Nasal cavity	Nasolacrimal duct

Clinical Remarks

Blunt force to the eyeball (e.g. center blow to the orbit) can result in a fracture of the base of the orbit *(blow-out fracture)* as shown on the right eye in the CT image (arrow shows normal condition). As a result, infraorbital structures (inferior rectus and inferior oblique) can be trapped in the fracture gap or be forced into the maxillary sinus entirely *(orbital hernia)*. Reduced mobility of the eye can cause double vision, enophthalmos, and/or the inability of this eye to look upwards. Involvement of the infraorbital nerve is likely if sensory dysfunction occurs in the dermal regions of the upper jaw because this nerve runs at the base of the orbit.
[E402]

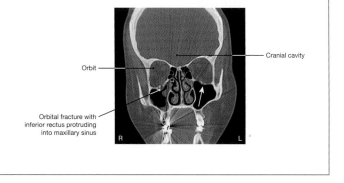

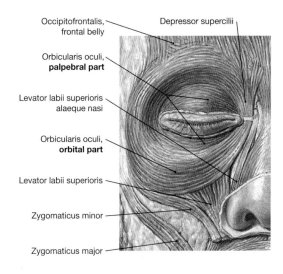

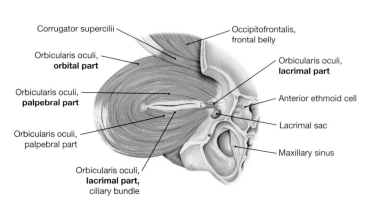

Fig. 9.11 Orbicularis oculi; frontal view.

The orbital part of the orbicularis oculi encircles the anterior opening of the orbit. The orbicularis oculi is innervated by zygomatic branches of the facial nerve.

Fig. 9.12 Orbicularis oculi, left side; posterior view. [L127]

The orbicularis oculi consists of three parts:
1. **Orbital part:** causes a voluntary firm eyelid closure;
2. **Palpebral part:** its contraction results in blinking of the eye (voluntarily and involuntarily);
3. **Lacrimal part:** also called HORNER's muscle; helps drain the tear fluid.

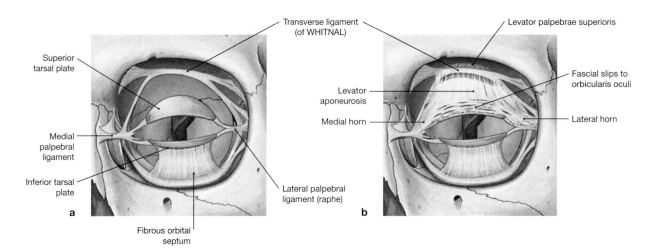

Fig. 9.13a and b Orbital septum. [G210]

The orbital septum is a fibrous membrane that connects the superior and inferior tarsus to the orbital margins. It is continuous with the periosteum of the orbit and keeps the orbital fat contained.

The **medial and lateral palpebral ligaments** (clin. term: canthal tendon) connect the superior and inferior tarsus to the orbital margins.

Clinical Remarks

A **retrobulbar hemorrhage** can cause an acute retrobulbar compartment syndrome and is a medical emergency. The pressure in the orbit can cause ischemia to the optic nerve and retina resulting in blindness. To release the pressure, a **lateral canthotomy** is performed. The inferior crus of the lateral palpebral ligament (lateral canthal tendon) is cut to relieve the orbital compression. A lateral canthotomy is performed because the lateral aspect of the orbital entrance is devoid of major blood vessels and nerves (➤ Fig. 9.14).
a [G740], b [F282]

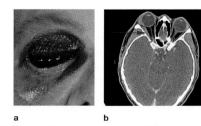

Right retrobulbar hemorrhage **(a)** with corresponding MRI **(b)**; the red arrow indicates an extensive retrobulbar hemorrhage within the right orbit.

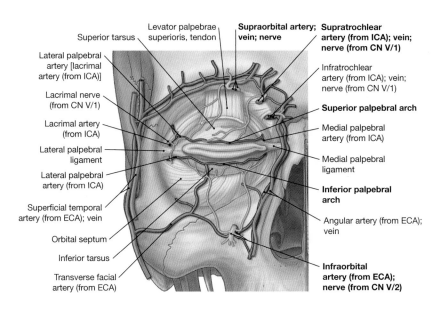

Levator palpebrae superioris, tendon
Superior tarsus
Supraorbital artery; vein; nerve
Supratrochlear artery (from ICA); vein; nerve (from CN V/1)
Lateral palpebral artery [lacrimal artery (from ICA)]
Infratrochlear artery (from ICA); vein; nerve (from CN V/1)
Lacrimal nerve (from CN V/1)
Superior palpebral arch
Lacrimal artery (from ICA)
Medial palpebral artery (from ICA)
Lateral palpebral ligament
Medial palpebral ligament
Lateral palpebral artery (from ICA)
Inferior palpebral arch
Superficial temporal artery (from ECA); vein
Angular artery (from ECA); vein
Orbital septum
Inferior tarsus
Transverse facial artery (from ECA)
Infraorbital artery (from ECA); nerve (from CN V/2)

Fig. 9.14 Arteries, veins, and nerves at the orbital opening and in the periorbital region, right side; frontal view. [E460]
The arterial circle is formed by arteries derived from the internal carotid artery (ICA) and external carotid artery (ECA). The periorbital innervation is supplied by supra- and infraorbital branches of the ophthalmic [CN V/1] and maxillary [CN V/2] nerves.

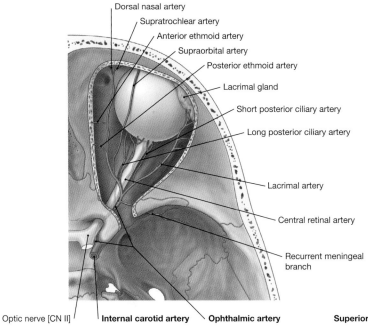

Dorsal nasal artery
Supratrochlear artery
Anterior ethmoid artery
Supraorbital artery
Posterior ethmoid artery
Lacrimal gland
Short posterior ciliary artery
Long posterior ciliary artery
Lacrimal artery
Central retinal artery
Recurrent meningeal branch
Optic nerve [CN II]
Internal carotid artery
Ophthalmic artery

Fig. 9.15 Arteries of the eye and of the orbit; superior view onto the opened orbit. [E460]
The ophthalmic artery is the main artery of the orbit and derives from the cerebral part of the internal carotid artery. It supplies blood to the eyeball and orbital structures. Arterial anastomoses exist with the external carotid artery. These include an orbital branch to the medial meningeal artery, the anterior and posterior ethmoid arteries, arteries supplying the nasal cavity, the facial artery and the temporal artery (supraorbital, supratrochlear, medial and lateral palpebral, angular, dorsal nasal arteries).

Fig. 9.16 Veins of the eye and of the orbit, right side; lateral view into the orbit; after removal of the lateral wall of the orbit. [E460]
The superior and inferior ophthalmic veins drain the venous blood from the orbit and eye. Venous anastomoses exist to the veins of the superficial and deep facial regions (pterygoid plexus) and to the cavernous sinus.

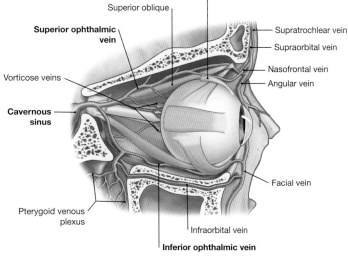

Superior rectus
Superior oblique
Superior ophthalmic vein
Supratrochlear vein
Supraorbital vein
Nasofrontal vein
Angular vein
Vorticose veins
Cavernous sinus
Facial vein
Pterygoid venous plexus
Infraorbital vein
Inferior ophthalmic vein

Clinical Remarks

An ascending spread of germs from the facial region to the intracranial cavernous sinus occurs through drainage of venous blood via the facial vein, the angular vein in the nasal part of the orbit and the inferior ophthalmic vein. This can lead to an infection and thrombosis of the cavernous sinus. The first cranial nerve to be impaired is often the abducens nerve [CN VI] be-cause of its central location within the sinus. Other cranial nerves affected are the oculomotor [CN III], trochlear [CN IV], ophthalmic [CN V/1] and maxillary [CN V/2] branches of the trigeminal nerve [CN V], resulting in paralysis of the extraocular muscles and facial sensory deficits.

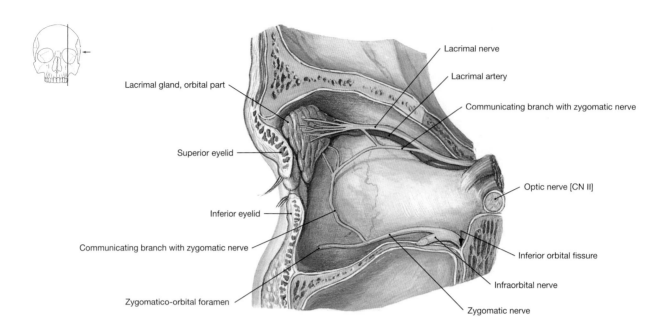

Fig. 9.17 Innervation of the lacrimal gland, right side; medial view onto the lateral wall of the orbit.

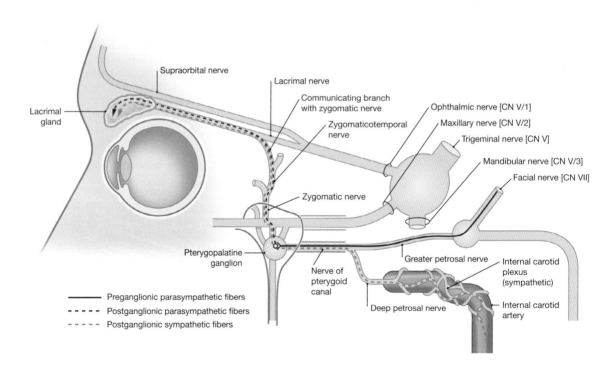

Preganglionic parasympathetic fibers
Postganglionic parasympathetic fibers
Postganglionic sympathetic fibers

Fig. 9.18 Sympathetic and parasympathetic innervation of the lacrimal gland; schematic drawing. [E460]

Preganglionic sympathetic (nerve) fibers synapse in the superior cervical ganglion. Postganglionic sympathetic fibers leave this ganglion and reach the lacrimal gland by accompanying the internal carotid, ophthalmic, and lacrimal arteries, or by parting from the internal carotid artery at the level of the foramen lacerum. The sympathetic fibers join the parasympathetic fibers on their way to the lacrimal gland.

Preganglionic parasympathetic (nerve) fibers originating from the lacrimal nucleus of the facial nerve [CN VII], run with the intermedi-

us portion of this cranial nerve, pass through the geniculate ganglion (sensory) without synapsing and reach the parasympathetic pterygopalatine ganglion via the greater petrosal nerve. Here the parasympathetic fibers synapse. The postganglionic parasympathetic fibers associate with the zygomatic nerve to reach the lacrimal nerve and the lacrimal gland via a communicating branch with the zygomatic nerve. The grey line delineates the pterygopalatine fossa, pterygoid canal and osseous canal with round foramen where the maxillary nerve [CN V/2] enters the pterygopalatine fossa.

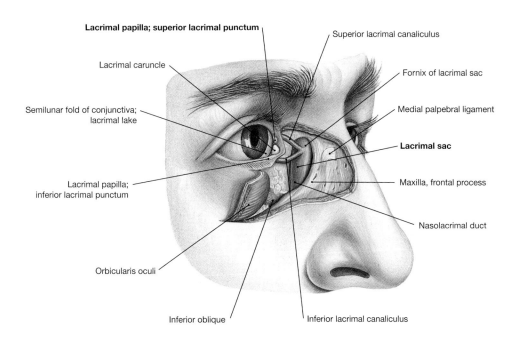

Lacrimal papilla; superior lacrimal punctum

Lacrimal caruncle

Superior lacrimal canaliculus

Fornix of lacrimal sac

Medial palpebral ligament

Semilunar fold of conjunctiva; lacrimal lake

Lacrimal sac

Lacrimal papilla; inferior lacrimal punctum

Maxilla, frontal process

Nasolacrimal duct

Orbicularis oculi

Inferior oblique

Inferior lacrimal canaliculus

Fig. 9.19 Lacrimal apparatus, right side; frontolateral view; after removal of skin, muscles, and orbital septum in the medial angle of eye.
Both **lacrimal canaliculi** originate as a **lacrimal punctum** and form approximately 10 mm long tubes. In the majority of cases (65–70 %), both canaliculi merge to form a common tube, which is approximately 1–2 mm (0.04–0.08 in) long and opens into the **lacrimal sac** about 2–3 mm (0.08–0.12 in) below the fornix of lacrimal sac.

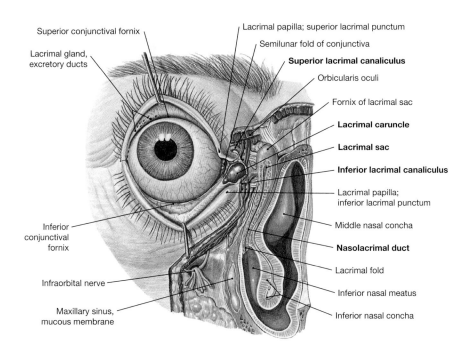

Superior conjunctival fornix

Lacrimal papilla; superior lacrimal punctum

Semilunar fold of conjunctiva

Lacrimal gland, excretory ducts

Superior lacrimal canaliculus

Orbicularis oculi

Fornix of lacrimal sac

Lacrimal caruncle

Lacrimal sac

Inferior lacrimal canaliculus

Lacrimal papilla; inferior lacrimal punctum

Middle nasal concha

Nasolacrimal duct

Inferior conjunctival fornix

Lacrimal fold

Inferior nasal meatus

Infraorbital nerve

Inferior nasal concha

Maxillary sinus, mucous membrane

Fig. 9.20 Lacrimal apparatus, right side; frontal view; the nasolacrimal duct has been opened up to the inferior nasal meatus.
A cavernous body of tissue surrounds the lumen of the lacrimal sac and functionally supports the transport of the tear fluid. Swelling of this cavernous tissue reduces or blocks the transport of fluid and this creates a tear-filled/wet eye.

Clinical Remarks

If an impaired function of the lacrimal gland is suspected, e.g. as part of a facial nerve palsy, the SCHIRMER's test is performed. A filter paper strip of standardized length, bent at one end, is hooked into the lower conjunctival sac. Absorbed tear fluid causes a change in color. At a normal rate of tear production, more than two thirds of the paper strip should be colored within 5 minutes. A shorter length of the moisturized (colored) paper strip suggests a reduced tear production.
[P310]

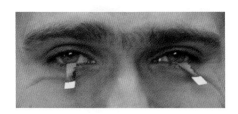

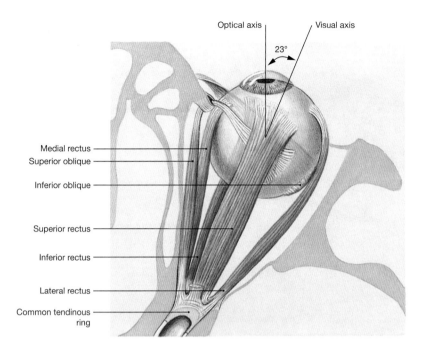

Fig. 9.21 Extraocular muscles, right side; superior view.

The visual axis (imaginary line from the mid-point of the visual field to the *fovea centralis*) and the optic axis (imaginary line through the center of the lens) differ by an angle of 23°. This is the reason why the fovea centralis (retinal location of focused central vision) is located lateral to the optic disc *(blind spot)*. The oval-shaped optic disc does not contain photoreceptors and marks the spot on the retina where the retinal fibers converge to form the optic nerve [CN II] (> Fig. 9.35).

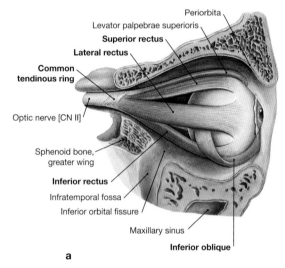

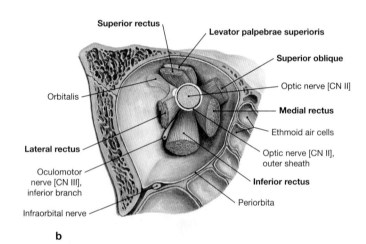

Fig. 9.22a and b Extraocular muscles, right side; lateral view **(a)**; after removal of the lateral wall of the orbit; frontal view **(b)** onto the posterior wall of the orbit.

The movement of the eyeball is controlled by six extraocular muscles in the orbit, four rectus and two oblique muscles. All rectus muscles originate from a common tendinous ring (anulus of ZINN) and insert at the sclera. The tendinous ring is also the origin of the levator palpebrae superioris which projects into the upper eyelid. A pulley-like tendinous trochlea attached to the frontal bone acts as hypomochlion for the superior oblique and redirects it backwards to its insertion area at the top of the eyeball.

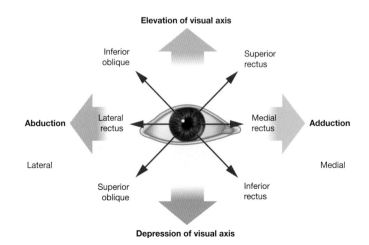

Fig. 9.23 Function of the extraocular muscles; right eye. [E402]

Testing the ability of the eyeball to move into the four main directions of the visual axis is part of a proper physical exam. Shown are the activated muscles during the movement of each eyeball into the four directions of the visual axis. The extraocular muscles receive very rich nerve supply and are distinct in fine structure from the normal striated muscles.

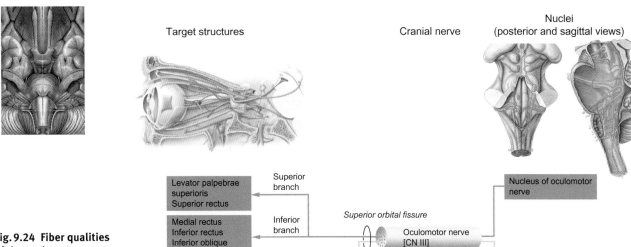

Fig. 9.24 Fiber qualities of the oculomotor nerve [CN III], left side; lateral view. [L127]

Target structures

Cranial nerve

Nuclei (posterior and sagittal views)

Levator palpebrae superioris
Superior rectus

Superior branch

Nucleus of oculomotor nerve

Medial rectus
Inferior rectus
Inferior oblique

Inferior branch

Superior orbital fissure

Oculomotor nerve [CN III]

Sphincter pupillae
Ciliary muscle

Ciliary ganglion

Accessory nucleus of oculomotor nerve

Clinical Remarks

Palsy of the oculomotor nerve [CN III] results in the paralysis of all extraocular muscles, except for the lateral rectus (abducens nerve [CN VI]) and the superior oblique (trochlear nerve [CN IV]). The non-paralyzed muscles pull the eye downward and outward (*down-and-out*; affected left eye in the image). At the same time, paralysis of the levator palpebrae superioris results in ptosis (drooping eyelid) which can result in the patient having difficulties in seeing with this eye. It is only when the drooping eyelid is pulled up manually that the patient complains about double vision (diplopia).
[E955]

Patient was asked to look straight ahead. Palsy of occulomotor nerve [CN III] on the left side.

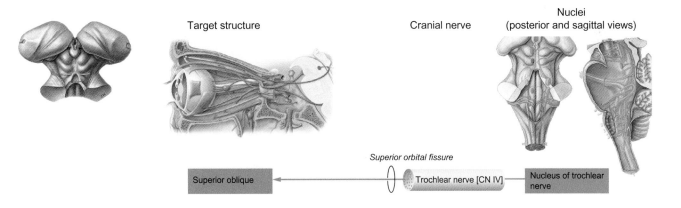

Target structure

Cranial nerve

Nuclei (posterior and sagittal views)

Superior orbital fissure

Superior oblique

Trochlear nerve [CN IV]

Nucleus of trochlear nerve

Fig. 9.25 Trochlear nerve [IV], left side; lateral view. [L127]

The trochlear nerve [CN IV] contains motor fibers for the superior oblique muscle. CN IV is the only cranial nerve that exits the brainstem dorsally and is easily damaged during dissection.

Clinical Remarks

Injury to the trochlear nerve [CN IV] can cause palsy of the trochlear nerve. Paralysis of the superior oblique causes the optic axis to point medially (nasal) and upward because the normal abduction and downward movement of the eyeball by the superior oblique muscle is absent and the action of the intact inferior oblique (innervated by CN III) dominates.
[G550]

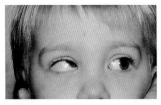

Patient was asked to look to the right side and upwards. Palsy of the trochlear nerve [CN IV] on the left side.

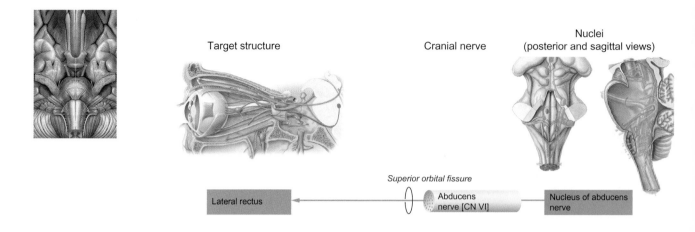

Target structure   Cranial nerve   Nuclei
(posterior and sagittal views)

Superior orbital fissure

| Lateral rectus | ← | Abducens nerve [CN VI] | Nucleus of abducens nerve |

Fig. 9.26 Abducens nerve [CN VI], left side; lateral view. [L127]

The abducens nerve [CN VI] contains motor fibers from the nucleus of abducens nerve for the lateral rectus.

Clinical Remarks

Abducens nerve palsies are the most frequent among palsies of the extraocular muscles, in part, because the abducens nerve [CN VI] runs through the central cavernous sinus and can be damaged more easily here than in the peripheral zone of the sinus where the oculomotor nerve [CN III] and trochlear nerve [CN IV] are located. Paralysis of the lateral rectus shifts the optic axis medially (nasally) due to the action of the medial rectus muscle. [E955]

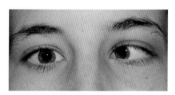

Patient was asked to look straight ahead. Palsy of left abducens nerve [CN VI] causes the left eye to turn medially.

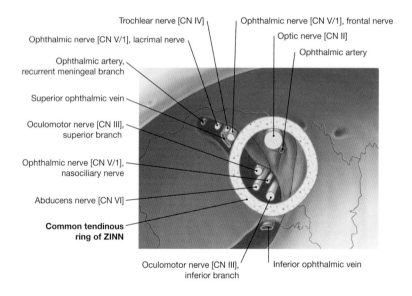

Trochlear nerve [CN IV]

Ophthalmic nerve [CN V/1], frontal nerve

Ophthalmic nerve [CN V/1], lacrimal nerve

Optic nerve [CN II]

Ophthalmic artery, recurrent meningeal branch

Ophthalmic artery

Superior ophthalmic vein

Oculomotor nerve [CN III], superior branch

Ophthalmic nerve [CN V/1], nasociliary nerve

Abducens nerve [CN VI]

Common tendinous ring of ZINN

Oculomotor nerve [CN III], inferior branch

Inferior ophthalmic vein

Fig. 9.27 Neurovascular structures passing through the optic canal and the superior orbital fissure, right side; frontal view. [E460]
The oculomotor [CN III], nasociliary and abducens nerves [CN VI], and the sympathetic root of ciliary ganglion enter the orbit through the superior orbital fissure and pass through the tendinous anulus of ZINN, as do the optic nerve [CN II] and the ophthalmic artery in the optic canal. The superior ophthalmic vein, the lacrimal nerve, frontal nerve, and trochlear nerve [CN IV] also pass through the superior orbital fissure outside of the common tendinous ring. The inferior orbital fissure contains the inferior ophthalmic vein as well as the infraorbital artery and nerve, and the zygomatic nerve (not shown).

Clinical Remarks

Incomplete or complete **ophthalmoplegia** (ophthalmoparesis) refers to the paralysis of one or more extraocular muscles. This often also includes sensory impairment in the upper facial region (ophthalmic nerve) when caused by fractures involving the superior orbital fissure. Destructive processes (e.g. tumors, trauma, chronic inflammation) at the tip of the orbit cause an *orbital apex syndrome* with ophthalmoplegia, facial hypoesthesia and progressive visual deficits. This requires an urgent surgical intervention.

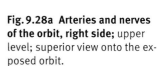

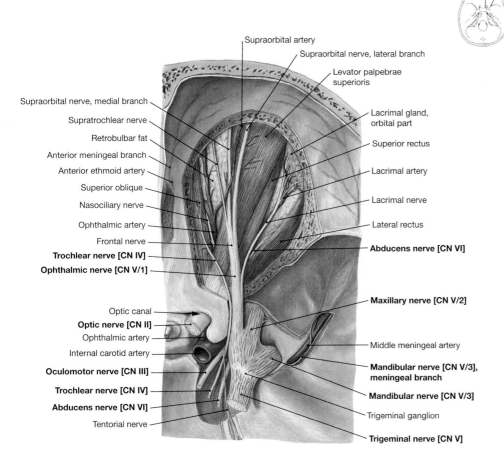

Supraorbital artery

Supraorbital nerve, lateral branch

Levator palpebrae superioris

Supraorbital nerve, medial branch

Supratrochlear nerve

Retrobulbar fat

Anterior meningeal branch

Anterior ethmoid artery

Superior oblique

Nasociliary nerve

Ophthalmic artery

Frontal nerve

Trochlear nerve [CN IV]

Ophthalmic nerve [CN V/1]

Lacrimal gland, orbital part

Superior rectus

Lacrimal artery

Lacrimal nerve

Lateral rectus

Abducens nerve [CN VI]

Maxillary nerve [CN V/2]

Optic canal

Optic nerve [CN II]

Ophthalmic artery

Internal carotid artery

Oculomotor nerve [CN III]

Trochlear nerve [CN IV]

Abducens nerve [CN VI]

Tentorial nerve

Middle meningeal artery

Mandibular nerve [CN V/3], meningeal branch

Mandibular nerve [CN V/3]

Trigeminal ganglion

Trigeminal nerve [CN V]

Fig. 9.28a Arteries and nerves of the orbit, right side; upper level; superior view onto the exposed orbit.

The upper level of the orbit is the space between the orbital roof and the levator palpebrae superioris. It contains the frontal nerve, trochlear nerve [CN IV], lacrimal nerve, supraorbital artery, supratrochlear artery, lacrimal artery and vein, and the superior ophthalmic vein.

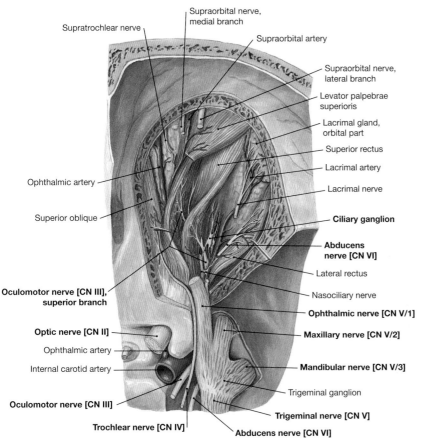

Supratrochlear nerve

Supraorbital nerve, medial branch

Supraorbital artery

Supraorbital nerve, lateral branch

Levator palpebrae superioris

Lacrimal gland, orbital part

Superior rectus

Lacrimal artery

Lacrimal nerve

Ciliary ganglion

Ophthalmic artery

Superior oblique

Abducens nerve [CN VI]

Lateral rectus

Nasociliary nerve

Ophthalmic nerve [CN V/1]

Oculomotor nerve [CN III], superior branch

Maxillary nerve [CN V/2]

Optic nerve [CN II]

Ophthalmic artery

Internal carotid artery

Mandibular nerve [CN V/3]

Oculomotor nerve [CN III]

Trigeminal ganglion

Trigeminal nerve [CN V]

Trochlear nerve [CN IV]

Abducens nerve [CN VI]

Fig. 9.28b Arteries and nerves of the orbit, right side; upper level; superior view onto the exposed orbit.

Positioned approx. 2 cm (0.8 in) lateral to the optic nerve [CN II] behind the eyeball, the ciliary ganglion contains perikarya of postganglionic parasympathetic neurons which synapse with the axons of preganglionic parasympathetic neurons located in the accessory nucleus of oculomotor nerve (EDINGER-WESTPHAL nucleus) of the brainstem. The postganglionic parasympathetic fibers innervate the inner muscles of the eye (ciliary and sphincter pupillae muscles, ➤ Fig. 9.31).

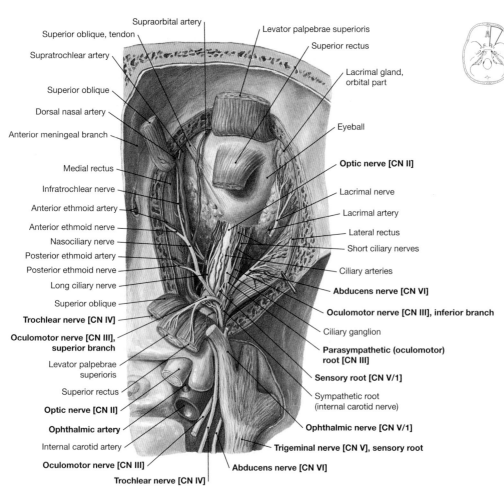

Supraorbital artery
Superior oblique, tendon
Supratrochlear artery
Superior oblique
Dorsal nasal artery
Anterior meningeal branch
Medial rectus
Infratrochlear nerve
Anterior ethmoid artery
Anterior ethmoid nerve
Nasociliary nerve
Posterior ethmoid artery
Posterior ethmoid nerve
Long ciliary nerve
Superior oblique
Trochlear nerve [CN IV]
Oculomotor nerve [CN III], superior branch
Levator palpebrae superioris
Superior rectus
Optic nerve [CN II]
Ophthalmic artery
Internal carotid artery
Oculomotor nerve [CN III]
Trochlear nerve [CN IV]

Levator palpebrae superioris
Superior rectus
Lacrimal gland, orbital part
Eyeball
Optic nerve [CN II]
Lacrimal nerve
Lacrimal artery
Lateral rectus
Short ciliary nerves
Ciliary arteries
Abducens nerve [CN VI]
Oculomotor nerve [CN III], inferior branch
Ciliary ganglion
Parasympathetic (oculomotor) root [CN III]
Sensory root [CN V/1]
Sympathetic root (internal carotid nerve)
Ophthalmic nerve [CN V/1]
Trigeminal nerve [CN V], sensory root
Abducens nerve [CN VI]

Fig. 9.28c Arteries and nerves of the orbit, right side; upper level; superior view onto the exposed orbit.
The middle level of the orbit extends between the extraocular rectus muscles. It contains the oculomotor nerve [CN III], nasociliary nerve, abducent nerve [CN VI], zygomatic nerve, ciliary ganglion, ophthalmic artery, superior ophthalmic vein, and the short and long posterior ciliary arteries.

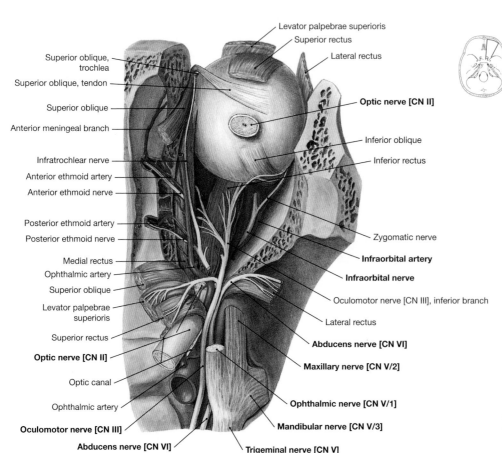

Superior oblique, trochlea
Superior oblique, tendon
Superior oblique
Anterior meningeal branch
Infratrochlear nerve
Anterior ethmoid artery
Anterior ethmoid nerve
Posterior ethmoid artery
Posterior ethmoid nerve
Medial rectus
Ophthalmic artery
Superior oblique
Levator palpebrae superioris
Superior rectus
Optic nerve [CN II]
Optic canal
Ophthalmic artery
Oculomotor nerve [CN III]
Abducens nerve [CN VI]

Levator palpebrae superioris
Superior rectus
Lateral rectus
Optic nerve [CN II]
Inferior oblique
Inferior rectus
Zygomatic nerve
Infraorbital artery
Infraorbital nerve
Oculomotor nerve [CN III], inferior branch
Lateral rectus
Abducens nerve [CN VI]
Maxillary nerve [CN V/2]
Ophthalmic nerve [CN V/1]
Mandibular nerve [CN V/3]
Trigeminal nerve [CN V]

Fig. 9.28d Arteries and nerves of the orbit, right side; middle and lower level; superior view onto the exposed orbit.
The lower level of the orbit extends from the inferior rectus and inferior oblique to the orbital floor. It contains the infraorbital nerve, infraorbital artery and inferior ophthalmic vein. The ethmoid cells at the medial (nasal) side have been opened up to demonstrate the course of the anterior and posterior ethmoid nerves and arteries from the orbit into the ethmoid bone. The infraorbital artery and nerve are located in the lower level of the orbit.

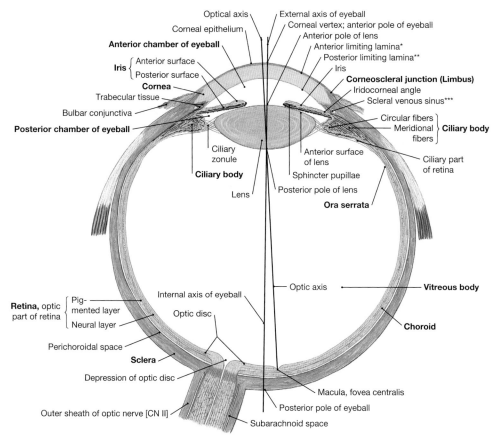

Optical axis
Corneal epithelium
Anterior chamber of eyeball
Iris { Anterior surface
       Posterior surface
Cornea
Trabecular tissue
Bulbar conjunctiva
Posterior chamber of eyeball

External axis of eyeball
Corneal vertex; anterior pole of eyeball
Anterior pole of lens
Anterior limiting lamina*
Posterior limiting lamina**
Iris
Corneoscleral junction (Limbus)
Iridocorneal angle
Scleral venous sinus***
Circular fibers
Meridional fibers } **Ciliary body**
Ciliary part of retina

Ciliary zonule
Ciliary body
Lens

Anterior surface of lens
Sphincter pupillae
Posterior pole of lens
Ora serrata

Internal axis of eyeball
Retina, optic { Pig-mented layer
part of retina { Neural layer
Optic disc
Perichoroidal space
Sclera
Depression of optic disc
Outer sheath of optic nerve [CN II]

Optic axis
Vitreous body

Choroid

Macula, fovea centralis
Posterior pole of eyeball
Subarachnoid space

Fig. 9.29 Eyeball, right side; schematic cross-section of the eye at the level of the exit of the optic nerve [CN II].
In the anterior part of the eye, the cornea forms the outer cover of the eyeball. The cornea does not contain blood vessels and is composed of five distinct layers:
• Epithelium (outermost layer),
• BOWMAN's membrane*,
• Stroma,
• DESCEMENT's membrane**,
• Endothelium (innermost layer).
Nourishment to the cornea derives from the tears and the aqueous humor in the anterior chamber of eye. At the corneal limbus (corneoscleral junction), the cornea merges into the sclera which forms the fibrous layer of the eyeball. The vascular layer of the eyeball (uvea) is located beneath the sclera. The anterior part of the uvea contains the iris and the ciliary body, while the choroid forms the posterior part. At the ora serrata, ciliary body and choroid meet. The inner space of the eyeball is filled with the vitreous body.

*** clin. term: canal of SCHLEMM

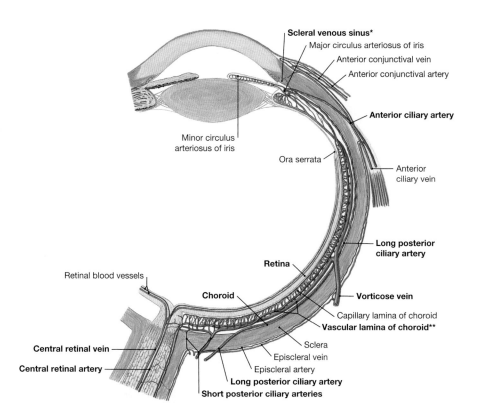

Scleral venous sinus*
Major circulus arteriosus of iris
Anterior conjunctival vein
Anterior conjunctival artery
Anterior ciliary artery

Minor circulus arteriosus of iris
Ora serrata

Anterior ciliary vein

Long posterior ciliary artery
Retina

Vorticose vein

Retinal blood vessels
Choroid
Capillary lamina of choroid
Vascular lamina of choroid**
Sclera
Episcleral vein
Episcleral artery
Long posterior ciliary artery
Short posterior ciliary arteries
Central retinal vein
Central retinal artery

Fig. 9.30 Blood vessels of the eyeball, right side; cross-section at the level of the optic nerve [CN II]; superior view.
The choroid is the most highly vascularized structure in the body. Its blood supply provides nutrients and oxygen to the adjacent retinal layer and is involved in thermoregulation of the eyeball. The retina is the innermost layer of the eyeball and contains the photoreceptors and pigment cells. The anterior retinal part constitutes the pigmented layer of the ciliary body and the epithelium of the iris. Arterial blood supply is via the central retinal artery, short and long posterior ciliary and the anterior ciliary artery. Venous drainage is through the central retinal vein and four to eight vorticose veins. The latter pierce the sclera posterior to the equator of the eyeball and join the superior and inferior ophthalmic veins.

* clin. term: canal of SCHLEMM
** uvea

Clinical Remarks

Occlusion of the central retinal artery by an embolus is referred to as **central retinal artery occlusion** (CRAO) and results in a painless and sudden complete loss of vision for the affected eye. It represents an ocular emergency similar to a cerebral stroke.

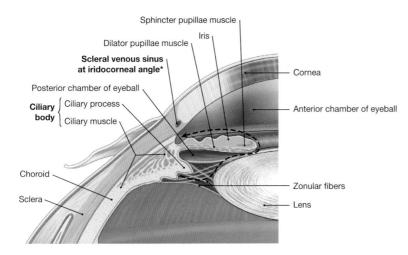

Fig. 9.31 Iridocorneal angle and adjacent structures; frontal view. [E402]

The cornea, iris, and sclera provide the borders for the iridocorneal angle. The epithelial layer of the ciliary body produces the aqueous humor that flows from the posterior to the anterior chamber of the eye. When this fluid reaches the trabecular meshwork at the iridocorneal angle (see dotted arrow indicating the direction of flow), it is collected in the canal of SCHLEMM (*) and drained into episcleral veins.

Clinical Remarks

Insufficient drainage of the aqueous humour from the iridocorneal angle leads to an increased intra-ocular pressure (normal 15 mmHg) and results in *glaucoma*, a leading cause of blindness in the Western world. Damage occurs primarily to the papilla of the optic nerve. Causes include blockage of the iridocorneal angle, for example by the impaired drainage through the trabecular meshwork of the canal of SCHLEMM in open-angle glaucoma (frequent) or the adhesion of the iris to the cornea (closed-angle glaucoma; rare). Medication that constricts pupil size (miotics) increases fluid drainage through the canal of SCHLEMM. This reduces the intraocular pressure and regulates the fluid production.

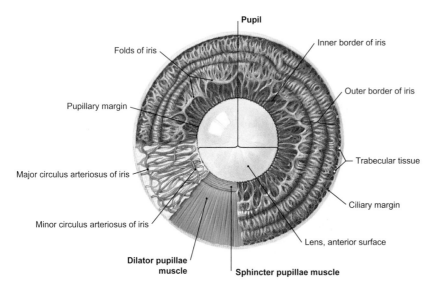

Fig. 9.32 Iris and ciliary body; frontal view. [L127]

The iris is composed of a dense vascular network and two smooth muscles for pupillary dilation (dilator pupillae) and constriction (sphincter pupillae). The dilator pupillae receives sympathetic innervation. Preganglionic cervical fibers synapse in the superior cervical ganglion and the postganglionic sympathetic fibers reach the dilator pupillae as long ciliary nerves. The sphincter pupillae receives parasympathetic innervation. Preganglionic fibers from the accessory nucleus of oculomotor nerve (EDINGER-WESTPHAL) travel with the oculomotor nerve [CN III], synapse in the ciliary ganglion and postganglionic parasympathetic short ciliary nerves reach the sphincter pupillae.

Clinical Remarks

The pupillary light reflex (PLR) controls the intensity of light that reaches the retina. Bright light triggers the pupillary constriction (*miosis*). Dim light dilates the pupils (*mydriasis*). Retina and optic nerve [CN II] are the afferent (sensory) and the pupillary muscles are the efferent (motor) limb of PLR. The PRL provides diagnostic information on the sensory (retina) and pupillary motor functions of the eye.
[L126]

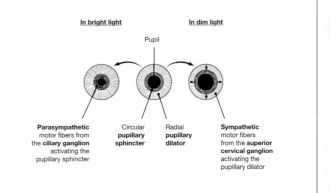

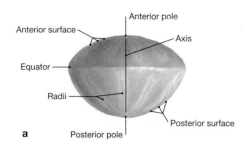

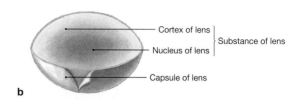

a

b

Fig. 9.33a and b Lens; viewed from the lens equator **(a)** and anterior oblique view **(b);** after meridional cut and partial detachment of the anterior capsule of lens.
The ciliary muscle is the major component of the ciliary body. Zonular fibers (suspensory ligaments of the lens) span the distance between the ciliary epithelium and the capsule of lens where they insert around the equator of the lens. Zonular fibers are important for accommodation.

Clinical Remarks

Accommodation relies on the lens to increase in diameter (round up) when the ciliary muscle circling the lens contracts and bulges out towards the lens. This releases tension on the zonular fibers that attach to the equator of the lens and leads to a change of up to 15 diopters in optical power in a young person. Reduced elasticity of the lens (starting at about 40 years of age) results in diminished accommodation, i.e. the inability to properly focus on objects at various distances (presbyopia) with either nearsightedness (myopia) or farsightedness (hyperopia). Both require correction through the use of appropriate eye glasses. [L275]

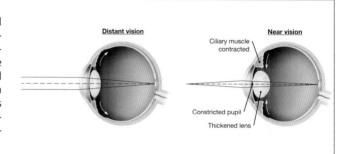

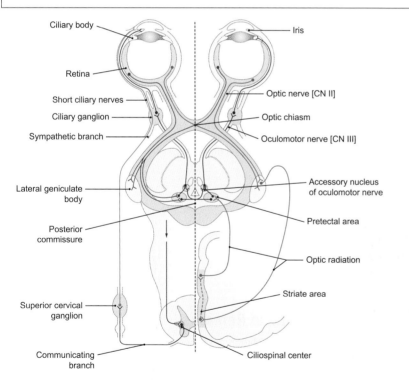

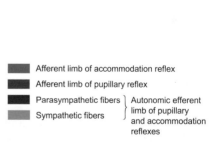

Fig. 9.34 Neuronal pathways for pupillary light reflex (left) and accommodation reflex (right). [L126]

Clinical Remarks

Reduction in intracellular water content causes alterations in proteins (crystallines) important for maintaining transparency of the lens. Slit lamp examination reveals the increase in lens opacity (senile cataract) as show in the image on the right. The white curved bar on the right side of the image constitutes the reflection of the cornea. Cataract surgery is one of the most frequently performed surgical procedures in Western industrialized countries. [P496]

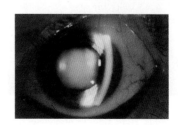

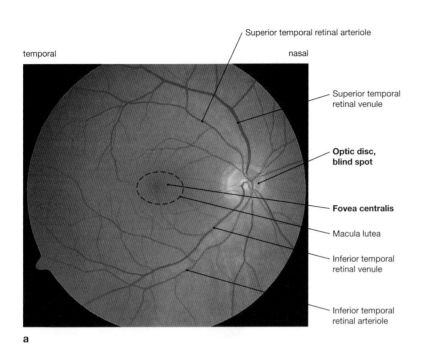

temporal

Superior temporal retinal arteriole

nasal

Superior temporal retinal venule

Optic disc, blind spot

Fovea centralis

Macula lutea

Inferior temporal retinal venule

Inferior temporal retinal arteriole

a

Normal optic disc

b

Glaucoma optic disc

c

Fig. 9.35a to c Ocular fundus, right side; frontal view; ophthalmoscopic image of the central region.
b Normal optic disc [E567],
c Glaucoma optic disc [E567].
Examination of the ocular fundus by direct ophthalmoscopy (*funduscopy or fundoscopy*) allows the clinical assessment of the condition of the retina, its blood vessels (in particular the central retinal artery and vein), the optic disc, and the macula lutea and the fovea centralis (point of central vision) in the center of the macula. Normally, the optic disc has a sharply delineated margin, a yellow to orange color, and contains a central depression (physiological cup; see enlarged image **b** and **c**). 3–4 mm (0.12 – 0.16 in) to the temporal side of the optic disc lies the macula lutea with the central fovea which contains the highest concentration of cone cells for color vision. Numerous branches of the central retinal blood vessels converge in a radial fashion onto the macula, but do not enter the center (fovea centralis) which is supplied by the underlying choroid. Glaucomatous changes to the optic nerve **(c)** can occur acutely or over time, include visible changes to the optic disc and lead to blindness if untreated.

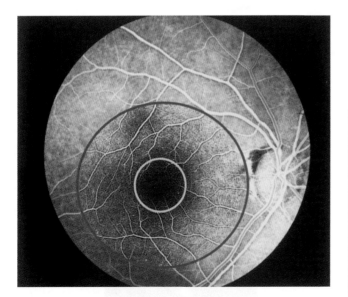

Fig. 9.36 Ocular fundus, right side; frontal view; fluorescence angiography during the arteriovenous phase with anatomic landmarks: macula (blue circle); fovea (yellow circle). [E282]

Clinical Remarks

Retinal ablation describes the detachment of the inner parts of the retina (neural layer, neuroretina) from its supplying retinal pigmented epithelium (pigmented layer). Symptoms include the sensation of flashes or colored spots. This may not occur if the macula (point of central vision) is unaffected. If the macula is detached from its supplying pigment epithelium for more than 48 hours, permanent loss of function of the corresponding retinal part will occur. After a successful re-attachment of the retina to the pigmented epithelium by laser therapy, the retina may partially recover, depending on the duration of the retinal ablation. In case of continued complete retinal ablation, blindness is inevitable.
Age-related macular degeneration (AMD) is a pathological age-dependent alteration of the macula and the most frequent cause of blindness in Western industrialized nations.

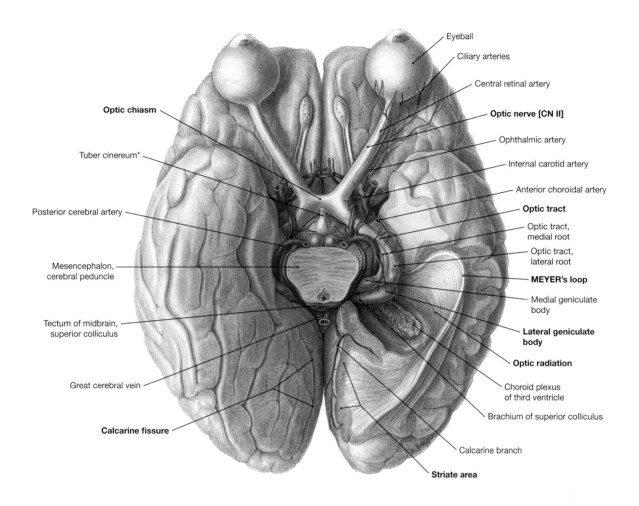

Eyeball

Ciliary arteries

Central retinal artery

Optic nerve [CN II]

Ophthalmic artery

Internal carotid artery

Anterior choroidal artery

Optic tract

Optic tract, medial root

Optic tract, lateral root

MEYER's loop

Medial geniculate body

Lateral geniculate body

Optic radiation

Choroid plexus of third ventricle

Brachium of superior colliculus

Calcarine branch

Striate area

Optic chiasm

Tuber cinereum*

Posterior cerebral artery

Mesencephalon, cerebral peduncle

Tectum of midbrain, superior colliculus

Great cerebral vein

Calcarine fissure

Fig. 9.37 The visual pathway; inferior view.
The pituitary gland has been removed at its infundibulum (*). The pituitary gland is located close to the optic chiasm.
The axons of the optic ganglionic cells (3rd neuron) within the retina form the optic nerve [CN II]. The optic nerves from both sides merge in the optic chiasm. From here the visual pathway continues as bilateral optic tract to the lateral geniculate body (lateral root). Several fibers also extend into the pretectal area and the superior colliculus (medial root) as well as to the hypothalamus. The axons within the optic nerve synapse at the 4th neuron located within the lateral geniculate body which is part of the hypothalamus. The ax-

ons of the 4th neuron form the optic radiation with an upper and lower division (MEYER's loop). The fibers of the upper division project to the upper bank of the calcarine fissure (cuneus). The lower division forms the MEYER's loop in the temporal lobe which projects into the lower bank of the calcarine fissure (lingual gyrus) of areas 17 and 18 of the cerebral cortex (striate area, primary visual cortex). The MEYER's loop can be injured during temporal lobe surgery and temporal lobe infarction or hemorrhage to cause superior quadrantanopia ('pie in the sky'; ➤ Fig. 9.38b) of the contralateral side.

Clinical Remarks

Diseases affecting the neuronal network of the retina can lead to impaired vision or blindness. Thrombosis of the central retinal vein *(central venous thrombosis)* is a relatively frequent retinal disease associated with significant reduction in vision. Diabetic patients often develop microvascular changes also involving

retinal blood vessels *(diabetic retinopathy)*. Affected blood vessels can rupture. Blood can enter the vitreous body and this impairs vision. If remnants of such bleeding into the vitreous body fail to resolve after 2–3 months, the resulting impairment in vision may require the removal of the vitreous body *(vitrectomy)*.

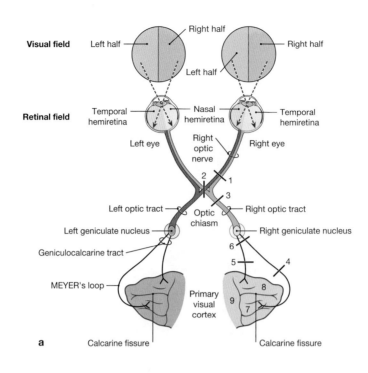

Fig. 9.38 Basic visual pathway; schematic overview. [L126]
a The medial (red) and lateral (blue) vision fields project to the lateral and medial retinal fields, respectively. Visual information from the left and right visual fields is projected to the opposite primary visual cortex.
b Lesions and their effects on vision.

Site of lesion (right side)	Left eye	Right eye	Name of the disorder
Optic nerve: 1			a. Total loss of vision in the right eye
Optic chiasm (midline): 2			b. Non-homonymous bitemporal hemianopia
Optic tract: 3			c. Contralateral (left) homonymous hemianopia
Temporal lobe (MEYER's loop): 4			d. Superior left homonymous quadrantanopia *(pie in the sky disorder)*
Parietal lobe: 5			e. Inferior left homonymous quadrantanopia *(pie in the floor disorder)*
Geniculocalcarine tract: 6			f. Contralateral (left) homonymous hemianopia
Inferior bank of calcarine fissure: 7			g. Superior left homonymous quadrantanopia (with macular sparing)
Superior bank of calcarine fissure: 8			h. Inferior left homonymous quadrantanopia (with macular sparing)
Both banks of calcarine fissure: 9			i. Contralateral (left) homonymous hemianopia (with macular sparing)

Deficit in the visual field

Clinical Remarks

Different lesions to the visual pathway cause distinct impairments of the visual field.

A severed optic nerve causes blindness (anopia) of the associated eye with total loss of vision of this side (see lesion 1).

Hemianopia (hemianopsia) usually affects both eyes and involves a loss of visual field on one side of the vertical midline. Sites of lesions can be the optic chiasm (see lesion 2), optic tract (see lesion 3), geniculocalcarine tract (see lesion 6) or both banks of the calcarine fissure (see lesion 9).

In homonymous hemianopsia, the loss of visual field affects the same side in both eyes (see lesions 3, 6 and 9).

Bitemporal hemianopsia is a non-homonymous loss of vision in the outer (temporal) half of both the right and left visual fields and can be caused by a lesion in the optic chiasm (see lesion 2). Patients with quadrantanopia (quadrantopsia or quadrant anopia) are blind in a quarter of their field of vision (see lesions 4, 5, 7 and 8). A lesion of the MEYER's loop (temporal lobe lesion) causes 'pie in the sky' quadrantanopia (see lesion 4).

Ear

Surface Anatomy 502

External Acoustic Meatus 503

Temporal Bone 504

Middle Ear – Tympanic Membrane .. 505

Middle Ear – Auditory Ossicles 506

Middle Ear –
Pharyngotympanic Tube 507

Middle Ear –
Neighboring Structures 508

Middle Ear –
Blood Supply and Innervation 509

Inner Ear –
Petrous Part of Temporal Bone 510

Inner Ear –
Bony and Membranous Labyrinth ... 511

Inner Ear – Cochlea 512

Inner Ear – Mechanoelectrical
Conduction 513

Central Auditory Pathways 514

Inner Ear – Vestibular Labyrinth 515

Central Vestibular Pathways 516

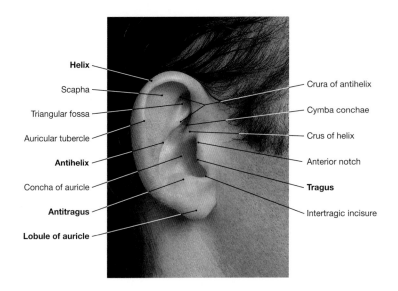

Helix
Scapha
Triangular fossa
Auricular tubercle
Antihelix
Concha of auricle
Antitragus
Lobule of auricle

Crura of antihelix
Cymba conchae
Crus of helix
Anterior notch
Tragus
Intertragic incisure

Fig. 10.1 Auricle, right side; lateral view.
The basic framework of the auricle consists of elastic cartilage. The earlobe is free of cartilage. The skin on the lateral surface of the auricle is directly attached to the perichondrium and cannot be moved. The skin on the posterior side of the auricle is movable. The auricle does not contain subcutaneous fat tissue.

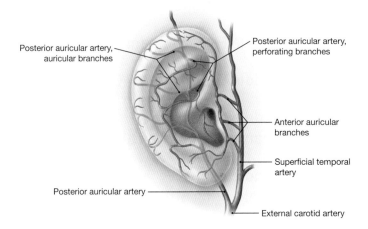

Posterior auricular artery, auricular branches

Posterior auricular artery, perforating branches

Anterior auricular branches

Superficial temporal artery

Posterior auricular artery

External carotid artery

Fig. 10.2 Arteries of the auricle, right side; lateral view. [L238]
The auricle is highly vascularized to protect it against freezing or to serve for heat convection. The supplying arteries branching off the external carotid artery are the **posterior auricular artery** and the **superficial temporal artery.**

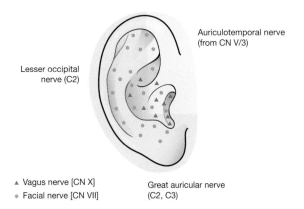

Lesser occipital nerve (C2)

Auriculotemporal nerve (from CN V/3)

▲ Vagus nerve [CN X]
● Facial nerve [CN VII]

Great auricular nerve (C2, C3)

Fig. 10.3 Sensory innervation of the auricle, right side; lateral view. [L126]
Sensory innervation of the auricle is provided by the:
1. **Auriculotemporal nerve,** a branch of the mandibular nerve [CN V/3] to the front of the ear
2. **Cervical plexus:** (C2, C3): great auricular nerve, lesser occipital nerve to the region behind and below the ear
3. **Facial nerve** [CN VII] to the auricle itself
4. **Vagus nerve** [CN X] to the entrance of the external acoustic meatus

Clinical Remarks

a Inherited external ear defects are common. Severe defects of the external ear and zygomatic bone, receding chin, and cleft palate are typical for the dominantly inherited FRANCESCHETTI's syndrome (mandibulofacial dysostosis). [E247-09]
b The cauliflower ear forms as a result of repeated blows to the ear, causing vascular damage and the collection of blood between cartilage and overlying perichondrium providing nutrients to the cartilage. If not drained, the cartilage dies and is replaced by fibrous tissue. [F217-003]

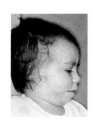

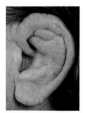

a   b

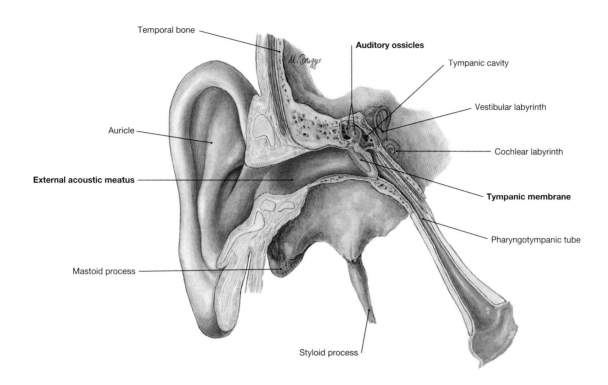

Fig. 10.4 Parts of the ear, right side; longitudinal section through the external acoustic meatus, middle ear, and pharyngotympanic tube (auditory tube); frontal view.
Sound waves initiate oscillation of the tympanic membrane (*aerotympanal conduction*). The auditory ossicles transmit the vibrations to the oval window of the inner ear and match the low impedance (resistance to acoustic waves) of air with the high impedance of the liquid-filled inner ear (= impedance matching). The inner ear converts sound energy into electric impulses which are transmitted via the cochlear nerve to specific regions of the brain. The inner ear can also sense vibrations of skull bones (*bone conduction*).

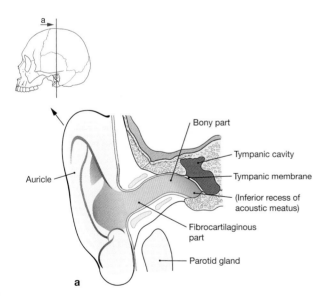

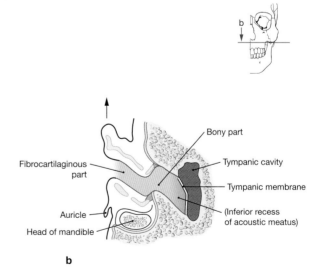

Fig. 10.5a and b External acoustic meatus, right side, frontal section **(a)**, horizontal section **(b)**; schematic drawing. [L126]
The external acoustic meatus is S-shaped and consists of an outer cartilaginous and inner bony part. To inspect the tympanic membrane with a reflecting otoscopic mirror or a microscope (*otoscopy*), the auricle must be pulled up and backwards (see arrow) to straighten the cartilaginous part of the external acoustic meatus. Sensory innervation of the external acoustic meatus is provided by the:

1. **Auriculotemporal nerve** [branch of CN V/3] (anterior and superior wall)
2. Auricular branch of the **vagus nerve** [CN X] (ARNOLD's nerve; posterior and partially inferior wall). In some individuals, physical stimulation of the auricular branch of CN X at the outer acoustic meatus can trigger coughing (ear-cough or ARNOLD's reflex)
3. Auricular branches of the **facial nerve** [CN VII]
4. **Glossopharyngeal nerve** [CN IX] (posterior wall and tympanic membrane)

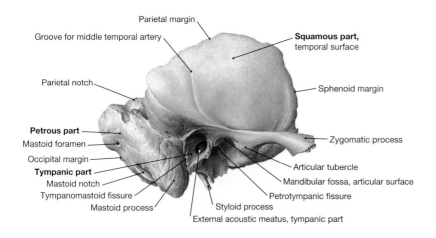

Parietal margin
Groove for middle temporal artery
Parietal notch
Petrous part
Mastoid foramen
Occipital margin
Tympanic part
Mastoid notch
Tympanomastoid fissure
Mastoid process
Squamous part, temporal surface
Sphenoid margin
Zygomatic process
Articular tubercle
Mandibular fossa, articular surface
Petrotympanic fissure
Styloid process
External acoustic meatus, tympanic part

Fig. 10.6 Temporal bone, right side; lateral view.
The paired temporal bone is part of the viscerocranium and neurocranium and consists of the squamous part, the tympanic part, and the petrous part. The petrous part of temporal bone contains the middle and inner ear.

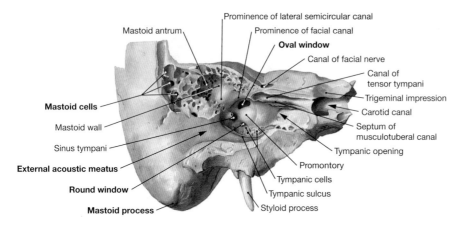

Prominence of lateral semicircular canal
Mastoid antrum
Prominence of facial canal
Oval window
Canal of facial nerve
Canal of tensor tympani
Trigeminal impression
Carotid canal
Septum of musculotuberal canal
Tympanic opening
Promontory
Tympanic cells
Tympanic sulcus
Styloid process
Mastoid cells
Mastoid wall
Sinus tympani
External acoustic meatus
Round window
Mastoid process

Fig. 10.7 Medial wall of the tympanic cavity, right side; vertical section in the longitudinal axis of the petrous part of temporal bone; frontolateral view.
Bone resorption within the temporal bone forms air-filled cavities lined with epithelium. This pneumatization process starts in week 22–24 of fetal life and continues until the age of 8 years. The pneumatized mastoid process connects with the tympanic cavity through the mastoid antrum.

Fig. 10.8 Temporal bone, right side; inner aspect.
The temporal bone forms part of the middle cranial fossa. The posterior surface of the petrous part shows the indentation by the sigmoid sinus. The cerebral surface of the squamous part shows arterial grooves of the medial meningeal artery.

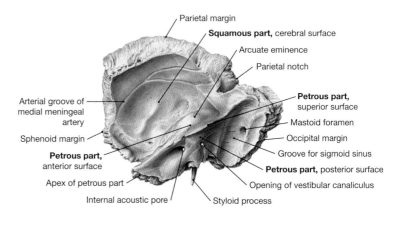

Parietal margin
Squamous part, cerebral surface
Arcuate eminence
Parietal notch
Petrous part, superior surface
Mastoid foramen
Occipital margin
Groove for sigmoid sinus
Petrous part, posterior surface
Opening of vestibular canaliculus
Arterial groove of medial meningeal artery
Sphenoid margin
Petrous part, anterior surface
Apex of petrous part
Internal acoustic pore
Styloid process

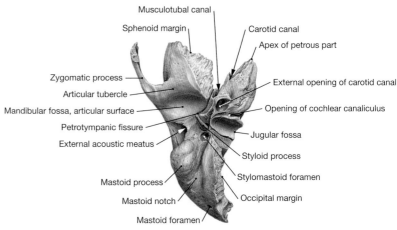

Musculotubal canal
Sphenoid margin
Carotid canal
Apex of petrous part
Zygomatic process
External opening of carotid canal
Articular tubercle
Mandibular fossa, articular surface
Opening of cochlear canaliculus
Petrotympanic fissure
Jugular fossa
External acoustic meatus
Styloid process
Stylomastoid foramen
Mastoid process
Occipital margin
Mastoid notch
Mastoid foramen

Fig. 10.9 Temporal bone, right side; inferior view.

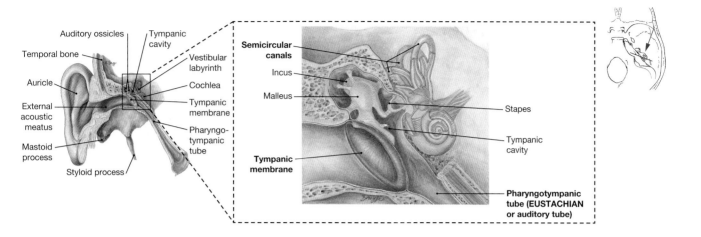

Fig. 10.10 Different levels of the tympanic cavity, right side; frontal section; frontal view.
The tympanic cavity is an air-filled space within the temporal bone which contains the auditory ossicles. The tympanic cavity is located directly behind the tympanic membrane and is aerated and drained by the auditory or pharyngotympanic tube (also named EUSTACHIAN tube) which also serves in pressure equalization. The auditory tube connects to the nasopharynx (➤ Fig. 10.15a).
The tympanic cavity divides into three sections:

- The epitympanum (red; epitympanic recess, 'attic') contains the suspension apparatus and the majority of the auditory os-

sicles and, through the mastoid antrum, connects with the mastoid cells.
- The mesotympanum (blue) contains the handle of malleus, the lenticular process of incus, and the tendon of the tensor tympani.
- The hypotympanum (green; hypotympanic recess) leads into the auditory tube.

The distance between the epitympanum and hypotympanum is 12–15 mm (0.5–0.6 in) and the depth is 3–7 mm (0.1–0.3 in), with an inner volume of the middle ear cavity of approximately 1 cm³ (0.06 in³).

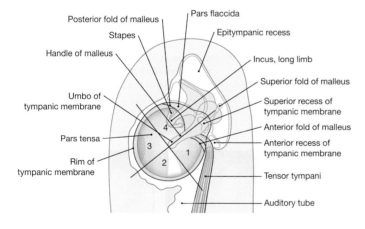

Fig. 10.11 Tympanic membrane and recesses of the tympanic cavity, right side; lateral view; schematic drawing with quadrants. [L126]
The quadrant scheme is of practical clinical relevance. The auditory ossicles are located in the upper anterior (1) and posterior (4) quadrants, as are the chorda tympani and the tendon of tensor tympani.

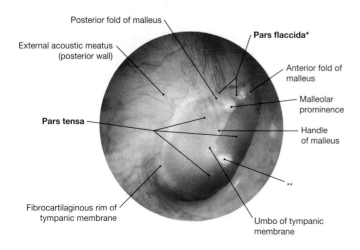

Fig. 10.12 Tympanic membrane, right side; lateral view; otoscopic image.
The tympanic membrane is composed of a small flaccid part (pars flaccida) and a larger tense part (pars tensa). In otoscopy, a healthy pars tensa typically shows a light reflex emanating from the umbo of tympanic membrane which is the deepest point in a healthy pars tensa.

* clin. term: SHRAPNELL's membrane
** typical position of light reflex

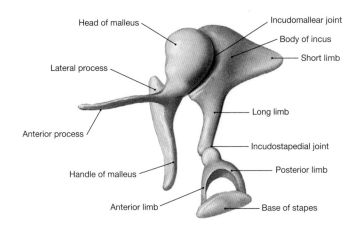

Fig. 10.13 Auditory ossicles, right side; supero-medial view.
The ossicle chain transmits the energy of sound waves from the tympanic membrane to the peri-lymph of the inner ear. This impedance match-ing is accomplished by the lever action of the auditory ossicles (1.3 times) and greatly en-hanced (17 times) by the size difference between the tympanic membrane (55 mm² [0.09 in²]) and the oval window (3.2 mm² [5 × 10⁻³ in²]). In total, the acoustic pressure amplifies 22-fold!

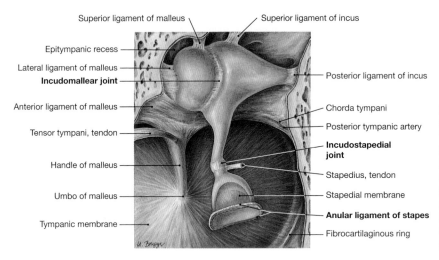

Fig. 10.14 Joints and ligaments of the auditory ossicles, right side; superomedial view.
The auditory ossicles are linked by true joints: the incudomallear joint (saddle joint) and the incudostapedial joint (spheroid joint). Liga-ments fasten the malleus and incus in the epit-ympanum. The base of stapes is secured to the oval window by the anular ligament of stapes (syndesmosis). All structures in the tympanic cavity, including the chorda tympani, are lined with mucosa of the middle ear.

Clinical Remarks

Spontaneous perforation and **defects in the conductive chain**
Spontaneous perforation of the tympanic membrane during pu-trid middle ear infection (otitis media) tends to occur more fre-quently in the pars flaccida which is the thinner part of the tym-panic membrane.
a Serous effusion or pus collecting in the middle ear is visible through the tympanic membrane which bulges outward and looses its light reflex.
b Tympanotomy (tympanostomy, myringotomy) drains liquid from behind the eardrum.
c Incision of the tympanic membrane after tympanotomy and drainage.
d A small tube (grommet) has been inserted into the tympanic membrane to ensure drainage and aeration of the middle ear. Once the middle ear infection is resolved, the grommet is re-moved and the opening of the tympanic membrane seals.
Defects in the conductive chain (tympanic membrane, auditory ossicles, occluded auditory tube) result in *conductive hearing loss.*
e In otosclerosis, the base of stapes progressively fixes to the oval window through ossification of the anular ligament of sta-pes causing slowly progressing conductive hearing loss. Wom-en at 20–40 years of age are affected two times more frequently than men. In 70% of cases, otosclerosis affects both ears.
a–d [E625], e [L126]

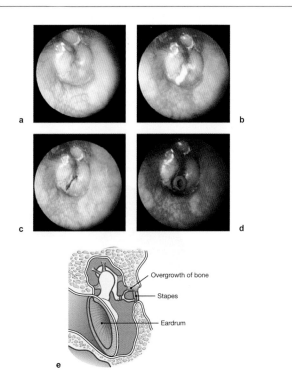

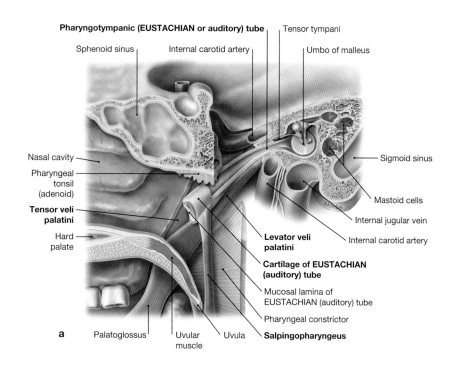

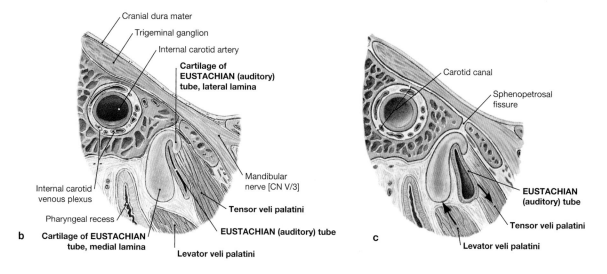

Fig. 10.15a to c Pharyngotympanic (auditory) tube, right side; medial view (**a**); schematic cross-sectional drawings (**b**, **c**) at the level of the lateral cartilaginous part of the (**b**) closed and (**c**) open auditory tube. a [L126]
The auditory tube connects the middle ear with the pharynx and is important for the aeration of the tympanic cavity. Two muscles facilitate the opening of the auditory tube: *tensor veli palatini* and *leva-*

tor veli palatini. The *salpingopharyngeus* closes the auditory tube. Opening of the auditory tube during swallowing involves pull at the membranous part of the auditory tube by the contracting tensor veli palatini (**c**). Simultaneously, the muscle belly of the contracting levator veli palatini thickens and widens the cartilaginous groove the auditory tube resides in, so the lumen of the auditory tube has space to expand (see arrows in **c**).

Clinical Remarks

Conductive hearing loss
In children, one of the most common causes of conductive hearing loss is the occlusion of the auditory tube caused by an inflammation of the tube or restricted nasal breathing due to enlarged pharyngeal tonsils (adenoids). This can lead to an inflammation of the middle ear (*otitis media*) with accumulation of fluid behind the tympanic membrane. The inflammation of the mastoid cells (*mastoiditis*) caused by an inflammatory process in the tympanic cavity is a frequent complication of otitis media. The inflammation can spread from the mastoid cells and affect the soft tissue behind and in front of the outer ear, the sternocleido-

mastoid, the inner ear (➤ Fig. 10.16a and b), the sigmoid sinus, the meninges, and the facial nerve [CN VII].
Cleft palate
Cleft palate coincides with a loss of function of the tensor veli palatini and levator veli palatini, as these muscles have lost their attachment (fixed end) at the hard and soft palate, respectively. As a result, the contraction of both muscles fails to open the auditory tube. Without treatment, children with cleft palate have a poorly aerated middle ear which results in mucosal adhesions. These children usually have major impairments in hearing and speech.

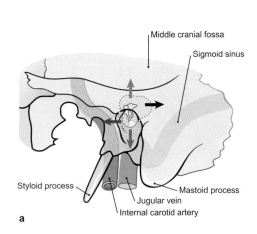

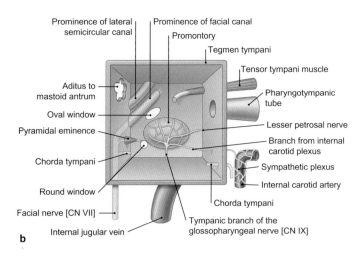

Fig. 10.16a and b Topographical relationship between the tympanic cavity and adjacent structures, right side; lateral view; schematic drawing. a [L126], b [E580]

Wall	Direction	Neighboring Structures
Tegmental	Superior	Middle cranial fossa
Carotid	Anterior	Internal carotid artery
Tympanic membrane	Lateral	External acoustic meatus
Mastoid	Posterior	Mastoid process
Labyrinthine	Medial	Inner ear
Jugular	Inferior	Bulb of jugular vein

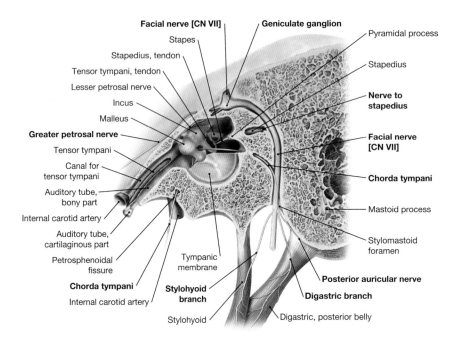

Fig. 10.17 Facial nerve [CN VII], tympanic cavity and auditory tube, right side; vertical section in the longitudinal axis of the petrous part of the temporal bone; frontal view; facial canal opened. [L238]
The facial nerve [CN VII] arches around the tympanic cavity. The stapedius is innervated by the facial nerve. The stapedius attenuates vibrations at the oval window by slightly tilting the stapes, thus, decreasing the transmission of sound waves and protecting the sensory cells of the inner ear from excessive noise.

Clinical Remarks

- The facial nerve [CN VII] courses through the bony mastoid process before exiting the temporal bone at the stylomastoid foramen. The facial nerve [CN VII] is at risk of injury during surgical access of the petrous part for cochlear implants as this involves opening of the mastoid process.
- The chorda tympani courses through the tympanic cavity and is vulnerable to injuries during operations in the middle ear. An isolated functional loss of the chorda tympani with dry

mouth and loss of taste sensation on the affected side is common during middle ear infections.
- Upon paralysis of the stapedius muscle as part of facial nerve palsy, normal sounds are perceived as unpleasantly loud (*hyperacusis*) due to the insufficient attenuation function of the stapedius muscle (no tilting of the base of stapes in the oval window).

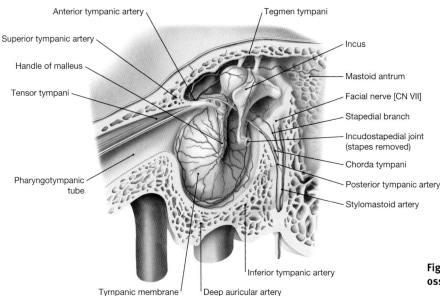

Fig. 10.18 Arteries of the middle ear: auditory ossicles and tympanic membrane. [L275]

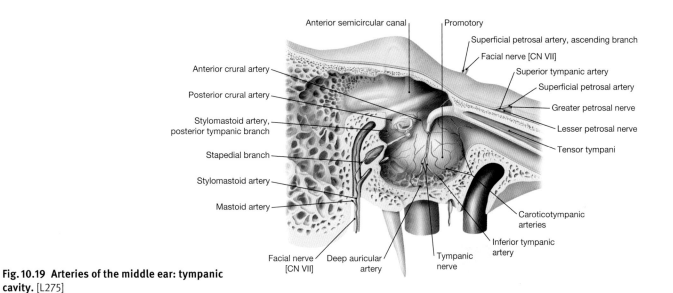

Fig. 10.19 Arteries of the middle ear: tympanic cavity. [L275]

Sensory and Parasympathetic

Tympanic nerve with the glossopharyngeal nerve [CN IX]

↓ *Tympanic canaliculus*

Tympanic plexus
Lesser petrosal nerve

↓ *Sphenopetrosal fissure*

Otic ganglion

Auriculotemporal nerve

Parotid gland

Sympathetic

Sympathetic plexus of internal carotid artery

↓ *Multiple small openings*

Caroticotympanic nerve branches	*Tympanic cavity*

Fig. 10.20 Schematic representation of the sensory and autonomic innervation of the middle ear. [L126]

The tympanic nerve contains preganglionic fibers from the inferior salivatory nucleus which is the parasympathetic nucleus of the glossopharyngeal nerve [CN IX]. The tympanic nerve courses through the inferior ganglion of CN IX without synapsing and generates the tympanic plexus of the middle ear.

Preganglionic parasympathetic fibers form the lesser petrosal nerve. It leaves the tympanic cavity through the sphenopetrosal fissure to synapse in the otic ganglion. Postganglionic parasympathetic fibers from the otic ganglion anastomose with the auriculotemporal (from [CN V/3]) and facial nerves [CN VII] to reach the parotid gland and regulate its secretory function. This course of the postganglionic parasympathetic fibers is known as JACOBSON's anastomosis.

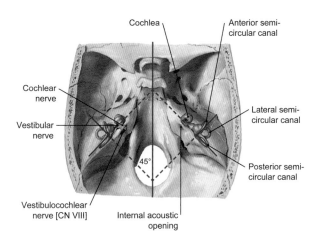

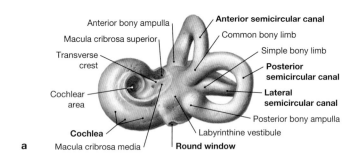

Fig. 10.21 Inner ear and vestibulocochlear nerve [CN VIII]; superior view; inner ear projected onto the petrous part of temporal bone illustrating its natural position.

The semicircular canals position in a 45° angle in relation to the main planes of the skull. This is important information to know when examining CT scans of the skull.

Fig. 10.22 Inner ear with facial nerve [CN VII] and vestibulocochlear nerve [CN VIII], right side; superior view onto the petrous part of temporal bone.

When entering the internal acoustic opening, the facial nerve [CN VII] and its intermediate part are located on top of the vestibulocochlear nerve [CN VIII] which is composed of the cochlear and vestibular nerves (in clinical terms often referred to as *statoacoustic nerve*).

Clinical Remarks

Magnetic resonance image (MRI) of an **acoustic neurinoma** (alias vestibular schwannoma, acoustic neuroma, acoustic neurilemmoma, acoustic neurofibroma, *arrow*). This is a benign tumor of the SCHWANN's cells and most frequently affects the vestibular part of the vestibulocochlear nerve [CN VIII]. It originates in the internal acoustic meatus, grows into the posterior cranial fossa and presses on adjacent structures (*cerebellopontine angle tumor*). Early symptoms include asymmetric hearing impairment, dizziness, and loss of balance. [F276-006]

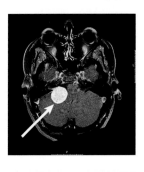

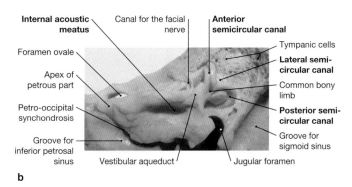

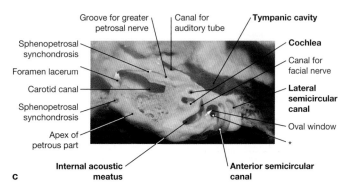

Fig. 10.23a to c Bony labyrinth, right side; osseous lining of the membranous labyrinth, from an oblique posterior angle **(a), partially hollowed out of the petrous part of temporal bone;** posterior and superior view **(b),** superior view **(c).**

The inner ear consists of bony canals and ampullary extensions in the petrous part of temporal bone. This *bony labyrinth* contains within it a system of similarly shaped membranous tubes and sacs, known as the *membranous labyrinth.* It harbors the vestibular and cochlear sensory organs.

* opening of the posterior canaliculus

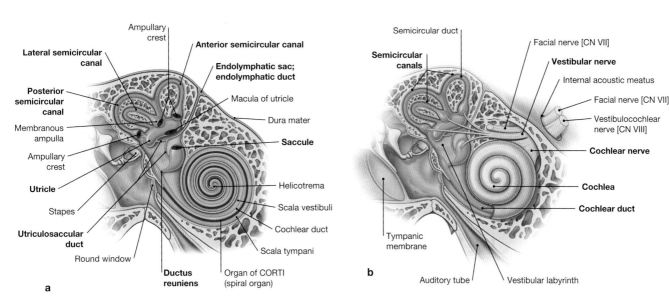

a

b

Fig. 10.24a and b Membranous labyrinth (a); part of the bony cochlear cast and nerves, right side; longitudinal section through the petrous part of temporal bone (b); frontal view, schematic drawing. [E402]

The membranous labyrinth contains potassium-rich and sodium-poor *endolymph*. The *perilymphatic space* filled with perilymph separates the membranous labyrinth from the bony labyrinth. The membranous labyrinth divides into a vestibular and cochlear compart-

ment **(a)** with corresponding nerves **(b)**. The vestibular labyrinth includes the saccule and utricle, the utriculosaccular duct, three semicircular canals, and the endolymphatic duct with the endolymphatic sac. The latter represents an epidural sac for the resorption of the endolymph. The cochlear labyrinth forms the cochlear duct. The ductus reuniens connects the vestibular and cochlear labyrinths.

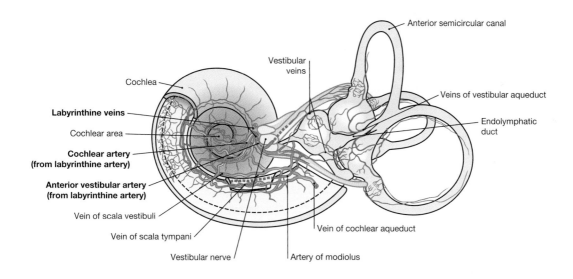

Fig. 10.25 Blood supply and innervation of the inner ear, right side; medial view. [L126]

The labyrinthine artery and labyrinthine veins from the anterior inferior cerebellar artery and vein, respectively, provide blood supply

to the labyrinth. The labyrinthine artery is a terminal artery and its occlusion can cause labyrinthine infarction.

┌─ Clinical Remarks ─────────────────────────────

Being a terminal artery, thrombotic occlusion of the labyrinthine artery or its contributing branches can cause labyrinthine infarction with loss of balance (vertigo) and sensorineural hearing impairment. MENIERE's disease presents with attacks of vertigo, unilateral hearing loss, and unilateral tinnitus. Its etiology is not

clear but hydropic swelling of the membranous labyrinth due to impaired resorption of endolymph (cochlear hydrops) is discussed. The increase in pressure due to the increased volume of endolymph causes damage to the sensory cells of the vestibulocochlear system.

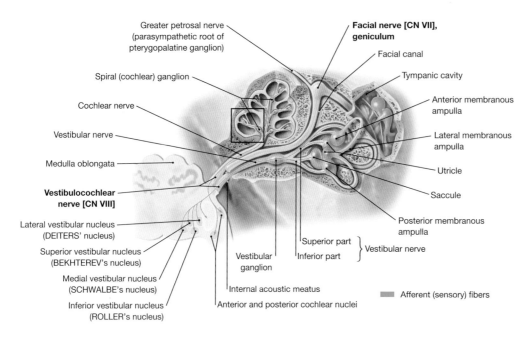

Fig. 10.26 Section through the petrous part of temporal bone; view from above. [L238]
Location of the cochlea (boxed), vestibular labyrinth, vestibulocochlear nerve [CN VIII] and facial nerve [CN VII] within the petrous part of temporal bone. The cochlea and middle ear have been opened. The boxed area is shown enlarged in ➤ Fig. 10.27.

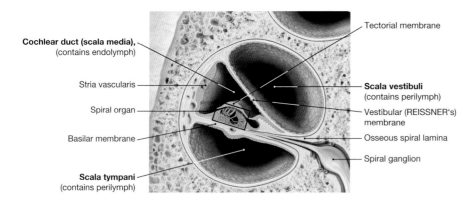

Fig. 10.27 Cross-section of the cochlea. [L238]
Schematic cross-sectional drawing shows the spiral canal of cochlea and cochlear organ (organ of CORTI). The REISSNER's membrane and the basilar membrane divide the spiral canal of cochlea into three spaces:

- **Scala vestibuli:** from the vestibulum to the helicotrema; filled with perilymph
- **Scala media** (cochlear duct): contains endolymph
- **Scala tympani:** from helicotrema to round window; filled with perilymph

Scala vestibuli and scala tympani join at the helicotrema.

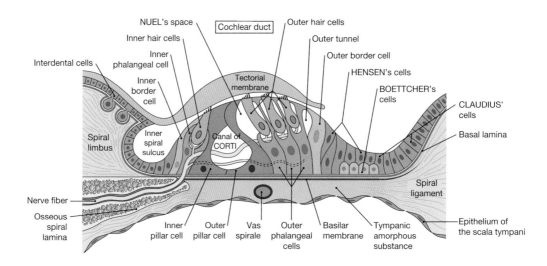

Fig. 10.28 Section through the cochlear duct and spiral organ. [L107]
The basilar membrane supports the cochlear organ. The stria vascularis at the lateral bony wall of the cochlea produces the endolymph.

The cochlear organ stretches along the whole length of the cochlear duct and is composed of cochlear sensory cells (hair cells) and different supporting cell types. A gelatinous membrane (tectorial membrane) covers the apical cell surface.

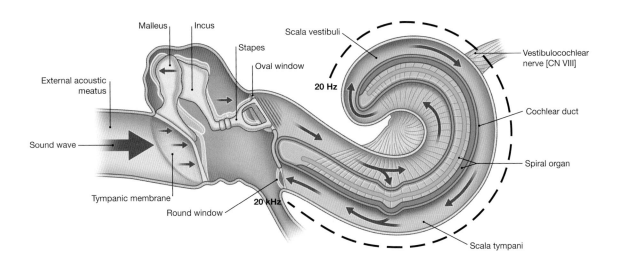

Fig. 10.29 Mechanoelectrical sound conduction. [E402]
Sound propagates by sound waves which reach the outer ear (auricle and external acoustic meatus) and are transmitted by the tympanic membrane and the chain of auditory ossicles through the base of stapes to the perilymph. At the oval window, piston-like movements of the stapes initiate a perilymph wave. This wave migrates along the cochlear duct and causes a deflection of the basilar membrane and the cochlear organ. This movement bends the stereocilia of the hair cells which insert in the stiff gelatinous tectorial membrane. This biomechanic event generates a receptor potential (mechanoelectrical transduction) by the hair cells. The apical wider and more compliant basilar membrane towards the helicotrema responds most efficiently to low frequencies, whereas its stiffer basal part resonates best at high frequencies (see dashed black line reflecting the frequency band). When the perilymph wave hits the round window its covering membrane bulges out to release the remaining energy of the wave.

The inner hair cells are mainly responsible for hearing, whereas the outer hair cells have a modulatory role. The excitatory hair cells synapse with primary bipolar sensory neurons. Their perikarya constitute the spiral ganglion along the central rim of cochlea and their axons form the cochlear nerve. Different locations along the basilar membrane resonate best to certain frequencies (➤ Fig. 10.29). This tonotopic organization of the cochlear organ is reflected in the organization of the cochlear nerve and the entire central auditory pathway up to the primary auditory cortex at the HESCHL's transverse convolutions (area 41).

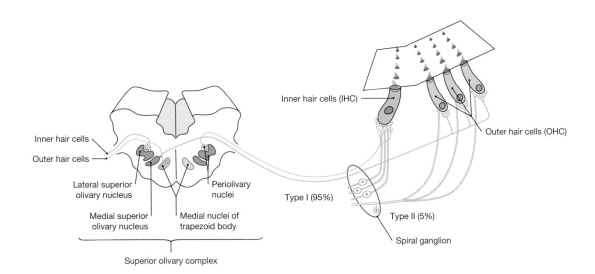

Fig. 10.30 Schematic drawing of the neural pathway connecting the hair cells with the superior olivary nuclei of the central auditory pathway in the rostral medulla. [L126]
The cochlear part of CN VIII contains afferent and efferent fibers. Afferent fibers derived from bipolar ganglionic cells connect to the inner hair cells (IHC) and outer hair cells (OHC) and transmit their impulses to the CNS. As part of a central descending pathway, efferent fibers within CN VIII connect with the IHC and OHC. This olivonuclear bundle originates in the superior olivary nuclear complex. Exiting the medulla, these fibers first course with the vestibular nerve before switching to the cochlear nerve in the inner ear canal (OORT anastomosis). The IHC receive fibers from ipsilateral nuclei, whereas the OHC receive fibers from the contralateral nuclei of the superior olivary complex. Olivonuclear efferences protect hair cells against loud noise and help in the detection and discrimination of sounds in a noisy environment.

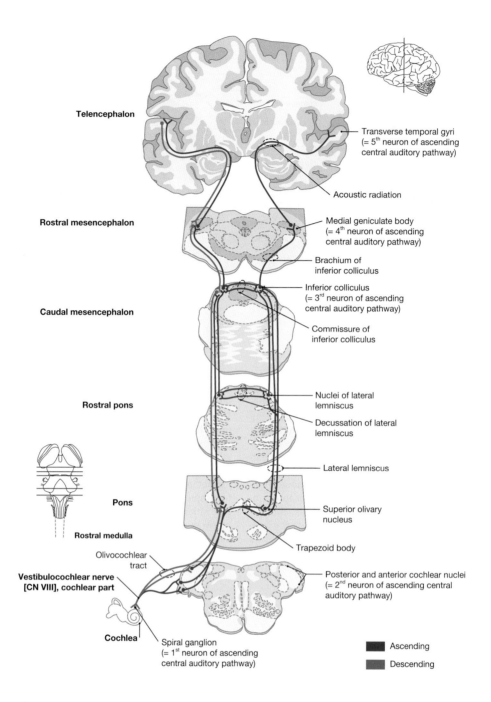

Telencephalon

Transverse temporal gyri
(= 5th neuron of ascending
central auditory pathway)

Acoustic radiation

Rostral mesencephalon

Medial geniculate body
(= 4th neuron of ascending
central auditory pathway)

Brachium of
inferior colliculus

Inferior colliculus
(= 3rd neuron of ascending
central auditory pathway)

Caudal mesencephalon

Commissure of
inferior colliculus

Nuclei of lateral
lemniscus

Rostral pons

Decussation of lateral
lemniscus

Lateral lemniscus

Pons

Superior olivary
nucleus

Rostral medulla

Trapezoid body

Olivocochlear
tract

Posterior and anterior cochlear nuclei
(= 2nd neuron of ascending central
auditory pathway)

**Vestibulocochlear nerve
[CN VIII], cochlear part**

Cochlea

Spiral ganglion
(= 1st neuron of ascending
central auditory pathway)

Ascending

Descending

Fig. 10.31 Auditory pathway; overview. [L127]
The *ascending central auditory pathway* (red) transmits acoustic signals
to the cortex to create acoustic awareness.
1. Neuron: bipolar cells in the spiral ganglion of cochlea
- At the internal acoustic meatus, fibers of the cochlear and vestibular nerves unite to form the vestibulocochlear nerve [CN VIII].
- Fibers from the basal and apical cochlear parts traverse to the posterior and anterior cochlear nuclei, respectively.
2. Neuron: multipolar cells of cochlear nuclei
- The lateral lemniscus connects the olivary nuclei with the inferior colliculus. Fibers that reach the olivary nuclei on the same side, either ascend to the nuclei of lateral lemniscus, synapse,

cross to the opposite side, synapse again, and then reach the
inferior colliculus or they ascend directly in the lateral lemniscus to reach the inferior colliculus.
3. or 4. Neuron: connecting the inferior colliculus with the medial
geniculate body
4. or 5. Neuron: The acoustic radiation connects the medial geniculate body of thalamus with the transverse temporal **HESCHL's gyri**
and the **WERNICKE's area** in the temporal lobe.
Descending fiber tracts (blue) are likely to affect auditory adaptive
processes by contributing to the dynamic reorganization of subcortical auditory networks.

Clinical Remarks

Tinnitus is frequently the consequence of damage to the hair
cells, e.g. after exposure to loud music or an explosion. Tinnitus
aurium, or Tinnitus for short ('ringing of the ears'), is a symptom

where the affected individual perceives sounds in the absence
of real sounds.

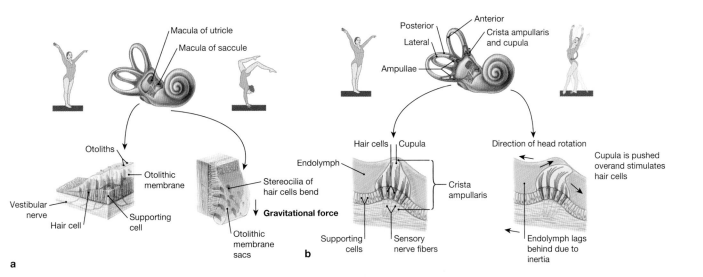

Fig. 10.32a and b The vestibular labyrinth registers rotational and linear movements. [L285]
The vestibular labyrinth is filled with endolymph and consists of the **(a)** saccule and utricle (macula of saccule and utricle) for vertical and horizontal linear acceleration, respectively, and **(b)** three semicircular canals (ampullary crests with their cupula) for rotational acceleration.

The vestibular sensory cells possess a long kinocilium and stereocilia which extend into a gelatinous substance. Movement results in the deflection of these cellular processes and triggers synaptic activation of afferent fibers of the vestibular nerve. The gelatinous matrix of the macula of saccule and utricle is covered with otoliths that assist in sensing linear motions.

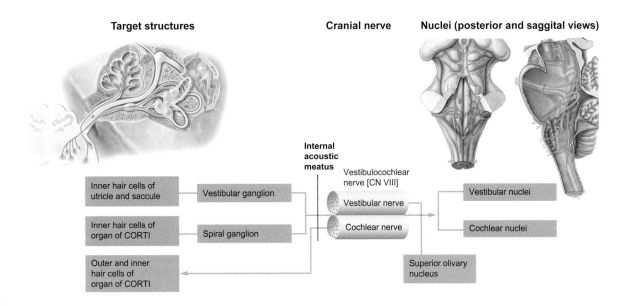

Fig. 10.33 The vestibulocochlear nerve [CN VIII] connects sensory cells of the inner ear with the central auditory and vestibular pathways. [L127]

Clinical Remarks

Labyrinthitis with dysequilibrium and/or dizziness, nystagmus, nausea, and anxiety can accompany skull trauma or infections of the middle ear. Entry ports for infectious germs are the round and oval windows, breaches in the bony labyrinth (caused by trauma or bone erosion due to infected pneumatic spaces), or ascending inflammation of the meninges via nerves and vessels, cochlear duct or vestibular ducts. The result is *sensorineural hearing impairment* with destruction of the vestibular organ.

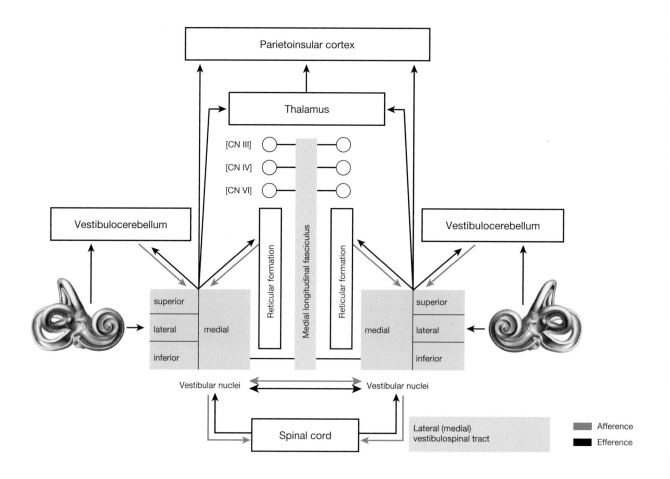

Fig. 10.34 The equilibrium (balance) pathway coordinates eye movements and movements of trunk, neck, and extremities. [L126]

1ˢᵗ Neuron:
- Afferent fibers of the vestibular ganglion mainly project into the medial vestibular nucleus (SCHWALBE's nucleus), the superior vestibular nucleus (nucleus of BEKHTEREV), and the inferior vestibular nucleus (ROLLER's nucleus).
- Afferent fibers of the ampullary crests of the semicircular canals mainly connect with the medial and superior nuclei and the vestibulocerebellum via the direct sensory cerebellar pathway.
- Afferent fibers of the utricle and saccule project into the medial and lateral vestibular nuclei, respectively.

- The lateral vestibular nucleus (DEITERS' nucleus) also receives collateral fibers from the vestibular pathways and, in particular, cerebellar afferences.

2ⁿᵈ Neuron: from the vestibular nuclei efferent fibers project to the:
- cerebellum (vestibulocerebellar tract)
- spinal cord (vestibulospinal tract)
- nuclei controlling the extraocular muscles (medial longitudinal fasciculus to the oculomotor nerve [CN III], trochlear nerve [CN IV], and abducens nerve [CN VI])
- thalamus via the vestibulothalamic tract to the inferior posterior ventral nucleus and from here via the thalamic radiation to the postcentral gyrus

Clinical Remarks

Commonly used tests to assess the body's sense of positioning or examine a tendency to fall to one side are the **ROMBERG test** (patient stands upright with feet together, eyes closed, and arms stretched forward) and the **UNTERBERGER stepping test** (patient walks on the spot with eyes closed). FRENZEL's lenses (FRENZEL's glasses) are used for the **nystagmus test** (nystagmus = involuntary rapid eye movements). This test is performed with the patient holding the head in different positions.

A caloric nystagmus test examines the responses by the labyrinth on one side. The patient is lying in a supine position (elevated head) in a room with dimmed light and the ear on each side is irrigated with cold and warm water. Cold water will initiate a physiological nystagmus to the opposite side. Warm water will stimulate a nystagmus to the same side of the labyrinth tested. A reduced or lacking nystagmus is pathological and suggests a peripheral functional impairment.

Neck

Surface Anatomy of the Neck 519

Triangles of the Neck 520

Cervical Fascia 521

Retropharyngeal Space 522

Anterior and Posterior Cervical
Region – Superficial Layer 523

Anterior and Posterior Cervical
Region – Vessels and Nerves 524

Anterior and Posterior Cervical
Region – Deep Layer 525

Cervical Plexus 526

Subclavian and Vertebral Arteries .. 527

Anterior Cervical Region – Surface
Anatomy and Superficial Layer 528

Anterior Cervical Region –
Neurovascular Structures 529

Pharyngeal Spaces 530

Pharyngeal Muscles 532

Pharyngeal Neurovascular Structures
and Parapharyngeal Space 533

Swallowing (Deglutition) 535

Larynx and Laryngeal Cartilages 536

Laryngeal Cartilages 537

Laryngeal Cartilages and
Vocal Cords 539

Laryngeal Muscles 540

Laryngoscopy 541

Endotracheal Procedures 542

Laryngeal Spaces 543

Laryngeal Neurovascular
Structures 544

Development of the Thyroid Gland .. 545

Thyroid Gland 546

Neurovascular Structures
of the Thyroid Gland 547

Topography of the Thyroid Gland ... 548

Parathyroid Glands 549

Lymphatic Drainage of the Neck 550

Superior Thoracic Aperture 551

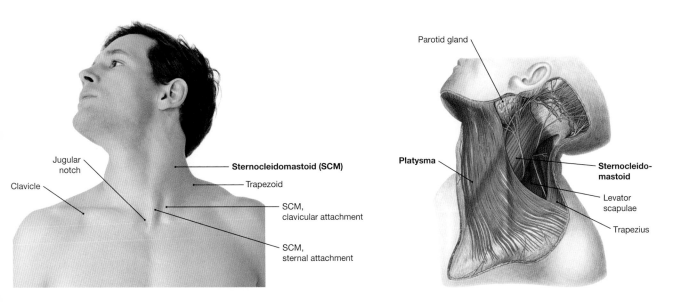

Fig. 11.1 Surface anatomy of the neck, left side; lateral view. [K340] The sternal and clavicular origins and the body of sternocleidomastoid are visible.

Fig. 11.2 Superficial muscles of the neck, left side; lateral view. The platysma inserts directly into the skin. The upper part of the sternocleidomastoid is a reference point during surgical interventions.

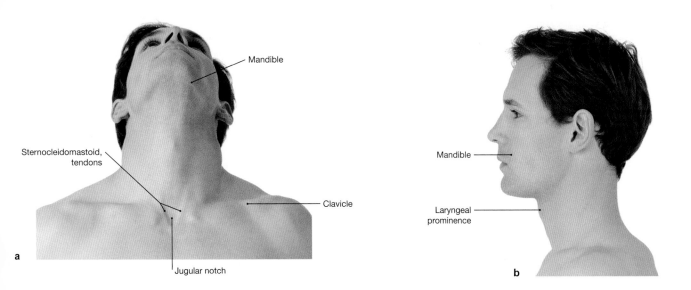

Fig. 11.3a and b Surface anatomy of the neck; anterior view **(a)**; **left side;** lateral view **(b).** [K340]

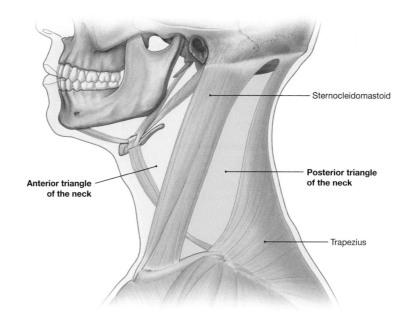

Fig. 11.4 Anterior and posterior triangles of the neck, left side; lateral view. [E402]
Boundaries of the anterior triangle (anterior cervical region) of the neck are the lower rim of the mandibular bone (mandible), the anterior border of the sternocleidomastoid, and the median cervical line (midline of the neck). Boundaries of the posterior triangle (posterior cervical region) of the neck are the posterior border of the sternocleidomastoid, the anterior border of the trapezius, the upper rim of the clavicle and the occipital bone.

Content of the Anterior and Posterior Triangles of the Neck		
Content	**Anterior Triangle of the Neck**	**Posterior Triangle of the Neck**
Arteries	• External carotid artery with branches • Internal carotid	• Occipital • Transverse cervical • 3rd part of subclavian • suprascapular
Veins	• External jugular • Anterior jugular • Internal jugular • Facial • Retromandibular	• Subclavian • External jugular

Nerves	• Mylohoid (branch of CN VIII)
	• Ansa cervicalis (cervical plexus)
	• Vagus [CN X]
	• Recurrent laryngeal (branch of CN X)
	• Hypoglossal [CN XII]
		• Greater occipital (C2)
		• Four cutaneous branches of the cervical plexus
		  – Lesser occipital
		  – Greater auricular
		  – Transverse cervical
		  – Supraclavicular nerves
		• Spinal accessory [CN XI]
		• Three trunks of the brachial plexus
		• Suprascapular

Muscles	• Suprahyoid • Infrahyoid • Superior belly of omohyoid	• Semispinalis capitis • Splenius capitis • Posterior scalene • Serratus anterior • Inferior belly of omohyoid
Other structures	• Lymph nodes • Submandibular gland • Thyroid gland • Parathyroid glands • Trachea • Larynx/Pharynx • Esophagus	• Lymph nodes

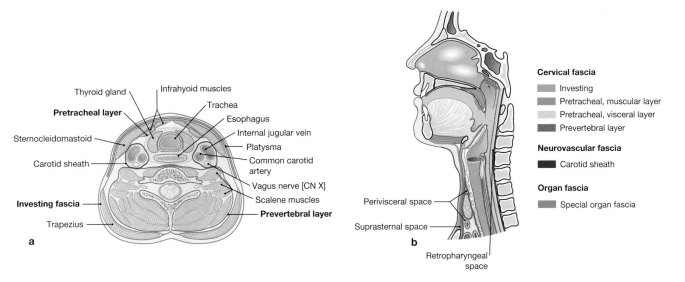

Fig. 11.5a and b Cervical fascia; transverse section (a) and sagittal section of the neck (b). a [E402], b [L126]
The **investing fascia (superficial layer)** encases the whole neck and ensheathes the sternocleidomastoid and trapezius muscles. The **pretracheal (muscular) layer**, covers the infrahyoid muscles. Its *visceral layer* encases pharynx, larynx, thyroid gland, parathyroid glands, the upper part of the trachea, and the cervical part of the esophagus. The **prevertebral (deep) layer** covers the scalene muscles, prevertebral muscles, the rectus capitis lateralis and merges with the fascia of the intrinsic [autochthonous] muscles of the back (➤ Fig. 2.34 and ➤ Fig. 2.35). The **carotid sheath** receives contributions from all three neck fascias and encapsulates the common, internal and external carotid arteries, the internal jugular vein, and the vagus nerve [CN X].

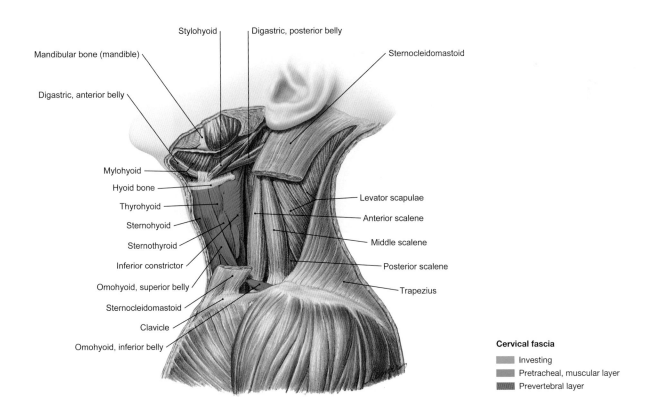

Fig. 11.6 Infrahyoid and neck muscles and their relationship to the cervical fascia; lateral view.
The same color scheme was used as shown in Fig. 11.5 to indicate the three different layers of the cervical fascia in relation to important neck structures. For details on the deep anterior neck (➤ Fig. 2.33) and the posterior region of neck (➤ Fig. 2.34 and ➤ Fig. 2.35).

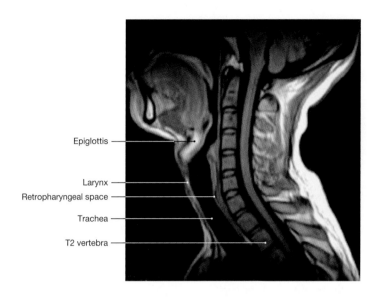

Fig. 11.7 Sagittal MRI image of the neck. [F589]

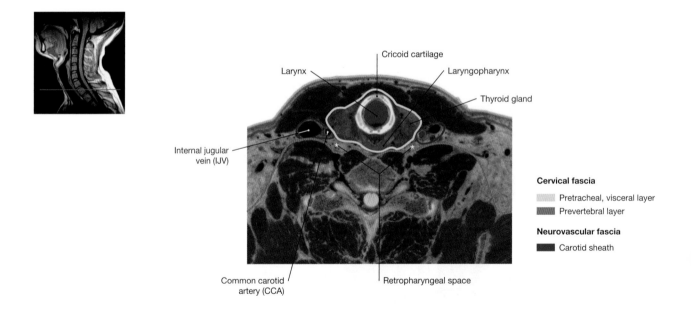

Fig. 11.8 Cross-sectional anatomy of the neck at the level of C7.
[F589, X338]

Structure/Function

Retropharyngeal Space
- Space denoted with (white *) between visceral part of the pretracheal fascia (yellow), prevertebral fascia (pink) and carotid sheath (purple) filled with loose connective tissue
- Largest interfascial space in the neck

- Allows movement of the pharynx, esophagus, larynx and trachea
- Major pathway for the spread of infections in the neck to base of skull cranially and mediastinum caudally
- Continues caudally into the superior mediastinum of the thorax

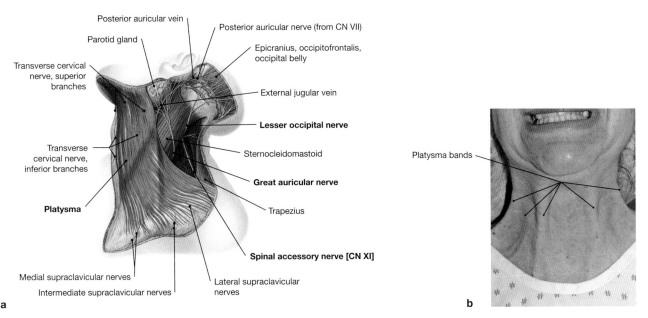

Fig. 11.9a and b **Superficial layer of the posterior cervical region:
a Vessels and nerves;** lateral view. b [E990]
The superficial fascia of the neck was removed dorsal to the platysma. The great auricular nerve and the lesser occipital nerve are sensory nerves derived from the cervical plexus (C1–C4). They in-

nervate the skin in front of and below the auricle.
b Platysma muscle contraction at both sides of the neck.
The platysma is innervated by the facial nerve [CN VII]. Platysma contractions create the typical muscle bands as shown.

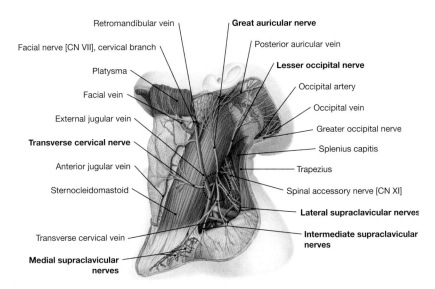

Fig. 11.10 **Superficial blood vessels and nerves of the posterior cervical region, left side;** lateral view.
Parts of the platysma were deflected upwards, and the investing layer of the cervical fascia was largely removed. The greater occipital nerve provides sensory cutaneous innervation to the occipital region. It is the dorsal branch of the spinal nerve C2.

The four sensory nerves of the cervical plexus emerge in a confined area, called *nerve point of the neck* (ERB's point, circled), midway of the posterior margin of the sternocleidomastoid. They are:
• Greater auricular nerve
• Lesser occipital nerve
• Transverse cervical nerve
• Supraclavicular nerves (medial, intermediate, lateral)

Structure/Function

Sensory innervation of the skin in the cervical region is provided by cutaneous nerves: the supraclavicular nerves, transverse cervical nerve, great auricular nerve, lesser occipital nerve, greater occipital nerve and third occipital nerve (not shown). [L126]

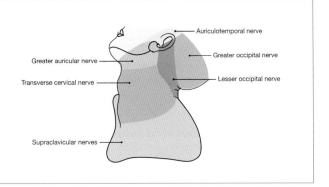

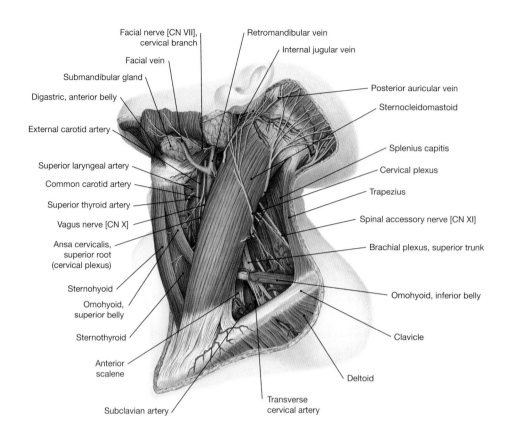

Facial nerve [CN VII], cervical branch
Facial vein
Submandibular gland
Digastric, anterior belly
External carotid artery
Superior laryngeal artery
Common carotid artery
Superior thyroid artery
Vagus nerve [CN X]
Ansa cervicalis, superior root (cervical plexus)
Sternohyoid
Omohyoid, superior belly
Sternothyroid
Anterior scalene
Subclavian artery
Retromandibular vein
Internal jugular vein
Posterior auricular vein
Sternocleidomastoid
Splenius capitis
Cervical plexus
Trapezius
Spinal accessory nerve [CN XI]
Brachial plexus, superior trunk
Omohyoid, inferior belly
Clavicle
Deltoid
Transverse cervical artery

Fig. 11.11 Muscles, vessels and nerves of the anterior and posterior cervical region, left side; lateral view; after removal of the superficial and middle fascia of the neck.

In the posterior triangle of the neck the brachial plexus and subclavian artery are shown in the scalene hiatus, the gap between the anterior and middle scalene muscles.

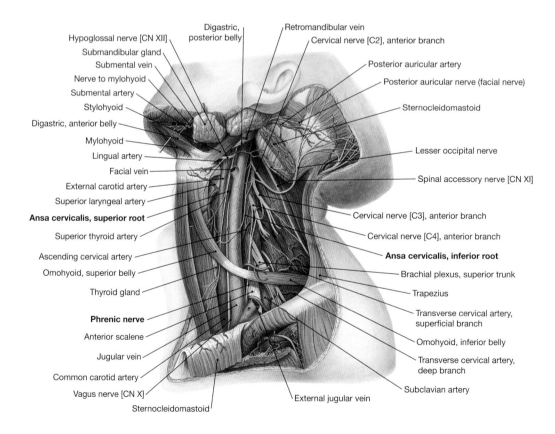

Hypoglossal nerve [CN XII]
Submandibular gland
Submental vein
Nerve to mylohyoid
Submental artery
Stylohyoid
Digastric, anterior belly
Mylohyoid
Lingual artery
Facial vein
External carotid artery
Superior laryngeal artery
Ansa cervicalis, superior root
Superior thyroid artery
Ascending cervical artery
Omohyoid, superior belly
Thyroid gland
Phrenic nerve
Anterior scalene
Jugular vein
Common carotid artery
Vagus nerve [CN X]
Sternocleidomastoid
Digastric, posterior belly
Retromandibular vein
Cervical nerve [C2], anterior branch
Posterior auricular artery
Posterior auricular nerve (facial nerve)
Sternocleidomastoid
Lesser occipital nerve
Spinal accessory nerve [CN XI]
Cervical nerve [C3], anterior branch
Cervical nerve [C4], anterior branch
Ansa cervicalis, inferior root
Brachial plexus, superior trunk
Trapezius
Transverse cervical artery, superficial branch
Omohyoid, inferior belly
Transverse cervical artery, deep branch
Subclavian artery
External jugular vein

Fig. 11.12 Vessels and nerves of the posterior cervical region, left side; lateral view; deeper layer; sternocleidomastoid removed. The superior and inferior roots of the ansa cervicalis enclose the internal jugular vein (IJV). The phrenic nerve originates from the cervical plexus (C3–C5), crosses the anterior scalene muscle and enters the upper thoracic aperture to reach the diaphragm which it innervates.

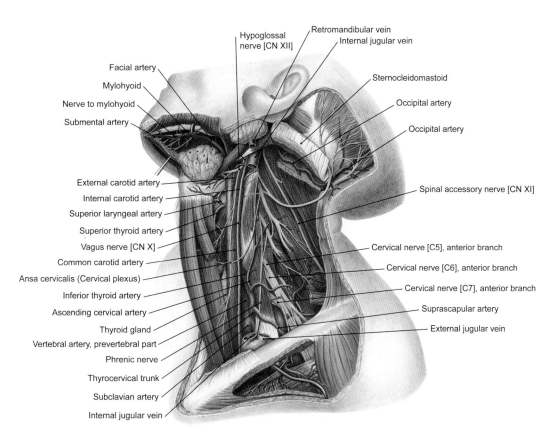

Fig. 11.13 Vessels and nerves of the posterior cervical region; deep layer, left side.

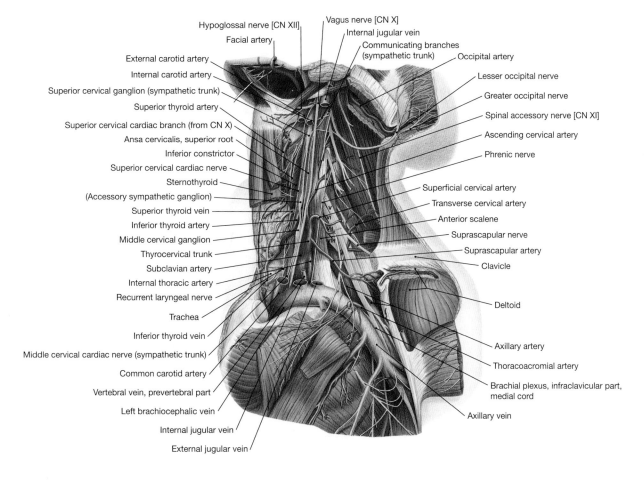

Fig. 11.14 Vessels and nerves of the anterior and posterior cervical region; deep layer, left side; after removal of the clavicle. Numbers V to VIII mark the ventral branches (rami) of the corresponding cervical nerves. The ventral rami of the C5–T1 spinal nerves form the brachial plexus. Together with the subclavian artery, the brachial plexus passes through the scalene hiatus between the anterior and middle scalene muscles. The subclavian vein courses in front of the anterior scalene across rib I.

525

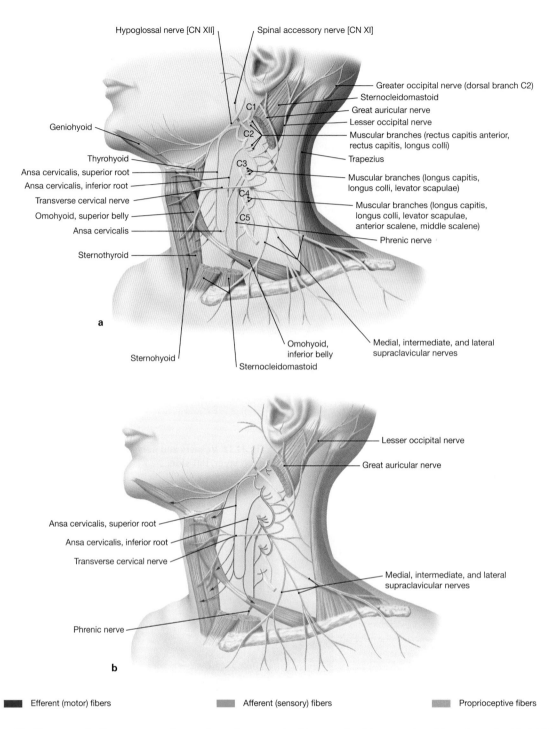

Fig. 11.15a and b   Plexus cervicalis, sensory and motor branches. [L127]

a The ansa cervicalis and the phrenic nerve constitute the motor branches of the cervical plexus. The ansa cervicalis consists of a superior root from segment C1 and an inferior root from segments C2 and C3. The two roots innervate the infrahyoid muscles: thyro-

hyoid, sternohyoid, sternothyroid, and omohyoid. Additional motor branches innervate the suprahyoid, geniohyoid, the prevertebral muscles, the rectus capitis anterior, the anterior and middle scalene muscles as well as parts of the levator scapulae.

b Schematic drawing of motor (red) and sensory fiber qualities (blue).

Fig. 11.16   Sensory innervation of the skin in the head and neck region and segmental mapping of the cutaneous areas. [E402]

The cervical segments C2, C3, and C4 provide the innervation to the skin in the neck region. The ventral branches of the spinal nerves innervate the anterior cervical region, while the posterior branches provide the sensory innervation to the posterior cervical region.

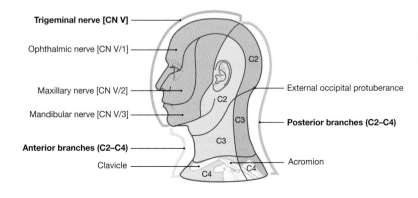

Structure/Function

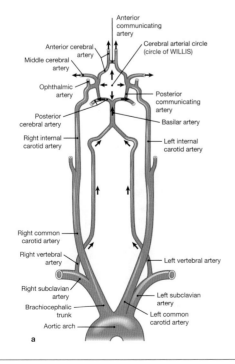

Variations in the level of entry of the vertebral artery into the foramina transversaria.

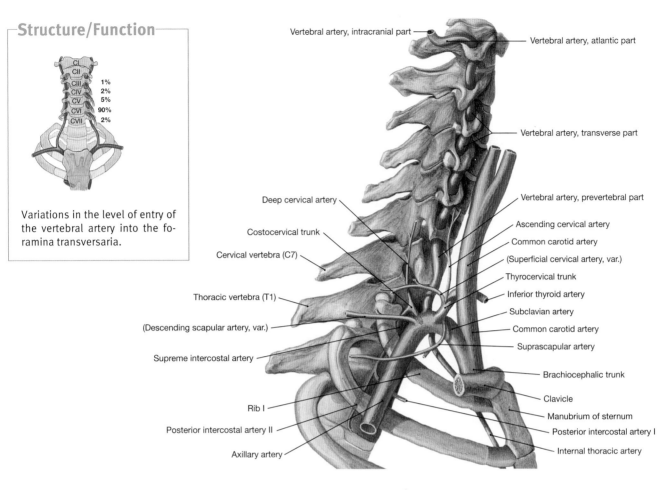

Fig. 11.17 Branches of the subclavian artery and the vertebral artery; lateral view.

Clinical Remarks

Schematic drawings of the arterial blood supply to the circle of WILLIS at the brainstem.

Blood flow (black arrows) in a healthy patient (**a**) and in a patient with subclavian steal syndrome (SSS, **b**). A proximal high-grade stenosis (narrowing) of the left subclavian artery can result in a retrograde (reversed) flow in the vertebral artery of the affected side (red arrows, **b**) during intense physical activity of the arm. The resulting reduction in the blood perfusion of the brain (thin arrow, **b**) can cause dizziness and headaches. SSS is more commonly observed in the left subclavian artery. [L126]

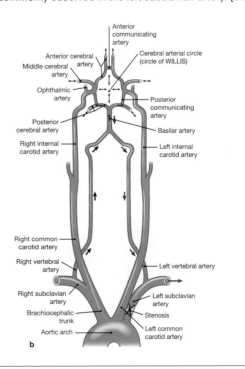

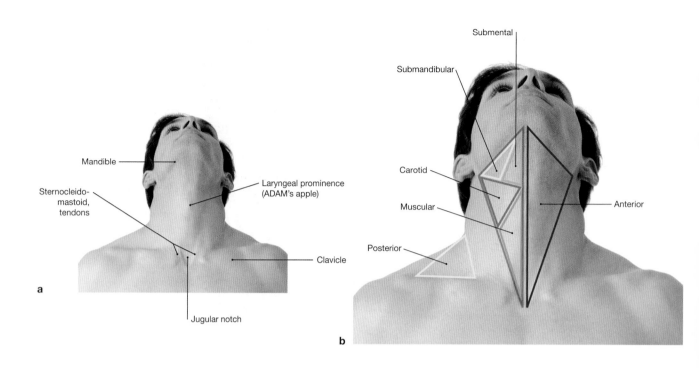

Mandible

Sternocleido-
mastoid,
tendons

Laryngeal prominence
(ADAM's apple)

Clavicle

a

Jugular notch

Submental

Submandibular

Carotid

Muscular

Posterior

Anterior

b

**Fig. 11.18a and b Anterior cervical region.
a Surface anatomy;** frontal view. [K340]

**b Location of the anterior and posterior triangles of the neck and
triangular subdivisions of the anterior cervical region.** [L126, K340]

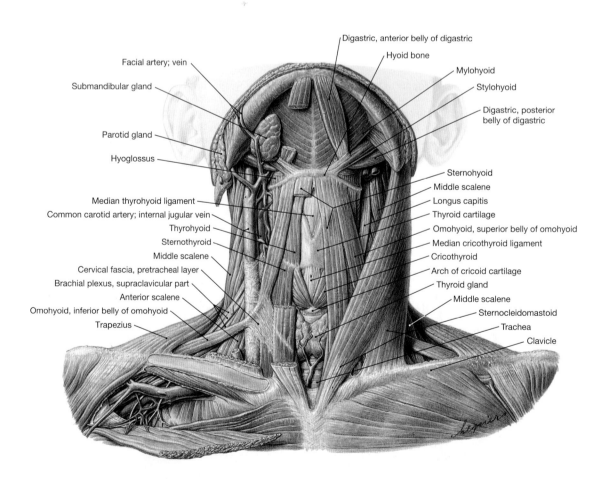

Facial artery; vein

Submandibular gland

Parotid gland

Hyoglossus

Median thyrohyoid ligament

Common carotid artery; internal jugular vein

Thyrohyoid

Sternothyroid

Middle scalene

Cervical fascia, pretracheal layer

Brachial plexus, supraclavicular part

Anterior scalene

Omohyoid, inferior belly of omohyoid

Trapezius

Digastric, anterior belly of digastric

Hyoid bone

Mylohyoid

Stylohyoid

Digastric, posterior
belly of digastric

Sternohyoid

Middle scalene

Longus capitis

Thyroid cartilage

Omohyoid, superior belly of omohyoid

Median cricothyroid ligament

Cricothyroid

Arch of cricoid cartilage

Thyroid gland

Middle scalene

Sternocleidomastoid

Trachea

Clavicle

Fig. 11.19 Anterior cervical region; frontal view.

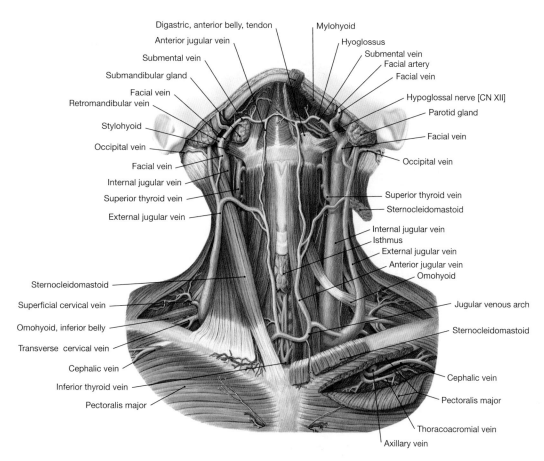

Fig. 11.20 Superficial veins of the neck; frontal view. The course of the superficial veins is highly variable.

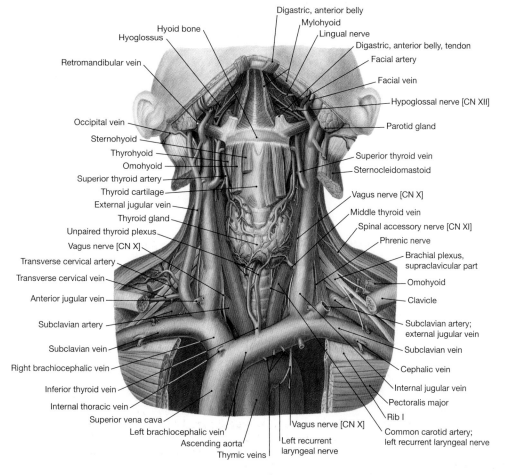

Fig. 11.21 Neurovascular structures of the neck and the upper thoracic aperture; frontal view.

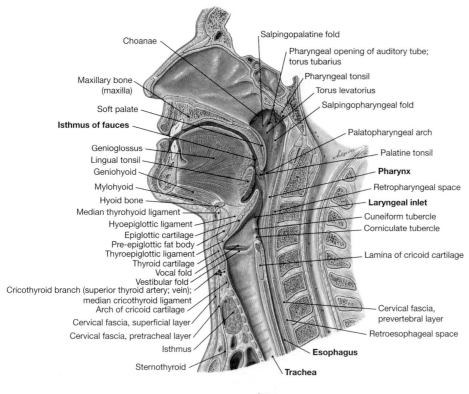

Choanae

Maxillary bone (maxilla)

Soft palate

Isthmus of fauces

Genioglossus
Lingual tonsil
Geniohyoid
Mylohyoid
Hyoid bone
Median thyrohyoid ligament
Hyoepiglottic ligament
Epiglottic cartilage
Pre-epiglottic fat body
Thyroepiglottic ligament
Thyroid cartilage
Vocal fold
Vestibular fold
Cricothyroid branch (superior thyroid artery; vein);
median cricothyroid ligament
Arch of cricoid cartilage
Cervical fascia, superficial layer
Cervical fascia, pretracheal layer
Isthmus
Sternothyroid

Salpingopalatine fold

Pharyngeal opening of auditory tube;
torus tubarius

Pharyngeal tonsil

Torus levatorius

Salpingopharyngeal fold

Palatopharyngeal arch

Palatine tonsil

Pharynx

Retropharyngeal space

Laryngeal inlet

Cuneiform tubercle

Corniculate tubercle

Lamina of cricoid cartilage

Cervical fascia, prevertebral layer

Retroesophageal space

Esophagus

Trachea

Fig. 11.22 Topographical relationship between nasal cavity, oral cavity, pharynx, and larynx; midsagittal section.

- The **nasopharynx** connects with the nasal cavity and the middle ear through the choanae and the auditory tube, respectively.
- The **oropharynx** connects with the oral cavity through the isthmus of fauces.
- The **laryngopharynx** has an anterior connection with the larynx through the laryngeal inlet and transitions caudally into the esophagus. Airways and alimentary passage cross within the pharynx.

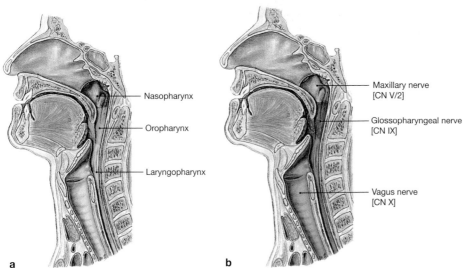

Nasopharynx

Oropharynx

Laryngopharynx

Maxillary nerve
[CN V/2]

Glossopharyngeal nerve
[CN IX]

Vagus nerve
[CN X]

a

b

Fig. 11.23a and b Pharynx.
a Levels of the pharynx; midsagittal section.
b Sensory innervation of the pharynx; midsagittal section.
Sensory and sympathetic nerve fibers form the pharyngeal plexus. Afferent and efferent fibers of this pharyngeal plexus are part of the vital swallowing and choking reflexes which remain active during sleep. The coordination of these complex reflexes takes place in the medulla oblongata.

Clinical Remarks

Different spaces in the neck are interconnected. This allows infections to spread. In the case of palatine tonsillitis, bacteria can enter the parapharyngeal space (area around the pharynx).

From here, germs can spread to other spaces in the neck indicated in the schematic diagram to cause abscesses and/or sepsis. [L126]

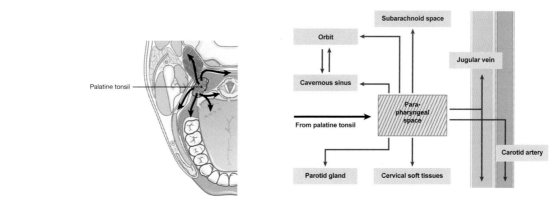

Palatine tonsil

Subarachnoid space

Orbit

Cavernous sinus

From palatine tonsil

Parotid gland

Cervical soft tissues

Para-pharyngeal space

Jugular vein

Carotid artery

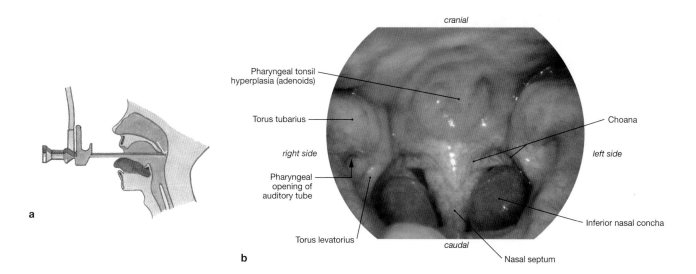

a

b

cranial

Pharyngeal tonsil
hyperplasia (adenoids)

Torus tubarius

right side

Pharyngeal
opening of
auditory tube

Torus levatorius

Choana

left side

Inferior nasal concha

caudal

Nasal septum

Fig. 11.24a and b Nasopharynx – endoscopy of the nasopharynx.
b [T720]
a Schematic of an indirect laryngoscopy of the posterior space of
the nasal cavity with choanae, the opening of the auditory tubes
and the pharyngeal tonsil (adenoids).

b An endoscopic view into the nasopharyngeal space reveals the
posterior tips of the inferior nasal conchae on both sides and the
pharyngeal opening of the auditory tube. The pharyngeal tonsil,
clinically known as adenoids, is located at the roof of the pharynx.

Clinical Remarks

The paired palatine tonsils are located at the entrance of the
oropharynx and are part of the WALDEYER's lymphatic ring of
mucosa-associated lymphatic tissue (MALT; see also ➤ chapter 8,
➤ Fig. 8.95). Often, streptococcal pharyngitis *(strep throat,* **a**) includes swollen palatine tonsils which present with white exudate deposited on their surface and inflamed throat (redness).
Strep throat causes pain when swallowing.
Hyperplasia of the pharyngeal tonsil **(adenoids, b)** occurs frequently in children. It can lead to the occlusion of the pharyngeal opening of the auditory tube, and cause recurring middle ear
infections. In young children, this condition can result in hearing impairment and subsequently can cause a delay in development. In these cases, the surgical removal (adenoidectomy) of
the pharyngeal tonsil (adenoids) is indicated.
a [F654], b [L275]

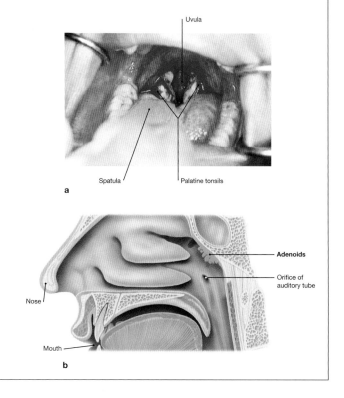

Uvula

Spatula

Palatine tonsils

a

Adenoids

Orifice of
auditory tube

Nose

Mouth

b

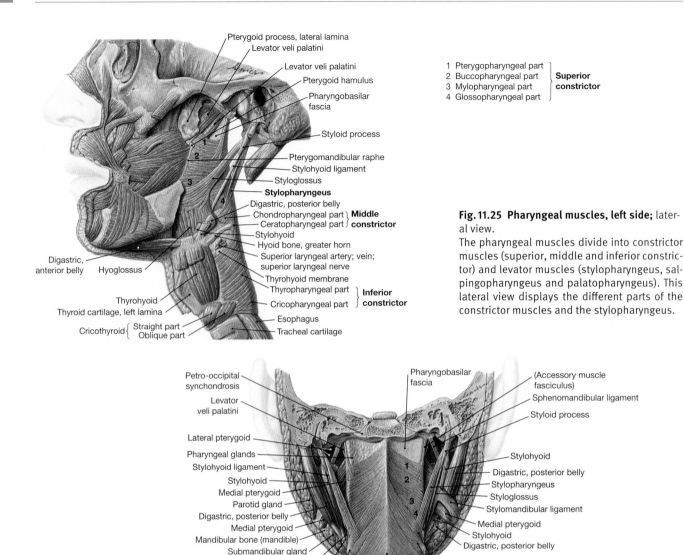

1 Pterygopharyngeal part
2 Buccopharyngeal part   **Superior**
3 Mylopharyngeal part   **constrictor**
4 Glossopharyngeal part

Pterygoid process, lateral lamina
Levator veli palatini
Levator veli palatini
Pterygoid hamulus
Pharyngobasilar fascia
Styloid process
Pterygomandibular raphe
Stylohyoid ligament
Styloglossus
Stylopharyngeus
Digastric, posterior belly
Chondropharyngeal part   **Middle**
Ceratopharyngeal part   **constrictor**
Stylohyoid
Hyoid bone, greater horn
Superior laryngeal artery; vein; superior laryngeal nerve
Thyrohyoid membrane
Thyropharyngeal part   **Inferior**
Cricopharyngeal part   **constrictor**
Esophagus
Tracheal cartilage
Digastric, anterior belly
Hyoglossus
Thyrohyoid
Thyroid cartilage, left lamina
Cricothyroid { Straight part / Oblique part }

Fig. 11.25 Pharyngeal muscles, left side; lateral view.

The pharyngeal muscles divide into constrictor muscles (superior, middle and inferior constrictor) and levator muscles (stylopharyngeus, salpingopharyngeus and palatopharyngeus). This lateral view displays the different parts of the constrictor muscles and the stylopharyngeus.

Petro-occipital synchondrosis
Levator veli palatini
Lateral pterygoid
Pharyngeal glands
Stylohyoid ligament
Stylohyoid
Medial pterygoid
Parotid gland
Digastric, posterior belly
Medial pterygoid
Mandibular bone (mandible)
Submandibular gland
Styloglossus
Stylohyoid
Hyoid bone, greater horn
Pharyngeal raphe

Pharyngobasilar fascia
(Accessory muscle fasciculus)
Sphenomandibular ligament
Styloid process
Stylohyoid
Digastric, posterior belly
Stylopharyngeus
Styloglossus
Stylomandibular ligament
Medial pterygoid
Stylohyoid
Digastric, posterior belly
Chondropharyngeal part   **Middle constrictor**
Ceratopharyngeal part
Thyropharyngeal part
Cricopharyngeal part   **Inferior constrictor**
Thyroid gland, left lobe
Superior and inferior parathyroid glands
Transverse part***
Thyroid gland, right lobe
Superior and inferior parathyroid glands
Trachea
Esophagus, muscular layer

1 Pterygopharyngeal part
2 Buccopharyngeal part   **Superior**
3 Mylopharyngeal part   **constrictor**
4 Glossopharyngeal part

Fig. 11.26 Pharyngeal muscles; dorsal view.
The cricopharyngeal part of the inferior constrictor muscle forms a triangle weak in muscle fibers (KILLIAN's dehiscence or KILLIAN's triangle). At the transition from inferior constrictor muscle to esophagus, muscle fibers projecting upwards from the esophagus form a muscular triangle (LAIMER's triangle). LAIMER's and KILLIAN's triangles form a rhombus. The transverse fibers of the cricopharyngeal part of inferior constrictor form the base of both triangles.

*   KILLIAN's triangle
**   LAIMER's triangle
*** transverse section of cricopharyngeal part, inferior constrictor (KILLIAN's muscle)

Clinical Remarks

The KILLIAN's triangle or dehiscence marks a weak spot in the pharyngeal muscles and often creates a problem in aged men. The increased intraluminal pressure forces the pharyngeal mucosal wall to bulge out through the muscular weak spot to form a pharyngoesophageal diverticulum (ZENKER's diverticulum). This ZENKER's diverticulum extends into the retropharyngeal space and can cause regurgitation of ingested food and bad breath.
[L126]

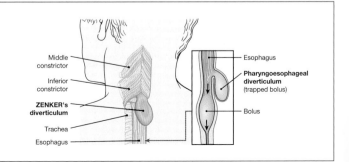

Middle constrictor
Inferior constrictor
ZENKER's diverticulum
Trachea
Esophagus
Esophagus
Pharyngoesophageal diverticulum (trapped bolus)
Bolus

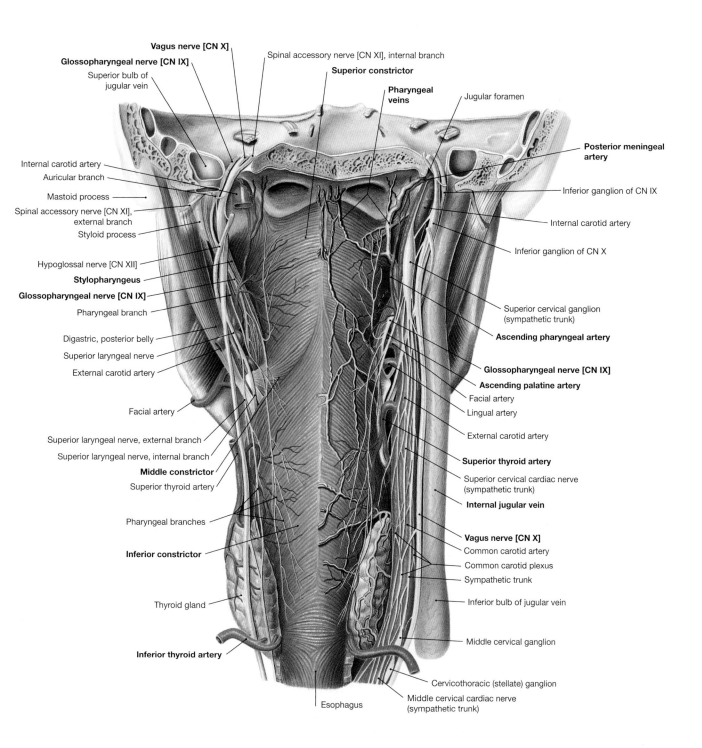

Fig. 11.27 Vessels and nerves of the pharynx and the parapharyngeal space; posterior view.
Arteries: The ascending pharyngeal artery is the main source of blood supply to the pharynx and ascends to the skull base in the parapharyngeal space medial of the neurovascular bundle of the neck. Its terminal branch, the posterior meningeal artery, enters the posterior cranial fossa through the jugular foramen. Additional blood supply comes from the ascending palatine artery and from the superior and inferior thyroid arteries.

Veins: The submucosa of the pharynx contains a plexus of pharyngeal veins which drain the blood into the internal jugular vein and meningeal veins.
Nerves: In addition to the cervical plexus (see sensory innervation of pharynx, ➤ Fig. 11.15), the glossopharyngeal nerve [CN IX] provides motor innervation for the superior constrictor, upper part of the middle constrictor and the stylopharyngeus. The vagus nerve [CN X] innervates the lower part of the middle constrictor and the inferior constrictor.

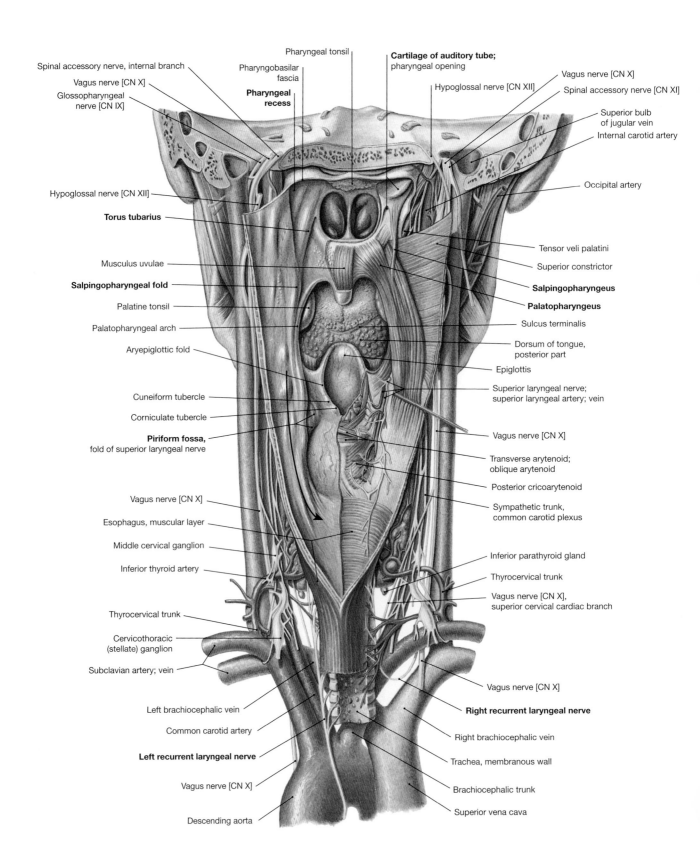

Spinal accessory nerve, internal branch

Vagus nerve [CN X]

Glossopharyngeal nerve [CN IX]

Pharyngeal tonsil

Pharyngobasilar fascia

Pharyngeal recess

Cartilage of auditory tube; pharyngeal opening

Hypoglossal nerve [CN XII]

Vagus nerve [CN X]

Spinal accessory nerve [CN XI]

Superior bulb of jugular vein

Internal carotid artery

Hypoglossal nerve [CN XII]

Torus tubarius

Musculus uvulae

Salpingopharyngeal fold

Palatine tonsil

Palatopharyngeal arch

Aryepiglottic fold

Cuneiform tubercle

Corniculate tubercle

Piriform fossa, fold of superior laryngeal nerve

Vagus nerve [CN X]

Esophagus, muscular layer

Middle cervical ganglion

Inferior thyroid artery

Thyrocervical trunk

Cervicothoracic (stellate) ganglion

Subclavian artery; vein

Left brachiocephalic vein

Common carotid artery

Left recurrent laryngeal nerve

Vagus nerve [CN X]

Descending aorta

Occipital artery

Tensor veli palatini

Superior constrictor

Salpingopharyngeus

Palatopharyngeus

Sulcus terminalis

Dorsum of tongue, posterior part

Epiglottis

Superior laryngeal nerve; superior laryngeal artery; vein

Vagus nerve [CN X]

Transverse arytenoid; oblique arytenoid

Posterior cricoarytenoid

Sympathetic trunk, common carotid plexus

Inferior parathyroid gland

Thyrocervical trunk

Vagus nerve [CN X], superior cervical cardiac branch

Vagus nerve [CN X]

Right recurrent laryngeal nerve

Right brachiocephalic vein

Trachea, membranous wall

Brachiocephalic trunk

Superior vena cava

Fig. 11.28 Vessels and nerves of the pharynx and the parapharyngeal space; posterior view; pharynx opened dorsally.
The pharyngeal opening of the auditory tube is positioned at the level of the inferior nasal meatus. The torus tubarius is a mucosal fold at the posterior and superior margin of the auditory tube opening. Caudally, the torus tubarius extends into the longitudinal salpingopharyngeal fold created by the salpingopharyngeus muscle. This orifice is the entrance to the auditory tube (EUSTACHIAN tube) and connects the nasal part of the pharynx with the tympanic cavi-

ty. The pharyngeal recess (fossa of ROSENMÜLLER) lies posterior to the torus tubarius and extends upwards to the roof of pharynx. The palatopharyngeus muscle is the lateral margin of the isthmus of fauces, the connection between oral cavity and oropharynx. On either side of the posterior laryngeal wall lies the piriform recess (black arrow). Note the side difference in the course of the recurrent laryngeal nerve; on the left side the nerve winds around the aortic arch, whereas on the right side the recurrent laryngeal nerve bends around the subclavian artery.

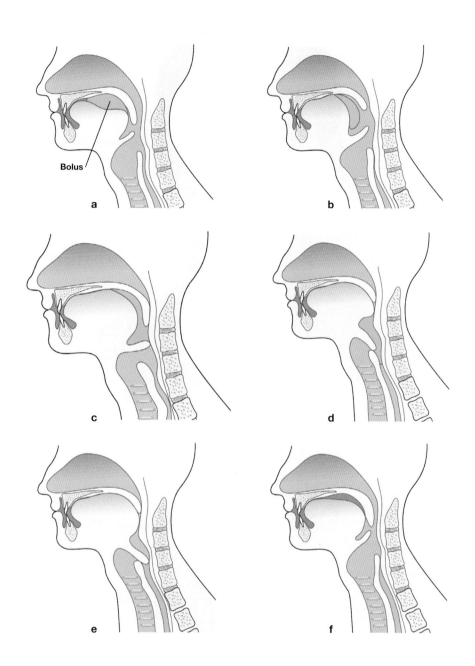

Bolus

a

b

c

d

e

f

Fig. 11.29a to f The act of swallowing (deglutition) involves a series of coordinated and complex muscular functions that include the tongue, floor of the oral cavity, muscles of the soft palate and the pharynx. [L106, R389]

The swallowing act can be divided into three phases: an oral **(a)**, pharyngeal **(b, c)**, and esophageal phase **(d to f)**. Proper swallowing (deglutition) is the result of a choreographed sequence of carefully timed steps. Each phase consists of multiple steps:

The voluntary **oral phase** includes food uptake into the mouth, salivation, mastication, trough-forming of the tongue, and the tongue moving the food bolus towards the pharynx.

Involuntary swallowing is triggered when the food bolus or fluids reach the back of the throat to initiate the **pharyngeal phase**. This reflex includes the reflexive closure of all passageways other than

the pharyngeal passage to the esophagus. This includes closure of the nasopharynx, oropharynx and larynx to prevent reflux or food/fluids entering the bronchial tree and lungs. Simultaneously with the nasopharyngeal closure, the pharynx and hyoid bone are elevated, sliding the pharynx over the bolus. Through sequential cranial to caudal constrictor actions of the pharyngeal muscles, the bolus is transported towards the esophagus. The closure of the nasopharynx and swallowing act will open the auditory tube for areation of the middle ear.

The last phase in the swallowing act is the involuntary **esophageal phase** which is composed of an esophageal peristalsis and relaxation step. Pharyngeal and esophageal muscle peristalsis pushes food/fluids towards the cardia of the stomach.

Dysphagia describes the difficulty of swallowing properly.

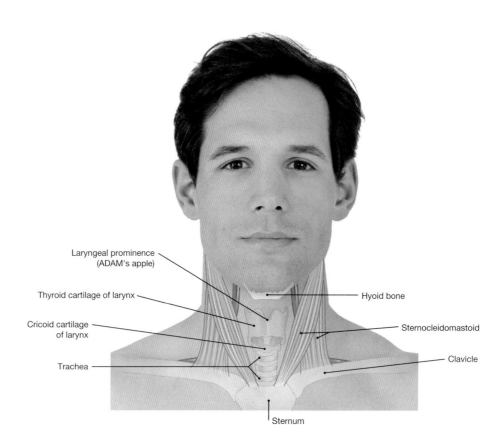

Laryngeal prominence
(ADAM's apple)

Thyroid cartilage of larynx

Cricoid cartilage
of larynx

Trachea

Hyoid bone

Sternocleidomastoid

Clavicle

Sternum

Fig. 11.30 Location of the hyoid bone and larynx in the anterior cervical region. [L126, K340]

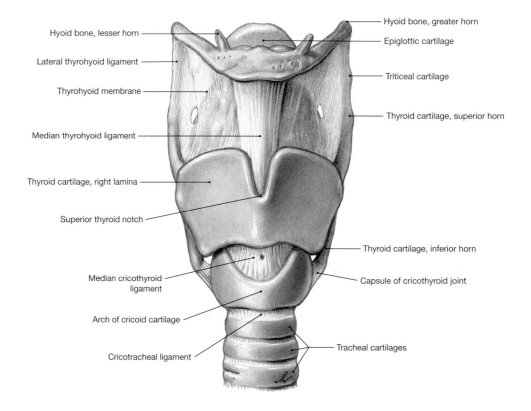

Hyoid bone, lesser horn

Lateral thyrohyoid ligament

Thyrohyoid membrane

Median thyrohyoid ligament

Thyroid cartilage, right lamina

Superior thyroid notch

Median cricothyroid
ligament

Arch of cricoid cartilage

Cricotracheal ligament

Hyoid bone, greater horn

Epiglottic cartilage

Triticeal cartilage

Thyroid cartilage, superior horn

Thyroid cartilage, inferior horn

Capsule of cricothyroid joint

Tracheal cartilages

Fig. 11.31 Larynx and hyoid bone; anterior view.
The individual parts of the laryngeal skeleton are connected by
fibrous joints (syndesmoses) and true joints (diarthroses).

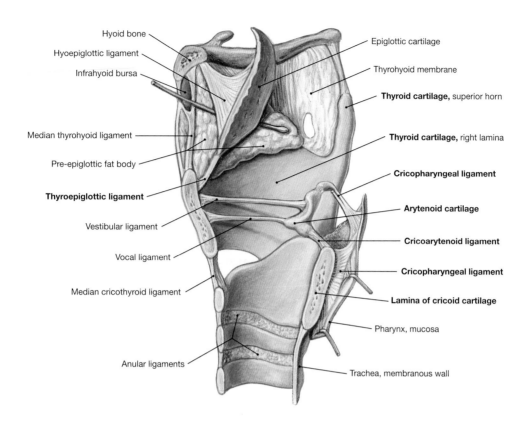

Fig. 11.32 Laryngeal cartilages and hyoid bone; median view.
The arytenoid and thyroid cartilages are connected by the vestibular ligament and the vocal ligament.

The thyroepiglottic ligament attaches the stalk of epiglottis to the inside of the thyroid cartilage.

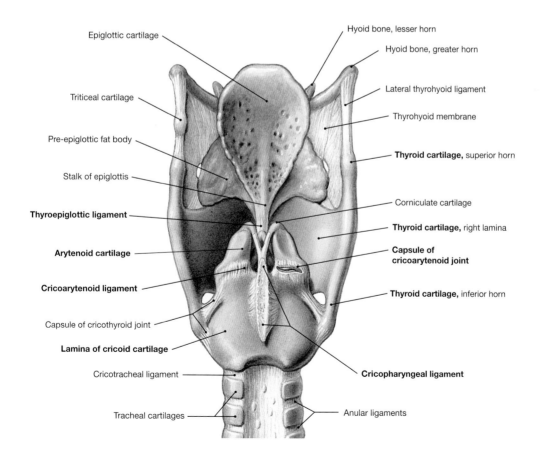

Fig. 11.33 Laryngeal cartilages and hyoid bone; posterior view.
True joints of the larynx are the cricothyroid joint, the paired joint between the cricoid cartilage and the inferior horns of the thyroid cartilage, as well as the cricoarytenoid joint between the cricoid and arytenoid cartilages. The cricoarytenoid ligament and the cricopharyngeal joint act as dorsal reins for the arytenoid cartilage.

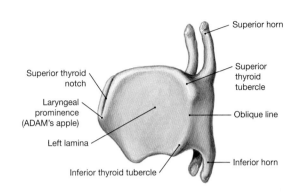

Fig. 11.34 Thyroid cartilage; view from the left side.

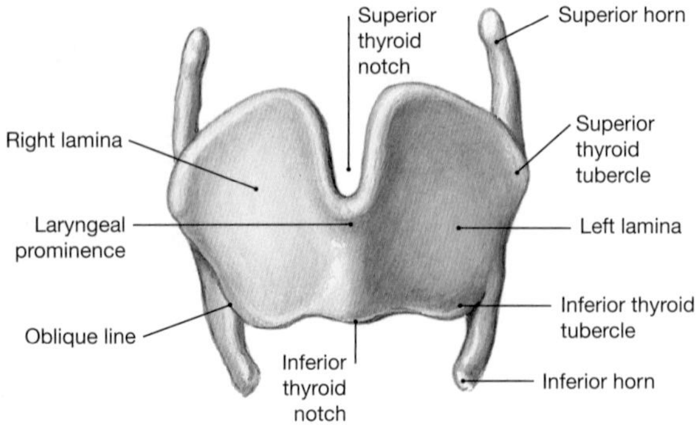

Fig. 11.35 Thyroid cartilage; anterior view.
Both laminae of the thyroid cartilage join at an angle of 90° and 120° in men and women, respectively.

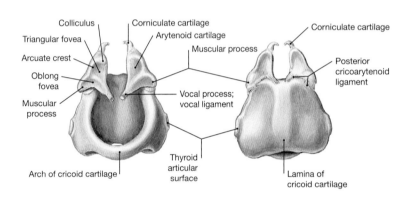

Fig. 11.36 Cricoid cartilage and arytenoid cartilages; anterior and posterior views.

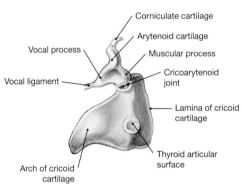

Fig. 11.37 Cricoid cartilage and arytenoid cartilages; view from the left side.

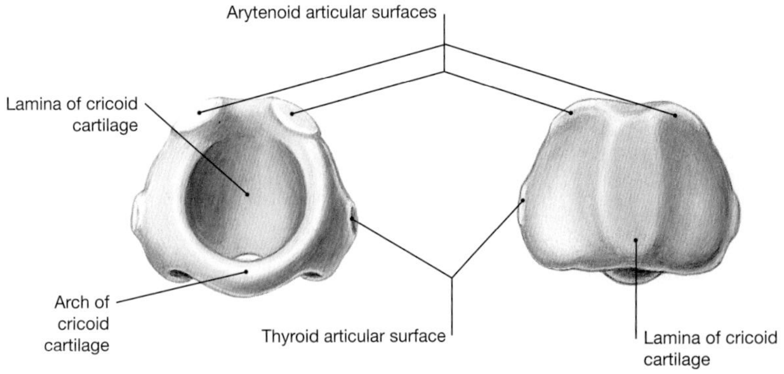

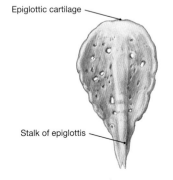

Fig. 11.38 Cricoid cartilage; anterior and posterior views.

Fig. 11.39 Epiglottic cartilage; posterior view.
Other than the major hyaline laryngeal cartilages, the epiglottis is made of elastic cartilage.

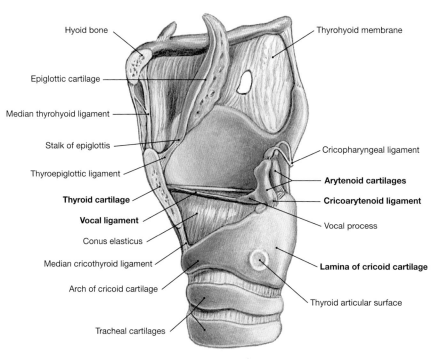

Fig. 11.40 Larynx and hyoid bone; view onto the vocal ligament and the arytenoid cartilage from the left side; the left lamina of thyroid cartilage has been removed.

The cricoid and arytenoid cartilages articulate in the cricoarytenoid joint. This joint is secured by the cricoarytenoid ligament which serves to guide the arytenoid cartilage and counteract the forces of the vocal ligament.

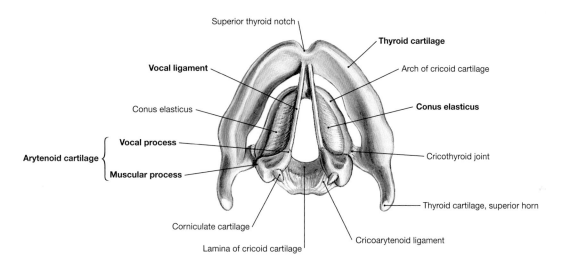

Fig. 11.41 Laryngeal cartilages and vocal ligament; view from above.

The paired vocal ligament stretches between the vocal process of the arytenoid cartilage and the inside of the thyroid cartilage. The conus elasticus (cricovocal membrane) is an elastic membrane and directs the airflow from the lungs passed the vocal ligaments.

Clinical Remarks

Surgical access to the ventral aspect of the trachea is best achieved upon dorsal hyperextension of the neck. During coniotomy, an incision or puncture through the median cricothyroid ligament located between the thyroid and cricoid cartilages provides access to the laryngeal lumen beneath the vocal folds. Upper and lower tracheotomy are defined as accesses to the airways above and below the isthmus of the thyroid gland, respectively.

*   coniotomy
**   upper tracheotomy
*** lower tracheotomy

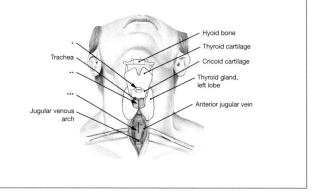

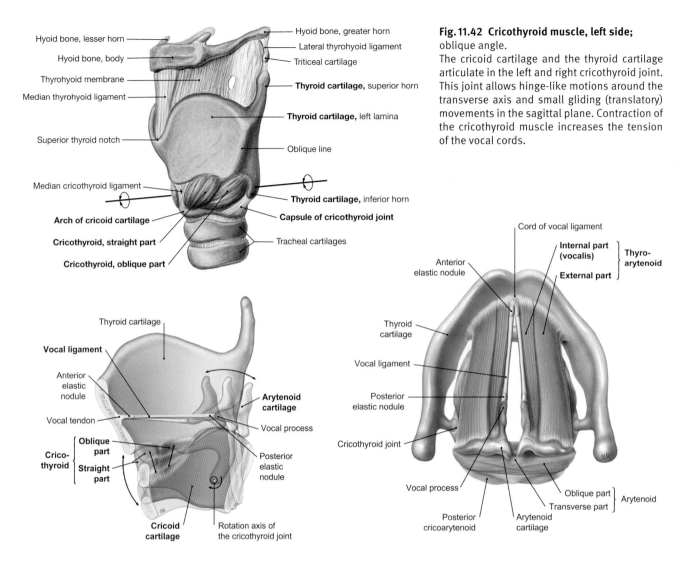

Hyoid bone, lesser horn
Hyoid bone, body
Thyrohyoid membrane
Median thyrohyoid ligament
Superior thyroid notch
Median cricothyroid ligament
Arch of cricoid cartilage
Cricothyroid, straight part
Cricothyroid, oblique part

Hyoid bone, greater horn
Lateral thyrohyoid ligament
Triticeal cartilage
Thyroid cartilage, superior horn
Thyroid cartilage, left lamina
Oblique line
Thyroid cartilage, inferior horn
Capsule of cricothyroid joint
Tracheal cartilages

Fig. 11.42 Cricothyroid muscle, left side; oblique angle.
The cricoid cartilage and the thyroid cartilage articulate in the left and right cricothyroid joint. This joint allows hinge-like motions around the transverse axis and small gliding (translatory) movements in the sagittal plane. Contraction of the cricothyroid muscle increases the tension of the vocal cords.

Thyroid cartilage
Vocal ligament
Anterior elastic nodule
Vocal tendon
Crico-thyroid
Oblique part
Straight part
Arytenoid cartilage
Vocal process
Posterior elastic nodule
Cricoid cartilage
Rotation axis of the cricothyroid joint

Cord of vocal ligament
Internal part (vocalis) **Thyro-arytenoid**
External part
Anterior elastic nodule
Thyroid cartilage
Vocal ligament
Posterior elastic nodule
Cricothyroid joint
Vocal process
Oblique part Arytenoid
Transverse part
Posterior cricoarytenoid
Arytenoid cartilage

Fig. 11.43 Cricothyroid muscle, left side; medial view. [L238]
Contraction of the cricothyroid muscle tilts the cricoid cartilage upwards and the arytenoid cartilages backwards which increases tension of the vocal cords. Airflow causes the vocal cords to vibrate at a higher frequency which increases the pitch of the voice.

Fig. 11.44 Vocalis muscle; view from above. [L238]

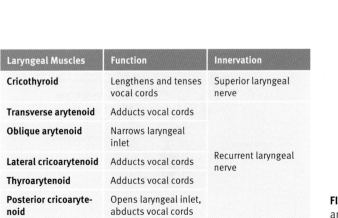

Laryngeal Muscles	Function	Innervation
Cricothyroid	Lengthens and tenses vocal cords	Superior laryngeal nerve
Transverse arytenoid	Adducts vocal cords	
Oblique arytenoid	Narrows laryngeal inlet	
Lateral cricoarytenoid	Adducts vocal cords	Recurrent laryngeal nerve
Thyroarytenoid	Adducts vocal cords	
Posterior cricoarytenoid	Opens laryngeal inlet, abducts vocal cords	

Corniculate cartilage (SANTORINI)
Superior horn
Thyroid cartilage
Cord of vocal ligament
Anterior elastic nodule
Apex
Cord of vocal ligament
Internal part (vocalis) **Thyro-arytenoid**
External part
Lateral cricoarytenoid
Cricoid cartilage
Posterior cricoarytenoid
Oblique part Transverse part
Arytenoid

Fig. 11.45 Laryngeal muscles; posterior view from an oblique angle. [L238]

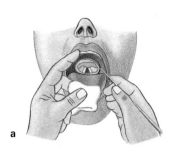

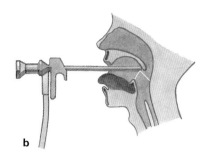

Fig. 11.46a and b Laryngoscopy. a Indirect laryngoscopy; **b** direct, endoscopic laryngoscopy.

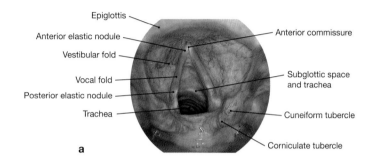

Epiglottis

Anterior elastic nodule

Vestibular fold

Vocal fold

Posterior elastic nodule

Trachea

Anterior commissure

Subglottic space and trachea

Cuneiform tubercle

Corniculate tubercle

a

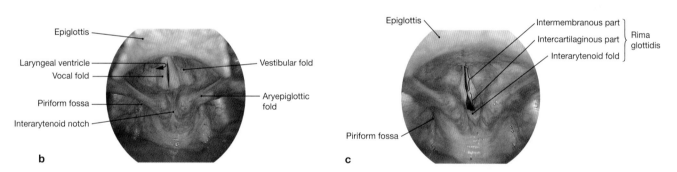

Epiglottis

Laryngeal ventricle

Vocal fold

Piriform fossa

Interarytenoid notch

Vestibular fold

Aryepiglottic fold

b

Epiglottis

Intermembranous part

Intercartilaginous part

Interarytenoid fold

Rima glottidis

Piriform fossa

c

Fig. 11.47a to c Direct laryngoscopy; respiratory position **(a);** phonation position **(b);** whispering position **(c).** [T719]
Normal breathing requires the action of the posterior cricoarytenoid. It is the only intrinsic laryngeal muscle that can separate the vocal cords. In case of recurrent laryngeal nerve damage, hoarseness (damage on one side) or difficulty breathing (bilateral injury) can occur due to impaired abduction of the vocal cords.

Clinical Remarks

People who stress their voice in a strenuous or abusive manner are at risk of developing vocal cord or singer's nodules located at the free margin of the vocal ligament. Weakness of the arytenoid muscle may result in an incomplete occlusion of the intercartilaginous part of the glottis (open whisper triangle), resulting in a weak and breathy voice.

a The most frequently observed benign tumors of the vocal fold are **polyps.** [G748]
b Malignant tumors of the larynx are most frequently **squamous cell carcinomas** (delineated by arrows). [H082-001]

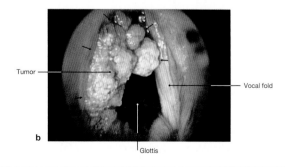

Polyp on vocal fold

Vocal fold

Vocal fold

a

Tumor

Vocal fold

b

Glottis

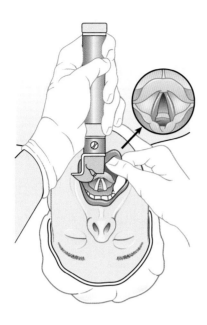

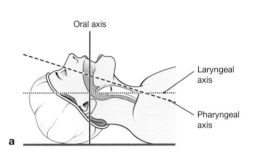

Fig. 11.48 View of the larynx by using a laryngoscope in preparation for endotracheal intubation. [L126]

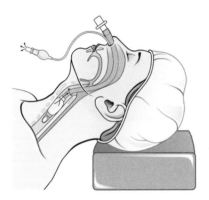

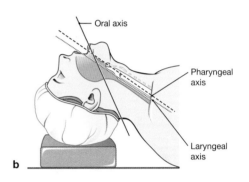

Fig. 11.49a and b Head position during endotracheal intubation. [L126]
Endotracheal intubation requires the head to be re-adjusted from a normal **(a)** to an extended **(b)** position for the pharyngeal, laryngeal and oral axes to line up. This way, the endotracheal tube can be inserted with minimal damage to the laryngx and upper airways.

Fig. 11.50 Proper placement of the endotracheal tube with inflated balloon in the trachea below the larynx. [L126]

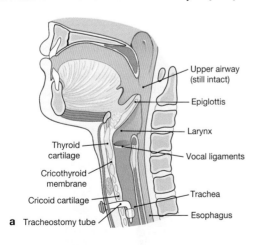

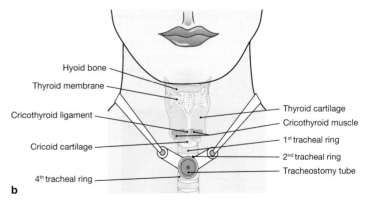

Fig. 11.51a and b Result of a tracheotomy. [L126]
Positioning of a tracheostomy tube below the larynx **(a)** at the level of the 3rd and 4th tracheal rings **(b)**. A tracheostoma is required when the upper airways are obstructed (e. g., by a laryngeal carcinoma) or in case of assisted ventilation of the lungs.

Structure/Function

Head of an infant; midsagittal section at the level of the nose and larynx. Contrary to adults and children, a young infant can drink and breathe simultaneously. This becomes possible because the larynx locates high in the neck and the epiglottis reaches the nasopharynx. Fluids (e.g. the breast milk from the mother) pass through the piriform recess of the larynx into the esophagus without entering the lower airways.
[E402]

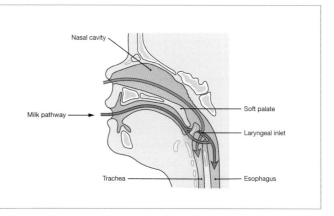

Fig. 11.52 / 11.53

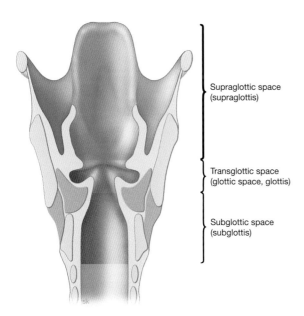

Fig. 11.52 Compartments of the larynx. [L238]

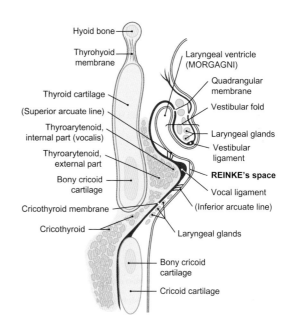

Fig. 11.53 Enlarged view of the glottis with transglottic space; frontal view. [L126]

Clinical Remarks

Laryngoscopic view of a normal larynx **(a)** and a larynx with REINKE's edema **(b)**.

An accumulation of fluid in the REINKE's space (REINKE's edema) creates a swelling of the vocal folds, which extends into the glottis and results in hoarseness and dyspnea (difficulty breathing). The REINKE's edema must be distinguished from a (supra) glottic edema. In the latter, fluid collects in the mucosa of the supraglottic space (e.g. due to allergic reactions or a result of in/extubation). Thus, the (supra)glottic edema is located above the glottis and restricts the airflow through the glottis. Its symptoms can range from stridor (pitched wheezing sound) to hoarseness, dyspnea and potential asphyxia (lack of gas exchange due to the inability to breath).
[H083-001]

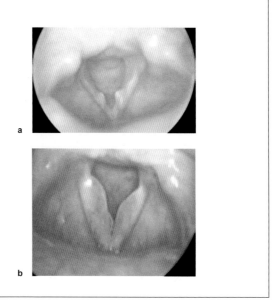

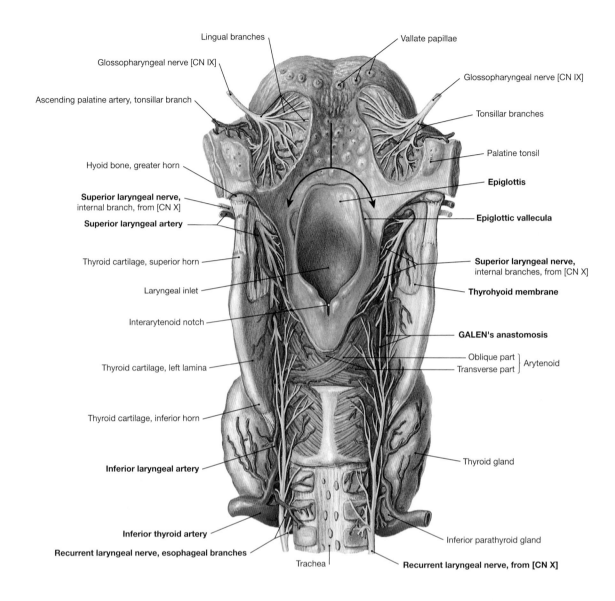

Fig. 11.54 Arteries and nerves of the larynx and root of the tongue; dorsal view.

The superior laryngeal artery branches off the superior thyroid artery and, together with the inferior laryngeal artery, supplies the mucosa of the piriform recess (black arrows). The larynx receives bilateral innervation through two branches of the vagus nerve [CN X]: The superior laryngeal nerve divides into an internal and an external branch. The latter innervates the cricothyroid muscle. Jointly with the superior laryngeal artery, the internal branch passes through the thyrohyoid membrane into the larynx. The internal branch of the laryngeal nerve provides sensory fibers for the mucosa of the epiglottic valleculae, and the epiglottis. The superior laryngeal nerve also contains parasympathetic fibers for innervation of the laryngeal glands.

The recurrent (inferior) laryngeal nerve derives from the vagus nerve [CN X] and innervates the inner laryngeal muscles. The connection between the superior laryngeal nerve and the inferior laryngeal nerve is called GALEN's anastomosis.

Clinical Remarks

Croup is a respiratory infection commonly caused by viruses and involves inflammation of the larynx, trachea and bronchi (laryngotracheobronchitis). Croup occurs mainly in younger children who present with a barking cough (seal's bark), stridor, hoarseness, fever, and cold symptoms. A milder form of croup is spasmotic croup which can be allergic, occur as part of a common cold, and frequently does not involve a fever.

Acute bacterial infections of the epiglottis occur most frequently in children and can cause an acute and life-threatening obstruction of the airways.

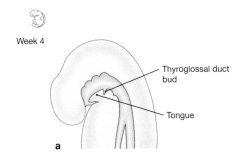

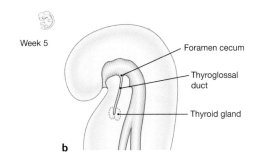

Fig. 11.55a and b Development of the thyroid gland. [E838]
a From day 24 after fertilization, epithelium from the ektodermal stomodeum grows caudally past the hyoid bone and larynx to form the thyroglossal duct.
b When the thyroglossal duct has reached its destination at the thyroid cartilage of larynx in week 7, it forms the isthmus and the two lobes of the thyroid gland. The cranial part of the thyroglossal duct regresses. The proximal opening of the thyroglossal duct per-

sists as foramen cecum behind the terminal sulcus of the tongue. Frequently a pyramidal lobe of thyroid tissue is found along the passageway of the primitive thyroglossal duct. Protruding from the fifth pharyngeal pouch, the ultimobranchial body gives rise to calcitonin-producing C-cells which migrate into the thyroid gland. The parathyroid glands derive from the third and fourth pharyngeal pouches and produce parathyroid hormone.

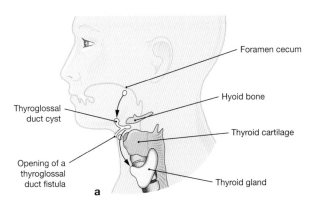

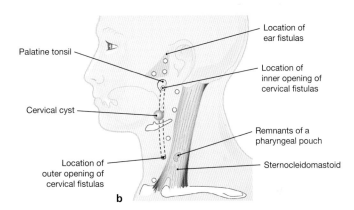

Fig. 11.56a and b Cervical cysts and cervical fistulas. [E247-09]
a Possible locations of cysts derived from the thyroglossal duct. Arrows show the location of the thyroglossal duct during the de-

scent of the thyroid gland from the foramen cecum to its final position in the anterior cervical region;
b Possible locations of cervical cysts and cervical fistulas.

Clinical Remarks

Persistence of parts of the thyroglossal duct can lead to a median cervical cyst as seen in the CT image **(a)** or a median cervical fistula. Both only become a concern when infected.
A lateral cervical fistula or cyst **(b)** is caused by the imperfect obliteration of the lateral aspects of the branchial clefts or the

cervical sinus. Lateral cervical fistulas usually open at the anterior margin of the sternocleidomastoid. The accumulation of fluid within the lateral cervical cysts results in a swelling at the side of the neck.
[E247-09]

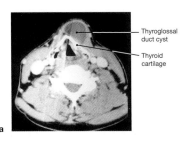

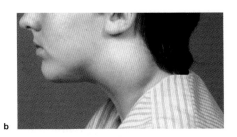

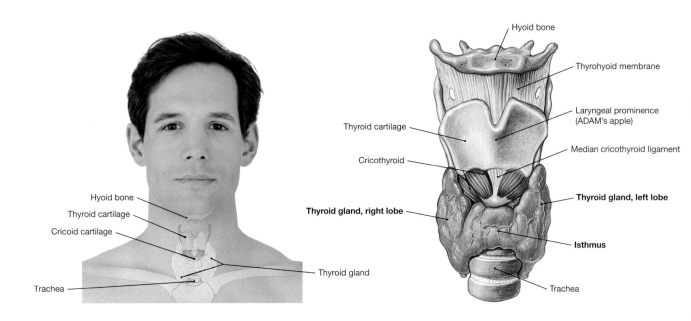

Fig. 11.57 Surface anatomy of the anterior neck region. [L126, K340]
The location of the thyroid gland is shown in relation to the hyoid bone and larynx with its thyroid and cricoid cartilages.

Fig. 11.58 Position of the thyroid gland; anterior view.
The thyroid gland (weight in an adult 20–25 g [0.71–0.88 oz]) is located below the larynx and surrounds the upper part of the trachea with two (right and left) lobes and an anterior isthmus.

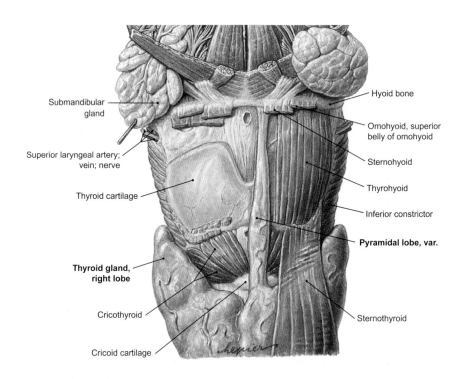

Fig. 11.59 Pyramidal lobe of the thyroid gland; anterior view.

Clinical Remarks

The pyramidal lobe of the thyroid gland, sometimes referred to as the third lobe, marks the passageway of the thyroglossal duct, can contain functional thyroid tissue and extends up from the isthmus towards the hyoid bone.

Thyroid surgery involves two strategies:
1. **lobectomy** removes one half of the thyroid gland and is the preferred surgical approach to remove thyroid nodules;
2. **total thyroidectomy** removes all identifiable thyroid tissue and is done in patients with thyroid cancer.

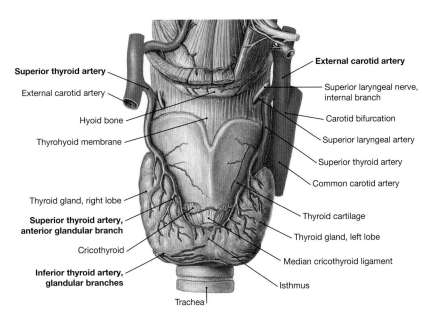

Fig. 11.60 Arteries of the thyroid gland; anterior view.

The thyroid gland has an exquisite blood supply through the superior thyroid artery from the external carotid artery and through the inferior thyroid artery from the thyrocervical trunk. A small thyroid ima artery from the brachiocephalic trunk or the aortic arch can also be present (not shown). The arteries also supply blood to the parathyroid glands.

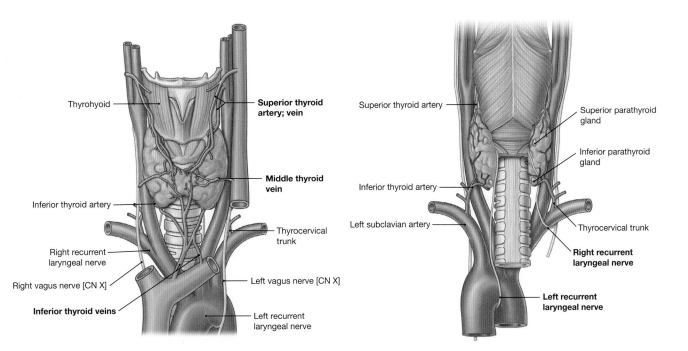

Fig. 11.61 Veins of the thyroid gland; anterior view. [E402]
The superior and medial thyroid veins drain into the internal jugular vein. The inferior thyroid vein drains into the left brachiocephalic vein.

Fig. 11.62 Left and right recurrent laryngeal nerve in relation to the thyroid gland; posterior view. [E402]
The thyroid gland has a close topographical relationship with the paired recurrent laryngeal nerves, also known as inferior laryngeal nerves, which is a branch of the vagus nerve [CN X].

Structure/Function

In most cases the recurrent laryngeal nerve ascends in the tracheo-esophageal groove and crosses the inferior thyroid artery near the lateral border of the thyroid gland. Thus, the inferior thyroid artery can serve as landmark to find the nerve during thyroid surgery.

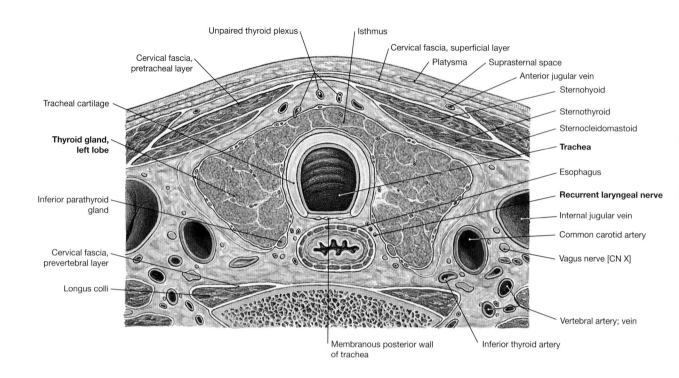

Unpaired thyroid plexus
Isthmus
Cervical fascia, superficial layer
Platysma
Suprasternal space
Cervical fascia, pretracheal layer
Anterior jugular vein
Sternohyoid
Tracheal cartilage
Sternothyroid
Sternocleidomastoid
Thyroid gland, left lobe
Trachea
Esophagus
Recurrent laryngeal nerve
Inferior parathyroid gland
Internal jugular vein
Common carotid artery
Cervical fascia, prevertebral layer
Vagus nerve [CN X]
Longus colli
Vertebral artery; vein
Membranous posterior wall of trachea
Inferior thyroid artery

Fig. 11.63 Thyroid gland; transverse section.
The recurrent laryngeal nerve courses bilaterally in a groove between the trachea and esophagus in close proximity to the thyroid gland. Extreme caution must be taken during thyroid surgery for removal of a lobe (lobectomy) or the whole thyroid gland (thyroidectomy) to avoid damage to the recurrent laryngeal nerve.

Clinical Remarks

The pathology of the thyroid gland is complex and includes diffuse and focal alterations. Both types may have multiple causes.
a The shape, size and function of the thyroid gland becomes visible with thyroid scintigraphy upon intravenous injection of Tc-99 m pertechnetate which is taken up by the thyroid gland. A thyroid region which incorporates less radiopharmaceutical (as indicated by the arrows) is a cold nodule and can hide a thyroid cancer. [M467, R132]
Deficiency or overproduction of the thyroid hormones thyroxine (T4 prohormone) and triiodothyronine (T3; > 10-fold more active than T4) causes hypothyroidism and hyperthyroidism, respectively.

b Goiter is a surplus of thyroid tissue. Resection of a goiter is a frequent cause of paralysis of the laryngeal muscles. The enlargement of the thyroid gland disrupts the normal topography of the recurrent laryngeal nerve. Although in case of goiter the nerve maintains close relationships with the thyroid gland and the inferior thyroid artery, the recurrent nerve is more difficult to localize and can be injured easily. An enlarged thyroid gland can compress the trachea. In advanced stages, localized pressure can weaken the tracheal cartilage rings and result in dyspnea. This often requires surgical intervention. [T908]

c A frequent cause of hyperthyroidism is GRAVES' disease, also known as toxic diffuse goiter. GRAVES' disease is frequently associated with orbitopathy which likely results from circulating antibodies against an antigen derived from the extraocular muscles. These autoimmune antibodies cross-react with the microsomal fraction of the thyroid follicular epithelial cells. An exophthalmos can result from a retro-orbital edema, deposition of glycosaminoglycans, lymphocytic infiltrates and progressive fibrosis. GRAVES' disease is more common in women than men. [T127, R104-05]

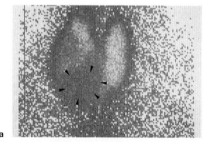
a

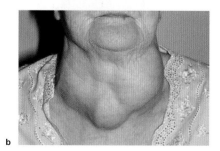
b

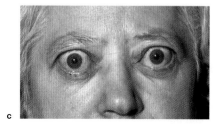
c

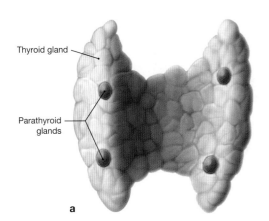

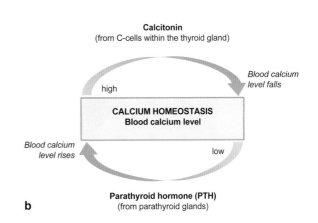

Calcitonin
(from C-cells within the thyroid gland)

Blood calcium level falls

high

CALCIUM HOMEOSTASIS
Blood calcium level

Blood calcium level rises

low

Parathyroid hormone (PTH)
(from parathyroid glands)

a   b

Fig. 11.64a and b Thyroid gland with parathyroid glands; posterior view. a [L275], b [L126]
a Four lentil-shaped parathyroid glands are located at the upper and lower pole of each thyroid lobe.
b Schematic diagram showing the endocrine regulation of blood calcium levels. Parathyroid glands secrete parathyroid hormone (PTH) which increases blood calcium levels. Calcitonin secreted by C-cells located within the thyroid gland antagonizes PTH and reduces calcium blood levels. PTH and calcitonin contribute to blood calcium homeostasis.

Clinical Remarks

Hyperplasia, adenoma, or carcinoma of the parathyroid glands can result in a hyperfunction with the development of a primary hyperparathyroidism. The increased secretion of parathyroid hormone (PTH) causes an increase of the serum calcium levels and is associated with complications affecting the bones, kidneys, and gastrointestinal tract. The inferior parathyroid glands develop from the 3rd pharyngeal pouch and may, together with the thymus, descend further into the mediastinum.

Key Features of the Thyroid and Parathyroid Endocrine System					
Endocrine Organ	**Endocrine Cells**	**Developmental Origin**	**Hormones***	**Target Organs***	**Disease***
Thyroid gland	Thyrocytes	Endoderm at foramen cecum	Triiodthyronin (T3) Thyroxine (T4) (80% T4, 20% T3) (Systemic regulator of metabolism)	Heart Brain Sexual organs Uterus	Hypothyrodism Hyperthyrodism GRAVES' disease
	Parafollicular C-cells	Ultimobranchial body 4th pharyngeal pouch	Calcitonin (Decreases blood calcium levels)	Bone	Medullary thyroid carcinoma
Parathyroid glands	Parathyroid cells	3rd and 4th pharyngeal pouch	Parathyroid hormone (PTH) (Increases blood calcium levels)	Nervous system Bones and joints Muscles GI-tract Kidney	Primary hyperpara-thyrodism

* denotes major hormones, main target organs, frequently associated diseases; does not represent a complete list

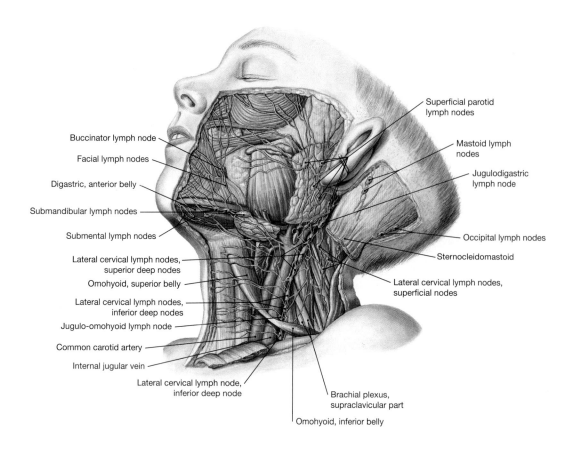

Fig. 11.65 Superficial lymphatic vessels and lymph nodes in the head and neck region of a child.
The neck region contains 200 to 300 lymph nodes, the majority assembled in groups along the neurovascular bundles of the neck.

Both major lymphatic ducts drain into the right or left jugular-subclavian angle of veins.

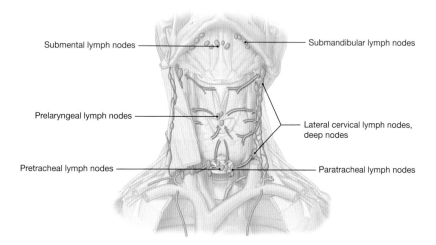

Fig. 11.66 Lymphatic vessels and lymph nodes of the tongue, larynx, thyroid gland, and trachea; anterior view. [E460]
These organs drain into the deep lymph nodes of the neck. These are the same lymph nodes stations palpated during a routine physical examination of a patient.

Clinical Remarks

According to the classification of the American Joint Committee of Cancer (AJCC), lymph node metastases of the neck are divided into six zones or compartments I–VI. These compartments serve as reference zones for the elective surgical removal of metastases in lymph nodes due to the lymphogenic spread of malignant tumors of the head and neck region *(neck dissection)*. Injuries to the thoracic duct during surgical interventions in the neck region can lead to the development of a chylous fistula. [L126]

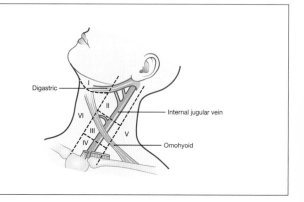

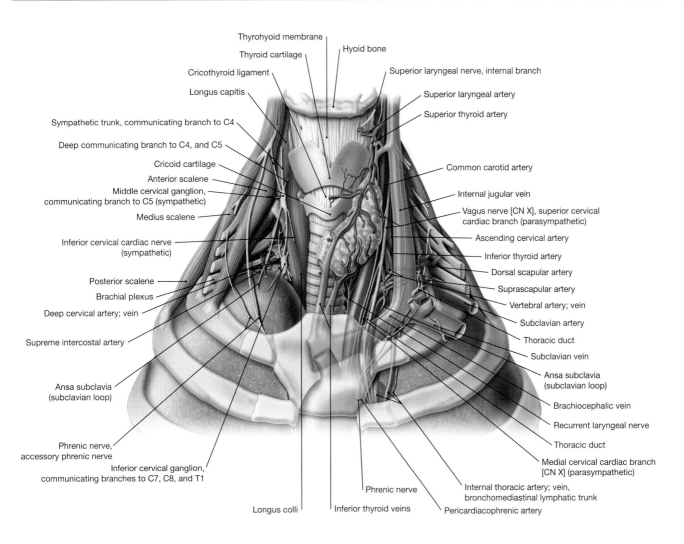

Thyrohyoid membrane
Thyroid cartilage
Cricothyroid ligament
Longus capitis
Sympathetic trunk, communicating branch to C4
Deep communicating branch to C4, and C5
Cricoid cartilage
Anterior scalene
Middle cervical ganglion, communicating branch to C5 (sympathetic)
Medius scalene
Inferior cervical cardiac nerve (sympathetic)
Posterior scalene
Brachial plexus
Deep cervical artery; vein
Supreme intercostal artery
Ansa subclavia (subclavian loop)
Phrenic nerve, accessory phrenic nerve
Inferior cervical ganglion, communicating branches to C7, C8, and T1
Longus colli

Hyoid bone
Superior laryngeal nerve, internal branch
Superior laryngeal artery
Superior thyroid artery
Common carotid artery
Internal jugular vein
Vagus nerve [CN X], superior cervical cardiac branch (parasympathetic)
Ascending cervical artery
Inferior thyroid artery
Dorsal scapular artery
Suprascapular artery
Vertebral artery; vein
Subclavian artery
Thoracic duct
Subclavian vein
Ansa subclavia (subclavian loop)
Brachiocephalic vein
Recurrent laryngeal nerve
Thoracic duct
Medial cervical cardiac branch [CN X] (parasympathetic)
Internal thoracic artery; vein, bronchomediastinal lymphatic trunk
Pericardiacophrenic artery
Inferior thyroid veins
Phrenic nerve
Inferior thyroid veins

Fig. 11.67 Structures of the neck and the superior thoracic aperture; anterior view. [L238]
On the right side of the body, the great blood vessels were removed to show the pleural cupula and the sympathetic trunk. On the left side, the great blood vessels and the left lobe of the thyroid gland were left in place.

Clinical Remarks

The term **PANCOAST's tumor** (apical sulcus tumor) describes a rapidly growing peripheral bronchial carcinoma at the apex of lung (**a** schematic, **b** MRI, **c** X-ray) which quickly expands and infiltrates the ribs, soft tissues of the neck, brachial plexus, and vertebrae.

Other structures affected may involve the phrenic nerve, the recurrent laryngeal nerve, the subclavian artery and vein, and the stellate ganglion. Damage to the latter can cause **(d)** HORNER's syndrome with the trias: enophthalmos, miosis, ptosis (drooping of upper eyelid, ➤ Fig. 12.71a and ➤ Fig. 12.71b).
a [L275], b [H084-001], c [E329], d [E538]

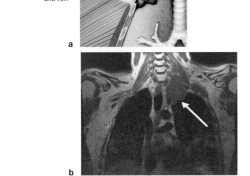

Vertebral body
Phrenic nerve
Brachial plexus (arm and shoulder pain)
Subclavian artery and vein
Sympathetic trunk (HORNER's syndrome)
Vagus nerve
PANCOAST tumor

a

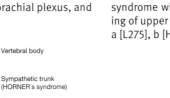
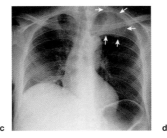
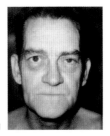

b   c   d

Neuroanatomy

Major Parts of the Brain
and Orientation 556

Structure of the Brain 557

Meninges of the Brain 558

Arterial Blood Supply
to the Meninges of the Brain 559

Venous Sinuses 560

Venous Sinuses and Diploic Veins .. 561

Venous Drainage of the Brain 562

Arterial Blood Supply of the Brain .. 563

Internal Carotid Artery 564

Circle of WILLIS 565

Cerebral and Cerebellar Arteries 566

Cerebral Arteries 567

Vascular Territories of Cerebral
and Cerebellar Arteries 568

Meninges of the Spinal Cord 569

Arterial Blood Supply
of the Spinal Cord 570

Spinal Cord within
the Vertebral Canal 571

Ventricular System 572

Blood-Brain/CSF-Barrier
and Circumventricular Organs 575

Cranial Nerves – Overview 576

Cranial Nerves –
Topography and Fiber Qualities 577

Cranial Nerves – Location of Cranial
Nerve Nuclei in the Brainstem 578

Cranial Nerves – Summary
of Nuclei of Cranial Nerves 579

Cranial Nerves – Sensory
and Parasympathetic Ganglia 580

Fila olfactoria [CN I] 582

[CN III], [CN IV], [CN VI] 583

Trigeminal Nerve [CN V] 585

Ophthalmic Branch [CN V/1] 587

Maxillary Branch [CN V/2] 588

Mandibular Branch [CN V/3] 589

Facial Nerve [CN VII] 590

Glossopharyngeal Nerve [CN IX] 594

Vagus Nerve [CN X] 597

Special Senses: Sensory
System of Tongue and Taste 600

Spinal Accessory Nerve [CN XI] 601

Hypoglossal Nerve [CN XII] 602

Autonomic Nervous System –
General Principles 603

Autonomic Outflow
and Target Organs 604

Sympathetic Outflow 605

Relationship of Sympathetic
Outflow with Spinal Nerves 606

Autonomic Nervous System –
HORNER's Syndrome 607

Spinal Cord – Segments
and Nomenclature 608

Spinal Cord – Function 609

Spinal Nerves 610

Spinal Cord – Reflexes 612

Spinal Cord –
Segmental Organization 613

Spinal Cord – Sensory Pathways ... 616

Spinal Cord – Motor Pathways 618

Spinal Cord Lesions 619

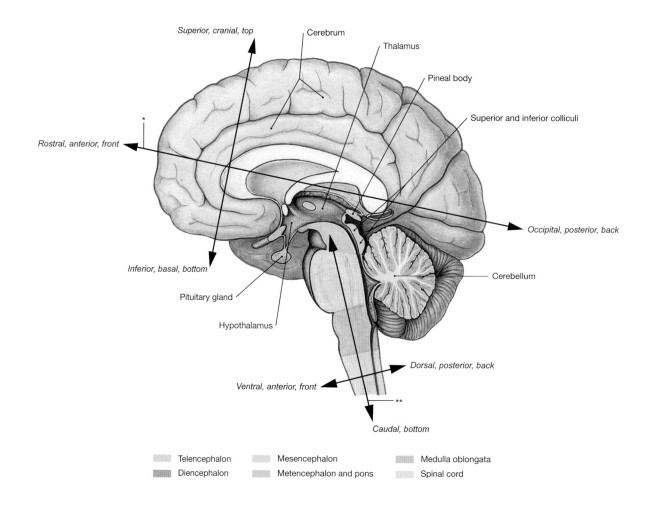

Telencephalon
Diencephalon
Mesencephalon
Metencephalon and pons
Medulla oblongata
Spinal cord

Fig. 12.1 Positional information and organization of the central nervous system (CNS; brain and spinal cord); median section.
The brain develops from three primary brain vesicles (forebrain [prosencephalon], midbrain [mesencephalon], and hindbrain [rhombencephalon]) which form the telencephalon, diencephalon, mesencephalon, pons and cerebellum [metencephalon], and medulla oblongata [myelencephalon].

During brain development, the neural tube bends and, thus, the longitudinal axis of the forebrain (prosencephalon = diencephalon and telencephalon) tilts forward. The FOREL's axis (*) refers to the topographical axis between the telencephalon and diencephalon, while the axis projecting through the center of the brainstem is called MEYNERT's axis (**).

Structure/Function

Development of the brain; a, b schematic frontal sections; **c** median section; **d** view from the left side.
Week 4: formation of three primary brain vesicles (forebrain [prosencephalon], midbrain [mesencephalon], and hindbrain [rhombencephalon]).
Week 5: formation of six secondary brain vesicles (the paired vesicles of the telencephalon and the di-, mes-, met-, and myelencephalon); optic cups are formed.

Week 8: Thalamus and oculomotor nerve [CN III] are visible. The metencephalon with pons and cerebellum and the medulla oblongata [myeloencephalon] derive from the rhombencephalon.
Week 20 (fetal crown-rump length 20 cm [7.9 in]): fast growth of the telencephalon.
a, b [E838]

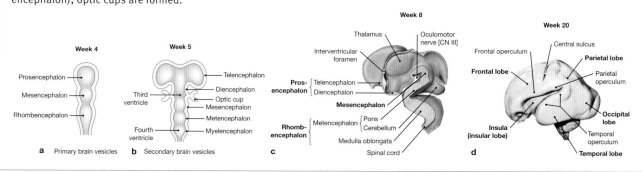

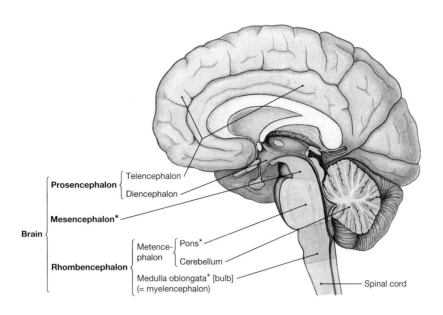

Fig. 12.2 Basic structure of the human CNS. The different sections of the brainstem (*) and the spinal cord are highlighted in color.

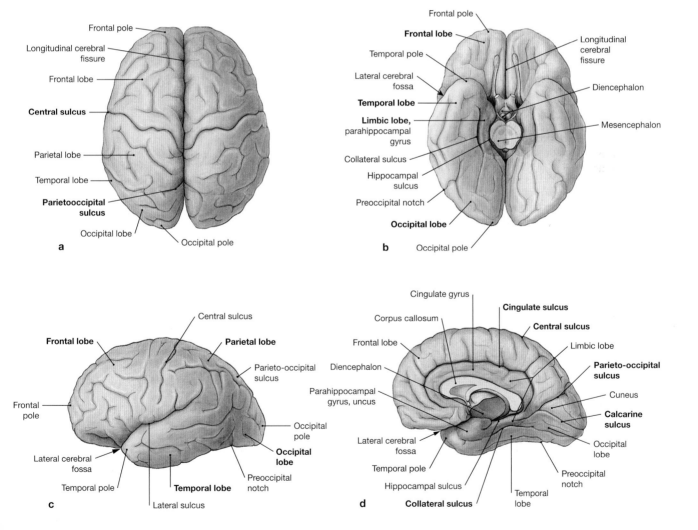

Fig. 12.3a to d Major parts of the human cerebrum. Cerebral lobes are colored and their topographical relationship to other cerebral structures is shown; superior view **(a)**, inferior view **(b)**, view at the lateral surface of the left hemisphere **(c)**, midsagittal view at the inner aspect of the right hemisphere **(d)**.

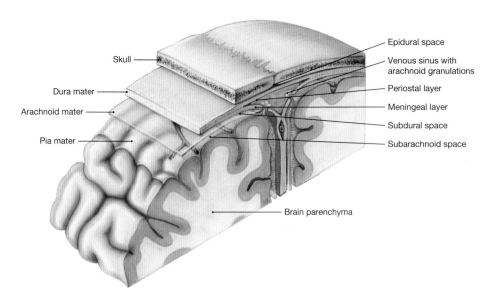

Skull

Dura mater

Arachnoid mater

Pia mater

Epidural space

Venous sinus with arachnoid granulations

Periostal layer

Meningeal layer

Subdural space

Subarachnoid space

Brain parenchyma

Fig. 12.4 Meninges of the brain; superior oblique view. [L285]
The brain is covered by three meninges. The **dura mater** forms a thick durable outermost layer. The cranial dura divides into an outer periosteal layer close to the bony skull and an inner meningeal layer. In the skull, the *epidural space* between the skull and the periostal layer of the dura mater is a potential space and contains the middle meningeal artery with its branches. The term peridural is a synonym of epidural. In the spinal canal, the *epidural space* contains connective tissue with fat deposits, the roots of spinal nerves, small lymphatic and arterial vessels, and the internal vertebral venous plexus. The dura mater encloses the arachnoid mater and pia mater which form the middle and innermost meningeal membranes, respectively. The latter two membranes constitute the leptomeninges.

The *subdural space* is a potential space between the meningeal layer of dura mater and the arachnoid mater. Bridging veins cross the subdural space. The bridging veins connect superficial veins in the subarachnoid space with the venous sinuses.
The side of the **arachnoid mater** facing the pia mater of the brain has a spider web-like appearance and delineates the subarachnoid space which is filled with circulating cerebrospinal fluid (CSF). The CSF is absorbed through arachnoid granulations into the venous sinuses.
The **pia mater** tightly associates with the surface of the brain. The meninges contain pain receptors which are absent in the brain parenchyma.

Clinical Remarks

Schematic presentation of Cranium bifidum formation and various types of herniation of the brain and/or meninges.
a Head of a newborn with an extensive herniation in the occipital region. The red circles mark defects at the posterior fontanelle and foramen magnum, respectively.
b Meningocele: the hernial sac is formed by skin and meninges and is filled with cerebrospinal fluid.

c Meningoencephalocele: the hernial sac comprises prolapsed parts of the cerebellum and is covered by meninges and skin.
d Meningohydroencephalocele: the hernial sac consists of prolapsed parts of the occipital lobe and of the posterior horn of the lateral ventricle.
[E247-09]

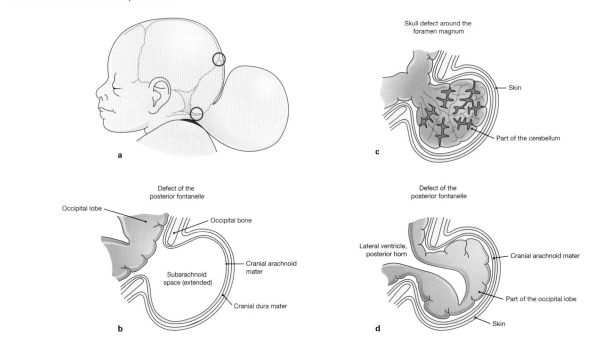

Skull defect around the foramen magnum

Skin

Part of the cerebellum

a

c

Defect of the posterior fontanelle

Occipital lobe

Occipital bone

Subarachnoid space (extended)

Cranial arachnoid mater

Cranial dura mater

b

Defect of the posterior fontanelle

Lateral ventricle, posterior horn

Cranial arachnoid mater

Part of the occipital lobe

Skin

d

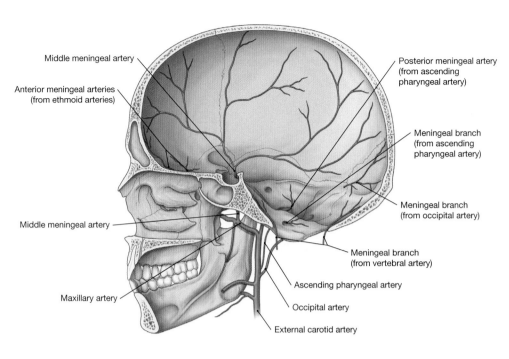

Middle meningeal artery

Anterior meningeal arteries
(from ethmoid arteries)

Middle meningeal artery

Maxillary artery

Posterior meningeal artery
(from ascending
pharyngeal artery)

Meningeal branch
(from ascending
pharyngeal artery)

Meningeal branch
(from occipital artery)

Meningeal branch
(from vertebral artery)

Ascending pharyngeal artery

Occipital artery

External carotid artery

Fig. 12.5 Meningeal arteries;
median view. [E580]
The arterial supply of the meninges derives from branches
of the external carotid artery.
These meningeal arteries course
in the epidural space between
the skull and dura mater. The
middle meningeal artery is most
vulnerable to injury.

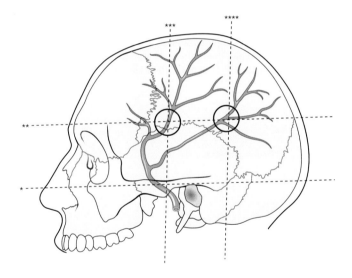

**Fig. 12.6 Circles mark the projections of the main
frontal and parietal branches of the middle meningeal artery onto the side of the skull.** [L126]
Anterior circle marks the craniometric point named
pterion which is the thinnest part of the skull. External
force to the side of the head can cause injury to the
branches of the middle meningeal artery. This results
in potentially fatal rupture with arterial bleeding and
the formation of an epidural hematoma.

*   FRANKFORT horizontal line
**   Supraorbital horizontal line
***   Vertical line through the middle of the zygomatic
       arch
**** Vertical line through the posterior mastoid pro-
       cess

Clinical Remarks

An **epidural hematoma** contains arterial blood due to injury to
the middle meningeal artery. The ensuing pressure caused by
the epidural hematoma can cause the midline to deviate side-
ways and results in parts of the temporal lobe being squeezed
underneath the tentorium cerebelli through the tentorial notch.
Compressed intracranial structures may also include CN III. As a
result, on the side of the injury the eye is positioned 'down and
out' and the pupil is fixed and dilated (see ➤ chapter 9 (Eye) for
more detail).
[L238]

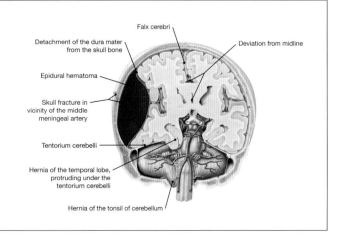

Falx cerebri

Detachment of the dura mater
from the skull bone

Deviation from midline

Epidural hematoma

Skull fracture in
vicinity of the middle
meningeal artery

Tentorium cerebelli

Hernia of the temporal lobe,
protruding under the
tentorium cerebelli

Hernia of the tonsil of cerebellum

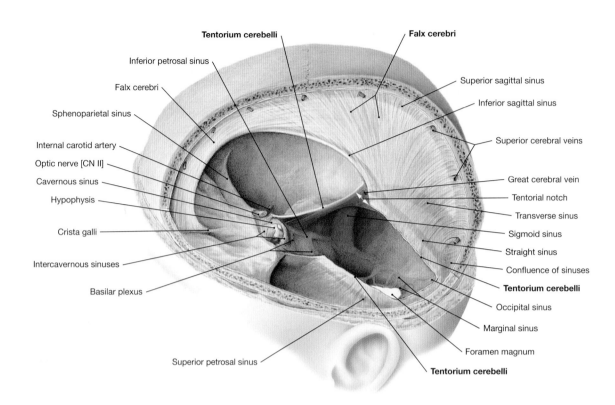

Tentorium cerebelli

Inferior petrosal sinus

Falx cerebri

Sphenoparietal sinus

Internal carotid artery

Optic nerve [CN II]

Cavernous sinus

Hypophysis

Crista galli

Intercavernous sinuses

Basilar plexus

Superior petrosal sinus

Falx cerebri

Superior sagittal sinus

Inferior sagittal sinus

Superior cerebral veins

Great cerebral vein

Tentorial notch

Transverse sinus

Sigmoid sinus

Straight sinus

Confluence of sinuses

Tentorium cerebelli

Occipital sinus

Marginal sinus

Foramen magnum

Tentorium cerebelli

Fig. 12.7 Cranial dura mater and dural venous sinuses; superior oblique view; tentorium cerebelli partially removed.
The cranial dura mater lines the cranial cavity completely and tightly adheres to the skull bones. The dural venous sinuses course within the dura. The sickle-shaped falx cerebri protrudes in the sagittal plane and extends from the crista galli to the ridge of the tentorium cerebelli. The latter spans the posterior cranial fossa and is attached along the transverse sinus and the pyramidal edge. The falx cerebri and the tentorium cerebelli divide the cranial cavity into three spaces that contain the two cerebral hemispheres and the cerebellum.

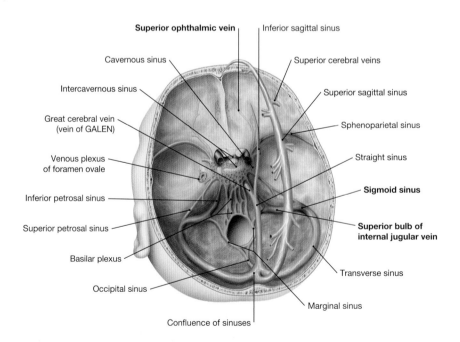

Superior ophthalmic vein

Cavernous sinus

Intercavernous sinus

Great cerebral vein
(vein of GALEN)

Venous plexus
of foramen ovale

Inferior petrosal sinus

Superior petrosal sinus

Basilar plexus

Occipital sinus

Confluence of sinuses

Inferior sagittal sinus

Superior cerebral veins

Superior sagittal sinus

Sphenoparietal sinus

Straight sinus

Sigmoid sinus

**Superior bulb of
internal jugular vein**

Transverse sinus

Marginal sinus

Fig. 12.8 Dural venous sinuses; superior view.
The dural venous sinuses are rigid canals devoid of valves that drain the venous blood from the brain via bridging veins. The main drainage from within the skull occurs via the paired sigmoid sinuses into the internal jugular veins initially forming the superior bulb of jugular vein. In addition, the paired superior ophthalmic veins drain venous blood from within the orbit, and highly variable emissary veins (➤ Fig. 12.9) form smaller valveless venous connections between the intra- and extracranial regions.

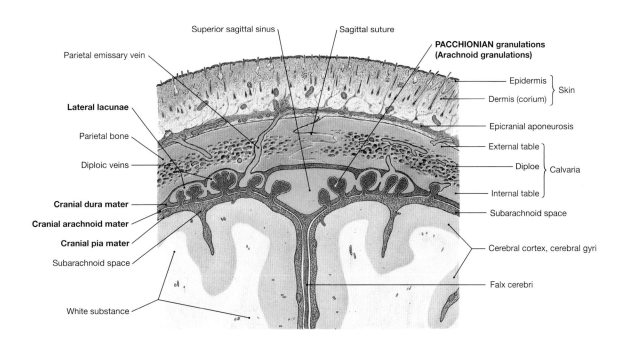

Fig. 12.9 Calvaria, meninges, and dural venous sinuses; frontal section.
In the adult, the cerebrospinal fluid is mainly reabsorbed into the venous system through the PACCHIONIAN granulations (arachnoid granulations, arachnoid protrusions into the superior sagittal sinus or the lateral lacunae) along the superior sagittal sinus. Reabsorption also occurs through the lymphatic sheaths of small vessels of the cranial pia mater as well as the perineural sheaths of the cranial and the spinal nerves (not shown).
Outer layers of the scalp depicted here are shown in more detail in ➤ chapter 8 (Head), ➤ Fig. 8.3 a and ➤ Fig. 8.3 b.

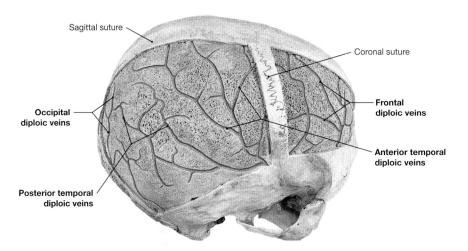

Fig. 12.10 Diploic canals and diploic veins of the calvaria, right side; superior oblique view; after the external layer of the compact bone has been removed from the calvaria.
Passing through the diploic space are diploic canals which harbor the diploic veins. They communicate with the emissary veins and the dural venous sinuses.

Clinical Remarks

Traumatic brain injuries, e.g., car accidents, concussion, or even milder injuries to the head in elderly) can cause subdural hematomas which are caused by the rupture of bridging veins (connecting veins between cranial veins and dural venous sinuses). Acutely or in a more subtle way (sometimes over weeks!), venous blood collects between the dura mater and the arachnoid mater in the subdural space (left side). Patients show general and uncharacteristic symptoms like dizziness, headache, fatigue, listlessness, or confusion. Subdural hematoma can also coincide with intracerebral bleeding and corresponding acute neurological deficits (right side).
[L238]

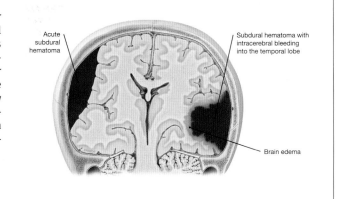

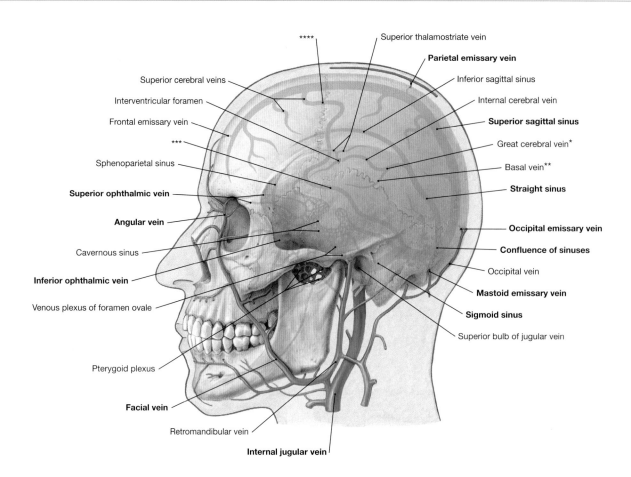

Fig. 12.11 Intra- and extracranial veins of the head.
The intra- and extracranial veins of the head communicate via numerous anastomoses. This includes the emissary veins, ophthalmic veins and the venous plexuses.

*	Vein of GALEN
**	ROSENTHAL's vein
***	Vein of LABBÉ
****	TROLARD's vein

Clinical Remarks

Injuries to the scalp can result in the spread of germs via the emissary veins and the diploic veins (➤ Fig. 12.9 and ➤ Fig. 12.10) into the dural venous sinuses and the intracranial space.

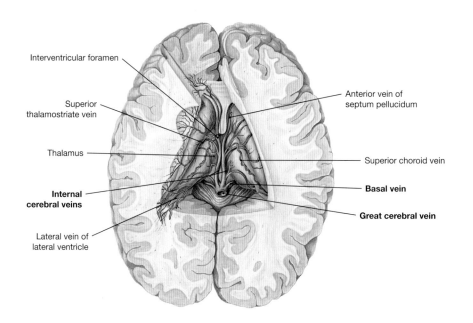

Fig. 12.12 Deep veins of the brain;
superior view.
The veins of the ventricular system, the basal ganglia, and the internal capsule belong to the deep veins of the brain. The blood from these structures is drained through the superior thalamostriatal veins into the internal cerebral veins and from here into the great cerebral vein (vein of GALEN). The internal cerebral veins run in the choroid membrane of the third ventricle.

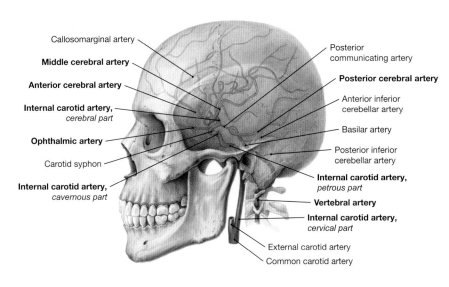

Fig. 12.13 Intracranial arteries to the brain.
Four large arteries supply blood to the brain: the paired internal carotid arteries and the paired vertebral arteries. These four blood vessels feed into the cerebral arterial circle of WILLIS (➤ Fig. 12.14 and ➤ Fig. 12.17) located at the base of the brain.

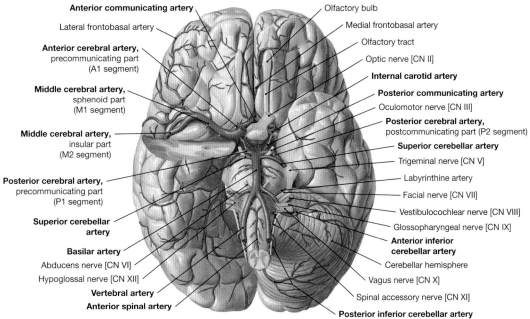

Fig. 12.14 Arteries of the brain; inferior view.
The vertebral arteries at the cranial base converge to form the basilar artery which releases the posterior cerebral arteries (PCA) and branches for the brainstem, the cerebellum, and the inner ear (*vertebral tributary*). Small posterior communicating arteries connect the posterior cerebral arteries with the internal carotid arteries. Each of the latter contributes one middle cerebral artery (MCA) and one anterior cerebral artery (ACA) which collectively provide the major part of the blood for the hemispheres (*carotid tributary*). The anterior communicating artery connects both anterior cerebral arteries. Clinically, the anterior, middle, and posterior cerebral arteries are divided into segments (see below).

Clinical Description of Segments of the Cerebral Arteries (used to describe the Location of Aneurysms)				
Cerebral Artery	**Relation to Communicating Artery**	**Segment**	**Topographical Relationship**	**Tributary**
ACA	Precommunicating	A1	Precommunicating	Carotid
	Postcommunicating	A2	Infracallosal	
		A3	Precallosal	
		A4	Supracallosal	
MCA	Precommunicating	M1	Sphenoid/horizontal	
	Postcommunicating	M2	Insular	
		M3	Opercular	
		M4	Terminal	
PCA	Precommunicating	P1	Precommunicating	Vertebral
	Postcommunicating	P2	Postcommunicating	
		P3	Quadrigeminal	
		P4	No name	

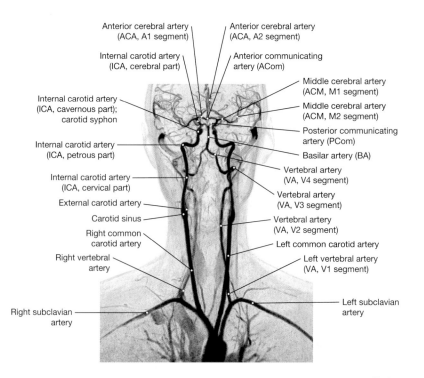

Fig. 12.15 Magnetic resonance (MR) angiogram of the arterial supply to the brain. [T786]
Contrary to the external carotid artery (not shown), the internal carotid artery (ICA) has no extracranial branches but only branches after entering the cranial cavity.
With courtesy of Dr. Stefanie Lescher, Prof. Dr. Joachim Berkefeldt, Neuroradiology, Clinic of Goethe University, Frankfurt.

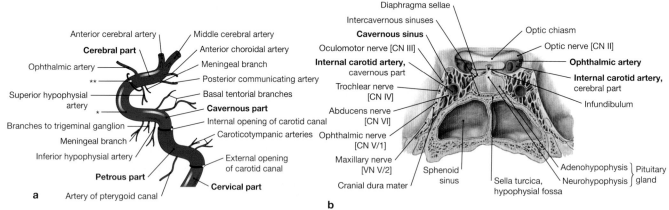

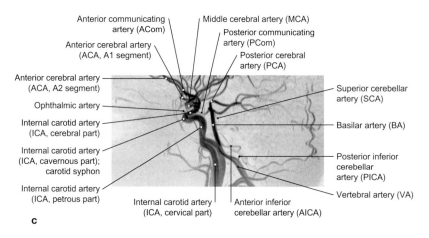

Fig. 12.16a to c Parts of the internal carotid artery. a [E402], c [T786]

a Upon entering the cranial cavity, the internal carotid artery (ICA) divides into the cervical, petrous, cavernous, and cerebral parts shown here in a lateral view.

b The ICA passes through the cavernous sinus, the external and internal openings of the carotid canal, and through the dura mater.

c Magnetic resonance angiogram depicting a lateral view of the intracranial course of the ICA and its branches.

With courtesy of Dr. Stefanie Lescher, Prof. Dr. Joachim Berkefeldt, Neuroradiology, Clinic of Goethe University, Frankfurt.

*   Carotid artery siphon
** Passage through the cranial dura mater into the region of the diaphragma sellae

---

Clinical Remarks

A **cavernous sinus syndrome** (CSS) can have multiple causes (cavernous sinus thrombosis, tumor, metastasis, aneurysm and fistulas of the internal carotid artery, inflammatory infiltration). CSS coincides with palsy of the abducens [CN VI], oculomotor [CN III], and ophthalmic [CN V/1] cranial nerves. A venous throm-bosis and/or fistula between the ICA and the cavernous sinus (carotid-cavernous or C-C fistula) coincides with acute onset of these palsies and signs of impaired venous drainage: venous stasis in the orbit with swelling of eyelids and conjunctiva, and/or protrusion of the eyeball (proptosis, exophthalmus).

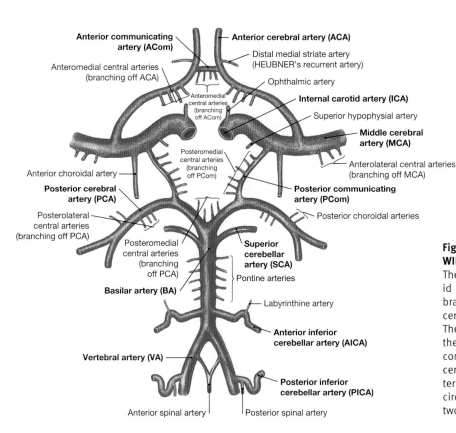

Anterior communicating artery (ACom)

Anterior cerebral artery (ACA)

Anteromedial central arteries (branching off ACA)

Distal medial striate artery (HEUBNER's recurrent artery)

Anteromedial central arteries (branching off ACom)

Ophthalmic artery

Internal carotid artery (ICA)

Superior hypophysial artery

Middle cerebral artery (MCA)

Anterior choroidal artery

Posteromedial central arteries (branching off PCom)

Anterolateral central arteries (branching off MCA)

Posterior cerebral artery (PCA)

Posterior communicating artery (PCom)

Posterolateral central arteries (branching off PCA)

Posterior choroidal arteries

Posteromedial central arteries (branching off PCA)

Superior cerebellar artery (SCA)

Pontine arteries

Basilar artery (BA)

Labyrinthine artery

Anterior inferior cerebellar artery (AICA)

Vertebral artery (VA)

Posterior inferior cerebellar artery (PICA)

Anterior spinal artery

Posterior spinal artery

Fig. 12.17 Arterial circle of the brain (circle of WILLIS); superior view.
The circle of WILLIS connects the internal carotid and vertebral arteries and releases paired branches of the anterior, middle, and posterior cerebral arteries.
The anterior communicating artery connects the two anterior cerebral arteries. The posterior communicating artery connects the posterior cerebral artery with the cerebral part of the internal carotid artery on both sides. This arterial circle provides an anastomosis between the two internal carotid and vertebral arteries.

Structure/Function

Angiogram after unilateral injection of a contrast enhancing medium into the internal carotid artery (ICA) followed by digital subtraction angiography (DSA). The ICA and its two major branches – anterior cerebral artery (ACA) and middle cerebral artery (MCA) – are shown. The contrast medium distributes to the vessels of the contralateral side via the cerebral arterial circle of WILLIS.
a A/P radiograph;
b Lateral radiograph
[T913]

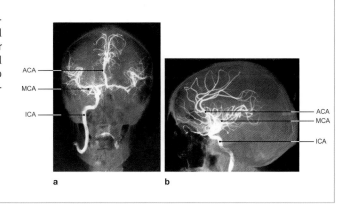

Clinical Remarks

More than 90 % of all **cerebral aneurysms** involve the arteries of the circle of WILLIS. The anterior communicating artery (ACA), internal carotid artery (ICA), and middle cerebral artery (MCA) are frequently affected. Most cerebral aneurysms are the result of congenital defects in the vascular wall close to branching points. While most cerebral aneurysms are asymptomatic, they can compress neighboring cranial nerves and have a tendency to rupture. Cerebral aneurysms are the most frequent cause of subarachnoid bleedings. Rupture of a cerebral aneurysm causes immediate and strong headaches combined with vomiting and changes in consciousness.
[G749]

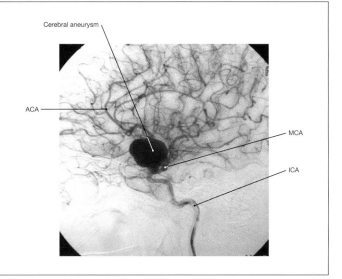

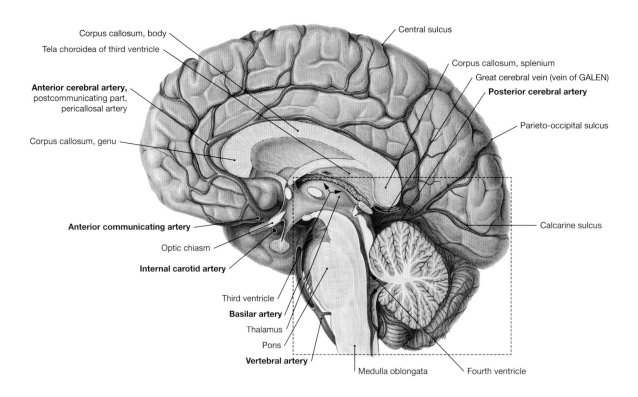

Fig. 12.18 Medial surface of the brain, diencephalon, and brainstem; median section; view from the left side.
Once the anterior communicating artery has branched off the anterior cerebral artery (ACA), the postcommunicating part (pericallosal [A2–A4] artery) of the ACA passes around the rostrum and genu of the corpus callosum and runs alongside the upper surface of the corpus callosum. Its extensions reach the parieto-occipital sulcus. The anterior cerebral artery supplies the medial area of the frontal and parietal lobes as well as the hemispheral rim and a small area alongside thereof at the cerebral convexity.
Blood supply to the posterior brain region is shown in ➤ Fig. 12.19 (boxed area in ➤ Fig. 12.18).

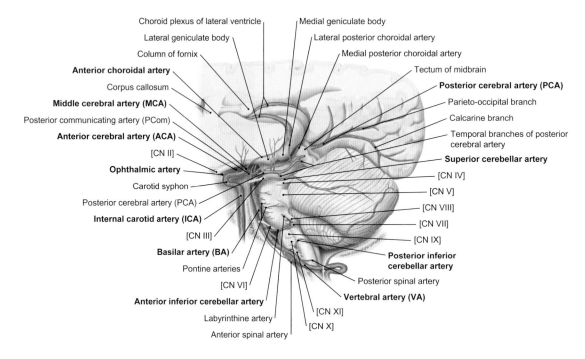

Fig. 12.19 Vertebral arteries, basilar artery, posterior cerebral arteries. Magnified from the dotted box in ➤ Fig. 12.18. [L127]
The vertebral arteries, the basilar artery, and the posterior cerebral arteries (PCA) supply arterial blood to the occipital lobe, the basal part of the temporal lobe, the lower part of the striatum and thalamus, and the cerebellum. Arterial branches are shown in relation to the cranial nerves.

Clinical Remarks

Paralysis of the lower extremity versus brachiofacial paralysis can indicate the affected cerebral blood vessel. A blockage of the anterior cerebral artery results in paralyses predominantly of the lower extremities. An impaired perfusion by the middle cerebral artery causes predominantly brachiofacial paralyses.

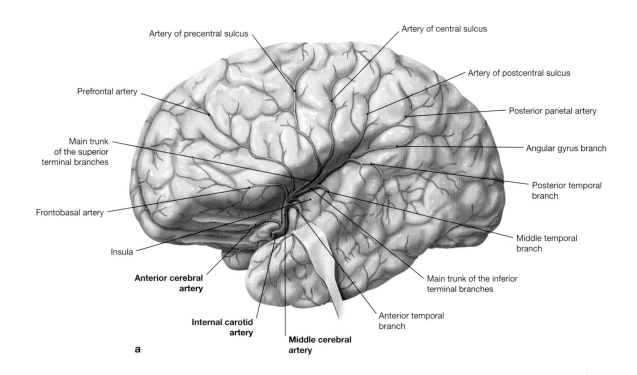

Artery of precentral sulcus

Artery of central sulcus

Prefrontal artery

Artery of postcentral sulcus

Posterior parietal artery

Main trunk
of the superior
terminal branches

Angular gyrus branch

Posterior temporal
branch

Frontobasal artery

Middle temporal
branch

Insula

**Anterior cerebral
artery**

Main trunk of the inferior
terminal branches

**Internal carotid
artery**

Anterior temporal
branch

**Middle cerebral
artery**

a

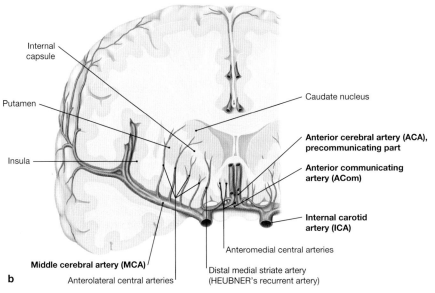

Internal
capsule

Caudate nucleus

Putamen

**Anterior cerebral artery (ACA),
precommunicating part**

**Anterior communicating
artery (ACom)**

Insula

**Internal carotid
artery (ICA)**

Anteromedial central arteries

Middle cerebral artery (MCA)

b

Anterolateral central arteries

Distal medial striate artery
(HEUBNER's recurrent artery)

**Fig. 12.20a and b Blood supply to the brain
by the middle cerebral artery (MCA);** lateral
view **(a)**, frontal view **(b)**. [L127]

a The right and left MCA are the main suppliers of arterial blood to the lateral side of each
cerebral hemisphere.

b The MCA also sends branches to deeper
brain structures, including the striatum.
These branches penetrate the brain and are
terminal arteries. Their blockage will result in
infarction of the brain tissue that depends on
the arterial supply by this artery.

Clinical Remarks

The projections of functional regions of the cerebral surface *(Homunculus)* are shown in this frontal view of a coronal section of
the brain. Occlusion of the middle cerebral artery shortly after
branching off the internal carotid artery results in cerebral infarction (ischemic stroke) and can damage these functional regions of the brain. This explains the severe symptoms which include a contralateral, predominantly brachiofacial hemiplegia
with weakness and loss of sensation (hypesthesia, local or general decrease in touch and pressure sensation of the skin). If the
dominant hemisphere is affected, additional symptoms include
aphasia (speech impairment), agraphia (inability to write words
or text, despite existing motor and intellectual capabilities), and
alexia (inability to read).

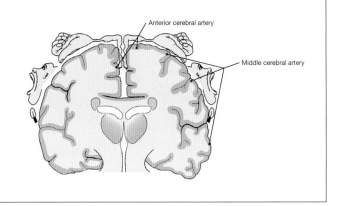

Anterior cerebral artery

Middle cerebral artery

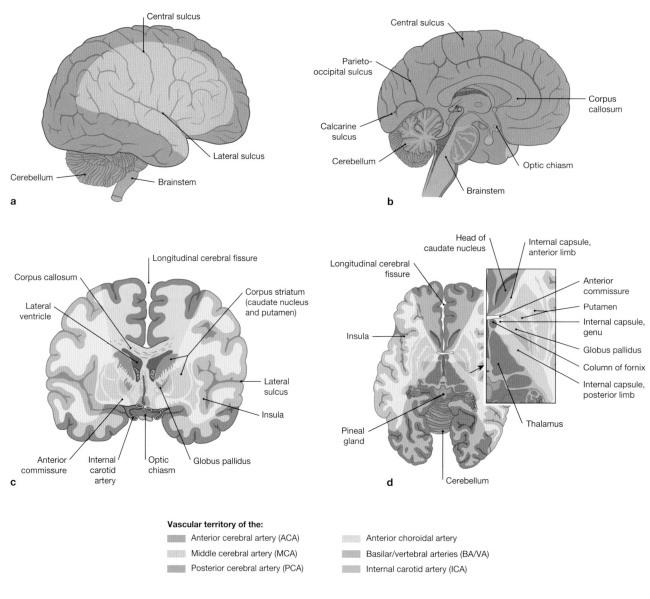

Vascular territory of the:

Anterior cerebral artery (ACA)

Middle cerebral artery (MCA)

Posterior cerebral artery (PCA)

Anterior choroidal artery

Basilar/vertebral arteries (BA/VA)

Internal carotid artery (ICA)

Fig. 12.21a to d Arterial blood supply to the brain; lateral view **(a)**, medial view **(b)**, frontal **(c)** and horizontal **(d)** sections. [L126] Vascular territories of the anterior cerebral artery (ACA), middle cerebral artery (MCA), posterior cerebral artery (PCA), basilar/vertebral arteries (BA/VA), internal carotid artery (ICA), and anterior choroidal artery are shown in different colors.

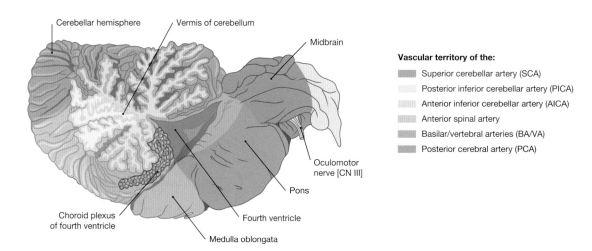

Vascular territory of the:

Superior cerebellar artery (SCA)

Posterior inferior cerebellar artery (PICA)

Anterior inferior cerebellar artery (AICA)

Anterior spinal artery

Basilar/vertebral arteries (BA/VA)

Posterior cerebral artery (PCA)

Fig. 12.22 Arterial blood supply to the cerebellum and brainstem; sagittal view. [L126]

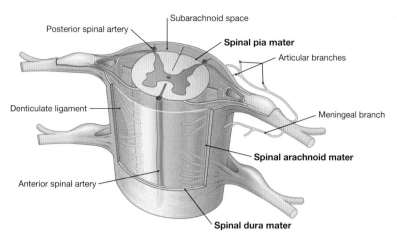

Fig. 12.23 Meninges of the spinal cord; oblique ventral view. [E402]
Like the brain, the spinal cord is surrounded by the three meninges, which provide protection and suspension of the spinal cord within the vertebral canal.
The outermost spinal dura mater forms a tubular dural sheath around the spinal nerve roots which fuses with the nerve sheath (epineurium) of the spinal nerves. The spinal pia mater is rich in blood vessels, tightly attached to the surface of the spinal cord,

and extends deeply into the anterior median fissure. The pia mater creates a sheath-like lining around the anterior and posterior spinal nerve roots on their way through the subarachnoid space.
Along both sides of the spinal cord, lateral extensions of the spinal pia mater, called denticulate ligaments, connect with the arachnoid mater and dura mater. They attach the spinal cord in the center of the subarachnoid space which is filled with CSF.

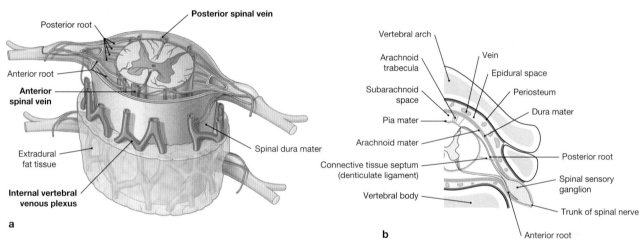

Fig. 12.24a and b Veins of the vertebral canal; oblique ventral view **(a)**; schematic cross-section of a spinal cord segment **(b)**.
a [E402], b [L126]
The veins draining the spinal cord mainly form longitudinal collecting vessels running alongside the spinal cord. Two pairs of longitudinal veins group around the exit and entry points of the anterior and posterior spinal nerve roots. In addition, unpaired anterior and

posterior spinal veins course alongside the anterior median fissure and the posterior median sulcus, respectively. These veins drain into the internal vertebral venous plexus in the epidural space of the vertebral canal. This venous plexus connects with segmental veins which drain into the large collecting veins of the body. Veins of the internal vertebral venous plexus communicate with intracranial veins.

Clinical Remarks

Spina bifida is a congenital defective closure of the vertebral column and spinal cord caused by teratogenic factors (e.g. alcohol, medication) or missing induction of the chorda dorsalis.
a The **spina bifida occulta** is the mildest form and exclusively involves the vertebral arches. In most cases, unfused arches are found in one or two vertebrae. The corresponding overlying skin is often covered with hair and is more intensely pigmented. Usually, these patients show no symptoms.
b In the case of a **spina bifida cystica,** the vertebral arches of a number of neighboring vertebrae are not closed; a cyst-like protrusion of the spinal meninges extends into the defect (*meningocele*). A *meningomyelocele* exists if the meningeal cyst contains spinal cord and nerves. This coincides with functional deficits.
Spina bifida aperta (*rachischisis, myeloschisis*) is the most severe form of spina bifida with underlying defect in the proper closure of the neural folds. With no skin cover to protect it, the undifferentiated neural plate is exposed on the back. Newborns with such defects usually die shortly after birth.
[E247-09]

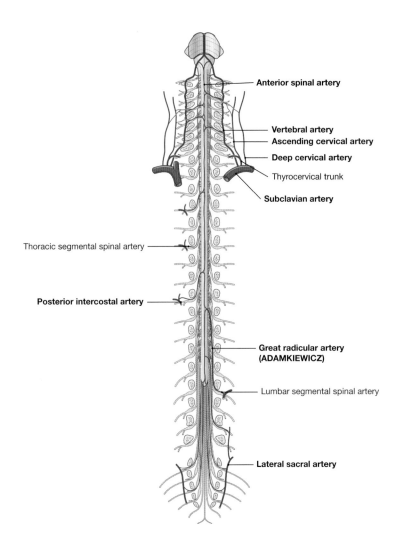

Anterior spinal artery

Vertebral artery
Ascending cervical artery

Deep cervical artery

Thyrocervical trunk

Subclavian artery

Thoracic segmental spinal artery

Posterior intercostal artery

Great radicular artery
(ADAMKIEWICZ)

Lumbar segmental spinal artery

Lateral sacral artery

Fig. 12.25 Arteries of the spinal cord; anterior view; not all segmental spinal arteries are shown. [E402]
The following major arteries provide branches for the arterial supply of the spinal cord:
- **cervical part:** the **subclavian artery** via the the vertebral artery, the ascending cervical artery and the deep cervical artery
- **thoracic part:** the **thoracic aorta** via the supreme intercostal artery and the posterior intercostal arteries supplying spinal arteries
- **lumbosacral part:** the **abdominal aorta** (lumbosacral part) via lumbal arteries
- the **internal iliac artery** supplies the cauda equina with segmental spinal arteries via the iliolumbar artery (not shown) and lateral sacral artery.

The largest spinal branch is the great radicular artery of ADAMKIEWICZ; vertebrae T12–L2 which is usually found on the left side of the body.

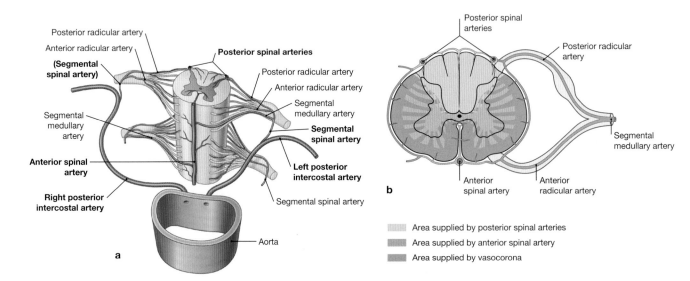

Posterior radicular artery

Anterior radicular artery

(Segmental spinal artery)

Segmental medullary artery

Anterior spinal artery

Right posterior intercostal artery

Posterior spinal arteries

Posterior radicular artery

Anterior radicular artery

Segmental medullary artery

Segmental spinal artery

Left posterior intercostal artery

Segmental spinal artery

Aorta

a

Posterior spinal arteries

Posterior radicular artery

Segmental medullary artery

Anterior spinal artery

Anterior radicular artery

b

░░ Area supplied by posterior spinal arteries
▓▓ Area supplied by anterior spinal artery
▓▓ Area supplied by vasocorona

Fig. 12.26a and b Segmental arterial supply of the spinal cord.
a [E402], b [L126]
a Blood supply to the spinal cord is achieved through the anterior spinal artery and the paired posterior spinal arteries which run alongside the spinal cord. Additional contributors are feeder arteries (segmental spinal arteries from the vertebral arteries, the deep cervical arteries, the intercostal arteries and the lumbar arteries) which enter the vertebral canal through the intervertebral foramina and divide into segmental medullary, anterior and posterior radicular branches at the level of each spinal cord plane. The anterior and posterior radicular branches follow the anterior and posterior

roots of the spinal nerves and supply them with blood. The spinal segmental arteries release segmental medullary arteries which are more prominent at the cervical and lumbar enlargements to ensure good blood supply. The segmental medullary arteries project to and anastomose with the anterior spinal artery.
b Schematic drawing of the arterial vascular territory of the anterior spinal artery (anterior two-thirds of spinal cord) and the posterior spinal arteries (posterior third of spinal cord) in the spinal cord. The vasocorona refers to the arterial blood supply to the spinal cord via anastomoses between anterior and posterior spinal arteries.

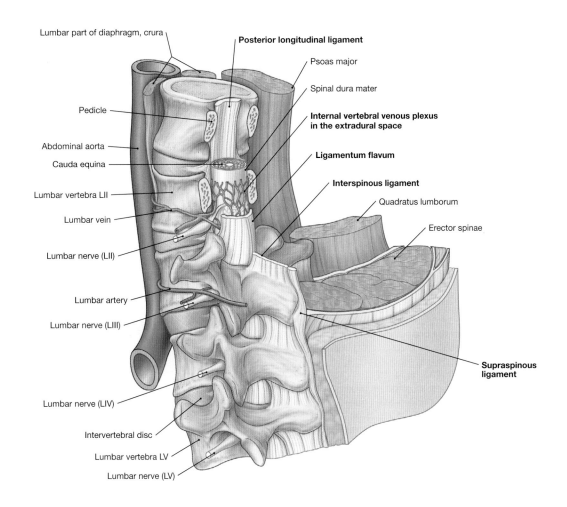

Fig. 12.27 Position of the spinal cord within the vertebral canal; dorsolateral view. [E402]
The posterior longitudinal ligament positions on the ventral side of the dural tube. The ligamentum flavum, vertebral arches and the interspinal and supraspinous ligaments provide the dorsal cover for the dural tube. Surrounding the dural tube is the internal vertebral venous plexus. The vertebral arches of the first two lumbar vertebrae have been removed. The topographical relationship of the spinal nerve root and the intervertebral disc below spinal nerve LII is shown.

Clinical Remarks

Epidural (peridural) anesthesia and spinal anesthesia

Anesthetics can be injected into the epidural space (epidural or peridural anesthesia) to anesthetize individual spinal nerves. In spinal anesthesia, the anesthetics are applied directly into the subarachnoid space. The medication mixes with the cerebrospinal fluid (CSF) but, as a result of g-force, anaesthetizes only nerve fibers located below the injection site.

a For lumbar puncture, the back must be maximally bent forward. The needle is inserted between the spinous processes of the lumbar vertebrae III and IV or IV and V and pushed forward carefully until the spinal dura mater is pierced and the tip of the needle rests in the subarachnoid (intrathecal) space. CSF can be drawn for diagnostic purposes or an anesthetic can be applied.

b The different tissue layers the needle passes through to reach the intrathecal space are indicated.
a [L126, R363], b [L126]

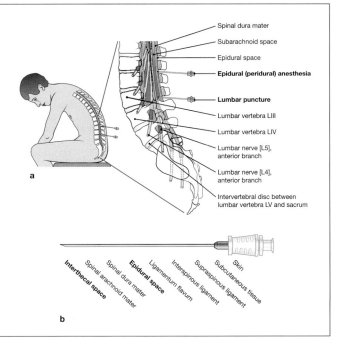

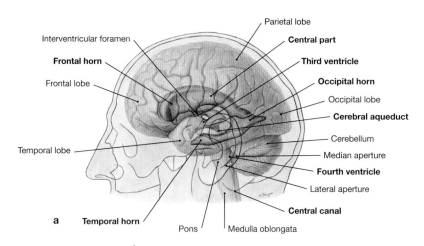

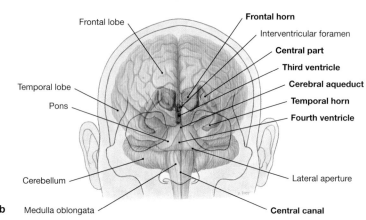

Fig. 12.28a and b Ventricles of the brain; view from the left side **(a)**, anterior view **(b)**.

In the brain, the ventricular system is composed of the paired lateral ventricles with frontal (anterior) horn, central part, occipital (posterior) horn, and temporal (inferior) horn, the third ventricle, the cerebral aqueduct, and the fourth ventricle. The spinal cord contains the central canal. The ventricles and the central canal contain cerebrospinal fluid (CSF).

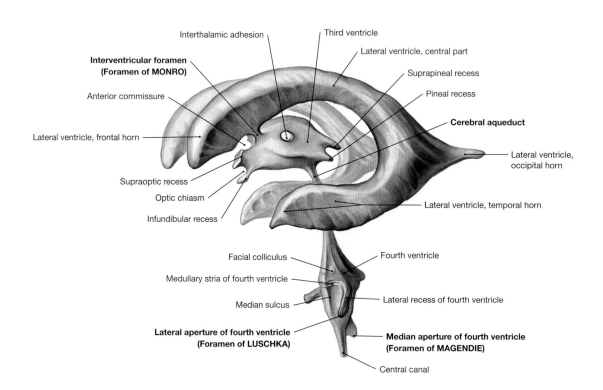

Fig. 12.29 Subarachnoid spaces; corrosion cast specimen; oblique view from the left side.

Each of the lateral ventricles connects with the third ventricle by a separate interventricular foramen (foramen of MONRO). The third ventricle communicates with the fourth ventricle through the cere-bral aqueduct. The fourth ventricle contains three openings to drain CSF to the subarachnoid space between the arachnoid and pia mater of brain and spinal cord: the median aperture (foramen of MAGENDIE) and the paired lateral apertures (foramina of LUSCHKA).

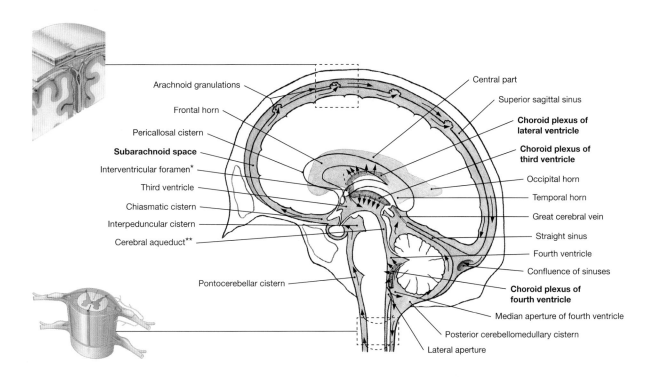

Fig. 12.30 Ventricles of the brain and subarachnoid spaces.
Schematic drawing showing the circulation (arrows) of the cerebrospinal fluid (green) within the ventricles and subarachnoid space in relation to venous blood flow in the sinuses (blue).
The subarachnoid space between the arachnoid and pia mater surrounds the brain and spinal cord. The choroid plexuses in the ventricles produce most of the cerebrospinal fluid (CSF). The circulating fluid volume (150 ml [5 fl oz]) is exchanged constantly, with a daily CSF production volume of approx. 500 ml [17 fl oz]. The CSF serves as a cushion to protect the CNS from mechanical forces, and

reduces the weight of the CNS (by creating a buoyancy which causes a 97 % weight reduction from 1,400 g to 45 g [49 oz to 1.6 oz]), supports the metabolism of the CNS, removes toxic substances, transports hormones (e.g. leptin), and facilitates electrical conductance.
Schematic inserts show the meningeal layers in the brain and spinal cord.

*   clin. term: foramen of MONRO
**   clin. term: aqueduct of SYLVIUS

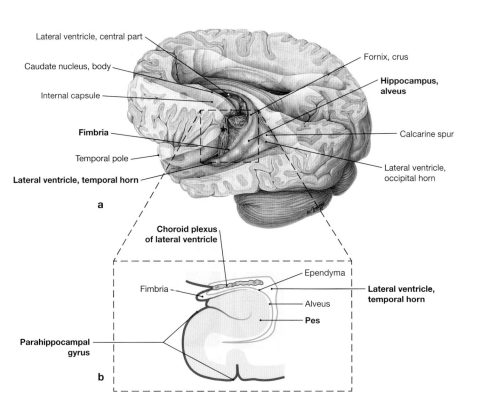

Fig. 12.31a and b Lateral ventricles; posterior superior view **(a)** from the left side; after removal of the upper parts of the cerebral hemispheres, schematic frontal section **(b)** of the temporal horn of lateral ventricle.
b [L126]
The choroid plexus (*) has been lifted up at the transition from the central part to the temporal part of the lateral ventricle. The schematic representation of this area **(b)** shows the topographical relationship between lateral ventricle and hippocampus formation. The choroid plexus protrudes into the lateral ventricle. The walls of the ventricle are lined with an ependymal cell layer.

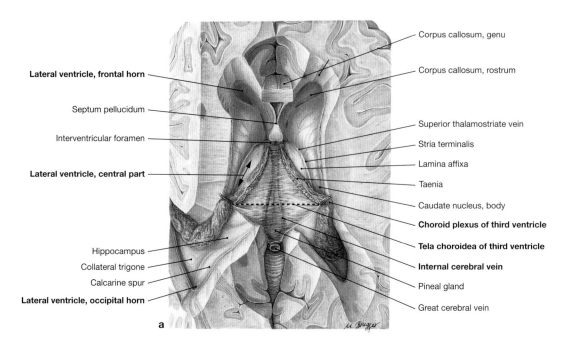

Corpus callosum, genu
Corpus callosum, rostrum
Lateral ventricle, frontal horn
Septum pellucidum
Interventricular foramen
Superior thalamostriate vein
Stria terminalis
Lamina affixa
Lateral ventricle, central part
Taenia
Caudate nucleus, body
Choroid plexus of third ventricle
Tela choroidea of third ventricle
Hippocampus
Collateral trigone
Internal cerebral vein
Calcarine spur
Pineal gland
Lateral ventricle, occipital horn
Great cerebral vein

a

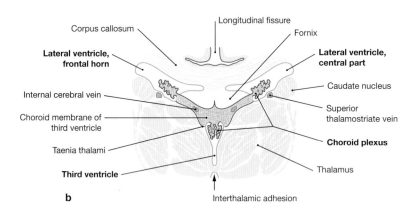

Corpus callosum
Longitudinal fissure
Fornix
Lateral ventricle, frontal horn
Lateral ventricle, central part
Caudate nucleus
Internal cerebral vein
Superior thalamostriate vein
Choroid membrane of third ventricle
Choroid plexus
Taenia thalami
Thalamus
Third ventricle
b
Interthalamic adhesion

Fig. 12.32a and b Lateral ventricles; superior view **(a)**; after removal of the central part of the corpus callosum and the columns of the fornix. Choroid plexuses in the lateral ventricles and in the third ventricle; schematic frontal section **(b)**. b [L126]

a The choroid membrane overarches the third ventricle. The internal cerebral veins drain into the great cerebral vein. On both sides, the choroid plexus runs alongside the hippocampus into the temporal horn. The dotted line marks the plane of the frontal section shown in ➤ Fig. 12.32b.

b The choroid plexus is present in the paired lateral ventricles, and in the third and fourth ventricles (not shown). In the choroid plexus, capillary blood and CSF space are separated by a blood-CSF barrier (➤ Fig. 12.33a and ➤ Fig. 12.33b).

Clinical Remarks

Impaired drainage of cerebrospinal fluid (CSF) can be the result of tumors, deformities, bleedings, or other causes.
a The increase in intracranial pressure results in headaches, nausea, and optic papilla protrusion (papilledema).
b When CSF cannot circulate into the outer subarachnoid space, it accumulates in the ventricles and causes a **non-communicating hydrocephalus** as shown in a computed tomographic (CT) cross-section of a patient with obstruction in the cerebral aqueduct (aqueduct of midbrain). Another form is the **communicating hydrocephalus** with obstruction of CSF flow in the subarachnoid space due to impaired CSF reabsorption.
c CT of a normal brain.
d Positron emission tomography (PET) scan of a normal brain.
e Hydrocephalus ex vacuo is not the result of a blockage of CSF flow but is caused by an increase in ventricular size due to a rarefication of brain matter. Positron emission tomography (PET) scan of a hydrocephalus ex vacuo shows greatly enlarged cerebral ventricles at the expense of the cerebral parenchyma. The patient showed massive mental disabilities and significantly impaired gait. Hydrocephalus ex vacuo occurs in ALZHEIMER's disease. Hydrocephalus ex vacuo results from an increase in ventricular size due to a rarefication of brain matter. This occurs in ALZHEIMER's disease as shown by positron emission tomography (PET) scan.
a [E761], b [E867], c [E602], d, e [F698-002]

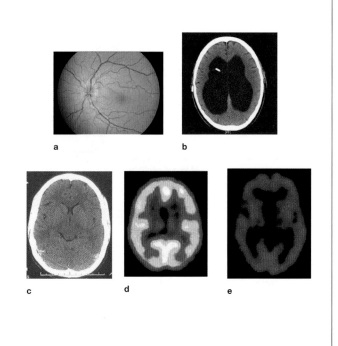

a   b

c   d   e

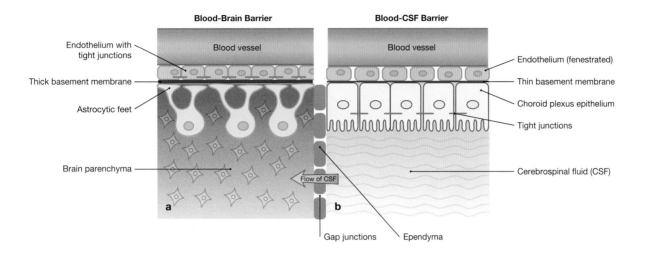

Fig. 12.33a and b Schematic drawings of the blood-brain barrier, the blood-CSF barrier and the ependymal cell layer between the brain and CSF. [L126]

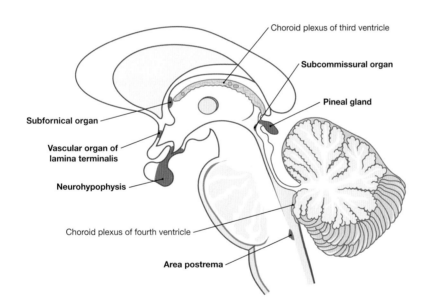

Fig. 12.34 Circumventricular organs; median sagittal section. [L126]

Characteristic features of the circumventricular organs are strong vascularization, a modified ependyma (tanycytes with tight junctions), and the formation of a blood-CSF barrier instead of a blood-brain barrier (BBB). Circumventricular organs include the neurohy-pophysis, the median eminence, the pineal gland, the vascular organ of lamina terminalis and the subfornical organ (the latter two regulate blood volume and blood pressure, secretion of hormones such as angiotensin and somatostatin), the subcommissural organ (present only in the fetus and newborn, secretion of a glycoprotein-rich product), and the area postrema (triggers vomiting).

Clinical Remarks

The circumventricular organs lack the blood-brain barrier and, thus, are capable of monitoring the plasma-blood milieu. This is not only of pharmacological interest. The area postrema contains numerous dopamine and serotonin receptors. Dopamine and serotonin antagonists are effective antiemetic drugs. In ad-dition, the activation of chemoreceptors in the area postrema presents a protective mechanism for the body as exemplified by centrally induced vomiting in response to the ingestion of spoiled food. This response will remove potentially harmful sub-stances from the body.

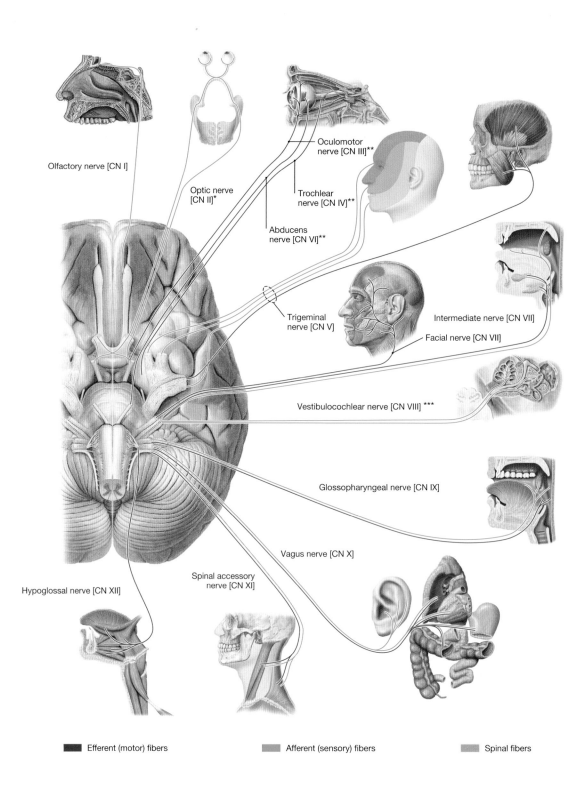

Olfactory nerve [CN I]

Optic nerve [CN II]*

Oculomotor nerve [CN III]**

Trochlear nerve [CN IV]**

Abducens nerve [CN VI]**

Trigeminal nerve [CN V]

Intermediate nerve [CN VII]

Facial nerve [CN VII]

Vestibulocochlear nerve [CN VIII] ***

Glossopharyngeal nerve [CN IX]

Vagus nerve [CN X]

Spinal accessory nerve [CN XI]

Hypoglossal nerve [CN XII]

■ Efferent (motor) fibers ■ Afferent (sensory) fibers ■ Spinal fibers

Fig. 12.35 Cranial nerves; functional overview of the telencephalon, brainstem and cerebellum; inferior view. [L127]
Twelve pairs of cranial nerves [CN I–XII] exit the brainstem from anterior to posterior. CN I and CN II have distinguishing features that separate them from the other cranial nerves. The afferent nerve fibers of the olfactory nerves [CN I] are very short and the terminal nuclei are located in the olfactory bulb, a part of the telencephalon that was rearranged cranially during development. The optic nerve [CN II] is exceptional as it includes the 3rd and possibly a 4th neuron

of the visual pathway. In contrast to all other cranial nerves, the optic nerve is actually not a nerve but a protrusion of the diencephalon.

* The optic nerve [CN II] is described in ➤ chapter 9 (Eye).
** The oculomotor nerve [CN III], trochlear nerve [CN IV], and abducens nerve [CN VI] functions are described in ➤ chapter 9 (Eye).
*** The vestibulocochlear nerve [CN VIII] is described in ➤ chapter 10 (Ear).

Overview of Fiber Qualities of the Twelve Cranial Nerves and Important Innervation Sites		
Cranial Nerve	**Quality**	**Important Innervation Sites**
Olfactory nerve [CN I]	SSA	Olfactory mucosa
Optic nerve [CN II]	SSA	Retina
Oculomotor nerve [CN III]	GSE, GVE	Intraocular and extraocular muscles
Trochlear nerve [CN IV]	GSE	Extraocular muscles
Trigeminal nerve [CN V]	SVE, GSA	Masticatory muscles, facial skin
Abducens nerve [CN VI]	GSE	Extraocular muscles
Facial nerve [CN VII]	GVE, SVE, SVA, GSA	Muscles of facial expression, gustatory organ, glands
Vestibulocochlear nerve [CN VIII]	SSA	Equilibrium and hearing
Glossopharyngeal nerve [CN IX]	GVE, SVE, GSA, GVA, SVA	Pharyngeal muscles, parotid gland, gustatory organ
Vagus nerve [CN X]	GVE, SVE, GSA, GVA, SVA	Pharyngeal and laryngeal muscles, gustatory and inner organs
Spinal accessory nerve [CN XI]	SVE	Trapezius and sternocleidomastoid
Hypoglossal nerve [CN XII]	GSE	Muscles of the tongue

SSA: specific somatic afferent; SVA: specific visceral afferent; GSA: general somatic afferent; GVA: general visceral afferent; GVE: general visceral efferent; GSE: general somatic efferent; SVE: specific visceral efferent

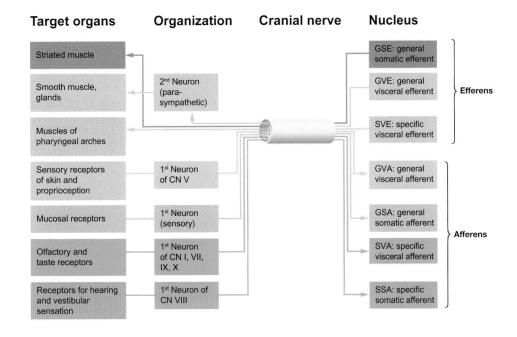

Fig. 12.36 Schematic representation of the composition and different fiber qualities of a cranial nerve. [L127]

Foramina of the skull where cranial nerves exit are listed in ➤ chapter 8 (Head).

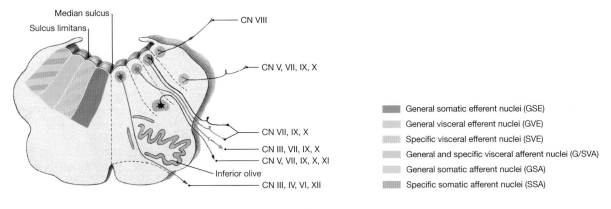

Fig. 12.37 Cranial nerves; schematic cross-section through the rhomboid fossa demonstrating the nuclei of cranial nerves.
In the brainstem, nuclei with similar functions are arranged in a column. There are four longitudinal nuclear columns arranged alongside each other. In a medial (efferents) to lateral (afferents)

direction. This includes a somatic efferent, a visceral efferent, a visceral afferent, and a somatic afferent column of nuclei. Within the visceral efferent, the visceral afferent, and the somatic afferent columns of nuclei, one can distinguish general and specific afferent nuclei.

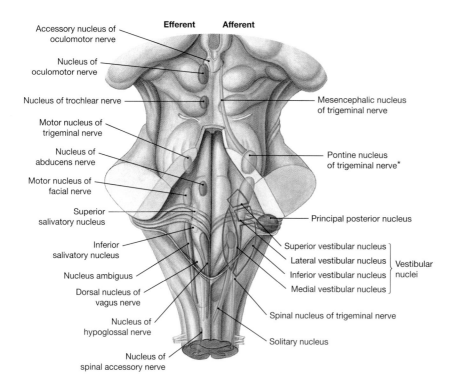

Accessory nucleus of oculomotor nerve

Nucleus of oculomotor nerve

Nucleus of trochlear nerve

Motor nucleus of trigeminal nerve

Nucleus of abducens nerve

Motor nucleus of facial nerve

Superior salivatory nucleus

Inferior salivatory nucleus

Nucleus ambiguus

Dorsal nucleus of vagus nerve

Nucleus of hypoglossal nerve

Nucleus of spinal accessory nerve

Efferent   **Afferent**

Mesencephalic nucleus of trigeminal nerve

Pontine nucleus of trigeminal nerve*

Principal posterior nucleus

Superior vestibular nucleus

Lateral vestibular nucleus

Inferior vestibular nucleus   Vestibular nuclei

Medial vestibular nucleus

Spinal nucleus of trigeminal nerve

Solitary nucleus

Fig. 12.38 Cranial nerves; topographical overview of the nuclei of CN III to CN XII; posterior view.
With the exception of CN I and CN II, the other cranial nerves [CN III–XII] have nuclei located in the brainstem:
- Mesencephalon: CN III and IV
- Pons: CN V/1–3, VI, VII
- Medulla oblongata: CN VII–XII

Topographically, the nuclei of CN III–XII are arranged in functional nuclear columns. On the left side are the nuclei of origin which contain the perikarya of the efferent neurons projecting into the periphery. In the terminal nuclei on the right side, the afferent fibers synapse onto the 2nd neuron of the sensory tract.

* clin. term: principal sensory nucleus of trigeminal nerve

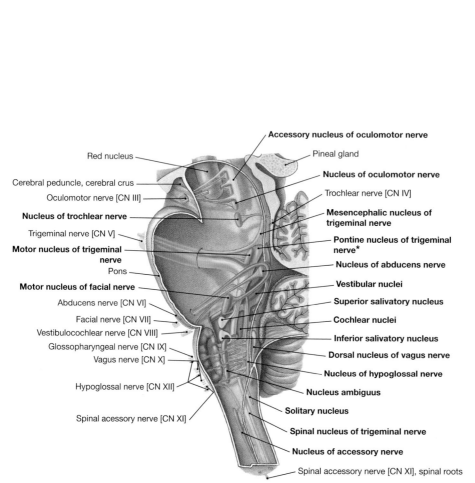

Red nucleus

Cerebral peduncle, cerebral crus

Oculomotor nerve [CN III]

Nucleus of trochlear nerve

Trigeminal nerve [CN V]

Motor nucleus of trigeminal nerve

Pons

Motor nucleus of facial nerve

Abducens nerve [CN VI]

Facial nerve [CN VII]

Vestibulocochlear nerve [CN VIII]

Glossopharyngeal nerve [CN IX]

Vagus nerve [CN X]

Hypoglossal nerve [CN XII]

Spinal acessory nerve [CN XI]

Accessory nucleus of oculomotor nerve

Pineal gland

Nucleus of oculomotor nerve

Trochlear nerve [CN IV]

Mesencephalic nucleus of trigeminal nerve

Pontine nucleus of trigeminal nerve*

Nucleus of abducens nerve

Vestibular nuclei

Superior salivatory nucleus

Cochlear nuclei

Inferior salivatory nucleus

Dorsal nucleus of vagus nerve

Nucleus of hypoglossal nerve

Nucleus ambiguus

Solitary nucleus

Spinal nucleus of trigeminal nerve

Nucleus of accessory nerve

Spinal accessory nerve [CN XI], spinal roots

■ General somatic efferent nuclei (GSE)

■ General visceral efferent nuclei (GVE)

■ Specific visceral efferent nuclei (SVE)

■ General and specific visceral afferent nuclei (G/SVA)

■ General somatic afferent nuclei (GSA)

■ Specific somatic afferent nuclei (SSA)

Fig. 12.39 Cranial nerves; topographical overview of the nuclei of CN III to CN XII in the median plane.
Nuclei of origin with perikarya of efferent/motor fibers divide into:
- **general somatic efferent nuclei:** CN III, IV, VI, XII
- **general visceral efferent nuclei:** accessory nuclei of oculomotor nerve [CN III], superior salivatory nucleus [CN VII], inferior salivatory nucleus [CN IX], dorsal (posterior) nucleus of vagus nerve [CN X]
- **special visceral efferent nuclei:** motor nucleus of trigeminal nerve [CN V], motor nucleus of facial nerve [CN VII], nucleus ambiguus [CN IX, X, cranial root of XI], nucleus of spinal accessory nerve [CN XI]

Terminal nuclei targeted by afferent/sensory fibers divide into:
- **general visceral afferent nuclei:** nuclei of solitary tract, inferior part [CN IX, X]
- **special visceral afferent nuclei:** nuclei of solitary tract, superior part [CN VII, IX, X]
- **general somatic afferent nuclei:** mesencephalic nucleus of trigeminal nerve [CN V], pontine (principal sensory) nucleus of trigeminal nerve [CN V], spinal nucleus of trigeminal nerve [CN V]
- **special somatic afferent nuclei:** superior, lateral, medial and inferior vestibular nuclei [CN VIII], anterior and posterior cochlear nuclei [CN VIII]

* clin. term: principal sensory nucleus of trigeminal nerve

Overview of Cranial Nerves and their Nuclei in the Brainstem.
The cranial nerves CN IV, VI, and XII only have one nucleus.

Cranial Nerve	Corresponding Nuclei
Oculomotor nerve [CN III]	Nucleus of oculomotor nerve
	Accessory nuclei of oculomotor nerve
Trochlear nerve [CN IV]	Nucleus of trochlear nerve
Trigeminal nerve [CN V]	Motor nucleus of trigeminal nerve
	Mesencephalic nucleus of trigeminal nerve
	Pontine (principal sensory) nucleus of trigeminal nerve
	Spinal nucleus of trigeminal nerve
Abducens nerve [CN VI]	Nucleus of abducens nerve
Facial nerve [CN VII]	Motor nucleus of facial nerve
	Superior salivatory nucleus
	Spinal nucleus of trigeminal nerve
	Nuclei of solitary tract
Vestibulocochlear nerve [CN VIII]	Vestibular nuclei
	Cochlear nuclei
Glossopharyngeal nerve [CN IX]	Inferior salivatory nucleus
	Nucleus ambiguus
	Spinal nucleus of trigeminal nerve
	Nuclei of solitary tract
Vagus nerve [CN X]	Dorsal (posterior) nucleus of vagus nerve
	Nucleus ambiguus
	Spinal nucleus of trigeminal nerve
	Nuclei of solitary tract
Spinal accessory nerve [CN XI]	Nucleus ambiguus (medulla oblongata)
	Nuclei of spinal accessory nerve (C1–C6)
Hypoglossal nerve [CN XII]	Nucleus of hypoglossal nerve

Structure/Function

Origin and cranial nerve innervation of muscles derived from the pharyngeal arches. [L127]

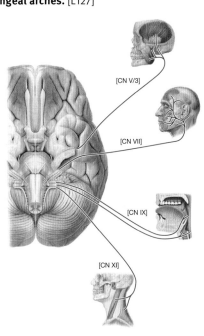

[CN V/3]
[CN VII]
[CN IX]
[CN XI]

Cranial Nerve	Pharyngeal Arch	Muscle
Trigeminal nerve [CN V/3] (mandibular branch)	1st	Masseter, temporalis, medial and lateral pterygoid
Facial nerve [CN VII]	2nd	Musculature of facial expression muscles, stylohyoid, digastric (posterior belly), stapedius
Glossopharyngeal nerve [CN IX]	3rd	Stylopharyngeus
Vagus nerve [CN X]	4th	Pharyngeal and laryngeal muscles
Spinal accessory nerve [CN XI]	5th (and cervical somites)	Sternocleidomastoid, trapezius

Structure/Function

Sensory ganglia harbor the perikarya of the 1st afferent neurons. Mostly, these are pseudo-unipolar neurons, with the exception of the vestibulocholear bipolar neurons. The afferent neurons conduct impulses from sensory receptors or systems towards the the brain where their fibers synapse with the 2nd neurons of the sensory pathway. The cranial nerves which have sensory ganglia are listed in the table below. Note that all dorsal root ganglia of the spinal nerves are also sensory ganglia.

Peripheral Sensory Ganglia of Cranial Nerves [CN V, VII, VIII, IX, X]			
Cranial Nerve	**Sensory Ganglia (Location of Primary Sensory Neuron)**	**Ganglionic Cell Type**	**Function**
Trigeminal nerve [CN V]	Trigeminal ganglion (GASSERIAN or semilunar ganglion)	Pseudo-unipolar	Sensations in the face, oral cavity, nasal cavity, sinuses, supratentorial meninges
Facial nerve [CN VII]	Geniculate ganglion	Pseudo-unipolar	Taste sensation of anterior two thirds of the tongue, skin sensation near outer ear canal
Vestibulocochlear nerve [CN VIII]	Spiral ganglion	Bipolar	Hearing
	SCARPA's vestibular ganglion	Bipolar	Balance/equilibrium
Glossopharyngeal nerve [CN IX]	Superior (jugular) ganglion of glossopharyngeal nerve	Pseudo-unipolar	External auditory meatus, middle ear, pharynx, posterior third of the tongue
	Inferior (petrosal) ganglion of glossopharyngeal nerve	Pseudo-unipolar	External auditory meatus, middle ear, pharynx, posterior third of the tongue, carotid body
Vagus nerve [CN X]	Superior (jugular) ganglion of vagus nerve	Pseudo-unipolar	Ear, pharynx, infratentorial meninges
	Inferior (nodose) ganglion of vagus nerve	Pseudo-unipolar	Epiglottis and larynx, heart and aortic arch, pulmonary system, abdominal organs up to CANNON-BOEHM point (left upper colon flexure)

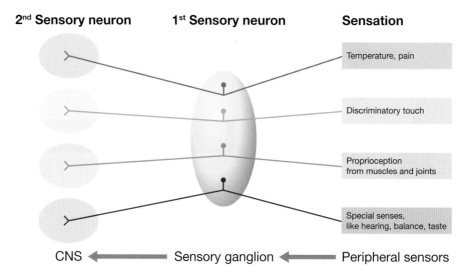

Fig. 12.40 Schematic drawing of the basic organization of sensory ganglia and their role in linking different peripheral sensory systems with defined sensory nuclei in the CNS (see individual cranial nerves for details). [L127]

Structure/Function

There is a key difference between ganglia of the autonomic nervous system and the sensory system. In **sympathetic and parasympathetic ganglia** of the autonomic system, preganglionic axons synapse onto postganglionic neurons.

In **sensory ganglia** no such synapsing occurs. Instead these sensory ganglia harbor the perikaryon of 1st afferent neurons.

Parasympathetic Ganglia of Cranial Nerves [CN III, VII, IX, X]			
Parasympathetic Nuclei in Brainstem (1st Neuron)	**Cranial Nerve Containing Parasympathetic Fibers**	**Parasympathetic Ganglia (2nd Neuron)**	**Function**
Accessory nuclei of oculomotor nerve (EDINGER-WESTPHAL)	Oculomotor nerve [CN III]	Ciliary ganglion	Miosis (sphincter pupillae), accommodation (ciliary muscle)
Superior salivatory nucleus	Intermediate nerve (of facial nerve [CN VII])	Sphenopalatine (pterygopalatine) ganglion	Lacrimal gland, mucosal glands of nose, palate, sinuses
		Submandibular ganglion	Submandibular gland, sublingual gland, anterior glands of the tongue
Inferior salivatory nucleus	Glossopharyngeal nerve [CN IX]	Otic ganglion	Parotid gland
Nucleus ambiguus*	Cardiac plexus	Heart	
Dorsal nucleus of vagus nerve	Vagus nerve [CN X]	• Intramural ganglia (AUERBACH), submucous ganglia (MEISSNER) • Organ-specific plexus, e. g. pulmonary plexus	Pulmonary system, esophagus, kidney, gastrointestinal tract up to left upper colon flexure (CANNON-BOEHM point)

* In addition to its motor neurons for the innervation of muscles of the soft palate, pharynx, larynx, the nucleus ambiguus (NA) also contains cholinergic parasympathetic neurons which form the parasympathetic plexus of the heart.

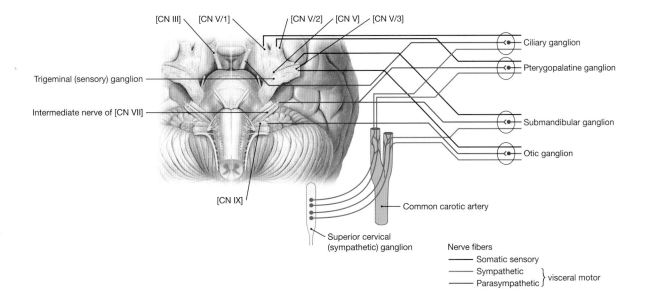

Fig. 12.41 In the four parasympathetic ganglia of the head, the preganglionic parasympathetic efferent fibers of cranial nerves [CN III, CN VII and CN IX] synapse onto the postganglionic parasympathetic neurons which extend their axons to the target organs (for details see table above). Somatic sensory fibers of the trigeminal nerve and fibers from the sympathetic superior cervical ganglion course through these ganglia but do not synapse in these parasympathetic ganglia. [L127]

Note: In the following pages, the cranial nerves [CN I, CN V, CN VII, CN IX, CN X, CN XI, and CN XII] are discussed in more detail. The functions of the optic nerve [CN II], oculomotor nerve [CN III], trochlear nerve [CN IV], and abducens nerve [CN VI] are discussed in ➤ chapter 9 (Eye). The vestibulochochlear nerve [CN VIII] is discussed in ➤ chapter 10 (Ear).

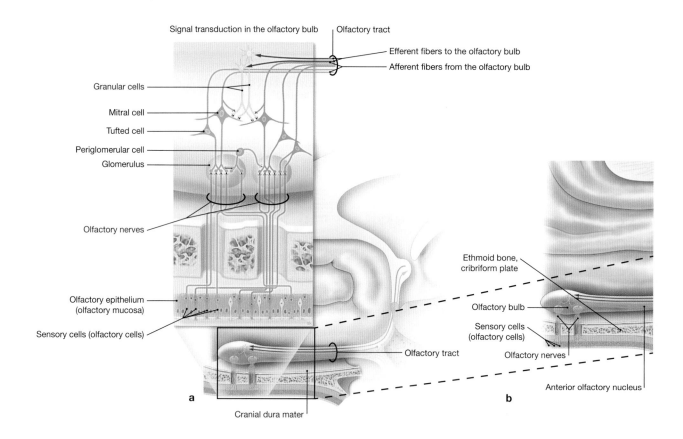

Fig. 12.42a and b Olfactory nerve [CN I] and olfactory tract; schematic projections of synaptic connections of the olfactory nerves; view from the left side. [L238]

An area of 3 cm² (0,5 in²) of olfactory mucosa locates to both sides at the roof of the nasal cavity. It contains approximately 30 million receptor cells (olfactory cells) which respond to chemical signals. These are bipolar neurons (olfactory neurons, 1st neurons, SSA) which respond to odorant molecules binding to olfactory receptors. The axons form the olfactory nerves [CN I]. Olfactory neurons are short-lived (30–60 days) and replaced by neuronal stem cells throughout life.

In each olfactory bulb, all olfactory nerve fibers converge onto approximately 1,000 glomeruli (two glomeruli are shown as an example; **a**). Multiple synapses within the glomeruli converge on the mitral cells (2nd neuron). The axons of all neurons possessing the identical odorant receptor reach a glomerulus that is specific for each of the approximately 1,000 different olfactory receptors. Mitral cells of the olfactory bulb project to different areas at the cranial base and the temporal lobe (primary olfactory cortex). Feedback mechanisms increase the discrimination of odorant stimuli and involve granular cells that connect back with different mitral cells. Secondary olfactory cortical areas and other brain regions, including the hypothalamus, ensure the conscious realization and complex sensory perception of olfactory stimuli.

Clinical Remarks

Viral infections, chronic sinusitis, obstruction of the nasal passage to the olfactory mucosa, e.g. due to allergy, side effects of medication, brain tumor or head trauma with injury to the olfactory nerves during their passage through the cribriform plate, can result in **hyposmia** (decreased ability to perceive odors) or **anosmia** (inability to perceive odors). Hyposmia and anosmia also affect taste perception.

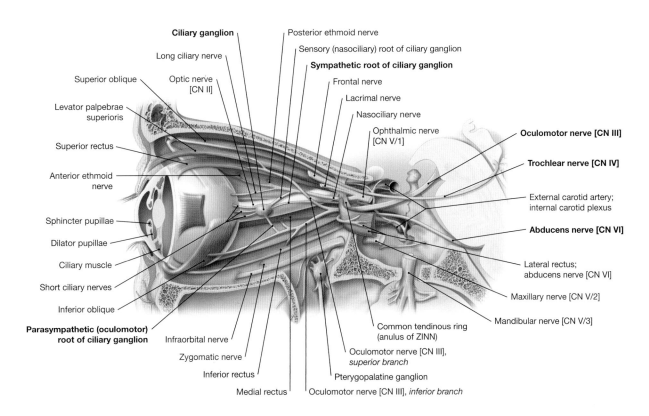

Fig. 12.43 **Oculomotor nerve [CN III], trochlear nerve [CN IV] and abducens nerve [CN VI], left side;** lateral view; orbit opened, and orbital fat body removed, the lateral rectus muscle was sectioned close to its insertion and deflected. [L238]

The oculomotor nerve [CN III] innervates the extraocular muscles with the exception of the superior oblique (trochlear nerve [CN IV]) and the lateral rectus muscles (abducens nerve [CN VI]). The parasympathetic part of CN III innervates the sphincter pupillae and the ciliary muscles. The dilator pupillae receives sympathetic innervation from the superior cervical ganglion.

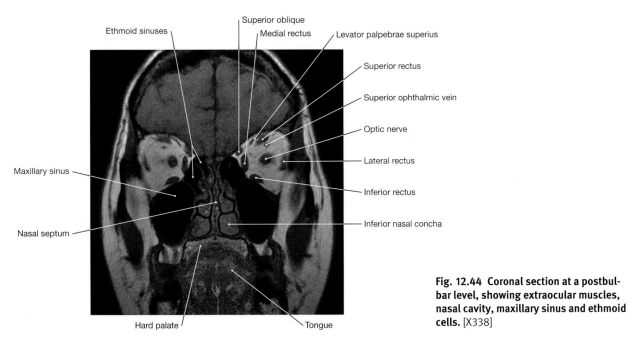

Fig. 12.44 **Coronal section at a postbulbar level, showing extraocular muscles, nasal cavity, maxillary sinus and ethmoid cells.** [X338]

Clinical Remarks

Lesions of individual cranial nerves that innervate extraocular muscles lead to the paralysis of the corresponding extraocular muscles with resulting deviations of the eyeball. The direction and extent of this deviation of the eye depends on the stronger action of the still intact extraocular muscles (and corresponding intact cranial nerves) as opposed to the paralyzed muscle(s). A complete paresis of the oculomotor nerve [CN III] results in pto-

sis, mydriasis, the inability to accommodate, and a bulbus turned down and outwards ('*down and out*' syndrome).

Paresis of the abducens nerve [CN VI] is particularly frequent due to the long extradural course of this nerve and its passage through the cavernous sinus. When the patient is asked to move the affected eye to the temporal side, the eyeball does not follow to the temporal side since the lateral rectus is paralyzed. For more details see ➤ chapter 9 (Eye).

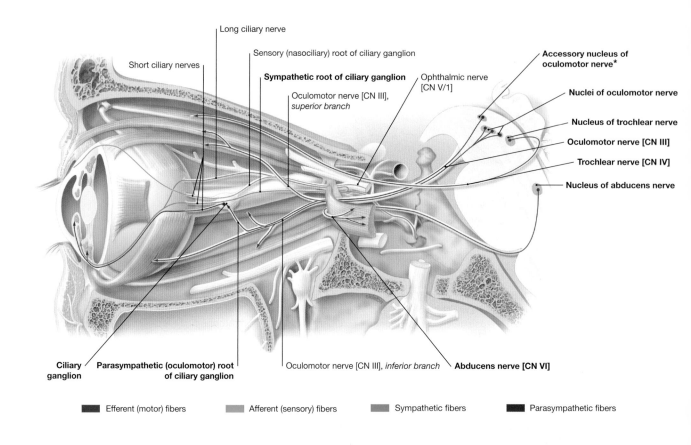

Fig. 12.45 Fiber qualities of the oculomotor [CN III], trochlear [CN IV] and abducens nerves [CN VI], left side; lateral view. [L238]
The oculomotor nerve [CN III] contains motor fibers (GSE) derived from the nucleus of oculomotor nerve for the majority of extraocular muscles. In the orbit, the nerve divides into a superior branch and an inferior branch which innervate specific extraocular muscles:
Superior branch:
• superior rectus
• levator palpebrae superioris
Inferior branch:
• medial rectus
• inferior rectus
• inferior oblique

The accessory nuclei of oculomotor nerve (EDINGER-WESTPHAL) contribute parasympathetic fibers (GVE) which reach the ciliary ganglion through the inferior branch and a parasympathetic root (oculomotor root). In the ciliary ganglion, only preganglionic parasympathetic fibers synapse onto postganglionic neurons, while sympathetic fibers pass through the ciliary region. The postganglionic parasympathetic fibers project alongside the short ciliary nerves to the eyeball, traverse its wall, and reach the intraocular sphincter pupillae and ciliary muscles which they innervate.
The trochlear nerve [CN IV] contains motor fibers (GSE) for the superior oblique muscle from the nucleus of trochlear nerve located in the mesencephalic brainstem.
The abducens nerve [CN VI] contains motor fibers (GSE) from the nucleus of abducens nerve for the lateral rectus.

* Nucleus of EDINGER-WESTPHAL

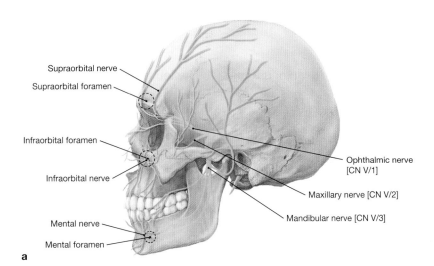

a

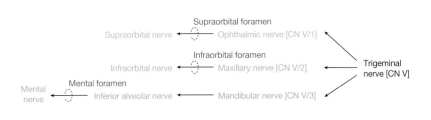

b

Fig. 12.46a and b Trigeminal nerve [CN V]; left side; lateral view **(a),** location of the three major trigeminal branches in the head; and schematic diagram **(b)** of the skull exit points of the three major trigeminal branches. a [L284], b [L126]

[CN V/1 and V/2] are sensory nerves and contain general somatoafferent (GSA) fibers. In addition to GSA fibers, the mandibular branch [CN V/3] also contains motor fibers (GSE) for the muscles of mastication.

Fig. 12.47 Innervation areas of the facial skin, exit points of nerves, and protopathic sensibility. [K340]

Left side: Concentric skin areas contain the afferent fibers for protopathic sensibility (pain, temperature) which project to the spinal nucleus of trigeminal nerve in a somatotopic order. This nucleus contains a ventral (oral, CN V/1), middle (maxillary, CN V/2) and dorsal (mandibular, CN V/3) division. The SOELDER's lines reflect the rostral to caudal organization of the spinal nucleus of trigeminal nerve.

Right side: Facial regions of general sensory innervation (GSA) plus exit points (circles) for [CN V/1–V/3]. These regions are the dermatomes of [CN V/1–V/3]. Loss of epicritical cutaneous sensitivity (fine discrimination of touch, temperature) in any of the three innervation areas of the facial skin indicates a peripheral trigeminal nerve lesion.

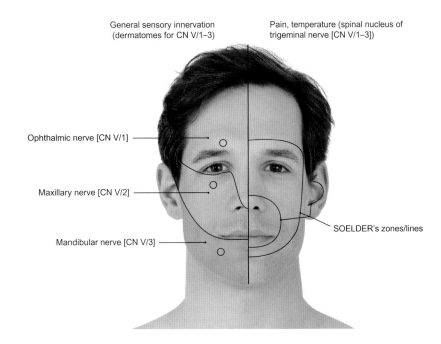

Clinical Remarks

Trigeminal neuralgia presents with hypersensitivity of the trigeminal nerve [CN V] and paroxysmal episodes of intense, stabbing pain in the sensory innervation area of the affected trigeminal branch. Even light touch to the area of the corresponding exit point of the branch can trigger pain.

Infections of the first trigeminal branch by varicella zoster virus can cause a post-zoster neuralgia of the ophthalmic nerve [CN V/1], known as opthalmic herpes zoster.
[E943]

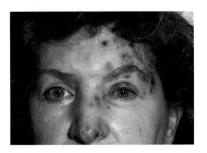

Target organs **Organization** **Cranial nerve** **Nucleus**

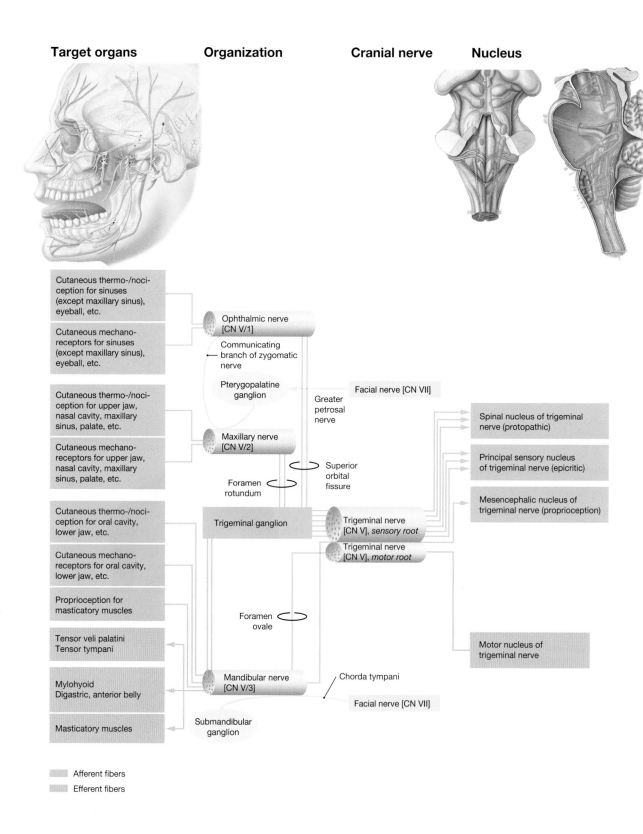

Cutaneous thermo-/noci-ception for sinuses (except maxillary sinus), eyeball, etc.

Cutaneous mechano-receptors for sinuses (except maxillary sinus), eyeball, etc.

Ophthalmic nerve [CN V/1]

Communicating branch of zygomatic nerve

Pterygopalatine ganglion

Facial nerve [CN VII]

Greater petrosal nerve

Cutaneous thermo-/noci-ception for upper jaw, nasal cavity, maxillary sinus, palate, etc.

Cutaneous mechano-receptors for upper jaw, nasal cavity, maxillary sinus, palate, etc.

Maxillary nerve [CN V/2]

Superior orbital fissure

Foramen rotundum

Spinal nucleus of trigeminal nerve (protopathic)

Principal sensory nucleus of trigeminal nerve (epicritic)

Mesencephalic nucleus of trigeminal nerve (proprioception)

Cutaneous thermo-/noci-ception for oral cavity, lower jaw, etc.

Cutaneous mechano-receptors for oral cavity, lower jaw, etc.

Proprioception for masticatory muscles

Trigeminal ganglion

Trigeminal nerve [CN V], *sensory root*

Trigeminal nerve [CN V], *motor root*

Tensor veli palatini Tensor tympani

Foramen ovale

Motor nucleus of trigeminal nerve

Mylohyoid Digastric, anterior belly

Mandibular nerve [CN V/3]

Chorda tympani

Facial nerve [CN VII]

Masticatory muscles

Submandibular ganglion

▨ Afferent fibers
▨ Efferent fibers

Fig. 12.48 Schematic representation of the trigeminal nerve [CN V]: key structures and their functions. [L127]

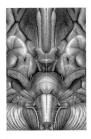

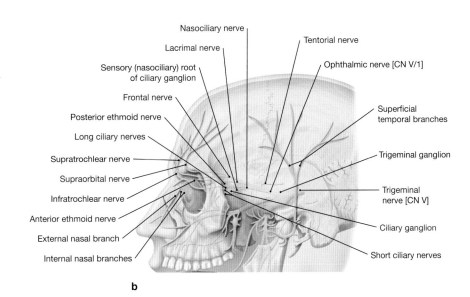

Fig. 12.49a and b Origin of the trigeminal nerve; ventral view **(a); trigeminal nerve, ophthalmic nerve branch [CN V/1], left side;** lateral view **(b).** b [L127]

The ophthalmic nerve [CN V/1] innervates the eye (including cornea and conjunctiva), the skin of the upper eyelid, forehead, back of the nose, the nasal and paranasal mucosa. Parasympathetic fibers innervate the lacrimal gland and associate with the peripheral course of the ophthalmic nerve [CN V/1].

Branches of the Ophthalmic Nerve [CN V/1]
They are exclusively somatic afferent; GSA.

Main Branch	Minor Branches	Innervation Area
Recurrent meningeal branch [tentorial branch]		Parts of the meninges
Frontal nerve	Supraorbital nerve	Skin of the forehead and mucosa of the frontal sinus
	Supratrochlear nerve	Skin and conjunctiva at the nasal corner of the eye
Lacrimal nerve		Lacrimal gland (postganglionic parasympathetic fibers from the zygomatic nerve for secretory innervation associate with the lacrimal nerve), skin and connective tissue of the nasal corner of the eye
Nasociliary nerve	(see below)	Nasal sinuses, anterior part of the nasal cavity and iris, ciliary body, cornea of the eye

Branches of the Nasociliary Nerve (derived from CN V/1)

Branch	Course/Function	Innervation Area
Sensory root of ciliary ganglion [communicating branch with ciliary ganglion]	Contributes the sensory component for the ciliary ganglion which generates the short ciliary nerves	Eyeball and conjunctiva (together with the long ciliary nerves)
Long ciliary nerves	Associate with the optic nerve and course with the short ciliary nerves from the ciliary ganglion to the eyeball; they also contain sympathetic fibers from the carotid plexus	Eyeball and conjunctiva; the sympathetic fibers innervate the dilator pupillae
Posterior ethmoid nerve	Passes through the identically named foramen to reach the posterior ethmoid cells and the sphenoid sinus	Mucosa of the posterior ethmoid cells and the sphenoid sinus
Anterior ethmoid nerve	Passes through the identically named foramen back into the anterior cranial fossa, courses through the cribriform plate into the nasal cavity; ends with external nasal branches in the skin of the dorsum of the nose	Mucosa of the anterior nasal cavity and the anterior ethmoid cells, skin of the dorsum of the nose
Infratrochlear nerve	Courses to the nasal corner of the eye inferior to the trochlea	Skin of the nasal corner of the eye

Structure/Function

The involuntary **corneal or blink reflex** instantly occurs upon stimulation of corneal receptors (e.g., by foreign objects or forced airflow) to protect the eye from injury. The blink reflex is consensual and usually affects both eyes. Other physical stimuli triggering a blink reflex include exposure to bright light (optical reflex) and sudden loud sounds (accustic reflex). The two limbs of the corneal/blink reflex include:

- *Sensory limb:* Nasociliary branch of [CN V/1] → pons in brainstem
- *Motor limb:* temporal and zygomatic branches of facial nerve [CN VII] → orbicularis oculi

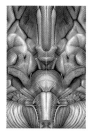

a

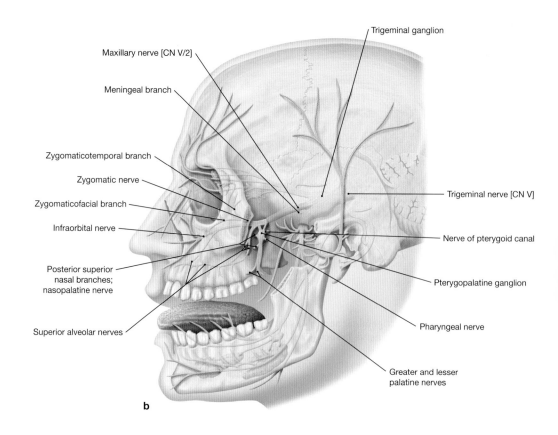

b

Fig. 12.50a and b Origin of the trigeminal nerve [V], ventral view **(a); trigeminal nerve, maxillary nerve [CN V/2], left side;** lateral view **(b).** b [L127]

The maxillary nerve [CN V/2] innervates the skin of the anterior temporal region and the upper cheek as well as the skin below the eye. This nerve also provides sensory fibers to the palate, the teeth of the upper jaw, the gingiva, and the mucosa of the maxillary sinus.

Branches of the Maxillary Nerve [CN V/2]
They are exclusively somatic afferent; GSA.

Main Branch	Minor Branches	Innervation Area
Meningeal branch		Parts of the meninges
Zygomatic nerve	Zygomaticofacial branch	Skin of the temporal region
	Zygomaticotemporal branch	Skin of the upper cheek region; for the secretory innervation of the lacrimal gland, postganglionic parasympathetic fibers associate with the zygomatic nerve which contributes to the lacrimal nerve
Ganglionic branches to pterygopalatine ganglion	(see below)	Contribute sensory fibers for the pterygopalatine ganglion, innervation of palate and nose, sympathetic and parasympathetic fibers for the nasal and palatine glands (specific visceral efferent) and taste fibers
Infraorbital nerve	Superior alveolar nerves with posterior, medial and anterior branches	Mucosa of the maxillary sinus, teeth and gingiva of the upper jaw Skin and conjunctiva of the lower eyelid, lateral skin area of the nasal wings, skin of upper lip and lateral cheek region between lower eyelid and upper lip

Branches to the Pterygopalatine Ganglion (from CN V/2)

Branch	Course	Innervation Area
Greater palatine nerve	Passes across the greater palatine canal and through the greater palatine foramen	Mucosa of the hard palate, palatine glands, palatine taste buds
Lesser palatine nerve	Exit the greater palatine canal through the lesser palatine foramina	Mucosa of the soft palate, palatine tonsil and glands, palatine taste buds
Posterior superior lateral and medial branches of maxillary nerve	Pass through the sphenopalatine foramen into the nasal cavity and branch off the nasopalatine nerve which reaches the hard palate through the incisive canal	Mucosa of the nasal conchae and nasal septum, mucosa of the anterior part of the hard palate, upper incisors and gingiva, nasal glands

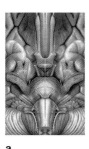

a

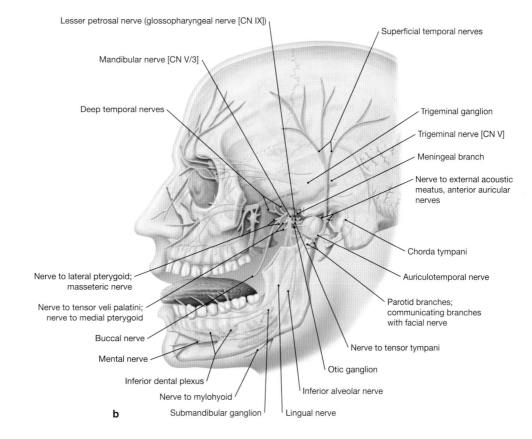

Lesser petrosal nerve (glossopharyngeal nerve [CN IX])

Superficial temporal nerves

Mandibular nerve [CN V/3]

Deep temporal nerves

Trigeminal ganglion

Trigeminal nerve [CN V]

Meningeal branch

Nerve to external acoustic meatus, anterior auricular nerves

Chorda tympani

Auriculotemporal nerve

Nerve to lateral pterygoid; masseteric nerve

Nerve to tensor veli palatini; nerve to medial pterygoid

Buccal nerve

Mental nerve

Inferior dental plexus

Nerve to mylohyoid

Submandibular ganglion

Parotid branches; communicating branches with facial nerve

Nerve to tensor tympani

Otic ganglion

Inferior alveolar nerve

Lingual nerve

b

Fig. 12.51a und b Origin of the trigeminal nerve [V]; ventral view **(a); trigeminal nerve, mandibular nerve branch [CN V/3], left side;** lateral view **(b).** b [L127]

The mandibular nerve [CN V/3] is the only trigeminal branch with motor fibers. It also contributes sensory fibers to the skin of the posterior temporal region, the cheek, and the chin, and innervates the teeth and gingiva of the lower jaw. Fibers with different quali-

ties from the facial nerve [CN VII] associate with branches of the mandibular nerve [CN V/3] to reach their targets. This includes parasympathetic fibers for the innervation of the large salivary glands (except parotid gland ⤳ see CN IX) as well as taste fibers for the tongue and sensory fibers for the anterior two-thirds of the tongue (see also ➤ Fig. 12.55).

Branches of the Mandibular Nerve [CN V/3] (somatic afferent and visceral efferent)		
Main Branch	**Minor Branches**	**Innervation Area**
Meningeal branch		Parts of the meninges
Masseteric nerve		Masseter muscle
Deep temporal nerves		Temporalis muscle
Nerve to lateral pterygoid		Lateral pterygoid muscle
Nerve to medial pterygoid		Medial pterygoid muscle
Nerve to tensor veli palatini		Tensor veli palatini muscle
Nerve to tensor tympani		Tensor tympani muscle
Buccal nerve		Mucosa of the cheek and gingiva of the lower jaw
Auriculotemporal nerve	Parotid branches	Associate with postganglionic parasympathetic fibers from the otic ganglion
	Communicating branches with facial nerve	Associate with postganglionic parasympathetic fibers from the otic ganglion
	Nerve to external acoustic meatus	External acoustic meatus, tympanic membrane
	Anterior auricular nerves	Skin anterior to the auricle
	Superficial temporal nerves	Skin of the posterior temporal region
Lingual nerve	Branches of lingual nerve to isthmus of fauces	Mucosa of the soft palate
	Sublingual nerve	Mucosa of the floor of mouth and sensory innervation of the anterior two-thirds of the tongue
Inferior alveolar nerve		Teeth and gingiva of the lower jaw
	Nerve to mylohyoid	Mylohyoid muscle and anterior belly of digastric muscle
	Mental nerve	Skin of the chin

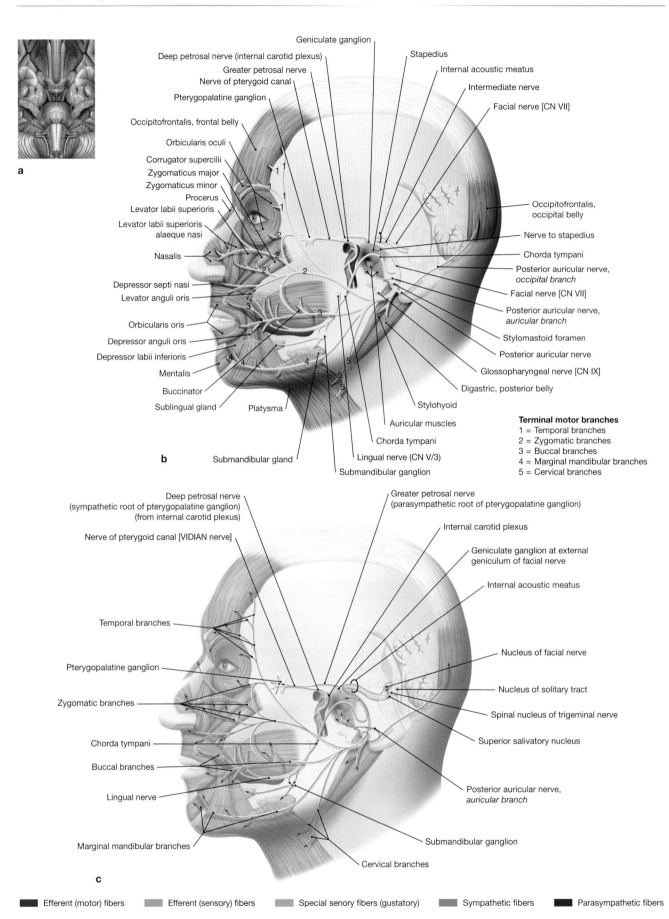

Geniculate ganglion
Deep petrosal nerve (internal carotid plexus)
Greater petrosal nerve
Nerve of pterygoid canal
Pterygopalatine ganglion
Occipitofrontalis, frontal belly
Orbicularis oculi
Corrugator supercilii
Zygomaticus major
Zygomaticus minor
Procerus
Levator labii superioris
Levator labii superioris alaeque nasi
Nasalis
Depressor septi nasi
Levator anguli oris
Orbicularis oris
Depressor anguli oris
Depressor labii inferioris
Mentalis
Buccinator
Sublingual gland
Platysma
Submandibular gland

Stapedius
Internal acoustic meatus
Intermediate nerve
Facial nerve [CN VII]
Occipitofrontalis, occipital belly
Nerve to stapedius
Chorda tympani
Posterior auricular nerve, occipital branch
Facial nerve [CN VII]
Posterior auricular nerve, auricular branch
Stylomastoid foramen
Posterior auricular nerve
Glossopharyngeal nerve [CN IX]
Digastric, posterior belly
Stylohyoid
Auricular muscles
Chorda tympani
Lingual nerve (CN V/3)
Submandibular ganglion

b

Terminal motor branches
1 = Temporal branches
2 = Zygomatic branches
3 = Buccal branches
4 = Marginal mandibular branches
5 = Cervical branches

Deep petrosal nerve (sympathetic root of pterygopalatine ganglion) (from internal carotid plexus)
Nerve of pterygoid canal [VIDIAN nerve]
Temporal branches
Pterygopalatine ganglion
Zygomatic branches
Chorda tympani
Buccal branches
Lingual nerve
Marginal mandibular branches

Greater petrosal nerve (parasympathetic root of pterygopalatine ganglion)
Internal carotid plexus
Geniculate ganglion at external geniculum of facial nerve
Internal acoustic meatus
Nucleus of facial nerve
Nucleus of solitary tract
Spinal nucleus of trigeminal nerve
Superior salivatory nucleus
Posterior auricular nerve, auricular branch
Submandibular ganglion
Cervical branches

c

■ Efferent (motor) fibers　　■ Efferent (sensory) fibers　　■ Special senory fibers (gustatory)　　■ Sympathetic fibers　　■ Parasympathetic fibers

Fig. 12.52a to c Origin of the facial nerve; ventral view **(a)**; **facial nerve [CN VII], left side;** lateral view (**b** and **c**). b, c [L127]
The facial nerve [CN VII] is the nerve of the second pharyngeal arch. The intermediate nerve (a part of CN VII), the facial nerve [CN VII], and the vestibulocochlear nerve [CN VIII] jointly exit at the cerebellopontine angle; then, intermediate nerve and facial nerve [CN VII] unite. [CN VII and CN VIII] enter the petrous part of temporal bone

through the internal acoustic meatus. The facial nerve [CN VII] enters the facial canal where it makes a posterior inferior turn in an almost right angle *(external geniculum of facial nerve)*. Upon exiting the cranial base through the stylomastoid foramen, [CN VII] turns rostral and enters the parotid gland where [CN VII] divides into its terminal motor branches (intraparotid plexus; ➤ Fig. 8.27 and ➤ Fig. 8.33 and table on p. 592).

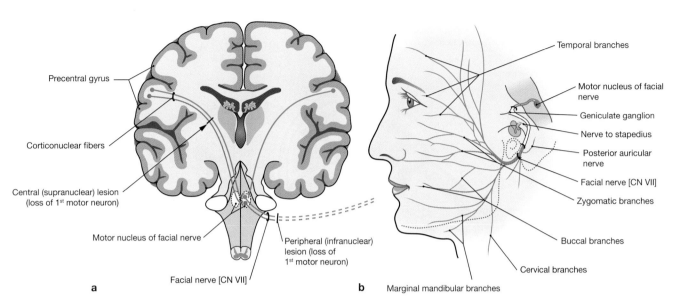

Fig. 12.53a and b Corticonuclear connections and peripheral course of the facial nerve [CN VII]. [L126]
On the left side **(a)**, the central connections to the motor nucleus of facial nerve are shown schematically. The corticonuclear tracts to the upper part of the nucleus (for temporal branches; green) derive from **both** hemispheres. The lower part of the nucleus (for the zygo-

matic, buccal, marginal mandibular, and cervical branches) connects exclusively with the **contralateral** hemisphere (red).
On the right side **(b)**, the peripheral efferent fibers derived from the upper and lower parts of the motor nucleus of facial nerve are shown.

Clinical Remarks

Central facial palsy (also named lower facial palsy) is caused by a supranuclear lesion (lesion of the corticonuclear fibers, e.g. through infarction in the internal capsule). In contrast to an infranuclear lesion and due to the bilateral innervation of the mimic muscles of the eye and forehead, only the lower contralateral part of the face displays motor defects (➤ Fig. 12.53a). An infranuclear lesion (inferior to the motor nucleus of facial nerve), e.g. caused by a malignant parotid tumor, results in the paralysis of **all** motor branches of the facial nerve [CN VII] on the affected side *(peripheral facial palsy)*.
An acoustic neuroma derives from SCHWANN's cells of the vestibulocochlear [CN VIII] or facial nerves [CN VII]. This benign tumor will slowly displace and damage both nerves causing a peripheral facial palsy. The diagnosis is concluded by MRI or CT imaging.

An example of a right-sided **peripheral facial palsy** or **BELL's palsy** is shown below.
a Admission status of the patient: skin folds on the right side of the face have disappeared.
b When asked to raise the eyebrows: only the left side of the patient's forehead displays wrinkles (paralysis of the right occipitofrontalis). This is evidence for a peripheral facial palsy.
c Patient is asked to shut both eyes: this is not accomplished on the side of the damaged facial nerve *(lagophthalmos)*. When the eyelids are closed, the eyeball automatically turns upwards and the white sclera of the eye becomes visible on the side of facial palsy *(BELL's phenomenon)*.
d Patient is asked to wrinkle his nose: this is impossible on the right side of the face.
e Patient is asked to whistle: no tone is produced but air escapes through the lips on the paralyzed side.
[T620]

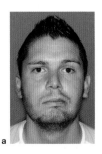
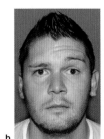
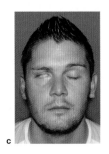
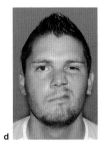
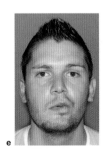

12

Neuroanatomy

Facial Nerve [CN VII]

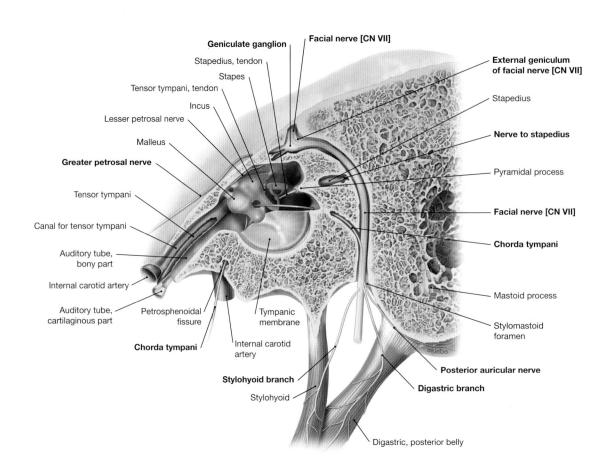

Fig. 12.54 Course of the facial nerve [CN VII]; vertical section through the facial canal; view from the left side. [L238]
Approximately 1cm (0.4 in) after the facial nerve [CN VII] enters the petrous part of temporal bone through the internal acoustic opening (not shown), it forms the external geniculum of facial nerve. The geniculate ganglion is located just before this bend of [CN VII].

The facial nerve [CN VII] runs within a bony canal and exits at the stylomastoid foramen. Along its way through the petrous part of temporal bone, [CN VII] releases the greater petrosal nerve, the nerve to stapedius, and the chorda tympani (from rostral to caudal).

Branches of the Facial Nerve [CN VII]		
Branch	**Course**	**Innervation Area**
Greater petrosal nerve [Parasympathic pterygopalatine root]	Exits at the external geniculum of facial nerve [CN VII] and courses through the canal of greater petrosal nerve into the middle cranial fossa; passes through the foramen lacerum to enter the pterygoid canal. Here, it forms the nerve of pterygoid canal together with the sympathetic deep petrosal nerve before projecting to the pterygopalatine ganglion, where the preganglionic parasympathetic fibers synapse.	GVE (via branches of the maxillary nerve [CN V/2]): lacrimal, nasal, palatine, pharyngeal glands SVA (via branches of the mandibular nerve [CN V/3]): taste buds of the palate
Nerve to stapedius	Exits in the lower part of the facial canal	SVE: stapedius muscle
Chorda tympani	Shortly before the distal end of the facial canal, it engages in a retrograde course through its own bony canal into the tympanic cavity which it traverses freely between the handle of malleus and the long limb of the incus behind the tympanic membrane; after passing through the petrotympanic fissure, it associates with the lingual nerve (from CN V/3)	GVE (via the lingual nerve, synapsing in the submandibular ganglion): submandibular and sublingual glands SVA (via the lingual nerve): anterior two-thirds of the tongue
Posterior auricular nerve	Branches off shortly after exiting the facial canal	SVE: occipitofrontalis, muscles of the outer ear
Digastric branch and stylohyoid branch	Small branches to the muscles	SVE: posterior belly of digastric muscle and stylohyoid muscle
Intraparotid plexus	Branches with motor fibers to the mimic muscles divide the parotid gland into a temporofacial part and a cervicofacial part; these motor branches subdivide into five terminal branches: temporal branches, zygomatic branches, buccal branches, marginal mandibular branches, cervical branches	SVE: facial (mimic) muscles, including buccinator and platysma

592

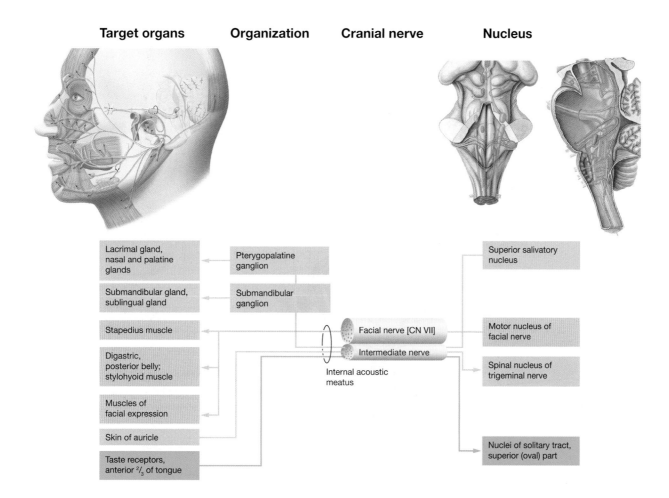

Target organs	**Organization**	**Cranial nerve**	**Nucleus**

Fig. 12.55 Fiber qualities of the facial nerve [VII], left side; lateral view. Yellow: parasympathetic fibers, purple: motor fibres, blue: sensory fibers, green: taste fibers. [L127]

The facial nerve [CN VII] has several fiber qualities. **Motor fibers** from its motor nucleus course around the nucleus of abducens nerve in a posterior arch (*internal geniculum of facial nerve*).

Preganglionic **parasympathetic fibers** from the superior salivatory nucleus run with the intermediate nerve, reach the pterygopalatine ganglion via the greater petrosal nerve or course with the chorda tympani to the submandibular ganglion via the lingual nerve (from CN V/3) where they synapse with postganglionic neurons. The postganglionic fibers project into the lacrimal, nasal, palatine (pterygopalatine ganglion) and sublingual and submandibular glands (submandibular ganglion).

Taste fibers for the anterior two-thirds of the tongue project into the superior part of the nuclei of solitary tract. These fibers reach the facial nerve [CN VII] via the lingual nerve and chorda tympani before entering the brainstem.

Sensory fibers innervate the posterior wall of the external acoustic meatus, an area behind the ear, the auricle, and the tympanic membrane. The perikarya of the sensory and taste fibers locate in the geniculate ganglion and the fibers reach the spinal nucleus of trigeminal nerve via the intermediate nerve, as a part of [CN VII].

Clinical Remarks

The close topographical relationship between the facial canal and the tympanic cavity puts the facial nerve [CN VII] at risk during petrous bone fractures, middle ear/mastoid infections, and surgical interventions involving the middle/inner ear. **Lesions** located close to or anterior to the **geniculate ganglion** result in paralysis of all mimic muscles and the stapedius muscle (*hyperacusis*), gustatory impairment, diminished tear production and reduced nasal and salivary secretion. A **lesion** located below the branching point of the **nerve to stapedius** causes paralysis of the mimic muscles and affects the chorda tympani fibers for taste and glandular secretion. Isolated injury to the chorda tympani occurs during middle ear infections or middle/inner ear surgery as the chorda tympani courses unprotected between malleus and incus in the tympanic cavity of the middle ear. The biggest problem of patients with peripheral facial palsy is *lagophthalmos*. Due to paralysis of the orbicularis oculi, the eye cannot be closed properly. This causes the cornea to dry out due to lack of blinking and reduced production of lacrimal fluid. This can lead to visual impairment or even blindness if left untreated.

Site of Lesion	Topodiagnostic Procedure	Examples for Cause of Lesion
Inferior to the nuclear area within the brainstem	MRI, CT, SCHIRMER's test (functional test for the lacrimal gland)	Acoustic neuroma
After greater petrosal nerve has branched off	Stapedius reflex test	Otitis media (middle ear infection)
After chorda tympani has branched off	Gustometry (testing taste perception)	Otitis media (middle ear infection)
After passing through the stylomastoid foramen	Testing facial motor functions	Malignant parotid tumor

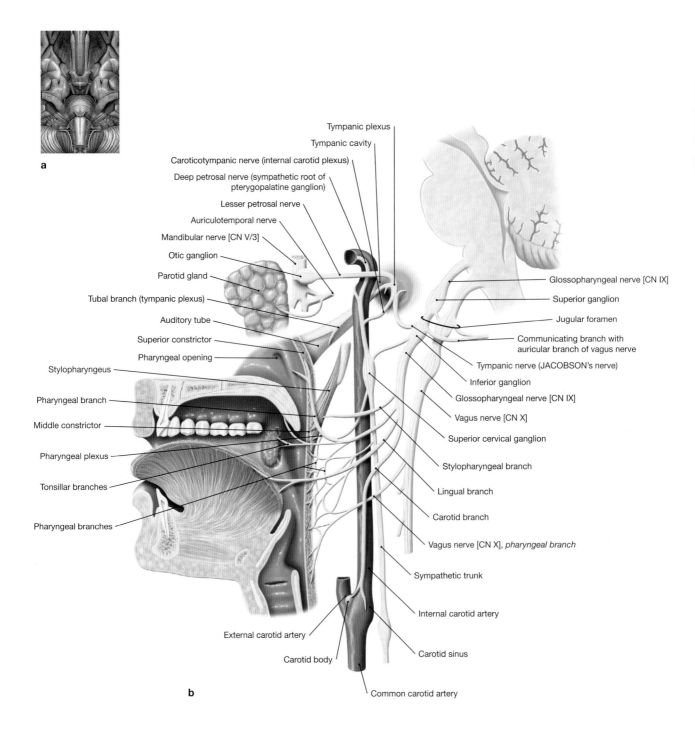

a

b

Tympanic plexus

Tympanic cavity

Caroticotympanic nerve (internal carotid plexus)

Deep petrosal nerve (sympathetic root of pterygopalatine ganglion)

Lesser petrosal nerve

Auriculotemporal nerve

Mandibular nerve [CN V/3]

Otic ganglion

Parotid gland

Tubal branch (tympanic plexus)

Auditory tube

Superior constrictor

Pharyngeal opening

Stylopharyngeus

Pharyngeal branch

Middle constrictor

Pharyngeal plexus

Tonsillar branches

Pharyngeal branches

External carotid artery

Carotid body

Common carotid artery

Glossopharyngeal nerve [CN IX]

Superior ganglion

Jugular foramen

Communicating branch with auricular branch of vagus nerve

Tympanic nerve (JACOBSON's nerve)

Inferior ganglion

Glossopharyngeal nerve [CN IX]

Vagus nerve [CN X]

Superior cervical ganglion

Stylopharyngeal branch

Lingual branch

Carotid branch

Vagus nerve [CN X], *pharyngeal branch*

Sympathetic trunk

Internal carotid artery

Carotid sinus

Fig. 12.56a and b Origin of the glossopharyngeal nerve [CN IX]; ventral view **(a); left side;** lateral view **(b).** b [L127]

The glossopharyngeal nerve [CN IX], the vagus nerve [CN X], and the spinal accessory nerve [CN XI] exit the brainstem in the retroolivary sulcus and pass through the jugular foramen at the cranial base. Located within the jugular foramen lies the smaller of two ganglia of [CN IX], the superior ganglion, followed immediately caudally by the inferior ganglion.

After exiting the skull, [CN IX] courses between internal jugular vein and internal carotid artery, then arches forward and passes in between the stylopharyngeus and styloglossus muscles to enter the root of tongue.

The glossopharyngeal nerve [CN IX] carries efferent, afferent, parasympathetic, and special sensory (gustatory) fiber qualities; ➤ Fig. 12.57.

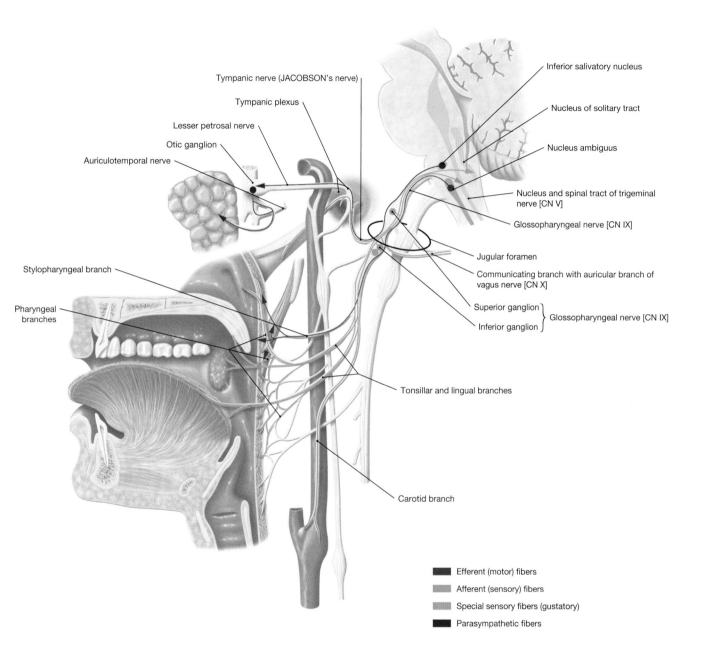

Fig. 12.57 Origin and fiber qualities of the glossopharyngeal nerve [CN IX]; ventral view. [L127]

The glossopharyngeal nerve [CN IX] provides different fiber qualities:

- **Motor efferents** project to the stylopharyngeus and pharyngeal branches innervate the superior constrictor, palatoglossus, and palatopharyngeus muscles.
- **Parasympathetic efferents** from the inferior salivary nucleus project as tympanic nerve into the tympanic cavity to form an intramucosal tympanic plexus. From this plexus generates the lesser petrosal nerve which exits the tympanic cavity through the foramen lacerum. Preganglionic parasympathetic fibers within the **lesser petrosal nerve** synapse in the otic ganglion. Post-ganglionic fibers exit the ganglion and form the JACOB-

SON's anastomosis by temporarily associating with the auriculotemporal nerve (from CN V/3) and facial nerve [CN VII] to provide parasympathetic innervation to the parotid gland.
- **Sensory afferent fibers** distribute within the pharyngeal mucosa and posterior third of the tongue. Together with the vagus nerve [CN X], sensory afferents from [CN IX] contribute to the pharyngeal plexus. **Tonsillar branches** from [CN IX] supply sensory fibers to the palatine tonsil and the mucosa of the isthmus of fauces. The **lingual branches** of [CN IX] provides sensory/gustatory (taste) fibers for the posterior third of the tongue. A **branch to the carotid sinus** transmits sensory input from mechano- and chemoreceptors at the carotid sinus and carotid body to the brainstem.

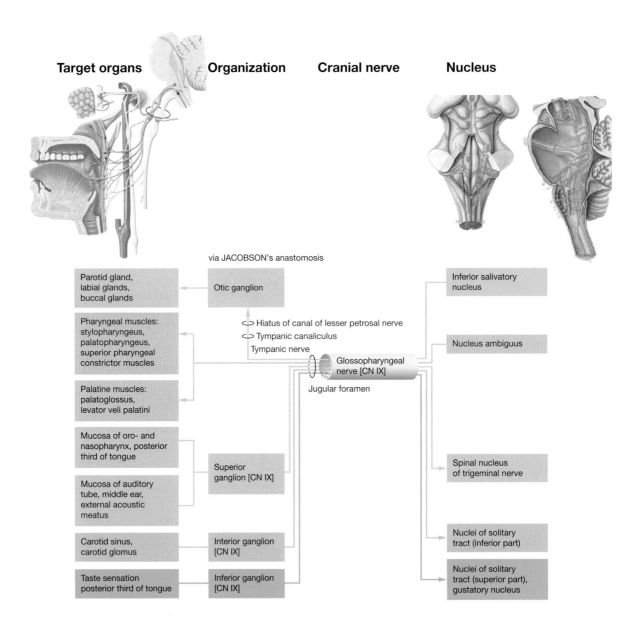

Target organs   Organization   Cranial nerve   Nucleus

via JACOBSON's anastomosis

Parotid gland, labial glands, buccal glands

Otic ganglion

Inferior salivatory nucleus

Hiatus of canal of lesser petrosal nerve
Tympanic canaliculus
Tympanic nerve

Pharyngeal muscles: stylopharyngeus, palatopharyngeus, superior pharyngeal constrictor muscles

Nucleus ambiguus

Palatine muscles: palatoglossus, levator veli palatini

Glossopharyngeal nerve [CN IX]

Jugular foramen

Mucosa of oro- and nasopharynx, posterior third of tongue

Superior ganglion [CN IX]

Spinal nucleus of trigeminal nerve

Mucosa of auditory tube, middle ear, external acoustic meatus

Carotid sinus, carotid glomus

Interior ganglion [CN IX]

Nuclei of solitary tract (inferior part)

Taste sensation posterior third of tongue

Inferior ganglion [CN IX]

Nuclei of solitary tract (superior part), gustatory nucleus

Fig. 12.58 Schematic representation of fiber qualities of the glossopharyngeal nerve [CN IX], left side; lateral view. Yellow: para- sympathetic fibers, purple: motor fibers, blue: mucosal sensory fibers, light green: visceral sensory fibers, green: taste fibers. [L127]

Structure/Function

The pharyngeal or gag reflex is activated by touch to the back of the mouth and throat and helps prevent choking.
Components of the **pharyngeal (gag) reflex:**

Sensory limb: predominantly glossopharyngeal nerve [CN IX], but also contributions from [CN V] ⟶ brainstem.
Motor limb: Vagus nerve [CN X] ⟶ soft palate and pharyngeal constrictor muscles.

Clinical Remarks

Lesions of the glossopharyngeal nerve [CN IX] can result in:
- swallowing difficulties (paralysis of the superior constrictor, failure to form the PASSAVANT's ridge),
- a deviation of the uvula to the healthy side (paralysis of the levator veli palatini, palatoglossus, palatopharyngeus, uvular muscles),
- an impaired sensibility of the pharyngeal region (lack of gag reflex),

- a lack of taste sensation at the posterior third of the tongue,
- dysfunctional secretion by the parotid gland.

Damage to the glossopharyngeal nerve [CN IX] is not an isolated event. Frequently, fractures, aneurysms, tumors, or thrombosis of cerebral blood vessels supplying the brain region around the jugular foramen also affect the vagus nerve [CN X] and the spinal accessory nerve [CN XI].

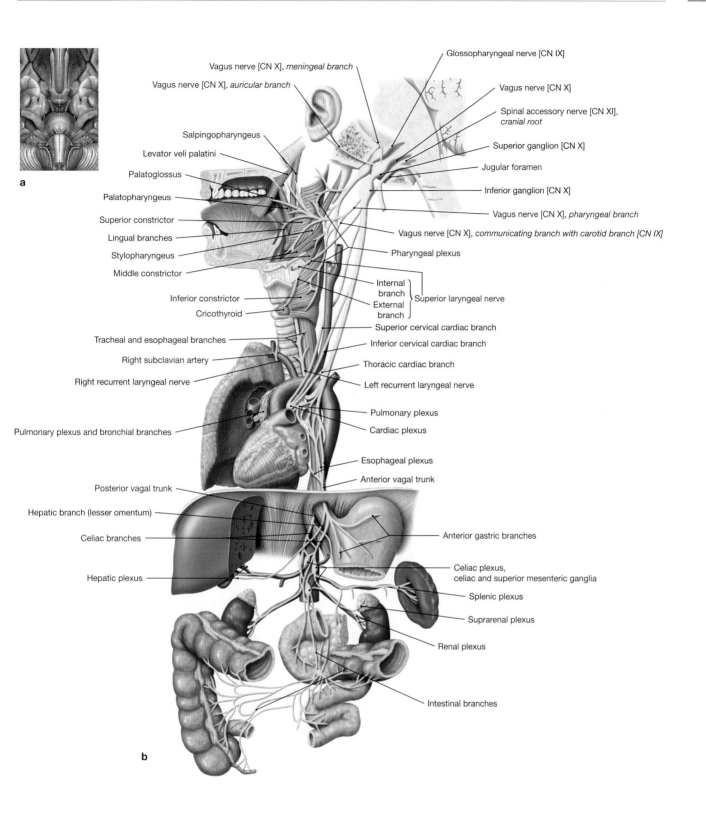

a

Glossopharyngeal nerve [CN IX]

Vagus nerve [CN X], *meningeal branch*

Vagus nerve [CN X], *auricular branch*

Vagus nerve [CN X]

Spinal accessory nerve [CN XI], *cranial root*

Salpingopharyngeus

Superior ganglion [CN X]

Levator veli palatini

Jugular foramen

Palatoglossus

Inferior ganglion [CN X]

Palatopharyngeus

Vagus nerve [CN X], *pharyngeal branch*

Superior constrictor

Vagus nerve [CN X], *communicating branch with carotid branch [CN IX]*

Lingual branches

Stylopharyngeus

Pharyngeal plexus

Middle constrictor

Internal branch

Superior laryngeal nerve

External branch

Inferior constrictor

Cricothyroid

Superior cervical cardiac branch

Inferior cervical cardiac branch

Tracheal and esophageal branches

Thoracic cardiac branch

Right subclavian artery

Left recurrent laryngeal nerve

Right recurrent laryngeal nerve

Pulmonary plexus

Cardiac plexus

Pulmonary plexus and bronchial branches

Esophageal plexus

Anterior vagal trunk

Posterior vagal trunk

Hepatic branch (lesser omentum)

Anterior gastric branches

Celiac branches

Celiac plexus, celiac and superior mesenteric ganglia

Splenic plexus

Hepatic plexus

Suprarenal plexus

Renal plexus

Intestinal branches

b

Fig. 12.59a and b Origin of the vagus nerve [CN X]; ventral view **(a)**; schematic median section in the region of the head **(b)**. b [L127]

Vagus Nerve [CN X], Parasympathetic Nuclei and Target Organs			
Cranial Nerve	**1st Neuron**	**2nd Neuron**	**Target Organ**
Vagus nerve [CN X]	Nucleus ambiguus	Cardiac plexus	Heart
	Dorsal (posterior) nucleus of vagus nerve	Organ-specific plexus, intramural ganglia	Pharynx, larynx, lungs, spleen, pancreas, liver, kidneys, blood vessels, GI-tract

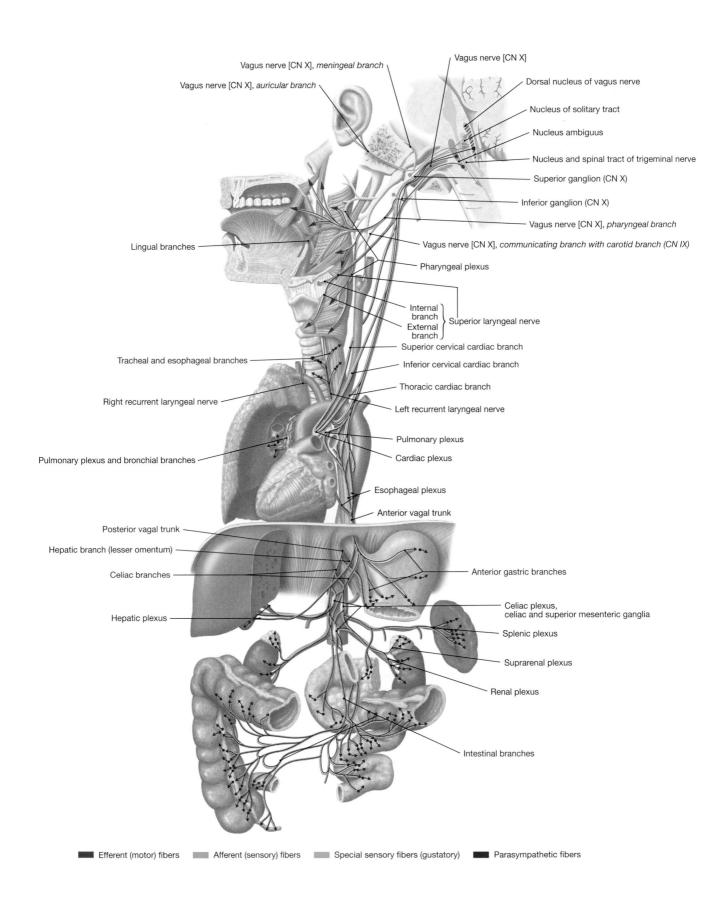

Vagus nerve [CN X], *meningeal branch*

Vagus nerve [CN X], *auricular branch*

Vagus nerve [CN X]

Dorsal nucleus of vagus nerve

Nucleus of solitary tract

Nucleus ambiguus

Nucleus and spinal tract of trigeminal nerve

Superior ganglion (CN X)

Inferior ganglion (CN X)

Vagus nerve [CN X], *pharyngeal branch*

Lingual branches

Vagus nerve [CN X], *communicating branch with carotid branch (CN IX)*

Pharyngeal plexus

Internal branch
External branch
} Superior laryngeal nerve

Superior cervical cardiac branch

Inferior cervical cardiac branch

Tracheal and esophageal branches

Thoracic cardiac branch

Right recurrent laryngeal nerve

Left recurrent laryngeal nerve

Pulmonary plexus

Cardiac plexus

Pulmonary plexus and bronchial branches

Esophageal plexus

Anterior vagal trunk

Posterior vagal trunk

Hepatic branch (lesser omentum)

Celiac branches

Anterior gastric branches

Celiac plexus, celiac and superior mesenteric ganglia

Splenic plexus

Hepatic plexus

Suprarenal plexus

Renal plexus

Intestinal branches

■ Efferent (motor) fibers ■ Afferent (sensory) fibers ■ Special sensory fibers (gustatory) ■ Parasympathetic fibers

Fig. 12.60 Origin of the vagus nerve [CN X], schematic median section in the region of the head. [L127]
Different nuclei in the brainstem contributing to the vagus nerve fiber qualities and parasympathetic ganglia (purple dots) where vagal preganglionic parasympathetic fibers synapse onto postganglionic fibers.

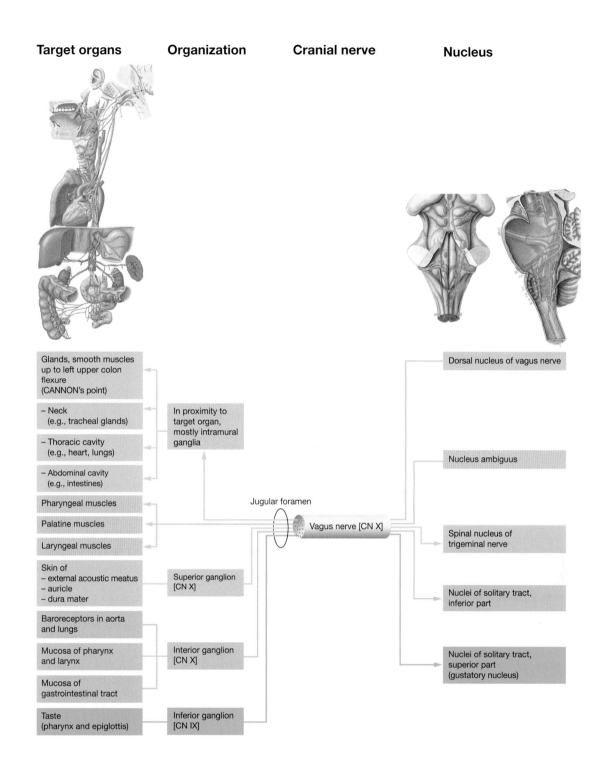

Target organs   **Organization**   **Cranial nerve**   **Nucleus**

Glands, smooth muscles up to left upper colon flexure (CANNON's point)

– Neck (e.g., tracheal glands)

– Thoracic cavity (e.g., heart, lungs)

– Abdominal cavity (e.g., intestines)

In proximity to target organ, mostly intramural ganglia

Pharyngeal muscles

Palatine muscles

Laryngeal muscles

Skin of
– external acoustic meatus
– auricle
– dura mater

Superior ganglion [CN X]

Baroreceptors in aorta and lungs

Mucosa of pharynx and larynx

Interior ganglion [CN X]

Mucosa of gastrointestinal tract

Taste (pharynx and epiglottis)

Inferior ganglion [CN IX]

Jugular foramen

Vagus nerve [CN X]

Dorsal nucleus of vagus nerve

Nucleus ambiguus

Spinal nucleus of trigeminal nerve

Nuclei of solitary tract, inferior part

Nuclei of solitary tract, superior part (gustatory nucleus)

Fig. 12.61 Fiber qualities of the vagus nerve [CN X], left side; lateral view. Yellow: parasympathetic fibers, purple: motor fibers, blue: sensory fibers, light green: visceral sensory fibers, green: gustatory (taste) fibers. [L127]

Clinical Remarks

Complete lesions of the vagus nerve [CN X] mainly occur at the jugular foramen. Frequently, the glossopharyngeal nerve [CN IX] and the spinal accessory nerve [CN XI] are affected as well. Depending on the location of the lesion, the symptoms can include:

* difficulty swallowing,
* deviation of the uvula to the healthy side (damage of the pharyngeal plexus),

* sensory deficits in the pharynx and the epiglottis (lack of gag reflex, gustatory impairment),
* hoarseness (paralysis of laryngeal muscles),
* tachycardia and arrhythmia (innervation of the heart).

The unilateral damage has little effect on autonomic vagal functions. However, bilateral damage of the vagus nerve [CN X] can result in severe respiratory and circulatory problems which can cause the death of a patient.

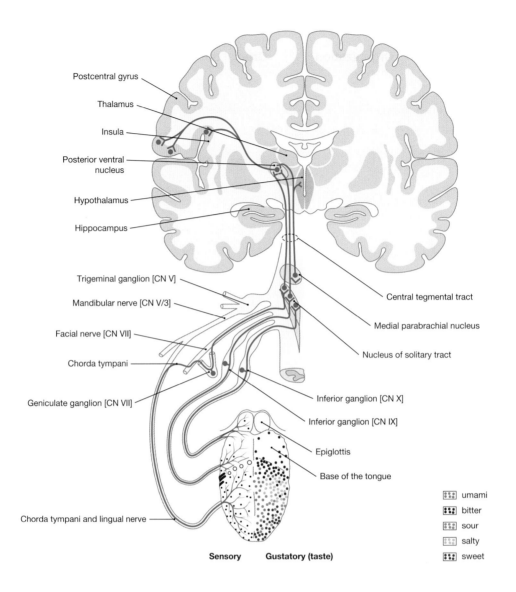

Postcentral gyrus
Thalamus
Insula
Posterior ventral nucleus
Hypothalamus
Hippocampus

Trigeminal ganglion [CN V]
Mandibular nerve [CN V/3]
Facial nerve [CN VII]
Chorda tympani
Geniculate ganglion [CN VII]

Chorda tympani and lingual nerve

Central tegmental tract
Medial parabrachial nucleus
Nucleus of solitary tract

Inferior ganglion [CN X]
Inferior ganglion [CN IX]
Epiglottis
Base of the tongue

Sensory   **Gustatory (taste)**

umami
bitter
sour
salty
sweet

Fig. 12.62 Sensory affects to the tongue: sensory and special sensory (gustatory/taste) systems with central pathways, nuclei and cranial nerves; schematic drawing of this special sensory system of the tongue. [L127]

The facial nerve [CN VII] is responsible for taste perception in the anterior two-thirds of the tongue. Taste fibers from the glossopharyngeal [CN IX] and vagus nerves [CN X] detect mainly bitter taste in the posterior third of the tongue and epiglottis, respectively. The first sensory neuron mediating taste perception of the facial nerve [CN VII] is located in the geniculate ganglion. In [CN IX and CN X], the corresponding sensory inferior ganglia serve a similar function. All taste fibers from [CN VII, CN IX, and CN X] converge onto the central nuclei of the solitary tract which contains the second sensory neurons of the central taste pathway. The lingual nerve is a branch of the mandibular nerve [CN V/3] and contains sensory fibers of the tongue and epiglottis area, respectively.

[CN IX and CN X] contribute sensory afferents to the posterior third of tongue and epiglottis area, respectively.

Structure/Function

A distortion in taste perception is called **dysgeusia** or **parageusia.** This can occur as a complete loss of taste *(ageusia)* or reduced taste sensitivity *(hypogeusia)*. Of all treatments, chemotherapy is a major cause of dysgeusia. This is the result of damage by the chemotherapeutic drug to the taste receptors and supportive cell system. Certain other drugs, head/neck radiation, zinc deficiency, or heavy smoking can also cause dysgeusia. Diseases include the common cold, dry mouth syndrome, inflammation in the mouth, traumatic head injuries, and BELL's palsy.
[L141, R170-4]

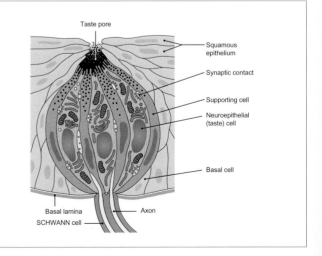

Taste pore
Squamous epithelium
Synaptic contact
Supporting cell
Neuroepithelial (taste) cell
Basal cell
Basal lamina
Axon
SCHWANN cell

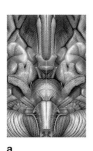

a

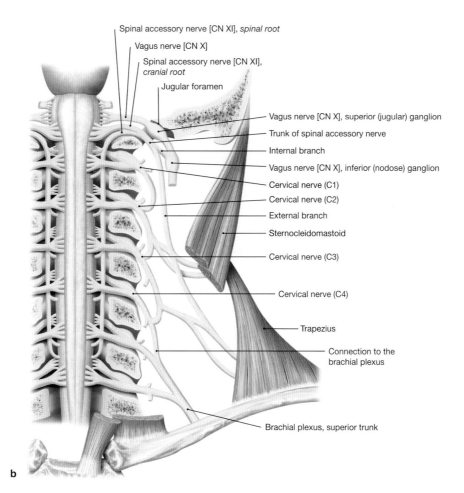

Spinal accessory nerve [CN XI], *spinal root*

Vagus nerve [CN X]

Spinal accessory nerve [CN XI], *cranial root*

Jugular foramen

Vagus nerve [CN X], superior (jugular) ganglion

Trunk of spinal accessory nerve

Internal branch

Vagus nerve [CN X], inferior (nodose) ganglion

Cervical nerve (C1)

Cervical nerve (C2)

External branch

Sternocleidomastoid

Cervical nerve (C3)

Cervical nerve (C4)

Trapezius

Connection to the brachial plexus

Brachial plexus, superior trunk

b

Fig. 12.63a and b Origin of the spinal accessory nerve [CN X]; ventral view **(a);** vertebral canal and skull have been opened **(b).** b [L127]

The spinal accessory nerve [CN XI] has two roots. Its cranial root originates from the nucleus ambiguus in the medulla oblongata. At the level of the jugular foramen, the cranial root joins the spinal root of the spinal accessory nerve [CN XI]. The latter consists of fibers derived from anterior and posterior segmental roots in the cer- vical spinal cord. Fibers of the cranial root form the internal branch which joins the vagus nerve [CN X] inferior to the jugular foramen. The cranial root participates in the innervation of the pharyngeal and laryngeal muscles and, strictly speaking, is not a part of the spinal accessory nerve [CN XI]. The fibers of the spinal root inner- vate both sternocleidomastoid and trapezius muscles (see also ➤ chapter 11 [Neck]). For lesions of [CN XI], see ➤ chapter 3 (Upper extremity).

Target organs   **Skull exit**   **Cranial nerve**   **Nucleus**

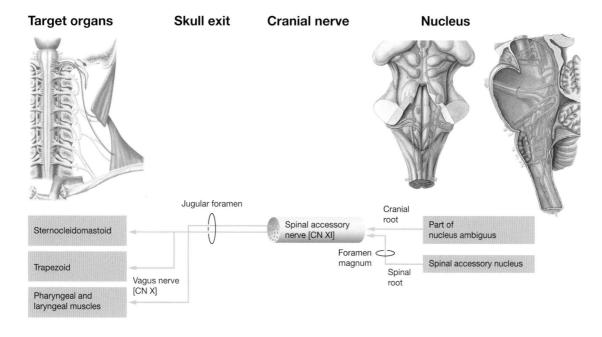

Jugular foramen

Cranial root

Sternocleidomastoid

Spinal accessory nerve [CN XI]

Part of nucleus ambiguus

Foramen magnum

Trapezoid

Spinal accessory nucleus

Vagus nerve [CN X]

Spinal root

Pharyngeal and laryngeal muscles

Fig. 12.64 Motor fibers of the spinal accessory nerve [CN XI]; ven- tral view; the vertebral canal and skull have been opened. [L127]

Purple: motor fibers.

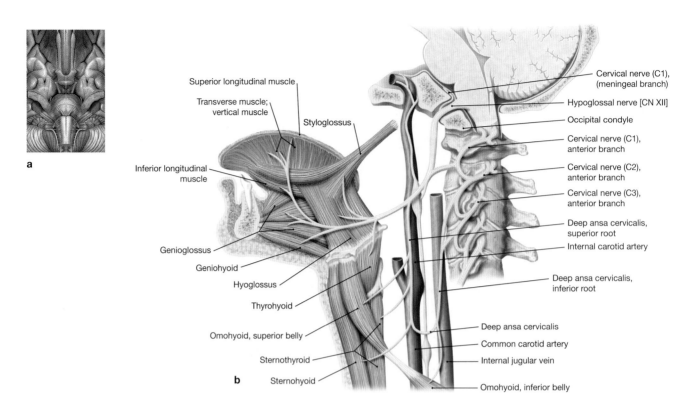

a

Superior longitudinal muscle

Transverse muscle; vertical muscle

Styloglossus

Inferior longitudinal muscle

Genioglossus

Geniohyoid

Hyoglossus

Thyrohyoid

Omohyoid, superior belly

Sternothyroid

b   Sternohyoid

Cervical nerve (C1), (meningeal branch)

Hypoglossal nerve [CN XII]

Occipital condyle

Cervical nerve (C1), anterior branch

Cervical nerve (C2), anterior branch

Cervical nerve (C3), anterior branch

Deep ansa cervicalis, superior root

Internal carotid artery

Deep ansa cervicalis, inferior root

Deep ansa cervicalis

Common carotid artery

Internal jugular vein

Omohyoid, inferior belly

Fig. 12.65a and b Origin of the hypoglossal nerve [CN XII], ventral view **(a);** schematic median section; view from the left side **(b).** b [L127]

The nucleus of hypoglossal nerve in the medulla oblongata provides the fibers for the hypoglossal nerve [CN XII] which exit the brainstem as multiple small bundles between the pyramid and olive in the anterolateral sulcus. The hypoglossal nerve [CN XII] exits the skull through the hypoglossal canal, associates briefly with the spinal nerves C1 and C2 as they form the superior root (limb) of ansa cervicalis. The inferior root created by C2 and C3 completes the ansa cervicalis which innervates most infrahyoid muscles. The hypoglossal nerve [CN XII] courses posterior to the vagus nerve [CN X] and pharynx, turns sharply rostral and medial and crosses the external carotid artery at the branching point of the lingual artery (upper margin of the carotid triangle) to reach the tongue between the hyoglossus and mylohyoid muscles. The hypoglossal nerve [CN XII] innervates all internal muscles of the tongue and the styloglossus, hyoglossus, and genioglossus (see also chapter 8 [Head]).

Target organs	Skull exit	Cranial nerve	Nucleus

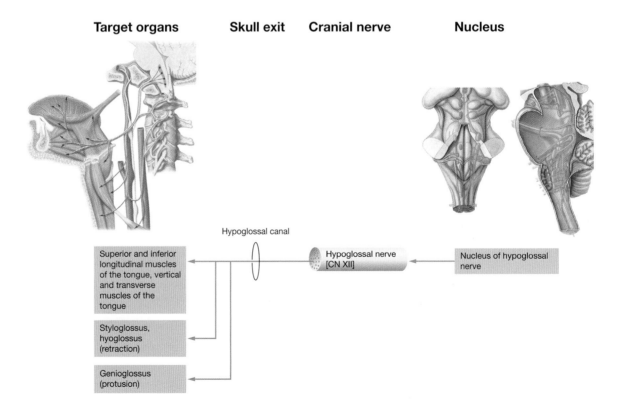

Hypoglossal canal

Superior and inferior longitudinal muscles of the tongue, vertical and transverse muscles of the tongue

Styloglossus, hyoglossus (retraction)

Genioglossus (protusion)

Hypoglossal nerve [CN XII]

Nucleus of hypoglossal nerve

Fig. 12.66 Motor fibers of the hypoglossal nerve [CN XII], schematic median section; view from the left side. [L127]

Purple: motor fibers.

Structure/Function

The autonomic nervous system can be divided into a general visceral efferent part (GVE; motor) and a visceral afferent part (GVA; sensory). The GVE part is divided further into the sympathetic and parasympathetic systems. No such partitioning exists for the viscerosensory system. GVA fibers conduct pain and reflex sensations (e.g., respiratory reflexes) from visceral or-

gans, blood vessels, and glands to the CNS. The corresponding GVA ganglionic cells reside in spinal root ganglia, the inferior ganglion of glossopharyngeal nerve [CN IX] (afferents from carotid body), and the inferior (nodose) ganglion of the vagus nerve [CN X] (afferents from neck, cardiopulmonary, and intestinal systems).

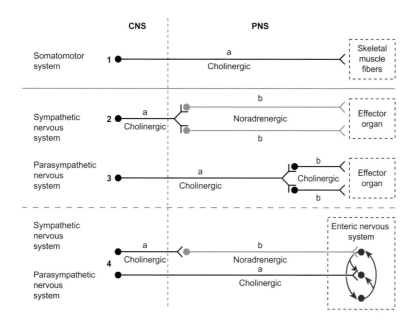

Fig. 12.67 Schematic drawing showing the specific neuronal connections between the central nervous system (CNS), the peripheral nervous system (PNS) and their target organs for the motor, sympathetic, parasympathetic, and enteric systems. [L141]

Exception: Sweat glands are innervated by the sympathetic system. The neurotransmitter of the postganglionic sympathetic fibers to sweat glands is acetylcholine and not norepinephrine!

Clinical Remarks

Excessive sweating is called hyperhidrosis. Local intradermal injection of Botulinum toxin A (Botox) reduces sweating by > approx. 80%. Botox blocks sympathetic cholinergic innerva-

tion of sweat glands. Botox is successfully used to treat axillary hyperhidrosis.

Major Differences between the Sympathetic and Parasympathetic Systems		
Neuron	**Sympathetic System**	**Parasympathetic System**
1st neuron	Short axon	Long axon
	Cholinergic	Cholinergic
	Perikarya located in the lateral column of thoracic and lumbar spinal cord	Perikarya located in parasympathetic nuclei of the brainstem and in sacral spinal cord
2nd neuron	Long axon	Short axon
	(Nor)adrenergic; exception: sweat glands (cholinergic)!	Cholinergic
	Perikarya located in ganglia of sympathetic chain, in prevertebral ganglia, and in ganglia of target organs	Perikarya located in ganglia at target organs and in parasympathetic ganglia of head

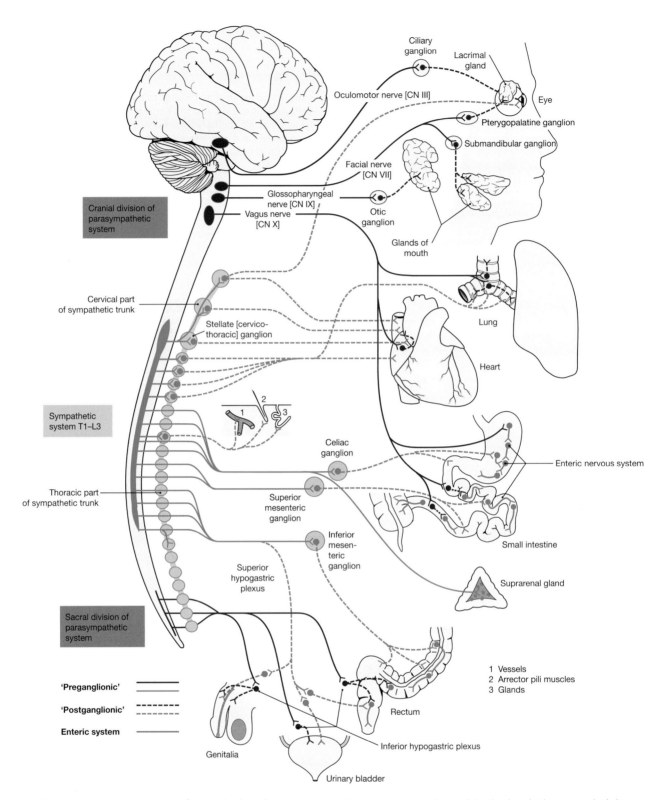

Fig. 12.68 Autonomic nervous system (sympathetic and para-sympathetic parts). [L106, S130-5]

The autonomic nervous system comprises the sympathetic (green), the parasympathetic (purple), and the enteric nervous systems (blue). The neurons of the **sympathetic** system are located in the intermediolateral horn of the thoracolumbar section of the spinal cord. Their axons project to the prevertebral chain of sympathetic ganglia and to ganglia of the enteric system. Here they synapse to postganglionic neurons which project to the target organs. The sympathetic activation serves to mobilize the body under physical and/or emotional stress. The adrenal medulla is part of the sympathetic system and secretes norepinephrine (noradrenaline) and epinephrine (adrenaline) into the bloodstream.

Parasympathetic nuclei are located in the brainstem and the sacral part of the spinal cord. Their axons project to ganglia adjacent

to the target organs located in the head, thorax, and abdomen. These preganglionic fibers synapse onto neurons that form parasympathetic ganglia. Their postganglionic fibers reach the target organs via short axons. The parasympathetic system has important roles in food intake, digestion, sexual arousal, and counteracts the sympathetic system.

The **enteric** nervous system regulates the intestinal activity and is modulated by sympathetic and parasympathetic influences.

Note: *Recent research in the mouse indicates a sympathetic, not parasympathetic, sacral autonomic outflow (Espinosa-Medina I, Saha O, Boismoreau F, Chettouh Z, Rossi F, Richardson WD, Brunet JF. The sacral autonomic outflow is sympathetic. Science 2016; 354: 893–7). Currently, these data have not been confirmed in the human.*

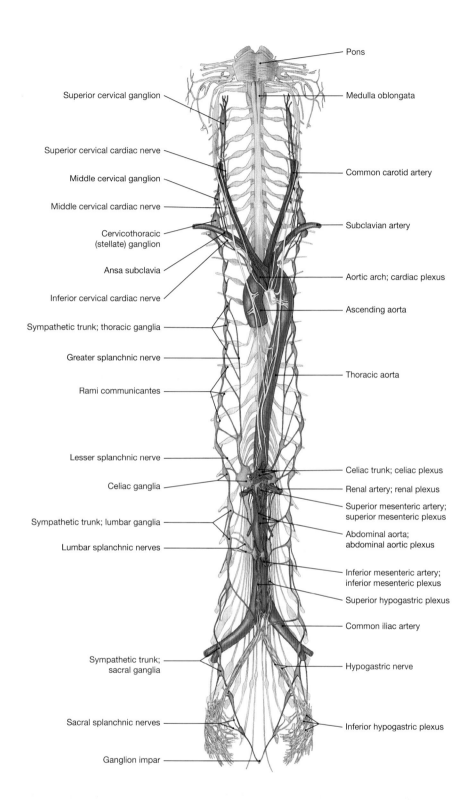

Superior cervical ganglion

Superior cervical cardiac nerve

Middle cervical ganglion

Middle cervical cardiac nerve

Cervicothoracic
(stellate) ganglion

Ansa subclavia

Inferior cervical cardiac nerve

Sympathetic trunk; thoracic ganglia

Greater splanchnic nerve

Rami communicantes

Lesser splanchnic nerve

Celiac ganglia

Sympathetic trunk; lumbar ganglia

Lumbar splanchnic nerves

Sympathetic trunk;
sacral ganglia

Sacral splanchnic nerves

Ganglion impar

Pons

Medulla oblongata

Common carotid artery

Subclavian artery

Aortic arch; cardiac plexus

Ascending aorta

Thoracic aorta

Celiac trunk; celiac plexus

Renal artery; renal plexus

Superior mesenteric artery;
superior mesenteric plexus

Abdominal aorta;
abdominal aortic plexus

Inferior mesenteric artery;
inferior mesenteric plexus

Superior hypogastric plexus

Common iliac artery

Hypogastric nerve

Inferior hypogastric plexus

Fig. 12.69 Schematic drawing of the sympathetic nervous system and its topographic relationship with the spinal cord and major arterial blood vessels. Sympathetic axons of the 1st neuron exit the spinal cord together with the spinal nerves and synapse with the 2nd sympathetic neuron in prevertebral ganglia and ganglia of the sympathetic chain. The postganglionic sympathetic fibers as-sociate with blood vessels and spinal nerves to reach their target organs. Ganglia of the sympathetic chain synapse to 2nd neurons for the sympathetic innervation of the skin. Prevertebral ganglia around aortic branches synapse to 2nd neurons for the sympathetic innervation of the viscera.

Structure/Function

Frequently, the inferior cervical ganglion fuses with the first thoracic sympathetic ganglion to create the cervicothoracic ganglion which is often referred to as **stellate ganglion**. The location of the stellate ganglion at the level of cervical vertebra CVII above the neck of the first rib is important to know for anesthesiologists when performing a stellate ganglion block.

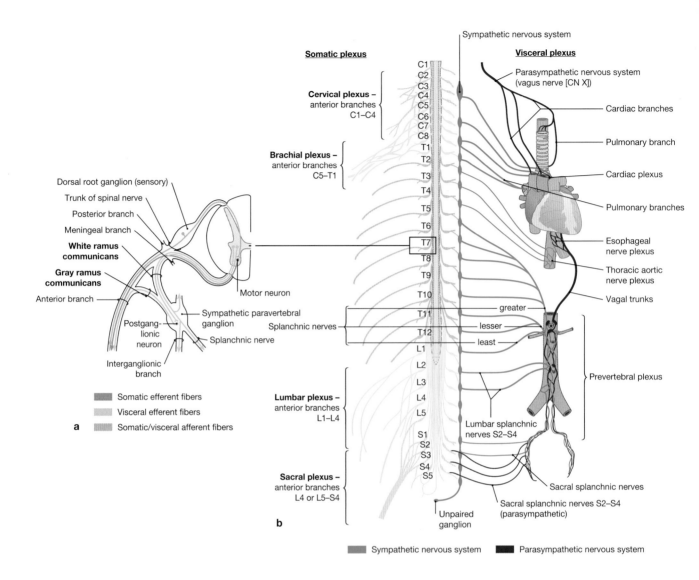

Fig. 12.70a and b The autonomic nervous system and its relationship to spinal nerves and somatic plexus. a [L126], b [E402]

a Composition, branching characteristics and autonomic nerve fibers of a spinal nerve of the thoracic segment (T7). The **white ramus communicans** contains preganglionic sympathetic fibers from the intermediolateral nuclear column of the spinal cord (T1–L2) for the sympathetic trunk. Thus, of the 30 spinal nerves, 14 contain white rami communicantes. Outside of T1–L2, preganglionic fibers ascend or descend through the sympathetic chain and synapse at a

ganglion located at the side of exit from the sympathetic chain to join the spinal nerve as gray ramus communicans. The **gray ramus communicans** contains postganglionic sympathetic fibers of the sympathetic trunk which project back to the spinal nerve. Grey rami communicantes are found at all levels of ganglia of the sympathetic outflow.

b The somatic plexus (left) and visceral (autonomic) plexus (right) are shown in comparison.

Splanchnic and Petrosal Nerves represent Preganglionic Autonomic Fibers which belong to the Parasympathetic or Sympathetic System		
Parasympathetic System	**Sympathetic System**	
• Greater petrosal nerve • Lesser petrosal nerve • Pelvic splanchnic nerves	• Deep petrosal nerve • Splanchnic nerves	 – Cardiopulmonary nerves – Thoracic splanchnic nerves – Lumbar splanchnic nerves – Sacral splanchnic nerves

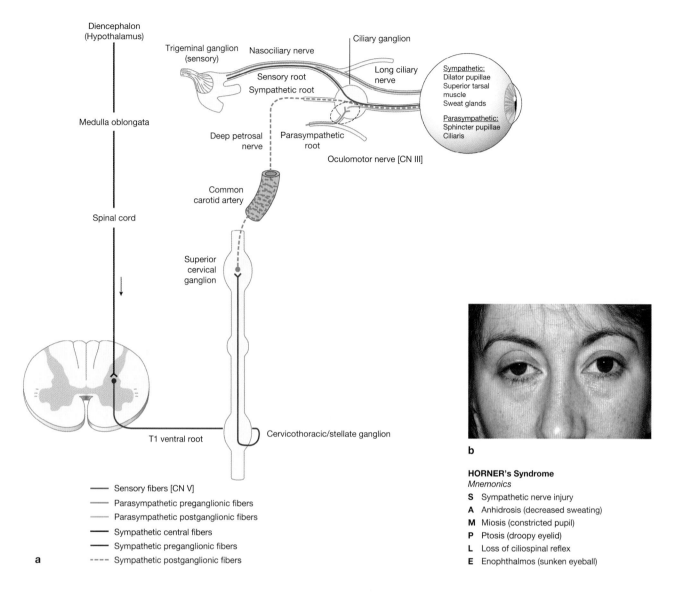

HORNER's Syndrome
Mnemonics

S Sympathetic nerve injury
A Anhidrosis (decreased sweating)
M Miosis (constricted pupil)
P Ptosis (droopy eyelid)
L Loss of ciliospinal reflex
E Enophthalmos (sunken eyeball)

Fig. 12.71a and b a Schematic diagram of sympathetic outflow to the eye; b patient with HORNER's syndrome (BERNARD-HORNER syndrome or oculosympathetic palsy) on the right side. a [L127], b [F276-007]

Clinical Remarks

HORNER's syndrome is caused by a nerve lesion of the sympathetic trunk. The trias of HORNER's syndrome includes: ptosis, miosis, enophthalmus. Typically, HORNER's syndrome occurs ipsilateral to the side of lesion to the sympathetic outflow and causes a loss of ciliospinal (pupillary-skin reflex): pain to one side of the neck, face, upper trunk and inability to cause dilation of the ipsilateral pupil (negative ciliospinal reflex). The location of the lesion to the sympathetic outflow determines the clinical appearance of HORNER's syndrome *(see also corresponding color coding in the above schematic diagram)*:

- **1st order neuron:** Central lesions in the hypothalamo-spinal tract (e.g. transection of the cervical spinal cord).
- **2nd order neuron:** Preganglionic lesions (e.g. compression of the sympathetic chain or stellate ganglion lesion by a lung tumor [PANCOAST's tumor that releases acetylcholine (see also Clinical Remarks on PANCOAST's tumor, ➤ chapter 11 Neck); stellate ganglion block by an anesthesiologist.

- **3rd order neuron:** postganglionic lesions at the level of the internal carotid artery (e.g. cavernous sinus tumor or carotid artery dissection) with release of norepinephrine.

Ptosis caused by HORNER's syndrome (loss of sympathetic eye innervation) coincides with miosis. By contrast, ptosis caused by a lesion to the oculomotor nerve [CN III] coincides with a dilated pupil due to a loss of innervation to the sphincter pupillae muscle.

Tests to confirm HORNER's syndrome include:

Apraclonidine (Lopidine) test: when applied to both eyes, this α2 sympathomimetic drug causes increased mydriasis (widened pupils) due to hypersensitivity on the affected side.

Paredrine test: this amphetamine determines whether the cause of HORNER's syndrome is a 3rd neuron disorder. If the latter is damaged, no mydriasis occurs. No pharmacological tests exist to differentiate 1st and 2nd neuron lesions.

Fig. 12.72 Spinal cord segments; schematic median section; view from the left side; regional segments highlighted in different colors.

The spinal cord is composed of cervical (C1–C8), thoracic (T1–T12), lumbar (L1–L5), sacral (S1–S5), and coccygeal (Co1–Co3) segments. The spinal cord does not keep up with the faster growth of the vertebral column. In the newborn, the spinal cord reaches down to the level of L3 or even L4, whereas in the adult the spinal cord extends only to the level of L1–L2 (ranging from T12 to L2/L3). This increases the distance between the roots of the spinal nerves and their corresponding intervertebral foramina from cranial to caudal within the vertebral canal. Inferior to the conus medullaris at the L1/L2 level, the anterior and posterior roots of the bundled lumbar, sacral, and coccygeal nerves extend caudally as cauda equina and exit the vertebral canal through their intervertebral foramina.

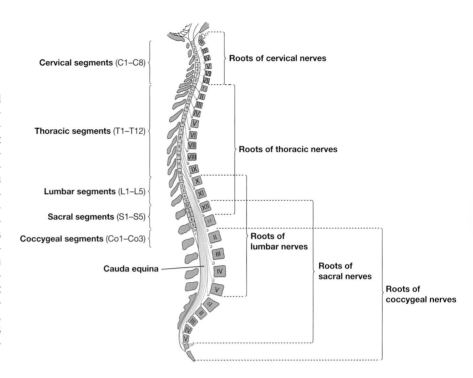

Cervical segments (C1–C8)

Roots of cervical nerves

Thoracic segments (T1–T12)

Roots of thoracic nerves

Lumbar segments (L1–L5)

Sacral segments (S1–S5)

Coccygeal segments (Co1–Co3)

Cauda equina

Roots of lumbar nerves

Roots of sacral nerves

Roots of coccygeal nerves

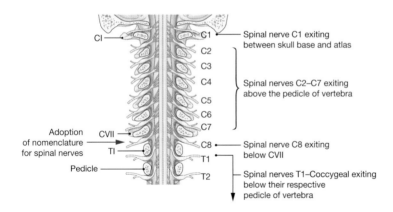

CI

Adoption of nomenclature for spinal nerves

CVII

TI

Pedicle

C1
C2
C3
C4
C5
C6
C7
C8
T1
T2

Spinal nerve C1 exiting between skull base and atlas

Spinal nerves C2–C7 exiting above the pedicle of vertebra

Spinal nerve C8 exiting below CVII

Spinal nerves T1–Coccygeal exiting below their respective pedicle of vertebra

Fig. 12.73 Nomenclature of the spinal nerves. [E402]

There are eight cervical nerves but only seven cervical vertebrae. The first pair of cervical nerves exits between the cranial base and the atlas (CI vertebra). The spinal nerve pairs C2–C7 each exit **superior** to the corresponding vertebral arch. At the transition from the 7th cervical (C VII) to the 1st thoracic (T I) vertebra, the nomenclature changes. The 8th spinal nerve (C8) exits **inferior** to the 7th cervical vertebra. All pairs of spinal nerves T1–coccygeal that follow will always exit **inferior** to the corresponding vertebral arch.

Fig. 12.74 Structure of a spinal nerve and spinal cord segment, exemplified by two thoracic nerves; oblique superior view.

Each spinal nerve is composed of an anterior and posterior root. The motor neurons are located in the gray matter of the spinal cord and exit through the anterior root. The perikarya of sensory neurons are located in the spinal sensory (posterior root) ganglion and their fibers enter the spinal cord via the posterior root. Rami communicantes connect the spinal cord with the sympathetic chain of ganglia. The dorsal branches of the spinal nerves are arranged in a segmental order. Except for the intercostal nerves 2 to 11, the other ventral branches create a plexus.

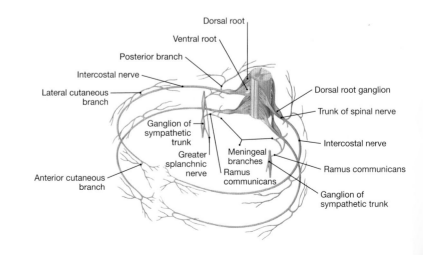

Dorsal root

Ventral root

Posterior branch

Intercostal nerve

Lateral cutaneous branch

Ganglion of sympathetic trunk

Greater splanchnic nerve

Anterior cutaneous branch

Meningeal branches

Ramus communicans

Dorsal root ganglion

Trunk of spinal nerve

Intercostal nerve

Ramus communicans

Ganglion of sympathetic trunk

Dermatomes

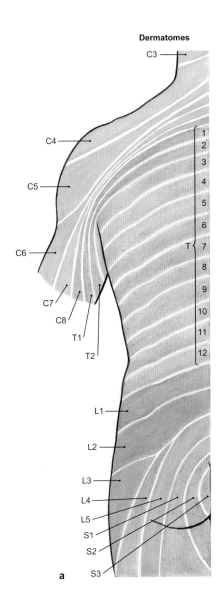

Spinal cord segments

Target regions and functions

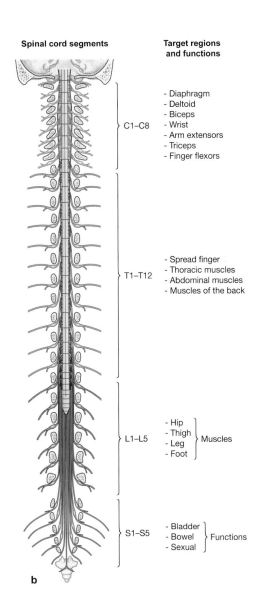

C1–C8
- Diaphragm
- Deltoid
- Biceps
- Wrist
- Arm extensors
- Triceps
- Finger flexors

T1–T12
- Spread finger
- Thoracic muscles
- Abdominal muscles
- Muscles of the back

L1–L5
- Hip
- Thigh
- Leg
- Foot
} Muscles

S1–S5
- Bladder
- Bowel
- Sexual
} Functions

Fig. 12.75a and b Dermatome chart (a) and corresponding spinal cord segments (b). b [E402]

The specific skin area innervated by the sensory fibers derived from a single spinal nerve root is called a **dermatome.** Dermatomes are overlapping. Injury to one spinal cord segment usually does not cause loss of sensitivity. Pain and rash can align with dermatomes. Some viruses lie dormant in sensory neurons (e.g., varicella zoster causing chickenpox or herpes zoster causing shingles). Once the virus is reactivated, pain and/or skin rash develop in the dermatomes corresponding to the infected sensory neurons. A group of muscles innervated by motor fibers of a spinal nerve are named a

myotome. Most muscles are innervated by more than one spinal nerve. Thus, paralysis of a muscle usually requires functional impairment of more than one spinal nerve or spinal cord segment. Both dermatome and myotome pattern show small interpersonal variability. **Specific spinal cord segments** are associated with specific functions. Major spinal cord lesions to the cervical region frequently result in severe functional impairments of spinal cord functions downstream of the lesion and affect the whole body.

Dermatomes of other body regions are depicted in ➤ Fig. 3.87, ➤ Fig. 4.87, ➤ Fig. 5.7, ➤ Fig. 5.8 and ➤ Fig. 6.3.

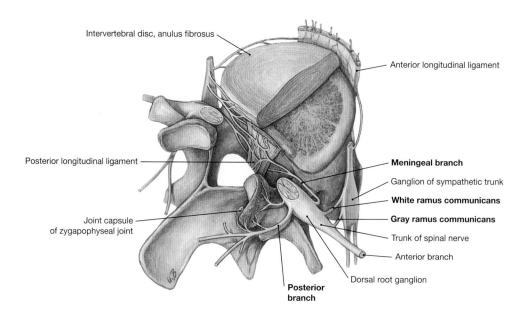

Fig. 12.76 **Nerves of the vertebral column;** view from the right side in an oblique angle.
Branches of the spinal nerve project to adjacent structures. These include the **meningeal branch** for the sensory innervation of the meningeal membranes of the spinal cord, smaller branches derived from the **posterior branch** for the joint capsule of the zygapophyseal joints, and the white and gray rami communicantes con-

necting with the sympathic trunk. The **white ramus communicans** contains preganglionic sympathetic fibers from the lateral column of the spinal cord. The **gray ramus communicans** consists of postganglionic sympathetic fibers from the sympathetic chain of ganglia which project back to the spinal nerve. Autonomic nerve fibers from the sympathetic trunk innervate the intervertebral discs and ligaments of the vertebral column.

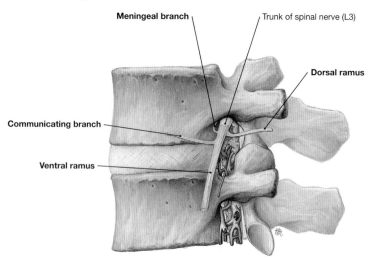

Fig. 12.77 **Spinal nerve in the lumbar region of the vertebral column;** view from the left side. [L240]
Upon its passage through the intervertebral foramen, the spinal nerve divides into the anterior ramus, posterior ramus, meningeal branch, and ramus communicans.

Clinical Remarks

The spinal nerve exits the vertebral canal through the intervertebral foramen (view from the top).
a Normal condition;
b Herniated vertebral disk ('slipped disk') pinching the spinal nerve at the site of the foramen. Frequent causes are age-related degeneration of the anulus fibrosus and injuries in the lum-

bar segment with the tear being located posterolaterally. The presence of the posterior longitudinal ligament prevents medial herniation and compression of the spinal cord.
c The spinal nerves L4, L5, and S1 are most frequently affected. a, b [L266]

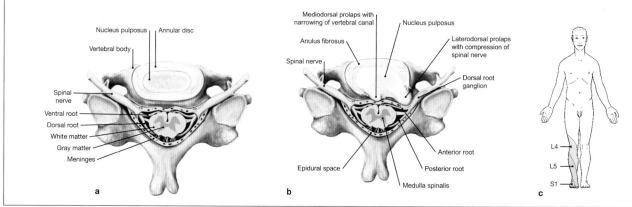

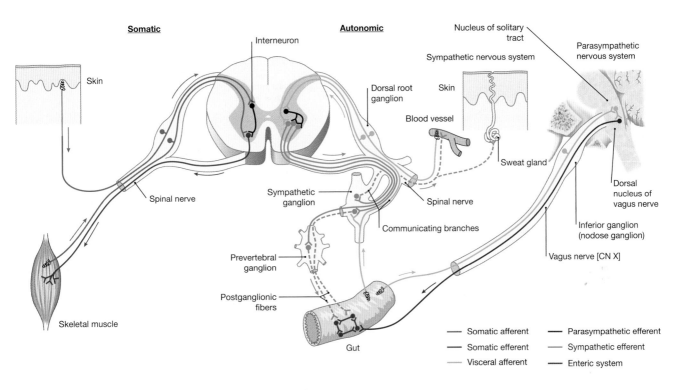

Fig. 12.78 Organization of the somatic nervous system (left) in comparison with the autonomic nervous system (right) in the spinal cord and the peripheral nervous system (PNS). [L127]
Somatic afferent fibers (dark blue) of neurons residing in the spinal root ganglia synapse either directly *(monosynaptic reflex arc)* or indirectly via interneurons *(polysynaptic reflex arc)* with α-motor neurons located in the anterior horn of the spinal cord. In the autonomic nervous system, visceral afferent fibers (light blue) connect with visceral efferent sympathetic (green, solid line) or parasympathetic (purple) neurons via interneurons. Preganglionic visceral efferent sympathetic axons (green, solid line) synapse in sympathetic ganglia and postganglionic fibers (green, dotted line) reach their target organs. The vagus nerve [CN X] receives visceral afferent information via neurons located in its inferior ganglion. Their axons synapse onto neurons in the solitary nucleus of vagus nerve via interneurons. Preganglionic parasympathetic visceral efferent fibers (purple) project into the vagus nerve [CN X], synapse in parasympathetic ganglia and the postganglionic fibers provide parasympathetic innervation to the target organs *(vasovagal reflex arc)*.

Clinical Remarks

Referred pain, sometimes also named reflective pain, is viewed as a misinterpretation of pain derived from inner organs by the brain. In the case of referred pain, visceral pain is not felt at the site of origin but is projected to a distant area of the skin **(HEAD's zone).** Normally, referred pain involves a region with a low number of sensory afferents, such as the intestine. These visceral afferents converge at the same level in the spinal cord with those of a specific cutaneous area that comprises a high number of sensory afferents. The brain erroneously localizes the visceral pain to the corresponding skin area. A typical example is the pain referred into the left shoulder and/or arm during angina pectoris or myocardial infarction. Referred pain is not associated with dermatomes. For further information on 'Referred Pain' see also ➤ chapter 6 (Abdomen).

Structure/Function

Key facts about reflexes

All reflexes are involuntary and stereotype responses to sensory input. Reflexes consist of a sensory/afferent and a motor/efferent arc to elicit a motor response to a sensory signal. The number of synapses required to elicit the reflex determines the complexity of a reflex. A muscle stretch reflex (➤ Fig. 12.79) is a simple monosynaptic reflex with a single synapse between the afferent sensory fiber and the efferent motor neuron (see ➤ Table for list of monosynaptic reflexes). The withdrawal reflex is a form

of polysynaptic reflexes which has interneurons interposed between the afferent and efferent arc. All superficial reflexes are polsynaptic reflexes and involve motor responses to scratching or pinching of the skin (see ➤ Table for list of polysynaptic reflexes). Upon repeated stimulation, reflexes can be increased (sensitization) or decreased (habituation). The reflex contraction of the bladder is a recruiting reflex evoked by increasing stimulation during filling of the urinary bladder. Higher centers of the CNS can alter or temporarily suppress reflexes.

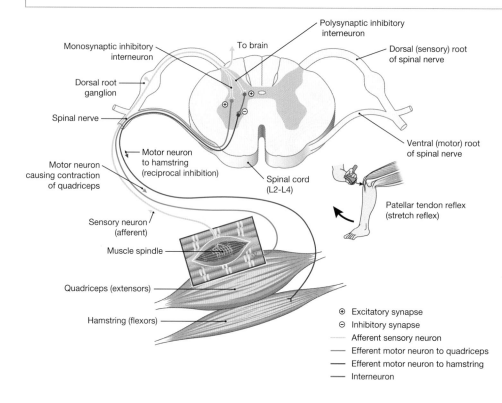

- ⊕ Excitatory synapse
- ⊖ Inhibitory synapse
- Afferent sensory neuron
- Efferent motor neuron to quadriceps
- Efferent motor neuron to hamstring
- Interneuron

Fig. 12.79 The monosynaptic reflex arc of a kneejerk/patellar reflex is shown. [L127]
Tapping the quadriceps femoris tendon below the patella causes an abrupt stimulation of muscle spindles. This generates a sensory/afferent signal which enters the spinal cord and directly synapses with motorneurons of the same spinal cord segment to elicit a contraction of the extensor muscle. Flexor activity is inhibited through a polysynaptic reflex arc which includes interneurons in the spinal cord.

List of clinically tested **stretch reflexes**. These *monosynaptic spinal reflexes* are triggered by tapping a muscle tendon. The resulting afferent stimuli are relayed to specific spinal cord segments and synapse directly (monosynaptic) onto α-motor neurons. They send efferent signals via specific spinal nerves to their target muscle(s) which cause instant muscle contraction.

Important Stretch Reflexes and Corresponding Spinal Cord Segments

Reflex	Spinal Cord Segments	Reflex Trigger	Targeted Muscles	Nerves (Afferent and Efferent Limb)
Biceps	C5, C6	Biceps tendon	Biceps brachii	Musculocutaneous nerve
Brachioradialis	C5, C6	Brachioradialis insertion, tendon or the periosteum	Brachioradialis, brachialis, biceps brachii	Radial nerve, musculocutaneous nerve
Triceps	C6–C8	Triceps tendon	Triceps brachii	Radial nerve
Kneejerk (patellar)	L2–L4	Patellar ligament	Quadriceps femoris	Femoral nerve
Anklejerk (ACHILLES)	L5–S2	ACHILLES tendon	Triceps surae	Tibial nerve

List of clinically tested **flexor reflexes**, also known as nociceptive, withdrawal, or flexor withdrawal reflex. These *polysynaptic spinal reflexes* are intended to protect the body from damaging events and are triggered by stroking specific skin regions. This sensory activation results in the activation of multiple neurons (polysynaptic), including α-motor neurons. Their efferent axons trigger the withdrawal movement by causing the contraction of specific muscles.

Important Flexor Reflexes and Corresponding Spinal Cord Segments

Reflex	Spinal Cord Segments	Reflex Trigger/ Stroking of:	Targeted Muscles	Afferent Limb	Efferent Limb
Abdominal	T8–T12	Abdominal skin	Abdominal muscles	Intercostal nerves (T8–T11), iliohypogastric nerve, ilioinguinal nerve	
Cremaster	L1, L2	Skin at the inside of the thigh	Cremaster	Femoral branch and genital branch of the genitofemoral nerve	
Foot sole/plantar	S1, S2	Lateral side of the foot sole	Flexor muscles of the toes (2–5)	Plantar nerves (of the tibial nerve)	Tibial nerve
Anal	S3–S5	Anal region	External sphincter ani	Anococcygeal nerves	Pudendal nerve

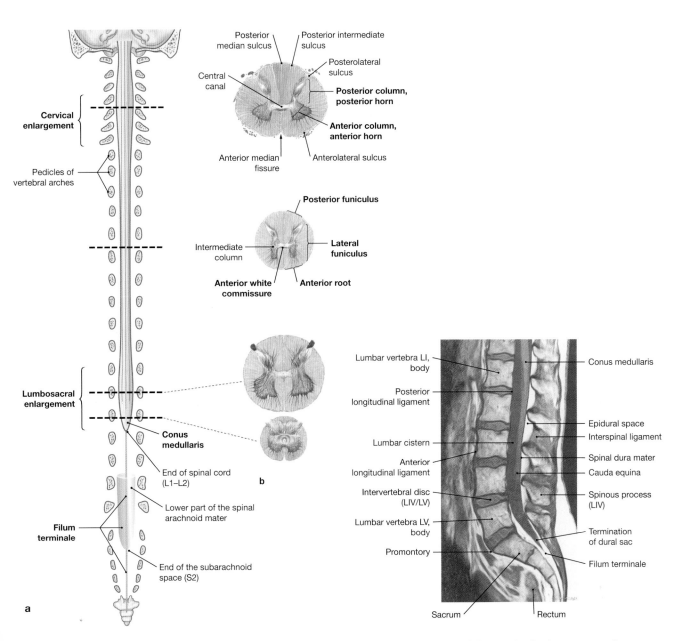

Posterior median sulcus
Posterior intermediate sulcus
Central canal
Posterolateral sulcus
Posterior column, posterior horn
Anterior column, anterior horn
Anterior median fissure
Anterolateral sulcus

Posterior funiculus
Intermediate column
Lateral funiculus
Anterior white commissure
Anterior root

Cervical enlargement
Pedicles of vertebral arches
Lumbosacral enlargement
Conus medullaris
End of spinal cord (L1–L2)
Lower part of the spinal arachnoid mater
Filum terminale
End of the subarachnoid space (S2)

a
b

Fig. 12.80a and b Spinal cord; ventral view **(a)**; and transverse sections **(b)**. a [E402]
The diameter of the spinal cord increases in the areas with spinal nerve roots dedicated for the innervation of the limbs. The upper (cervical) intumescentia (enlargement C5–T1) contains neurons for the innervation of the upper extremities, the lower (lumbosacral) intumescentia (enlargement L1–S3) serves for the innervation of the lower extremities.

Lumbar vertebra LI, body
Conus medullaris
Posterior longitudinal ligament
Epidural space
Interspinal ligament
Lumbar cistern
Spinal dura mater
Anterior longitudinal ligament
Cauda equina
Intervertebral disc (LIV/LV)
Spinous process (LIV)
Lumbar vertebra LV, body
Termination of dural sac
Promontory
Filum terminale
Sacrum
Rectum

Fig. 12.81 Lumbar part of the vertebral column; magnetic resonance imaging (MRI), T1-weighted scan; median section of the lumbar and lower thoracic parts of the vertebral column. [R316–007]
The border between the end of the spinal cord at the level of LI/LII and the beginning of the cauda equina is clearly visible. The cauda equina only partially occupies the vertebral canal allowing safe lumbar puncture in this region without the risk of injury to the spinal cord (see also ➤ p. 571).

Clinical Remarks

Tumors or median disc prolapse inferior to the spinal cord segment S3 can result in a *conus medullaris syndrome* (lesion of spinal cord segments S3–Co3) or *cauda equina syndrome* (CES; lesion of the spinal nerve roots in the area of the cauda equina). The symptoms are sensory deficiencies (saddle anesthesia), flaccid paralysis, incontinence, and impotence. In this MRI scan, a metastasis of a bronchial carcinoma presents as white mass against the surrounding spinal cord. The patient was admitted with complete paraplegia of the lower extremities and loss of all sensory functions below dermatome L2.
[R363]

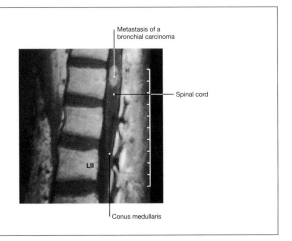

Metastasis of a bronchial carcinoma
Spinal cord
LII
Conus medullaris

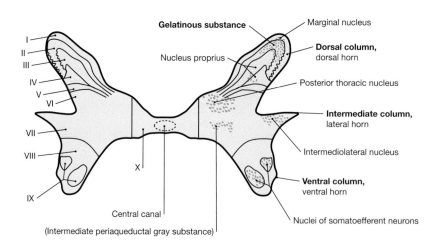

Fig. 12.82 Spinal cord; laminar organization of the gray matter [according to REXED, 1952], exemplified by the tenth thoracic segment (T10).

The gray matter of the spinal cord divides into ten spinal layers (REXED laminae I–X; from posterior to anterior). The extent and number of the layers vary in different segments of the spinal cord. Nuclei can stretch over more than one spinal layer. The paired **posterior horns** are composed of REXED laminae I–VI. Their neurons located in these laminae (e.g., posterior thoracic nucleus [CLARKE's column], nucleus proprius, gelatinous substance) transmit afferent sensory information from the skin, proprioceptive information, and perception of pain from the periphery. The two **lateral horns** contain REXED lamina VII with neurons for autonomic efferences (intermediolateral nuclei). The paired **anterior horns** with REXED laminae VIII and IX form the anterior columns and contain somatic efferent neurons for the innervation of muscles (e.g., motor neurons and interneurons).

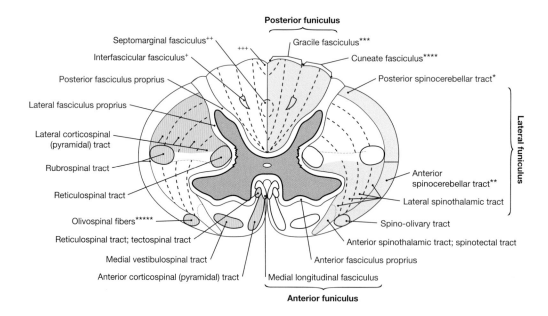

Fig. 12.83 Spinal cord; schematic organization of the white matter exemplified by a lower cervical segment.

Afferent (= ascending) pathways in blue; efferent (= descending) pathways in red.

The regions indicated with +, ++, and +++ designate descending collateral tracts of the posterior fasciculi.

+ SCHULTZE's comma tract (cervical part)
++ Oval bundle of FLECHSIG (thoracic part)
+++ Triangle of PHILIPPE and GOMBAULT (lumbar and sacral parts)

*	clin. term: FLECHSIG's tract
**	clin. term: GOWERS' tract
***	clin. term: GOLL's tract conducts sensations from below T6
****	clin. term: BURDACH's tract conducts sensation from T6 and above
*****	The actual existence of these fibers has not been documented definitively.

Structure/Function

There are **three major afferent/sensory tracts** ascending from the spinal cord:
1. Dorsal column tracts: Gracile and cuneate fasciculi conduct epicritic sensations (conscious proprioception to cerebrum, fine touch, pressure, vibration).
2. Anterolateral System: Anterior and lateral spinothalamic tracts conduct crude pressure, touch (anterior) and pain, temperature (lateral).

3. Spinocerebellar tracts: Anterior and posterior spinocerebellar tracts conduct non-conscious proprioception to the cerebellum.

There are **two major motor systems** descending in the spinal cord:
1. Pyramidal tracts with anterior and lateral corticospinal tracts.
2. Extrapyramidal tract system composed of the rubro-, reticulo, olivo- and vestibulospinal tracts.

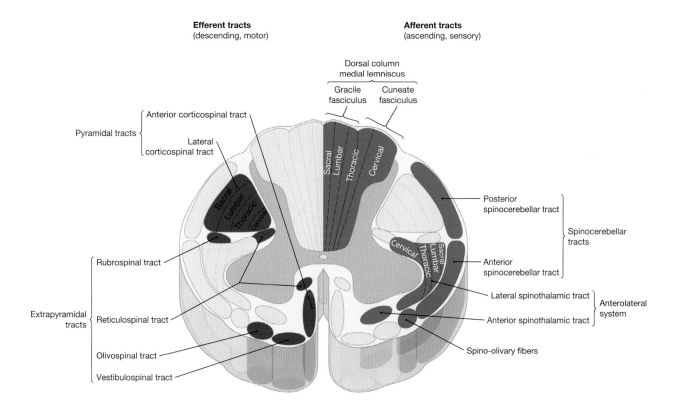

Fig. 12.84 Schematic representation of major ascending and descending white matter tracts in a cervical spinal cord segment.
[L127]
Afferent (= ascending) pathways in blue; efferent (= descending) pathways in red. The ascending dorsal column tract conducts epicritic sensations of the lower extremities up to T6 spinal segment (gracile fasciculus) and from T6 upwards (cuneate fasciculus). Protopathic sensations are conducted by the anterior and lateral spinothalamic tracts. Non-conscious proprioception is conducted by the anterior and posterior spinocerebellar tracts to the cerebellum. Motor efferences (= descending) are involved in muscle movements of the body.

Note the differences in the way the fiber tracks are layered in the pyramidal tract versus the afferents in the dorsal column (gracile and cuneate fasciculi). The efferent fibers of the descending pyramidal tract for the cervical region form the innermost layer. These fibers are the first to synapse with α-motoneurons in the ventral column for the innervation of cervical muscles. These are followed by fiber tracks for the thoracic, lumbar and sacral regions (see also ➤ Fig. 12.87). The opposite layering exists for the ascending afferent fibers in the dorsal column. Here, the cervical fibers are the last to join the column (see also ➤ Fig. 12.85).

Epicritic – Dorsal Column Tracts	Protopathic – Spinothalamic Tracts
Large, myelinated, rapidly conducting fibers	Small, lightly or unmyelinated, slowly conducting fibers
Type Aα and Aβ GSA fibers	Type Aδ and type C GSA fibers
High spatial and temporal resolution	Low spatial and temporal resolution
Fine touch, position, texture	Crude touch
Pressure, slippage, vibration	Temperature
Conscious proprioception	Pain

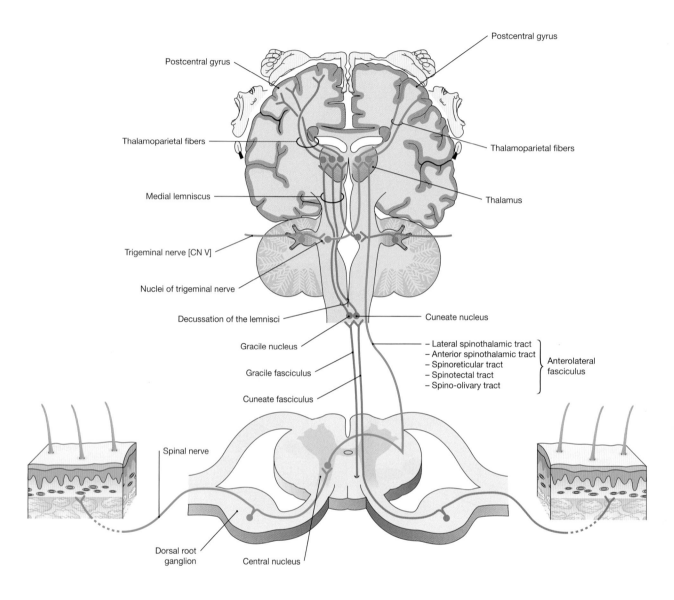

Fig. 12.85 Pathways of epicritic (blue) and protopathic (green) sensibility (afferent tracts).

The pathway of **epicritic sensibility** serves the perception of precise differentiation of pressure and touch as well as proprioception:

- **1ˢᵗ neuron (uncrossed):** from exteroceptors in the skin, mucosa, periosteum, joints and muscle spindles etc., to the gracile and cuneate nuclei in the medulla oblongata via the gracile and cuneate fasciculus, respectively, located in the posterior funiculus. The perikarya reside in the spinal ganglia.
- **2ⁿᵈ neuron (crossed):** from the medulla oblongata (gracile nucleus, cuneate nucleus) to the thalamus (medial lemniscus, perikarya in the gracile and cuneate nuclei).
- **3ʳᵈ neuron (uncrossed):** from the thalamus (posterolateral ventral nucleus) to the cerebral cortex, particularly to the postcentral gyrus (thalamocortical fibers, perikarya in the thalamus).

The pathway of **protopathic sensibility** serves pain, temperature and general pressure sensations:

- **1ˢᵗ neuron (uncrossed):** from exteroceptors in the skin and mucosa etc., to the posterior horn, REXED laminae I to V (perikarya in the dorsal root ganglia).
- **2ⁿᵈ neuron (crossed, some fibers possibly uncrossed):** from the posterior horn to the thalamus, in the reticular formation and to the tectum of midbrain (anterior and lateral spinothalamic tract, spinoreticular tract, spinotectal tract; perikarya in the posterior column).
- **3ʳᵈ neuron (uncrossed):** from the thalamus to the cerebral cortex, particularly to the postcentral gyrus (thalamocortical fibers, perikarya in the thalamus).

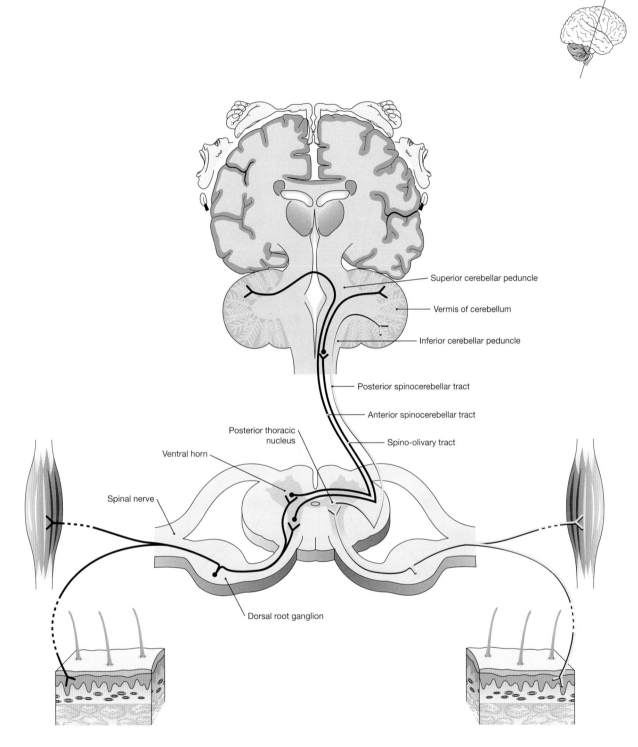

Superior cerebellar peduncle

Vermis of cerebellum

Inferior cerebellar peduncle

Posterior spinocerebellar tract

Anterior spinocerebellar tract

Spino-olivary tract

Posterior thoracic nucleus

Ventral horn

Spinal nerve

Dorsal root ganglion

Fig. 12.86 Pathways of involuntary proprioception (afferent tract).

Pathway of **involuntary proprioception** (involuntary but precise spatial differentiation as a prerequisite for movement coordination by the cerebellum) via the *anterior spinocerebellar tract* (black):

- **1ˢᵗ neuron (uncrossed):** from proprioceptors in muscles, tendons, and in the connective tissue to the nuclei in the intermediate zone and the anterior column (perikarya in the spinal ganglia).
- **2ⁿᵈ neuron (two times crossed):** from the anterior horn within the anterior spinocerebellar tract of the anterolateral tract via the superior cerebellar peduncle to the cerebellum (perikarya in the intermediate zone and the anterior horn).

Pathway of involuntary proprioception via the *posterior spinocerebellar tract* (yellow):

- **1ˢᵗ neuron (uncrossed):** from proprioceptors in muscles, tendons, and in the connective tissue to the nuclei of the posterior column and to the thoracic nucleus (perikarya in the dorsal root ganglia).
- **2ⁿᵈ neuron (uncrossed):** from the posterior horn and thoracic nucleus within the posterior spinocerebellar tract of the lateral tract via the inferior cerebellar peduncle to the cerebellum (perikarya in the thoracic nucleus and at the base of the posterior column).

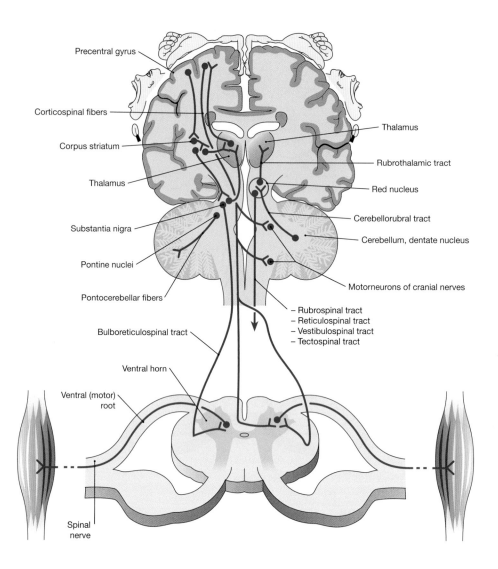

Fig. 12.87 Pathways of the motor system (efferent tracts).
The motor system comprises a large number of nuclear regions and tracts. Three major motor systems are:

Cranial nerves:

- In the brainstem, the motor nuclei of the cranial nerves [CN III, IV, VI, VII, IX, X, XI, XII] are connected with the pyramidal (corticonuclear and bulbar corticonuclear fibers) and extrapyramidal motor system.

Pyramidal (corticospinal) tract:

- **Central neuron (crossed):** from the cerebral cortex through the internal capsule and cerebral peduncles to interneurons in the anterior and posterior columns of spinal cord (lateral corticospinal tract, anterior corticospinal tract; perikarya in the precentral gyrus).
- **Peripheral neuron (α-motor neurons):** from the anterior horn to the motor end plates of the skeletal muscles (motor neuron perikarya in the anterior horn of spinal cord).

Extrapyramidal motor system:

- **Central neurons (crossed and uncrossed):** from the cerebral cortex, particularly the precentral gyrus and adjacent anterior cortical areas, including synapses to the basal ganglia, thalamus, subthalamic nucleus, red nucleus, substantia nigra, cerebellum, etc., feedback loops to interneurons in the anterior column (rubrospinal tract, reticulospinal tract, medial and lateral vestibulospinal tracts, tectospinal tract).
- **Peripheral neuron (α-motor neurons):** from the anterior horn of spinal cord to the motor end plates of the skeletal muscles (motor neuron perikarya in the anterior horn of spinal cord).
- **Motor nuclei of cranial nerves**

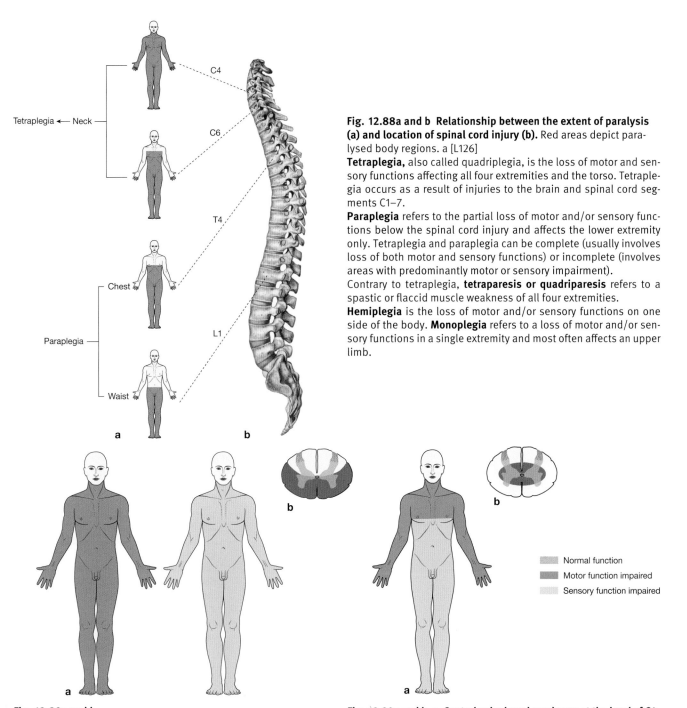

Fig. 12.88a and b Relationship between the extent of paralysis (a) and location of spinal cord injury (b). Red areas depict paralysed body regions. a [L126]

Tetraplegia, also called quadriplegia, is the loss of motor and sensory functions affecting all four extremities and the torso. Tetraplegia occurs as a result of injuries to the brain and spinal cord segments C1–7.

Paraplegia refers to the partial loss of motor and/or sensory functions below the spinal cord injury and affects the lower extremity only. Tetraplegia and paraplegia can be complete (usually involves loss of both motor and sensory functions) or incomplete (involves areas with predominantly motor or sensory impairment).

Contrary to tetraplegia, **tetraparesis or quadriparesis** refers to a spastic or flaccid muscle weakness of all four extremities.

Hemiplegia is the loss of motor and/or sensory functions on one side of the body. **Monoplegia** refers to a loss of motor and/or sensory functions in a single extremity and most often affects an upper limb.

Normal function
Motor function impaired
Sensory function impaired

Fig. 12.89a and b
a Anterior spinal cord syndrome at the level of C4; b cross-section of the spinal cord, highlighted (region of paralysis). [L126]
Below the spinal cord injury:
* Loss of motor function
* Loss of pain and temperature sensation
* Proprioception (postural sense), tactile and vibration senses remain functionally normal.

See also ➤ Fig. 12.85, ➤ Fig. 12.86 and ➤ Fig. 12.87 for course of fibers with specific qualities.

Fig. 12.90a and b a Central spinal cord syndrome at the level of C4; b cross section of the spinal cord, highlighted (region of paralysis). [L126]

Motor impairment of all four extremities but more pronounced in the upper extremities. Sensory impairment below the cervical level of spinal cord injury is variable.

Clinical Remarks

Occlusion of the anterior spinal artery results in an *anterior spinal artery syndrome* and damage of the anterior horns at the level of the occlusion. This causes a flaccid paresis of the muscles/muscle parts innervated by the corresponding spinal cord segment and damage to the tracts in the anterolateral funiculus which becomes nonfunctional in the spinal cord segments below the site of injury. This causes spastic parapareses (partial paralysis of lower extremities), loss of pain and temperature perception and deficits in micturition, defecation and sexual functions. Sensations of touch and vibration are preserved. *An anterior/great radicular artery syndrome* results from blockage of the blood supply from the largest of the anterior radicular vessels, the anterior/great radicular artery (artery of ADAMKIEWICZ; see also ➤ Fig. 12.25). This causes paraplegia in the lower thoracic or upper lumbar regions with complete loss of the entire caudally located spinal cord functions.

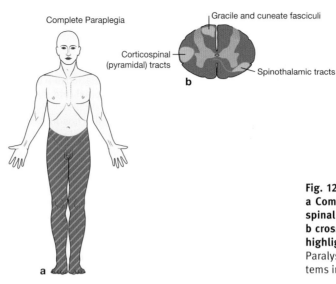

Complete Paraplegia

Gracile and cuneate fasciculi

Corticospinal (pyramidal) tracts

Spinothalamic tracts

b

Fig. 12.91a and b
a Complete paraplegia at the level of the T11 spinal segment;
b cross-section of the spinal cord, completely highlighted (region of paralysis). [L126]
Paralysis of the whole motor and sensory systems in the hatched area.

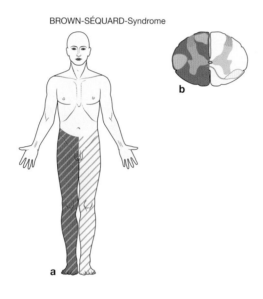

BROWN-SÉQUARD-Syndrome

b

Fig. 12.92a and b
a Hemiplegia (BROWN-SÉQUARD) due to a hemilateral right-sided disruption of the spinal cord at the level of T11;
b cross-section of the spinal cord, right side highlighted (region of paralysis). [L126]
On the right side (ipsilateral):
- Loss of motor function (hemiparaplegia; initially flaccid, later spastic)
- Loss of fine discriminative tactile sensation (epicritic)
- Loss of postural sense and vibration (proprioception; gross touch sensation remains functionally normal)
On the left side (contralateral):
- Loss of pain (hemianesthesia)
- Loss of temperature sensation

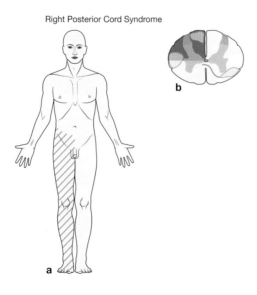

Right Posterior Cord Syndrome

b

Fig. 12.93a and b
a Paralysis of the tracts of the right posterior funiculus at the level of T11;
b cross-section of the spinal cord, half of right side highlighted (region of paralysis). [L126]
On the right side (ipsilateral):
- Loss of fine tactile sensation (epicritic)
- Loss of postural sense and vibration (proprioception; gross touch sensation remains functionally normal).

Index

A

Abdomen 3, 283
- 3-D CT angiography 28
- CT image 6
- horizontal planes 283
- lymphatic drainage 361
- surface orientation 284
Abdominal
- aorta 81, 237, 253, 273, 280, 329, 347, 351, 357, 358, 570, 605
-- branches 359
- aortic nerve plexus 605
- CT cross-section 316, 323, 343
- folds 290
- fossae 290
- intestinal tract
-- parasympathetic innervation 328
-- sympathetic innervation 328
- lymph nodes 307
- ostium of uterine tube 391
- part
-- of esophagus 253, 306, 307
-- of pectoralis major 101
-- of stomach 311
-- of ureter 355
- reflex 612
- region 4
- regions 283
- viscera
-- arteries 329
-- autonomic innervation 360
-- parasympathetic nerve fibers 360
-- position
--- in relation to the peritoneum 300
--- in the hypogastrium 299
-- projection onto the body surface 346
-- sympathetic nerve fibers 360
-- veins 336
- wall 77
-- anterior muscles 78, 79
-- arteries 285
-- blood vessels 285
-- layers 288
-- lymphatic drainage 287
-- muscles 77
-- posterior muscles 80
-- surface anatomy 77
-- surgical incisions 289
-- veins 286
Abdominopelvic viscera
- innervation 360
Abducens nerve [CN VI] 438, 491, 492, 493, 494, 516, 563, 564, 566, 576, 578, 579, 583, 584
- fiber qualities 492, 577, 584
- innervation 577
- palsy 492
- paresis 583
Abductor
- digiti minimi
-- of foot 207, 208
-- of hand 137
- hallucis 208, 209

Abductor
- pollicis
-- brevis 132, 134, 136, 139, 146
-- longus 128, 132, 136
Accessory
- hemiazygos vein 82, 239, 240, 252, 279
- inferior polar artery 352
- lacrimal glands 483
- nerve [CN XI] 437, 438, 444, 445, 520, 523, 524, 525, 526, 529, 533, 534, 563, 566, 576, 578, 579, 594, 597, 601
-- fiber qualities 577, 601
-- innervation 577
- nuclei of oculomotor nerve (EDINGER-WESTPHAL nucleus) 479, 491, 496, 497, 578, 579, 581, 584
- pancreatic duct (SANTORINI's duct) 341, 344
- parotid gland 441, 475
- phrenic nerves 142, 551
- process 44, 69
- renal arteries 352
- saphenous vein 221
- sex glands in man 380
- superior polar artery 352
- sympathetic ganglion 525
Accommodation 497
- reflex 497
Acetabular
- fossa 158, 159, 163, 164
- labrum 164
- margin 159
- notch 159
Acetabulum 158, 162
- position and shape 164
ACHILLES reflex (ankle-jerk reflex) 612
ACHILLES tendon (calcaneal tendon) 156, 190, 199, 204
- rupture 204
ACL (anterior cruciate ligament) 183, 184
Acoustic
- neuroma 591, 592
-- MRI 510
- radiation 514
Acromial end of clavicle 90
Acromioclavicular
- joint 86, 88, 89, 95
-- injury, radiograph 95
- ligament 95
-- injury 95
Acromion 41, 89, 91, 95, 96, 97, 102, 104
Acustic
- reflex 587
ADAMKIEWICZ, artery of (anterior/great radicular artery) 570, 619
ADAM's apple (laryngeal promi-nence) 528, 529, 536, 538, 546
ADDISON plane (transpyloric plane) 283, 310
Additional anatomical movements 10
Adductor
- brevis 172, 415
- canal 175, 220
- hallucis 208, 209
-- oblique head 209
-- transverse head 209

Adductor
- hiatus 172, 174
- longus 157, 172, 175, 415
- magnus 166, 172, 174, 188, 415
- pollicis 136, 138, 146
- tubercle 162, 179
Adductors of thigh 415
Adenohypophysis 564
Adenoids 471, 507, 531
Adipose tissue 22
Aditus to mastoid antrum 508
Adolescent kyphosis (SCHEUERMANN's disease) 65
Adrenal gland *see* Suprarenal gland 357
Aerotympanal conduction 503
Age-related macular degeneration (AMD) 498, 499
Ageusia 600
Aggregated lymphoid nodules
- of small intestine 322
- of vermiform appendix 322
Agraphia 567
AIIS (anterior inferior iliac spine) 158
Airways 27
Ala
- of crista galli 434
- of ilium 158, 159
- of nose 448
- of sacrum 74, 75, 76
- of vomer 450
Alar
- groove 448
- ligaments 59
ALCOCK's canal (pudendal canal) 411, 413, 414, 416, 417
Alexia 567
Alimentary tract 306
ALLEN's test 140
Alveolar
- arch 457
- part 457
- process of maxilla 427, 451, 452, 453
Alveoli of lung, capillary networks 248
Alveus of hippocampus 573
ALZHEIMER's disease
- hydrocephalus ex vacuo 574
Amacrine cells 499
Amastia 230
Ampulla
- of duodenum 317, 319
- of uterine tube 389, 391
- of vas deferens 380, 398, 418
- of VATER (major duodenal papilla) 317
Ampullary
- crest 511, 515
- cupula 511
Anal
- canal 369, 370, 371, 374, 375, 383, 384, 415
-- innervation 373
-- lymphatic drainage 375
-- projection onto the body surface 371
-- rectoscopy 374
-- segments 371
- carcinoma 373, 375
- column 374

Anal
- fistulas 416
- glands (proctodeal glands) 371
- hiatus 368
- nerves 373
- pecten 371, 375
- prolapse 371
- reflex 612
- region 364
- sinus 371, 374
- sphincter muscles 372
- triangle 405, 406, 413
- valves 371, 375
Anatomical
- axes 7
- conjugate 365
- dead space 247
- movements 10
- neck of humerus 92, 93
- planes 6
- regions 4
- systems 11
- terminology 5
Anconeus 115, 128, 131, 132
Anemic patient
- whitish pale conjunctiva 482
Angina pectoris 267
- referred pain 611
Angiogram/Angiography
- of internal carotid artery 565
- of kidney 34
Angiotensin 575
Angle
- of HIS (cardiac notch) 309
- of LOUIS (sternal angle) 226, 228, 233, 250
-- vertebral projection 228
- of mandible 457, 458, 460
- of rib 233
Angular
- artery 442, 444, 446, 447, 487
- gyrus
-- branches of middle cerebral artery 567
- incisure of stomach 311
- vein 443, 487, 562
Anhidrosis 607
Ankle
- anterior muscles 201, 202
- joint 191, 197, 198
-- ligaments 199
-- range of motion 9, 196
-- sprain 199
- lateral muscles 201, 203
- synovial sheaths 206
Ankle-jerk reflex (ACHILLES reflex) 612
Anococcygeal
- ligament 413, 416
- nerve 214
Anocutaneous line 371, 375
Anopia 500
Anorectal
- angle 368, 371
- flexure (perineal flexure) 371
- junction 371
- line 371, 375
Anosmia 582
Ansa
- cervicalis 520, 524, 525, 526
-- inferior root 524, 526
-- profunda 529
-- superior root 524, 525, 526

Ansa
- GALENI 544
- subclavia 280, 551, 605
- tendinis of digastric 474
Anteflexion of the uterus 386
Anterior 5
- abdominal wall
-- arteries 285
-- dermatomes 284
-- muscle-free weak areas 289
-- muscles 78, 79
- apical lingual gland 479
- arch of atlas 56
- arm 4
-- biceps region 114
- articular facet of dens 57
- atlanto-occipital membrane 59
- auricular
-- branches of superficial temporal artery 502
-- nerves 589
- axillary fold 87, 105, 226
- basal
-- segment
--- of left lung 247
--- of right lung 247
- belly of digastric 441, 474, 475, 477, 521, 524, 525, 528, 529, 532
- bony ampulla 510
- border
-- of fibula 193
-- of left lung 246
-- of right lung 245
-- of tibia 156, 190, 192
- branch/es
-- of cervical nerves (C2–C4) 524
-- of great auricular nerve 523
-- of medial cutaneous nerve of forearm 147
-- of spinal nerves (C2–C4) 526, 610
- cecal artery 324, 326
- cerebral artery 527, 563, 564, 565, 566, 567, 568
-- clinical segments 563
- cervical
-- region 4, 225, 425, 520, 528
--- blood vessels and nerves 524, 525, 529
--- muscles 524
--- surface anatomy 528, 546
--- triangular subdivisions 528
--- veins 529
- chamber of eyeball 495, 496
- choroidal artery 499, 564, 565, 566, 568
- ciliary
-- artery 495
-- vein 495
- circumflex humeral artery 107, 149
- clinoid process 434, 435, 436
- cochlear nucleus 512, 514
- column of spinal cord 613, 614
- commissure of diencephalon 568, 572
- communicating artery 527, 563, 564, 565, 566, 567
- compartment of forearm 128, 129, 130
- conjunctival
-- artery 495
-- vein 495
- cord syndrome 619
- corticospinal (pyramidal) tract 614, 615
- cranial fossa 434, 484, 485

Anterior
- cruciate ligament (ACL) 177, 183, 184
-- injury 183
-- MR imaging 183
- crural artery 509
- cusp
-- of left atrioventricular valve (mitral valve) 260, 261
-- of right atrioventricular valve (tricuspid valve) 259, 261
- cutaneous
-- branch/es
--- of iliohypogastric nerve 217
--- of intercostal nerve 229, 240
--- of subcostal nerve 284
--- of thoracic nerve 608
--- of thoracoabdominal nerve 284
- deep temporal artery 442
- dislocation of lower jaw, radiograph 459
- elastic nodule 540, 541
- ethmoid
-- artery 454, 487, 493, 494
-- cells 453, 486
-- foramen 484, 485
-- nerve 446, 454, 494, 583, 587
- external vertebral venous plexus 82
- fasciculus proprius of spinal cord 613, 614
- fold of malleus 505
- fontanelle 430, 431
- forearm 4
-- deep muscles 130
-- muscles 128
-- superficial muscles 129
- funiculus of spinal cord 614
- gastric branches of anterior vagal trunk 280, 307, 597, 598
- glandular branch of superior thyroid artery 547
- gluteal line 159
- horn
-- of lateral ventricle 572, 573
-- of spinal cord 613, 614, 618
- inferior
-- cerebellar artery 563, 565, 566, 568
-- iliac spine 158, 159
-- mediastinum 250
- intercondylar area 179, 192
- intercostal
-- arteries 239, 241
-- branch of intercostal artery 240
-- veins 239, 240, 241
- intermuscular septum of leg 201, 203
- internal vertebral venous plexus 82
- interosseous
-- artery 133, 139, 149
-- nerve 106, 133, 146
- interventricular
-- branch of left coronary artery 257, 260, 266, 267, 269
-- sulcus (groove) 257, 258
-- vein 257, 269
- jugular vein 520, 523, 529
- knee 4
- labial nerves 411
- lacrimal crest 484
- lateral malleolar artery 212, 213, 220
- ligament
-- of fibular head 183, 191
-- of malleus 506

Anterior
– limb
– – of internal capsule 568
– – of stapes 506
– limiting lamina of cornea (BOWMAN's membrane) 495
– longitudinal ligament 50, 59, 235, 279, 610, 613
– lower leg 4
– medial malleolar artery 213, 220
– median fissure of spinal cord 613
– mediastinal lymph nodes 255
– mediastinum 250
– – anatomical structures 250
– membranous ampulla 512
– meningeal
– – artery 559
– – branch of anterior ethmoid artery 493, 494
– meniscofemoral ligament 184
– meniscotibial ligament 184
– (motor) root of spinal cord 618
– nasal spine 427, 428, 448, 449, 450, 451, 453, 456
– notch of auricle 502
– olfactory nucleus 582
– palpebral margin 482, 483
– papillary muscle
– – of left ventricle 260
– – of right ventricle 259
– part of tongue 467
– pectoral cutaneous branches of intercostal nerve 147, 231
– pole
– – of eyeball 495
– – of lens 495, 497
– process
– – of calcaneus 198
– – of malleus 506
– radicular artery (artery of ADAMKIEWICZ) 570, 619
– radiculomedullary artery 81
– ramus of spinal nerve 240
– recess
– – of ischioanal fossa 417, 418
– – of tympanic membrane 505
– region
– – of arm 4, 86
– – of forearm 87
– – of neck 4
– root of spinal nerve 569, 570, 608
– sacral foramina 67, 75
– sacroiliac ligament 160
– scalene 61, 62, 141, 235, 238, 521, 524, 525, 528, 551
– scrotal
– – artery 414
– – branches of deep external pudendal artery 397
– segment
– – of left lung 247
– – of liver 330, 331
– – of right lung 247
– semicircular
– – canal 509, 510, 511
– – duct 510, 511
– semilunar cusp of pulmonary valve 261
– septal branch of anterior ethmoidal artery 454
– shoulder muscles 101
– spinal
– – artery 81, 563, 565, 566, 569, 570

Anterior spinal artery
– – – occlusions 619
– – – syndrome 619
– – vein 569
– spinocerebellar tract (GOWERS' tract) 614, 615, 617
– spinothalamic tract 614, 615, 616
– sternoclavicular ligament 94
– superior
– – alveolar
– – – artery 466
– – – nerves 461, 465
– – iliac spine 156, 157, 158, 159, 160, 186, 364
– – pancreaticoduodenal artery 325, 329, 345
– surface
– – of eyelid 483
– – of lens 495
– – of patella 185
– – of petrous part 434
– – of petrous part of temporal bone 504
– – of sacrum 75
– talofibular ligament 199
– temporal
– – branch of middle cerebral artery 567
– – diploic veins 443, 561
– thigh 4
– – muscles 171
– – sensory innervation 217
– thoracic wall
– – cutaneous nerves 229, 240
– – muscles 235
– – projections of the borders of lung and pleura 227
– – segmental innervation 229, 240
– – surface landmarks 226
– thoracoabdominal wall
– – dermatomes 229
– tibial
– – artery 189, 212, 213, 220
– – recurrent artery 212
– – veins 221
– tibiofibular ligament 191, 199, 206
– tibiotalar part of deltoid ligament 199
– torsion angle 181
– triangle
– – of cervical region 528
– – of neck 520
– tubercle
– – of atlas 56
– – of transverse process 55
– tympanic artery 446, 509
– vagal trunk 280, 307, 315, 328, 358, 597, 598
– veins
– – of right ventricle 269
– – of septum pellucidum 562
– vertebral line 53
– vestibular artery 511
– wall of stomach 310
– white commissure of spinal cord 613
Anterolateral
– central arteries 565, 567
– sulcus of spinal cord 613
– system of spinal cord 615
Anteromedial
– central arteries 565, 567
Anteroposterior axis 7
Anteversion of the uterus 386
Antihelix 502
Anti-MÜLLERIAN hormone 388, 399

Antitragus 502
Anular
– epiphysis 44
– ligament/s 247
– – of radius 111, 123
– – of stapes 506
– – of trachea 537
– pancreas 342
– part of flexor sheath 208
Anulus fibrosus 45, 47, 48
Anus 31, 406, 407, 412, 413, 415
Aorta 241, 262, 265, 274, 285, 316, 323, 343
– projection onto the thoracic wall 228
Aortic
– arch 81, 248, 253, 254, 256, 257, 266, 269, 273, 274, 275, 277, 307, 605
– – arterial branches 274
– bifurcation 326
– bulb 260
– coarctation 273, 285
– hiatus 237, 253, 306
– lymph nodes 358, 395
– nerve plexus 328
– ring 258
– sinus 260, 261
– sulcus 246
– valve 261, 262, 274
– – auscultation 254, 263
– – projection onto the anterior thoracic wall 254
– – projection onto the thoracic wall 228
Aorticorenal ganglia 358, 360
Apex
– head of fibula 193
– of arytenoid cartilage 540
– of bladder 376
– of heart 255, 257, 258, 259, 260
– – projection onto the anterior thoracic wall 254
– – projection onto the thoracic wall 228
– of lung 245, 246
– of nose 448
– of patella 185
– of petrous part of temporal bone 504, 510
– of urinary bladder 380
Aphasia 567
Apical
– axillary lymph nodes 231, 232
– foramen of tooth 462
– ligament of dens 59
– segment of right lung 247
Apicoposterior
– segment of left lung 247
APLEY's Test 8
Aponeurosis
– of external oblique 288
– of transversus abdominis 288
Apophyseal
– joints 49
– ossification 14
Appendicitis 320, 322, 369, 389
– McBURNEY's point 322
Appendicular
– artery 324, 326, 329
– lymph nodes 361
– vein 336
Appendix
– of epididymis 400
– of testis 400

Appendix
- vermiformis 299, 305, 319, 322, 324, 371, 389
- – positional variants 322
- – projection onto the anterior abdominal wall 322
Apraclonidine (Lopidine) test, HORNER's syndrome 607
Aqueduct of midbrain (aqueduct of SILVIUS) 572, 573, 574
Aqueous humour 496
Arachnoid
- granulations (PACCHIONIAN granulations) 561, 573
- mater 558
- trabecula 569
Arch of cricoid cartilage 528, 530, 536, 538, 539, 540
Arc of RIOLAN (RIOLAN's anastomosis) 324, 325, 326, 329
Arcuate
- arteries of kidney 354
- artery of foot 213, 220
- crest of arytenoid 538
- eminence 432, 504
- line 79, 158, 159, 288, 290, 365, 367
- – of rectus sheath 377
- popliteal ligament 188
- veins of kidney 354
Area postrema 575
Areola 230
Areolar
- artery 231
- glands 230
- venous plexus 231
Arm 3, 88, 115
- deep and superficial lymphatic vessels 150
- muscles 114
- posterior muscles 115
- surface anatomy 87
ARNOLD's nerve (auricular branch of vagus nerve [CN X]) 503
ARNOLD's reflex (ear-cough) 503
Arrector muscle of hair 25, 280
Arrhythmia 599
- electrocardiography (ECG) 271
Arterial
- grooves 435
- – of medial meningeal artery 504
- hypertension 272, 352
- structure 28
- vasocorona 570
Arteries 27, 28
Arteriosclerosis
- coronary artery disease (CAD) 267
Artery
- of bulb of penis 398, 414, 416
- of caudate lobe 331
- of central sulcus 567
- of modiolus 511
- of postcentral sulcus 567
- of precentral sulcus 567
- of pterygoid canal 466, 564
- to ductus deferens 292
- to tail of pancreas 329
- to vas deferens 401, 402, 420
Arthritis 18
Articular
- branch of descending genicular artery 175, 220
- capsule of knee joint 186

Articular
- circumference
- – of head of radius 110, 119, 121
- – of ulna 120
- disc
- – of distal radioulnar joint 123
- – of sternoclavicular joint 94
- – of temporomandibular joint 459
- facet
- – for head of fibula 192
- – for lateral malleolus 193, 197
- – for medial malleolus 192, 197
- pillar 55
- surface
- – of arytenoid 538
- – of head of fibula 193
- – of sacrum 75
- tubercle of temporomandibular joint 459
Aryepiglottic fold 534, 541
Arytenoid 540
- articular surface on cricoid 538
- cartilage 537, 538, 539, 540
- muscle weakness 541
Ascending
- aorta 81, 255, 256, 257, 264, 266, 269, 274, 275, 278, 280, 529, 605
- branch
- – of lateral circumflex femoral artery 220
- – of medial circumflex femoral artery 174
- – of superficial petrosal artery 509
- central auditory pathway 514
- cervical artery 524, 525, 527, 551, 570
- colon 299, 301, 305, 319, 321, 323, 326, 343
- lumbar vein 82, 279
- palatine artery 442, 447, 533, 544
- part of duodenum 317
- pharyngeal artery 442, 471, 533, 559
Ascites 301
ASIS (anterior superior iliac spine) 156, 157, 158, 159, 160, 364
Athelia 230
Atlantic part of vertebral artery 81, 527
Atlantoaxial joint 58
- movements 58
Atlanto-occipital joint 58, 59
- ligaments 59
- movements 58
Atlas 53, 55, 56, 57
Atrial branches
- of left coronary artery 267
- of right coronary artery 267
Atrial veins 269
Atrioventricular
- branches of right coronary artery 267
- bundle (bundle of HIS) 258, 266, 268, 270, 309
- nodal branch of right coronary artery 267, 268
- node (AV node, node of TAWARA) 259, 270
- – blood supply 268
Atypical pivot joint 196
Auditory
- ossicles 503, 505, 506, 509
- – arteries 509
- – defects 506
- – joints and ligaments 506
- pathway 514

Auditory
- tube (pharyngotympanic tube, EUSTACHIAN tube) 472, 503, 505, 507, 508, 509, 534, 592, 594
- – occlusion 506
AUERBACH's plexus (Plexus myentericus) 320, 581
Auricle 257, 502, 503, 505
- arteries 502
- sensory innervation 502
Auricular
- branch/es
- – of facial nerve [CN VII] 503
- – of posterior auricular artery 502
- – of posterior auricular nerve 533, 590
- – of vagus nerve [CN X] 437, 447, 503, 597, 598
- muscles 590
- region 425
- surface of ilium 159
- tubercle 502, 504
Auricularis
- anterior 440
- posterior 440
- superior 440
Auriculotemporal nerve 444, 445, 446, 447, 479, 502, 503, 509, 523, 589, 594
Autonomic nervous system 35, 604, 606, 611
- parasympathetic part 604
- sympathetic part 604
AV bundle of HIS (atrioventricular bundle) 258, 266, 268, 270, 309
AV node (atrioventricular node, node of TAWARA) 259, 270
- blood supply 268
Avulsion fracture of finger 126
AV-valve insufficiency 263
Axilla 4, 105
- contents 105
- lymph nodes 151
Axillary
- artery 81, 105, 106, 107, 108, 141, 149, 525, 527
- – angiogram 107
- – branches 149
- fascia 151, 232
- fat 105
- fossa 86
- – lymph nodes 232
- lymphatic vessels 105
- lymph nodes 30, 105, 150, 151, 231, 232, 287
- lymph vessels 232
- nerve 106, 108, 141, 144, 147, 229
- – injury 144
- process of mammary gland 232
- recess 97
- region 105, 225
- – angiogram 107
- sheath 105
- vein 105, 150, 151, 529
Axis 53, 55, 57
- of movement 7
Azygos
- system 239, 279
- vein 239, 240, 251, 252, 264, 265, 278, 279, 308, 337

B

Back
- bony landmarks 41
- deep muscles 73
- intermediate muscles 72
- muscles 71, 72, 73
- superficial muscles 71
- surface anatomy 41
Backpacker's palsy 142
BAKER's cyst 187
Ball and socket joint 17
- glenohumeral joint 98
- hip joint 163
Bare area of liver 331
Baroreceptors afferents 272
BARRETT's esophagus 309
BARTHOLIN's glands (greater vestibular glands) 406, 407, 417, 418
Basal
- lamina of spiral lamina 512
- skull fractures 433
- tentorial branch
-- of internal carotid artery 564
- vein (ROSENTHAL's vein) 562
Base
- of cochlea 510
- of lung 245, 246
- of mandible 457
- of metatarsal 194
- of occipital bone 56
- of patella 185
- of phalanx of foot 194
- of sacrum 75
- of skull
-- foramina 437
-- inner aspect 434, 438
-- nerve exit sites
--- inner aspect 438
--- outer aspect 437
-- outer aspect 437
- of stapes 506
Basilar
- artery 527, 563, 564, 565, 566, 568
- membrane of cochlear duct 512
- part of occipital bone 436
- plexus 560
- skull fractures 454
Basilic
- hiatus 150
- vein 109, 150, 151, 232
-- of forearm 150
BAUHIN's valve (ileocecal valve) 322
Bayonet like deformity 121
BEKHTEREV/BECHTEREW, nucleus of (superior vestibular nucleus) 512, 516
BELL's palsy 591, 600
BELL's phenomenon 439, 591
Benign prostatic hyperplasia (BPH) 370, 381
BERNARD-HORNER syndrome 607
Biceps
- brachii 87, 97, 108, 109, 114, 116, 117, 118, 128, 145
-- rupture of the proximal tendon 114
-- tendon 116, 119
- femoris 166, 167, 173, 176, 180, 181, 188, 189
- reflex 612
BICHAT's fat pad (buccal fat pad) 439, 441, 475

Bicipital groove 89, 92, 93
Bifid
- renal pelvis 355
- ureter 355
Bifurcate ligament 199
Bifurcation
- of aorta 81
- of pulmonary trunk 256
Bile duct 317, 331, 332, 334, 339, 341, 342, 344
- lymph nodes and vessels 338
- sphincter 341
- variations 340, 344
Bipennate muscle 21
Bipolar cell layer of retina 499
Bipolar cells 514
Bitemporal hemianopsia (hemianopia) 500
BLANDIN's gland (anterior/apical lingual gland) 479
Blepharitis 483
Blindness 498, 500, 593
- glaucoma 496
- macular degeneration 499
- retinal ablation 498
Blind spot 490, 498
Blink (corneal) reflex 587
Blister 24
Blood-brain-barrier 575
Blood-CSF-barrier 575
Blow-out fracture 485
Body
- of bladder 376
- of clavicle 90
- of epididymis 400, 401
- of fibula 191, 193
- of gallbladder 339, 341
- of hyoid bone 473, 546
- of incus 506
- of ischium 159
- of mandible 427, 457, 474
- of metatarsal 194
- of pancreas 305, 319, 342, 344
- of penis 397
- of phalanx of foot 194
- of sphenoid 435, 450
- of sternum 226, 233
-- vertebral projection 228
- of stomach 303, 310, 311, 333
- of talus 194, 197, 198
- of tibia 191, 192
- of tongue 467
- of uterus 369, 385, 391, 394, 418
- regions 4
BOETTCHER's cells 512
Bone conduction 503
Bone marrow, aspiration 233
Bones 12, 22
- development 14
- structure 15
- types 13
Bony
- cricoid cartilage 543
- labyrinth 510, 511
- nasal septum 427, 430, 450
- part
-- of auditory tube 508
-- of pharyngotympanic tube 503, 592
BOWMAN's membrane (anterior limiting lamina of cornea) 495
Boxer's fracture 122

Brachial
- artery 107, 108, 116, 117, 133, 149, 231
-- branches 149
- lymph nodes 287
- plexus 61, 106, 141, 238, 520, 524, 525, 529, 550, 551, 601, 606
-- branches 105, 106
-- compression 234
-- entrapment 139
- pulse 28
- vein 150
Brachialis 108, 114, 116, 117, 128, 130, 144, 145
Brachiocephalic
- artery 306
- trunk 81, 141, 239, 253, 257, 274, 276, 278, 527, 534
- vein 251, 252, 257, 274, 275, 277, 279, 525, 529, 534, 551
Brachiofacial
- hemiplegia 567
- paralysis 566
Brachioradialis 87, 109, 115, 116, 117, 128, 130, 131, 144
- reflex 612
Brachium
- of inferior colliculus 514
- of superior colliculus 499
Bradycardia 268
- electrocardiography (ECG) 271
Brain
- arterial blood supply 568
- arteries 563, 566, 567
- deep veins 562
- development 556
- edema 561
- internal arteries 563
- MR angiogram of arterial supply 564
- MRI 6
- positional information and organization 556
- schematic representation 36
- vesicles 556
Brainstem 36, 568
- arteries 566, 568
- blood supply 568
Branch/es
- of lingual nerve to isthmus of fauces 589
- of subclavian artery 527
- to angular gyrus 567
- to trigeminal ganglion 564
Branchial arch, remnants 545
Breast 230
- absence 230
- cancer
-- lumpectomy/mastectomy 232
-- sentinel lymph node 232
- lymph nodes 232
Bregma 429
Brittle nails 26
Broad ligament of uterus 369, 385, 389, 390, 391
Bronchial
- artery 248
- bifurcation
-- projection onto the thoracic wall 228
- blood vessels 248
- branches
-- of pulmonary artery 248
-- of thoracic aorta 251, 278
-- of vagus nerve 278, 280, 307, 597

Bronchial
- cartilages 247
- tree 247
- vein 251
Bronchoaortic (thoracic) constriction of esophagus 306
Bronchomediastinal
- lymphatic duct 550
- lymphatic trunk 551
- trunk 249, 307
Bronchopulmonary
- (hilar) lymph nodes 249
- segments 248
-- blood vessels 248
-- of left lung 247
-- of right lung 247
BROWN-SÉQUARD syndrome (hemiplegia) 619, 620
Buccal
- artery 442, 446, 447
- block 465
- branches of facial nerve 440, 591
- fat pad (BICHAT's fat pad) 439, 441, 475
- glands 596
- nerve 446, 447, 461, 589
- region 425
Buccinator 439, 441, 455, 475, 590
- lymph node 550
Buccopharyngeal
- part of superior constrictor 532
Bucket handle movement of rib cage during respiration 238
Buckle handle meniscal tear 184
Bulb
- of penis 378, 383, 384, 398, 415, 418
- of vestibule 407, 409, 411, 418
Bulbar conjunctiva 482, 495
Bulboreticulospinal tract 618
Bulbospongiosus 406, 407, 409, 411, 413, 416, 418
Bulbourethral glands (COWPER's glands) 370, 378, 380, 399, 403, 413, 418
Bundle of HIS 258, 266, 268, 270, 309
BURDACH's tract (cuneate fasciculus) 614, 615, 616, 620
Bursitis, knee joint 187
B zell zone of lymph node 287

C

Calcaneal
- anastomosis 213
- branches of posterior tibial artery 213
- tendon (ACHILLES tendon) 190, 199, 204
-- rupture 204
- tuberosity 195, 198, 200, 208
Calcaneocuboid
- joint 198, 200
- ligament 199
Calcaneofibular ligament 199
Calcaneonavicular ligament 199
Calcaneus 156, 190, 194, 195, 198, 199, 210
- lateral view 198
Calcarine
- branch of medial occipital artery 499, 566
- fissure 499, 500
- spur 573, 574
- sulcus 499, 557, 566, 568

Calcitonin 549
Callosomarginal artery 563
Callus 24
CALOT's triangle (cystohepatic triangle) 340
Calvaria 433, 561
CAMPER's fascia 288
Canal for
- auditory tube 510
- facial nerve [CN VII] 504, 510
- lacrimal nerve 510
- tensor tympani 504, 508, 592
Canal of CORTI 512
Canine tooth 461, 463
CANNON's point 599
Canthal tendon (lateral and medial palpebral ligaments) 486
Capillary
- lamina of choroid 495
- network of lung alveoli 248
Capitate 119, 122, 123, 124, 134
Capitulum of humerus 110
Capsule of lens 497
Capsulopalpebral fascia 486
Cardia 309, 310, 311
Cardiac
- branches of vagus nerve 606
- conducting system 259
- ganglia 272
- impression 245, 246
- muscle 19, 258
- nerve plexus 252, 280
- notch 227, 246
- plexus 272, 307, 597, 598, 605, 606
- skeleton 258
- valves
-- auscultation areas 254, 263
-- during systole and diastole 261, 262
-- projection onto the anterior thoracic wall 228, 254
-- stenosis 263
- veins 269
- wall structure 258
Cardial
- notch (angle of HIS) 309, 311
- orifice of esophagus 305, 311
Cardinal ligament (MACKENRODT's ligament, transverse cervical ligament) 391, 392
Cardiopulmonary nerves 606
Cardiorespiratory system 11, 27
Carinal
- lymph nodes (inferior tracheobronchial lymph nodes) 245, 249, 253
Caroticotympanic
- artery 509, 564
- nerve 509, 594
Carotid
- bifurcation 442, 547
- body 272, 594, 603
- branch of glossopharyngeal nerve 594, 595
- canal 437, 438, 504, 507, 510
-- external opening 564
- glomus 596
- pulse 28
- sheath 521
- sinus 564, 594, 595, 596
- sulcus 434, 435, 436
- syphon 563, 564, 566
- triangle 425, 528
- tributary of cerebral arteries 563

Carotid-cavernous or C-C fistula 564
Carpal
- articular facet 123
- bones 119, 123
-- fracture 122
-- radiograph 123
- tunnel 134, 136, 137, 139, 146
-- syndrome 134
Carpometacarpal
- joint of thumb 123, 124
-- range of motion 127
- joints (CMC) 88, 123
Carrying angle of elbow joint 112
Cartilage 12, 22
- of auditory tube 534
- of pharyngotympanic tube (auditory tube) 507
- types 18
Cartilaginous
- external acoustic meatus 441
- joints 16
- part
-- of auditory tube 508
-- of pharyngotympanic tube 592
Carunculae hymenales 406, 407
Cataract 497
Cauda equina 571, 608
- syndrome 613
Caudal
- epidural block 396
- part of mesencephalon 514
Caudate
- lobe of liver 303, 331, 332, 333
- nucleus 567, 568, 573, 574
Caval
- lymph nodes 358
- opening 237, 253
-- of diaphragm 306
Cavernous
- nerves of penis 375, 398, 403, 421
- part of internal carotid artery 510, 563, 564
- sinus 487, 560, 562
-- syndrome (CSS) 564
-- thrombosis 487, 564
Cavity
- of scrotal septum 400
- of septum of scrotum 294, 295
- of tunica vaginalis 400
C-cells of thyroid gland 549
Cecum 299, 305, 319, 322, 326
- projection onto the anterior abdominal wall 322
Celiac
- branches
-- of posterior vagal trunk 597
-- of vagal trunk 315
-- of vagus nerve 598
- ganglia 315, 328, 358, 373, 597, 598, 604, 605
- lymph nodes 307, 314, 318, 338, 345, 358, 361
- plexus 328, 373, 597, 598, 605
- trunk 307, 312, 318, 329, 334, 342, 343, 345, 358, 359, 605
-- branches 334
-- origin 325
Cement of tooth 462
Central
- auditory pathway 513, 514
- axillary lymph nodes 231, 232
- canal 572, 613, 614

Central
– compartment of hand, palmar muscles 138
– cord syndrome 619
– facial nerve palsy 439
– nervous system (CNS) 35
– – neuronal connections 603
– nucleus 616
– part of lateral ventricle 572, 573, 574
– retinal
– – artery 487, 495, 499
– – – occlusion (CRAO) 495
– – vein 495
– sulcus 556, 557, 566, 568
– (supranuclear) facial palsy 591
– tegmental tract 600
– tendon of diaphragm 237, 251, 256
– vein of liver 335
– venous thrombosis 499
– zone of prostate 380
Cephalic vein 105, 109, 118, 135, 150, 151, 232, 275, 286, 529
Ceratopharyngeal part of middle constrictor 469, 532
Cerebellar
– fossa 436
– hemisphere 563, 568
Cerebellopontine angle, tumor 510
Cerebellorubral tract 618
Cerebellum 36, 556, 557, 568, 572, 618
– arterial blood supply 568
Cerebral
– aneurysms 565
– aqueduct (aqueduct of midbrain, aqueduct of SILVIUS) 572, 573, 574
– arterial circle of WILLIS 527, 563, 565
– arteries 563, 567, 568
– hemisphere 36
– infarction 567
– part of internal carotid artery 563, 564
– peduncle 499
– pedunculi 578
– stroke 495
– surface of sphenoid bone 435
Cerebrospinal fluid (CSF) 558, 571, 573
– drainage 574
Cerebrum 36, 556, 557
Cervical
– branch of facial nerve [CN VII] 445, 523, 524, 590, 591
– canal 386, 391
– cysts 545
– enlargement of spinal cord 613
– fascia 439, 440, 441, 475, 478, 521, 530, 548
– fistulas 545
– lordosis 43
– lymph nodes 30, 307
– mandibular branch of facial nerve [CN VII] 444
– nerves 470, 524, 525, 601, 602, 608
– – roots 608
– part
– – of esophagus 253, 306, 307
– – of internal carotid artery 563, 564
– – of subclavian artery 570
– – of vertebral artery 81
– (pharyngoesophageal) constriction of esophagus 306
– pleura 227, 242, 243, 244
– plexus 229, 444, 502, 520, 524, 525, 606
– – sensory and motor branches 526

Cervical
– region
– – facet joints 49
– – muscles 62
– – range of motion 60
– – sensory innervation 523
– – spinal motion segments 49
– ribs 234
– rib syndrome 275
– segments of spinal cord 608
– septum 388
– spine 53, 60
– – lateral radiograph 46, 53
– – ligaments 59
– – radiograph 54
– – range of motion 60
– vertebrae 42, 53, 56, 57
– – distinguishing features 55
– – radiograph 54
Cervicofacial branch of facial nerve [CN VII] 440
Cervicothoracic
– ganglion (stellate ganglion) 272, 280, 533, 534, 604, 605, 607
– junction 41
Cervix 33
– of uterus 385, 386, 390, 391, 393
Chalazion 483
Cheek 455
Chemoreceptors afferents 272
Chest
– anterior/posterior (A/P) radiograph 6
– X-ray in posterior-anterior projection 236
Chiasma plantare 209
Chiasmatic cistern 573
Chickenpox 609
Choana 431, 530, 531
Cholangiocarcinomas 341
Cholecystocolic fistula 339, 347
Cholecystoduodenal fistula 339, 347
Cholecystolithiasis 339
Cholestasis 340
Chondroglossus 469
Chondropharyngeal part of middle constrictor 469, 532
CHOPART's region (transverse tarsal joint) 194, 195, 198
Chordae tendineae 259, 260, 262
Chorda tympani 437, 447, 467, 470, 477, 479, 506, 508, 509, 586, 589, 590, 592, 600
– branch of intermedius part of facial nerve [CN VII] 467
– injuries 508
Chorda urachi 294
Choroid 495, 496
– plexus
– – of fourth ventricle 568, 573, 575
– – of lateral ventricle 566, 573, 574
– – of third ventricle 499, 573, 574, 575
Chyle cistern (cisterna chyli) 361
Ciliary
– arteries 494, 499
– body 495, 496, 497
– bundle of palpebral part of orbicularis oculi (muscle of RIOLAN) 486
– ganglion 479, 491, 494, 497, 581, 583, 584, 586, 587, 604, 607
– – sympathetic root 492
– margin of iris 496
– muscle 479, 491, 495, 496, 583

Ciliary
– part of retina 495
– process 496
– zonule 495
Ciliospinal
– center 497
– reflex, loss 607
Cingulate
– gyrus 557
– sulcus 557
Circle of WILLIS (cerebral arterial circle) 527, 563, 565
Circular folds
– of small intestine (KERCKRING's valves) 317
– of stomach 311
Circumflex
– branch of left coronary artery 257, 266, 267, 269
– scapular artery 107, 108, 149
Circumventricular organs 575
Cisterna chyli (chyle cistern) 279, 361
CLARKE's column (posterior thoracic nucleus) 614, 617
Clavicle 89, 90, 226, 233, 519, 524, 525, 527
– fracture 90
Clavicular
– head
– – of pectoralis major 86, 101
– – of sternocleidomastoid 61
– notch 233
– region 4
Clavipectoral triangle 225
Cleft palate 464, 507
Clinical
– crown of tooth 462
– root of tooth 462
Clitoris 405
Clivus 434, 436, 450
CLOQUET's lymphe node (deep inguinal lymph node) 296, 395, 404
Closed-angle glaucoma 496
Closed kinetic chain movements 9
CNS (central nervous system)
– basic structure 557
– major parts 557
– organization and positional information 556
Coccygeal
– cornu 75, 76
– nerve 214
– – roots 608
– plexus 214
– region 76
– segments of spinal cord 608
– vertebrae 76
Coccygeus (ischiococcygeus) 367, 368, 420
Coccyx 42, 74, 75, 76, 157, 158, 405, 412, 413
– distinguishing features 76
Cochlea 505, 510, 511, 514
– tonotopic organization 513
Cochlear
– area 511
– artery 511
– duct 511, 512, 513
– ganglion 512, 513, 515
– hydrops 511
– implants 508
– labyrinth 503, 505
– nerve 510, 511, 512, 514, 515
– nuclei 515, 578, 579

Colic
- branch of ileocolic artery 324
- impression
-- on liver 331
-- on spleen 346
- lymph nodes 327, 361
Colitis ulcerosa 327
Collagen
- bundles or fascicles 23
- fibers 23
Collateral
- eminence 573
- ligaments 200
- sulcus 557
- trigone 573, 574
Collecting
- duct of kidney 354
- tubule of kidney 354
COLLES' fascia (deep perineal fascia) 288, 417
COLLES' fracture 121
Colliculus of arytenoid 538
Colon
- fluoroscopy after barium swallow test 31
- spatial relations 321
Colored spots, retinal ablation 498
Columella 448
Column
- of capsule 568
- of fornix 566, 568
Columnar zone 375
Commissural cusp
- of left atrioventricular valve (mitral valve) 261
Commissure/s of inferior colliculus 514
Common
- bile duct (ductus choledochus) 317, 342
- bony limb 510
- carotid
-- artery 81, 248, 252, 253, 257, 274, 275, 276, 280, 306, 307, 441, 442, 447, 470, 524, 525, 527, 528, 529, 533, 534, 547, 551, 563, 564, 594, 602, 605, 607
-- plexus 533, 534
- cold 544
- femoral artery 219
- fibular nerve 174, 189, 212, 214, 216, 217
-- lesions 211
- flexor sheath of hand 134
- hepatic
-- artery 312, 325, 329, 334, 340, 342, 345
-- duct 332, 334, 335, 339, 340
--- variations 340
- iliac
-- artery 219, 273, 347, 355, 359, 368, 414, 419, 421, 605
-- lymph nodes 358, 395, 404
-- vein 337, 347, 368
- interosseous artery 133, 149
- palmar digital
-- arteries 139, 140
-- nerves
--- of median nerve 139, 146, 147
--- of ulnar nerve 145, 147
- plantar digital nerves 213
- tendinous
-- ring (anulus of ZINN) 490, 492, 583
-- sheath of fibulares (peronei) 206
Communicating
- branch/es
-- of auriculotemporal nerve to with facial nerve 589

Communicating branch/es
-- of intermediate nerve 479
-- of spinal nerves 229, 240
-- of sympathetic trunk 551
-- of zygomatic nerve 586
-- with auricular branch of vagus nerve 594, 595
-- with carotid sinus branch 597, 598
-- with ciliary ganglion 587
-- with facial nerve 479
-- with ulnar nerve 139, 147
-- with zygomatic nerve 488
- hydrocephalus 574
Compartments
- of forearm 22
- of lower leg 22
- of peritoneal cavity 301
Compartment syndrome 201
- fasciotomy 201
Complete paraplegia 620
Compound skull fractures 433
Concentric contraction 20
Conchal crest 449
Concha of auricle 502
Conducting system of heart 268, 270
- blood supply 268
Conductive hearing loss 506
- in children 507
Condylar
- canal 434, 437, 438
- joint 17
- process 453, 457, 458
Cones of retina 499
Confluence of sinuses 560, 562
Congenital inguinal hernia 400
Congested renal pelvis 381
Coniotomy 539
Conjunctiva 482
- stratified squamous nonkeratinized epithelium 483
Conjunctival sac 482
Conjunctivitis 482
Connecting segment of nephron 354
Connective tissue 22
Conoid
- ligament 95
- tubercle of clavicle 90
Constrictor pharyngis 507
Contralateral abductors of hip 211
Contralateral homonymous
- hemianopsia (hemianopia) 500
- quadrantanopia (quadrantopsia, quadrant anopia) 500
Conus
- arteriosus 257, 266
- branch
-- of left coronary artery 267
-- of right coronary artery 267
- elasticus 539, 543
- medullaris 613
-- syndrome 613
Convoluted part
- of distal tubulus 354
- of proximal tubulus 354
COOPER's ligaments (suspensory ligaments of breast) 230
Coracoacromial ligament 95, 96, 104
Coracobrachialis 105, 108, 114, 145
Coracoclavicular ligament 95
Coracohumeral ligament 95, 96, 97
Coracoid process 89, 91, 95, 96, 104

Cord
- of umbilical artery 290, 294
- of vocal ligament 540
Cornea 495, 496
- stratified squamous nonkeratinized epithelium 483
Corneal
- (blink) reflex 587
- epithelium 495
- vertex 495
Corneoscleral junction 495
Corniculate
- cartilage (SANTORINI's cartilage) 537, 538, 539, 540
- tubercle 530, 534, 541
Coronal
- plane 6
- suture 427, 428, 429, 430, 431, 432, 433
Corona of glans 397, 398
Coronary
- arteries 266
-- angiogram 267
-- stenosis 267
- artery disease (CAD) 267
- bypass graft/surgery 268
- catheterization 267
- ligament of liver 297, 300, 301, 302, 330, 331, 333
- sinus 257, 269
-- opening 259
- sulcus (groove) 257, 269
Coronoid
- fossa 110
- process
-- of mandible 453, 457, 458
-- of ulna 110, 111, 120
Corpus
- callosum 36, 557, 566, 568, 574
- cavernosum
-- of clitoris 407
-- of rectum 371
-- penis 378, 383, 384, 398, 403, 413, 415
- luteum 391
- penis 397
- spongiosum penis 378, 384, 398, 403
- striatum 568, 618
Corrugator
- ani 372, 373
- supercilii 439, 441, 590
Cortex
- of kidney 353
- of lens 497
- of suprarenal gland 357
Cortical
- bone of femur 162
- radiate
-- arteries of kidney 354
-- veins of kidney 354
Cortical or compact bone 15
Corticonuclear fibers 591
Corticospinal fibers 618
Corticospinal tract 620
CORTI, organ of (spiral organ) 511, 512, 513
Costal
- arch 226, 233
- cartilage 233
- facet 66
- groove 234
- margin 226
- notch 233
- part of diaphragm 237
- pleura 242, 243, 244, 251

Costal
- process 44
- sulcus 234
- surface
-- of left lung 246
-- of right lung 245
- tubercle 234
Costocervical trunk 81, 239, 278, 527
Costoclavicular
- ligament 94
- syndrome 275
Costodiaphragmatic
- process 244
- recess 227, 236, 242
Costomediastinal recess 242
- projection onto the thorax 254
Costotransverse
- foramen 66
- joint 52, 66, 233, 234
- ligament 50, 51, 52
Costovertebral
- joints 51, 52, 234
- ligaments 51
COWPER's glands (bulbourethral glands) 370, 378, 380, 399, 403, 413, 417, 418
Coxa
- valga 165
- vara 165
Cranial
- arachnoid mater 561
- base 56
-- foramina 438
-- inner aspect 438
-- nerve exit sites
--- inner aspect 438
--- outer aspect 437
- bones 426
-- frontal view 427
-- inside view 433
-- lateral view 428
-- medial view 432
-- posterior view 429
-- superior view 429
- dura mater 507, 560, 561
- nerves 576
-- nuclei 577, 578, 579
-- parasympathetic ganglia 581
-- schematic representation and organization 37
-- sensory ganglia 580
- pia mater 561
- root of accessory nerve 601
- sutures 428
Cranium
- of a newborn 430, 431
- roof 433
Cremaster 291, 293, 294, 295, 399, 400
Cremasteric
- artery 293, 397, 401, 402, 419
- fascia 293, 294, 295, 399, 400
- reflex 291, 612
- vein 397, 402
Crest
- of greater tubercle 92
- of lesser tubercle 92
Cribriform
- area of kidney 353
- foramina 432, 434, 438, 448, 449, 450, 484
- plate 432, 434, 438, 448, 449, 450, 451, 484

Cricoarytenoid
- joint 538
-- capsule 537
- ligament 537, 539
Cricoid cartilage 247, 537, 538, 539, 540, 542, 543, 546, 551
Cricopharyngeal
- ligament 537, 539
- part of inferior constrictor 532
Cricothyroid 528, 532, 540, 542, 543, 546, 547, 597
- branch
-- of superior
--- thyroid artery 530
--- thyroid vein 530
- joint 539, 540
-- capsule 536, 537, 540
-- rotation axis 540
- ligament 542, 551
- membrane 543
Cricotracheal ligament 536
Cricovocal membrane 539
Crista
- galli 432, 434, 450, 451, 560
- terminalis 259, 270
CROHN's disease 327
Croup 544
Crown
- of tooth 462
- pulp 462
Cruciate ligament of atlas 59
Cruciform eminence 436
Crumbly nails 26
Crus
- of antihelix 502
- of clitoris 407, 408, 418
- of fornix 573
- of helix 502
- of penis 398, 415, 418
Cryptorchidism 399
Cubital
- fossa 4, 116, 118
- lymph nodes 150, 151, 232
- pulse 28
- region 88
- tunnel 117
Cuboid 194, 195, 198, 210
Culumnar zone
- anal canal 371
Cuneate
- fasciculus (BURDACH's tract) 614, 615, 616, 620
- nucleus 616
Cuneiform 194, 210
- part of vomer 450
- tubercle 530, 534, 541
Cuneonavicular joint 198
Cuneus 557
Cupula 515
Cutaneous
- branch of obturator nerve 217
- nerves of upper extremity 147
- zone 375
Cymba conchae 502
Cystic
- artery 312, 329, 331, 334
- duct 332, 334, 339, 340, 342
-- variations 340
- lymph nodes 338
- vein 336
Cystitis 379
Cystocele 386

Cystohepatic triangle (triangle of CALOT) 340

D

Dartos
- fascia 293, 294, 399, 400
- muscle 293, 294, 399
Deciduous teeth 463
- lower jaw 463
- upper jaw 463
Decussation
- of lateral lemniscus 514
- of lemnisci 616
Deep
- ansa cervicalis 447, 602
- artery
-- of arm 107
-- of clitoris 409
-- of penis 398, 414
-- of thigh 175, 219
- auricular artery 509
- branch/es
-- of lateral plantar nerve 213
-- of medial circumflex femoral artery 174
-- of posterior superior alveolar artery 446
-- of radial nerve 117, 133, 139, 144
-- of transverse cervical artery 524
-- of ulnar nerve 139, 145
- cervical
-- artery 81, 278, 527, 551, 570
-- lymph nodes 253, 307
-- vein 443, 551
- circumflex iliac artery 285, 359
- dorsal
-- artery of penis 398
-- vein of penis 397, 398, 413
- dorsal vein
-- of clitoris 407
-- of penis 420
- external pudendal
-- artery 397
-- vein 397
- facial vein 447
- fascia
-- of leg 201
-- of penis 397, 398
- femoral
-- artery 175, 220
-- vein 175, 221
- fibular nerve 212, 213, 216, 217
- infrapatellar bursa 187
- inguinal
-- lymph node (CLOQUET's or ROSEMUELLER's lymph node) 296, 395, 404
-- ring 290, 291, 292, 376
- lateral cervical lymph nodes 550
- lingual
-- artery 470
-- vein 470
- lymphatic vessels of arm 150
- palmar
-- arch 140, 149
-- branch of ulnar artery 140
- part
-- of masseter 441, 460
-- of parotid gland 478

Deep
- perineal
-- fascia (COLLES' fascia) 417
-- muscles
--- in man 413
--- in woman 407
-- nerve 410, 414
-- space (pouch) 417
--- in man 416, 418
--- in woman 416, 417, 418
- petrosal nerve 437, 466, 488, 590, 594, 606, 607
- plantar
-- arch 213, 220
-- artery 213
-- flexors 211
- posterior sacrococcygeal ligament 160
- temporal
-- artery 442
-- nerve 446, 447, 589
- transverse
-- metacarpal ligament 124, 126
-- metatarsal ligament 200
-- perineal muscle 379, 380, 413, 416, 418
- vein/s
-- of thigh 221
-- of upper extremity 150
- venous palmar arch 150
- venous thrombosis (DVT) 221
-- pulmonary embolism 249
-- ultrasonografic image 29
- vertebral artery 527
Deeper venous system 29
Deferential nerve plexus 403
Deglutition 535
DEITERS' nucleus (lateral vestibular nucleus) 512, 516
Deltoid 41, 86, 87, 101, 102, 103, 114, 115, 144, 524, 525
- ligament 199
-- anterior tibiotalar part 199
-- posterior tibiotalar part 199
-- tibiocalcaneal part 199
-- tibionavicular part 199
- region 4, 225, 425
- tuberosity 92
Deltopectoral lymph nodes 150
DENONVILLIER's fascia (rectoprostatic fascia) 366, 370, 375, 381
Dens axis 57, 60
Dental branches
- of posterior superior alveolar artery 446
Dentate
- line (pectinate line) 371, 373, 375
- nucleus 618
Denticulate ligament 569
Dentine 462
Depressed skull fractures 433
Depression of optic disc 495
Depressor
- anguli oris 439, 440, 441, 590
- labii inferioris 439, 440, 441, 590
- septi nasi 439, 590
- supercilii 439, 440, 441, 486
Dermatomes
- cholecystolithiasis 339
- corresponding spinal cord segments 609
- of lower extremity 218
- of the anterior abdominal wall 284

Dermatomes
- of the anterior thoracoabdominal wall 229
- of upper extremity 148
Dermis 24
DESCEMET's membrane (posterior limiting lamina of cornea) 495
Descending
- aorta 81, 253, 257, 264, 274, 275
- branch of lateral circumflex femoral artery 175, 220
- colon 299, 301, 305, 319, 321, 322, 326, 343
- genicular artery 189, 220
- palatine artery 442, 466
- part of duodenum 311, 317, 321, 342
- scapular artery (var.) 527
Descensus of uterus 386
Desmodontium 462
Detrusor 376
Diabetic retinopathy 499
Diagonal
- axis of the forearm 88
- conjugate 365, 387
Dial test 180
Diaphragm(a) 236, 238, 243, 251, 254, 255, 279, 306, 310, 316
- blood supply 237
- innervation 236
- lateral and inferior view 237
- oris 474
- sellae 564
Diaphragmatic
- constriction of esophagus 306
- dome 236
- paralysis 236
- pleura 243, 244
- surface
-- of heart 257
-- of left lung 246
-- of liver 310, 330, 331, 333
-- of spleen 346
Diaphyseal ossification 14
Diaphysis 15
Diastatic skull fractures 433
Diastole 262
- blood flow and valve position 262
- ventricular action 261, 262
Diastolic murmurs 263
Diencephalon 556, 557
- arteries 566
Digastric 61, 441, 474, 475, 477, 478, 508, 524, 525, 528, 529, 532, 586, 590, 592, 593
- branch of facial nerve [CN VII] 446, 447, 474, 508, 592
- fossa 457
Digestive
- system 11, 31
- tract 306
Dilator pupillae 496, 583, 607
Dinner fork like deformity 121
Diploe 425, 433, 561
Diploic
- canals 561
- veins 561
Diplopia (double vision) 491
Direct inguinal hernia 289, 295
- laparoscopic image 290
Direct laryngoscopy 541
- phonation position 541
- respiratory position 541
- whispering position 541

Direct ophthalmoscopy (funduscopy or fundoscopy) 498
Disc herniations, posterolateral 45
Disc injury 218
Distal 5
- interphalangeal joints (DIP) 88, 118, 126
-- range of motion 127
- medial striate artery (HEUBNER's recurrent artery) 565, 567
- phalanx 88
-- of foot 194, 195
-- of hand 118, 119, 122
- radioulnar joint 88, 119, 123
- tubule of kidney 354
Dithalamic joint 459
Dizziness 510, 515
Dopamine
- antagonists 575
- receptors 575
Dorsal 5
- aponeurosis of hand 135, 138
- artery
-- of clitoris 407, 409
-- of foot 212, 213, 220
-- of penis 397, 398, 413, 414, 416, 420
- branch/es
-- of C2 526
-- of posterior intercostal artery 240
-- of ulnar nerve 145
- carpal
-- arch 139
-- branch
--- of radial artery 139, 149
--- of ulnar artery 139, 140, 149
- carpometacarpal ligaments 124
- column of spinal cord 614, 615
- cuboideonavicular ligament 199
- cuneonavicular ligament 199
- digital
-- arteries
--- of foot 213
--- of hand 149
-- branches of radial nerve 147
-- nerves
--- of arm 144
--- of foot 212, 217
- horn of spinal cord 614
- intercarpal ligaments 124
- interossei
-- of foot 206, 207, 209
-- of hand 135, 137, 138
- lingual
-- branches of lingual artery 471
-- vein 470
- mesogastrium 297, 300
- mesohepaticum 297
- metacarpal
-- arteries 139, 149
-- ligaments 124
- metatarsal
-- arteries 212, 213, 220
-- ligament 199
- motor nucleus
-- of vagus nerve 272
- nasal artery 447, 487, 494
- nerve
-- of clitoris 407, 410, 411, 414
-- of penis 397, 398, 413, 414, 416, 421
- nucleus of vagus nerve 360, 578, 581, 597, 598, 611
- pancreatic artery 329, 345
- radiocarpal ligament 124

Dorsal
- ramus of spinal nerve 610
- root ganglion 606, 616, 617
- scapular
-- artery 551
-- nerve 106, 141, 142
- vein of penis 420
- venous netwerk of foot 221
Dorsalis pedis artery 212, 213, 220
- pulse 28
Dorsiflexion 196
Dorsolateral
- bundle of lymph collectors
-- in the upper arm 232
- collecting system 222
Dorsum 5
- of foot 4, 156
-- muscles 207
-- nerves and vessels 213
-- palpable pulse 213
- of hand 4, 87
-- arteries 139
-- nerves 139
- of nose 448
- of penis 397
- of tongue 455, 467, 471, 534
-- innervation 467
-- taste qualities 467
- sellae 432, 434, 435, 450
Double uterus 388
Double vision (diplopia) 491
DOUGLAS, pouch of (rectouterine
  pouch) 301, 319, 347, 366, 369, 387,
  389, 392
Down and out syndrome 583
Drop foot disability 211
Duct of bulbourethral gland 378
Ductus
- arteriosus 273
- choledochus (common bild duct) 317
- deferens 294, 295, 380
- reuniens 511
- venosus 273
Duodenal
- ampulla (duodenal cap) 317
- impression on liver 331
Duodenojejunal flexure 299, 317, 344, 347
Duodenum 297, 299, 304, 305, 311, 313,
  316, 321, 342, 343, 347
- arteries 318
- blood supply 318
- divisions 317, 341
- horizontal part 299
- inner relief 317
- posterior view 342
- projection onto the body surface 317
- radiograph 317
- topography 317
Dural
- part of filum terminale 613
- venous sinuses 560, 561
Dura mater 558
Dysequilibrium 515
Dysgeusia 600
Dysphagia 253

E

Ear
- congenital defects of external ear 502
- longitudinal section 503

Ear-cough or ARNOLD's reflex 503
Eccentric contraction 20
Ecchymoses 457
EDINGER-WESTPHAL nucleus (accessory
  nucleus of oculomotor nerve) 479, 491,
  496, 497, 578, 581, 584
Efferent ductules 399, 401
Ejaculation 403
Ejaculatory ducts 378, 380
Elastic cartilage 18
Elbow
- alignment 112
- conventional radiograph (X-ray) 12
- cubital fossa 116
- joint 88, 110
-- bones 110, 111
-- carrying triangle 112
-- dislocation 112
-- fractures 112
--- sail sign 110
-- hinge movements (extension and
   flexion) 113
-- HUETER's triangle 112
-- ligaments 111
-- radiograph 110
-- range of motion 113
-- rational movements (pronation and
   supination) 113
- lateral radiograph 6
- movements 8
- region 109
-- arteries and nerves 116, 117
- surface anatomy 109
Electrocardiogram (ECG).
- anatomical principles 271
Ellipsoid joint 17
Emissary veins 466
Emission 403
Endoabdominal fascia 288
Endocardium 258
Endocrine system 11, 32, 35
Endolymph 512, 515
Endolymphatic
- duct 511
- sac 511
Endomysium 20
Endoscopic (direct) laryngoscopy 541
Endoscopic retrograde cholangiopancrea-
  tography (ERCP) 344
Endosteum 15
Endothoracic fascia 241, 242, 243, 244
Endotracheal
- intubation 542
- tube, proper placement 542
Enophthalmus 607
Enteric nervous system 604
Entrapment of ulnar nerve 117
Ependyma 573, 575
Epicardium 255, 257, 258, 260
Epicranial aponeurosis 425, 439, 440,
  441, 561
Epicranius 439, 440, 441, 523
Epicritic sensibility 586, 615, 616
Epidemic parotitis (mumps) 475
Epidermis 24
Epididymis 293, 294, 370, 399, 400, 403
- blood vessels 401
Epidural
- anesthesia 396, 571
- hematoma 559
- space 558, 571, 613

Epifascial
- abdominal veins, anastomoses 286
- tributaries of the femoral vein 221
Epigastric
- fossa 226
- hernia 289
- region 225, 283
Epigastrium 299, 301
Epiglottic
- cartilage 471, 530, 536, 537, 538, 539
- vallecula 467, 544
Epiglottis 467, 471, 534, 541, 542, 544
Epimysium 20
Epinephrine 357
Epineurium 569
Epiorchium 399
Epipharynx 530
Epiphyseal
- growth plane 15
- line 15, 178, 197, 198
- ossification 14
Epiphysis 15
Epiploic foramen (omental foramen,
  foramen of WINSLOW) 302, 303
Episcleral
- artery 495
- vein 495
Episiotomy 412
Epistaxis (nose bleeding) 454
Epitympanic recess 505, 506
Epitympanum 505
Eponychium 26
Equilibrium (balance) pathway 516
ERCP (endoscopic retrograde cholangio-
  pancreatography) 344
Erectile dysfunction 403
Erection 403
Erector spinae 41, 70, 72, 77, 80
Erythropoietin (EPO) 354
Esophageal
- branch/es
-- of left gastric artery 307
-- of left gastric vein 308
-- of recurrent laryngeal nerve 544
-- of splenic artery 329
-- of thoracic aorta 278, 307
-- of vagus nerve 278, 597, 598
- hiatus 237, 253, 306, 307, 309
- impression of left lung 246
- impression on liver 331
- muscle fibers 309
- plexus 251, 256, 280, 307, 597, 598, 606
- submucosal venous plexus 309
- varices 308, 337
- veins 308, 313, 336, 337
- venous plexus 308
Esophagus 251, 252, 256, 264, 265, 276,
  277, 278, 279, 306, 309, 311, 530, 532, 533
- abdominal part 253
- arteries 307
- cervical part 253
- compression 253
- constrictions 306
- innervation 307
- lymphatic drainage 307
- thoracic part 253
- veins 308
Estrogens 388
Ethmoid
- bone 427, 432, 434, 448, 449, 450,
  452, 484, 485
- cells 451, 452, 453, 484, 485, 490, 583

Ethmoid
- crest 451
- foramina 485
- labyrinth 449, 484
-- fractures 484
- process 451
- sinuses 485, 583
EUSTACHIAN tube (auditory tube, pharyngotympanic tube) 472, 503, 505, 507,
  508, 509, 534, 592, 594
- occlusion 506
Excretory ducts (ductules)
- of lacrimal gland 489
- of tarsal glands 483
Exophthalmos 564
- GRAVES' disease 548
Expiration muscles 238
Extensor
- carpi
-- radialis
--- brevis 128, 131, 135
--- longus 118, 128, 131, 135
-- ulnaris 118, 128, 131, 135
- digiti minimi 128, 131, 135
- digitorum 128, 131, 135
-- brevis 206, 207
-- longus 201, 202, 206, 207
- hallucis
-- brevis 206, 207
-- longus 201, 202, 206, 207
- indicis 132
- lever arm 185
- pollicis
-- brevis 128, 132, 135
-- longus 128, 132, 135
- retinaculum
-- of foot 202, 206, 207
-- of hand 132, 135
External
- acoustic
-- meatus 437, 503, 504, 505, 513
-- pore 428, 458
- anal sphincter 372, 373, 374, 383, 407,
  408, 409, 411, 412, 413, 415, 416
- axis of eyeball 495
- branch of superior laryngeal nerve 533
- carotid artery 274, 442, 446, 447, 466,
  470, 478, 520, 524, 525, 533, 547, 559,
  563, 564, 594
- female genitalia 406, 407
-- lymph nodes and vessels 395
- geniculum of facial nerve 590, 591, 592
- iliac
-- artery 81, 175, 219, 273, 285, 321, 355,
  359, 374, 409, 414, 419
-- lymph nodes 358, 395, 404
-- vein 175, 221, 321, 355, 374, 420
- intercostal muscles 78, 235, 238, 241,
  242, 244, 278
- jugular vein 275, 443, 444, 445, 466,
  475, 520, 523, 524, 525, 529
- male genitalia 397
-- lymphatic drainage 404
-- lymph nodes and lymph vessels 404
-- neurovascular structures 397
- nasal
-- branch/es
--- of anterior ethmoid artery 454
--- of anterior ethmoid nerve 454
--- of infraorbital nerve 587
-- nerve 446

External
- oblique 70, 77, 78, 288, 289, 291, 292,
  294, 295, 349
-- aponeurosis 78
- occipital protuberance 41, 429, 432
- opening of carotid canal 437, 504, 564
- os of uterus 387, 391
- part of thyroarytenoid 540
- plate 433
- pudendal
-- artery 286, 414
-- vein 221, 286, 296
- spermatic fascia 293, 294, 295, 399,
  400
- table of calvaria 425, 433
- urethral
-- orifice 378, 379, 397, 406, 407, 418
-- sphincter 376, 379, 407, 413
Extradural space 571
Extrahepatic bile ducts 339
Extraocular muscles 490, 516, 583
- function 490
- innervation 491
- paralysis 487, 491, 492, 583
Extraperitoneal
- abdominal organs 300
- space of pelvis
-- in man 418
-- in woman 418
Extrapyramidal
- motor system 618
- tracts of spinal cord 615
Extrauterine (ectopic) pregnancies 391
Eye 482
- arteries 487
- structures producing the tear film 483
- veins 487
Eyeball 494, 495, 499
- blood vessels 495
Eyelashes 482, 483
Eyelids 482, 483

F

FABER muscle of the hip 169
Facet
- for dens 57
- joints 45, 47, 49
-- cervical region 49, 60
-- lumbar region 49
-- orientation 49
-- range of spinal motion 49
-- thoracic region 66
Facial
- area, inflammations via angular
  vein 443
- artery 442, 444, 445, 446, 447, 475,
  525, 528, 529, 533
- canal 512
- colliculus 572
- hypoesthesia 492
- lymph nodes 550
- muscles 439, 440
-- paralysis 593
-- superficial layer 441
- nerve [CN VII] 437, 438, 446, 447, 470,
  478, 479, 488, 502, 503, 508, 509, 510,
  511, 512, 523, 524, 563, 566, 576, 578,
  579, 586, 590, 591, 592, 600, 604
-- branches 592
-- corticonuclear connections 591

Facial nerve [CN VII]
-- course 592
-- fiber qualities 577, 593
-- innervation 577
-- innervation area 592
-- palsy 440, 489, 508, 593
-- peripheral course 591
-- peripheral palsy 439
-- sensory ganglion 580
-- terminal branches 440
- plane 428
- sensory deficits 487
- skin, innervation 585
- vein 443, 444, 445, 446, 447, 466, 475,
  487, 520, 523, 524, 528, 529, 562
Falciform ligament of liver 290, 297, 300,
  302, 305, 330, 333, 376
FALLOPIAN tube (uterine tube) 33, 369,
  385, 388, 389, 390, 391, 396
- peritoneal duplicatures 369
False ribs 233
Falx cerebri 560
Fanstrapped muscle 21
Farsightedness (hyperopia) 497
Fascia 22
- lata 168, 288, 296
- of forearm 22
- of lower leg 22
- of penis 398
Fascial slips to orbicularis oculi 486
Fasciotomy
- compartment syndrome 201
Fatty liver 330, 335
Fecal
- continence 368
- incontinence 371
Femoral
- anteversion 165
- artery 81, 175, 219, 220, 285, 290, 291,
  296, 382, 414
- branch of genitofemoral nerve 214, 217,
  296, 356, 612
- canal 296
- head 162, 163, 164, 219
-- avascular necrosis (AVN) 162
-- blood supply 162
-- position 164
- hernia 296
- neck 162, 163
-- angle of inclination 165
- nerve 170, 171, 172, 175, 214, 215, 217,
  296, 321, 356, 612
- pulse 28
- retroversion 165
- sheath 175
- triangle 156, 157, 175
- vein 175, 221, 290, 296, 382
Femoropatellar joint 178, 181
- radiograph 178
Femorotibial joint 178, 181
- radiograph 178
Femur 12, 162, 163, 165, 177, 178, 179, 181,
  182, 183, 184, 185, 188
- CT scan 15
- radiograph 162
- torsion angle 165
Fetal circulation 27
Fetus, ultrasound image 33
Fibrocartilage 16, 18
Fibrocartilaginous
- part of pharyngotympanic tube 503
- ring of tympanic membrane 505, 506

Fibrous
- appendix of liver 331
- joints 16
- membrane 16
- orbital septum 486
- pericardium 243, 252, 255, 256
- skeleton of heart 258
Fibula 12, 156, 177, 178, 179, 181, 182, 183, 184, 187, 188, 191, 193, 194, 197, 198, 199
- fracture 197
- proximal fractures 211
Fibular
- artery 189, 212, 220
- collateral ligament 181, 182, 187, 188
- head 178, 179, 181
- neck 178, 179, 181
- notch 192
- (peroneal) retinaculum 203, 204, 206
- shaft 191
- veins 221
Fibularis (peroneus)
- brevis 201, 203, 206, 207
- longus 190, 201, 203, 208, 209
- tertius 201, 202, 206, 207
Filiform papillae 467
Filum
- radiculare 613
- terminale 613
Fimbria/e
- of hippocampus 573
- of uterine tube 389, 391
Fimbriated fold of tongue 477
Finger joints 126
- ligaments 126
- range of motion 8, 127, 138
Fissura petrotympanica 437
Fissure for round ligament 331
Fistulas of anal canal 416
Flashes, retinal ablation 498
Flat bones 13
FLECHSIG, oval bundle of (septomarginal fasciculus) 614
FLECHSIG's tract (posterior spinocerebellar tract) 614, 615, 617
Flexor
- carpi
-- radialis 115, 116, 118, 128, 129, 134, 146
-- ulnaris 118, 128, 129, 134, 145
- digiti minimi brevis
-- of foot 208, 209
-- of hand 137
- digitorum
-- brevis 208
-- longus 205, 208, 209
-- profundus 130, 134, 138, 145, 146
-- superficialis 128, 129, 130, 134, 138, 146
- hallucis
-- brevis 208, 209
-- longus 205, 208, 209
- pollicis
-- brevis 136, 146
-- longus 128, 130, 134, 136, 138, 146
- reflexes 612
- retinaculum
-- of foot 204, 205, 213
-- of hand 134, 137, 138, 146
Flexors of toes 211
Floating ribs 233
Floor of mouth 474
- muscles 473

Fold/s
- of iris 496
- of superior laryngeal nerve 534
Foliate papillae 467
Foot 3
- anterior muscles 201, 202
- bones 194
- joints
-- ligaments 200
-- range of motion 200
- lateral muscles 201, 203
- muscles
-- on the dorsal surface 207
-- on the plantar surface 208, 209
- plantar arches 210
- plantar surface
-- arteries and nerves 213
- pronation 211
- skeleton, radiograph 194, 195
- sole (plantar) reflex 612
- supination 211
- synovial sheaths 206
- tension band system 210
Foramen
- caecum
-- of frontal bone 434
-- of tongue 467, 468, 545
- lacerum 434, 437, 438, 510
- magnum 56, 431, 434, 436, 437, 438, 560, 601
- of WINSLOW (omental foramen, epiploic foramen) 302, 303, 333
- ovale 259, 273, 434, 436, 437, 438, 507, 510, 586
- rotundum 434, 435, 436, 438, 510, 586
- spinosum 434, 436, 437, 438, 510
- transversarium 53, 55, 56, 57
Forearm 3, 88, 119, 120, 121, 133
- anterior compartment 128
- anterior deep muscles 130
- anterior muscles 128
- anterior superficial muscles 129
- arteries 133
- bones 119
- fascia 22
- movements 8
- nerves 133
- posterior compartment 128
- posterior deep muscles 132
- posterior superficial muscles 131
- surface anatomy 118
Forebrain 556
Foregut, blood supply 318
Foreign body aspiration 247
FOREL's axis 556
Fornix 573, 574
- of lacrimal sac 489
- of stomach 311
Fossa
- for lacrimal
-- gland 449
-- sac 428, 484
- of incus 504
- ovalis 259
Fourth ventricle 556, 566, 568, 572, 573
Fovea
- centralis 490, 495, 498
- for ligament of femoral head 162, 163
Fracture of fibula 197
FRANCESCHETTI's syndrome (mandibulo-facial dysostosis) 502
FRANKFORT horizontal line 428, 559

Free taenia 299, 321, 322
Frenulum
- of clitoris 406, 407
- of ileal orifice 322
- of labia minora 406, 407
- of lower lip 455, 461
- of prepuce 397
- of tongue 468, 476
- of upper lip 455, 461
FRENZEL's lenses (FRENZEL's glasses) 516
Frontal
- belly of occipitofrontalis 439, 440, 441, 486, 590
- bone 426, 430, 431, 432, 434, 441, 449, 450, 451, 484, 485
-- squamous part 484
- branch of superficial temporal artery 442, 444, 446
- crest 433, 434
- diploic veins 443, 561
- emissary vein 562
- horn of lateral ventricle 572, 573, 574
- lobe 36, 556, 557, 572
- margin of sphenoid bone 436
- nerve 492, 493, 583, 587
- operculum 556
- plane 6, 66
- pole 557
- process
-- of maxilla 427, 430, 448, 449, 450, 485, 489
-- of zygomatic bone 426, 453
- region 425
- sinus 432, 448, 450, 451, 452, 453, 484
-- development 452
- suture 430, 431
- tuber 429, 430
Frontobasal artery 567
Frontolacrimal suture 427, 428
Frontomaxillary suture 448, 484
Frontomental line 448
Frontonasal suture 426, 427, 448, 450
Frontozygomatic suture 427, 428, 453
Fulcrum 185
Functional occlusal plane 428
Fundiform ligament
- of penis 291, 397
Fundus
- of gallbladder 305, 319, 339, 341
- of stomach 302, 309, 310, 311
- of urinary bladder 347, 376
- of uterus 347, 369, 385, 387, 389, 391
-- level during pregnancy 387
Funduscopy or fundoscopy (direct ophthalmoscopy) 498
Fungiform papillae 467
Fusiform muscle 21

G

Gag (pharyngeal) reflex 596, 599
Gait 211
- cycle 211
Galea aponeurotica 425
GALEN's anastomosis 544
GALEN, vein of (great cerebral vein) 560, 562, 566
Gallbladder 31, 302, 303, 306, 310, 312, 313, 316, 330, 331, 332, 339
- arteries 334
- lymph nodes and vessels 338

GALT (gut-associated lymphoid tissue) 327
Ganglion
– impar 605, 606
– of sympathetic trunk 229, 240, 373, 608, 610, 611
Ganglionic
– branches
– – of maxillary nerve to pterygopalatine ganglion 588
– layer of retina 499
GASSERIAN ganglion (trigeminal or semi-lunar ganglion) 580, 607
Gastric
– arteries 312
– branches of vagal trunk 315
– canal 311
– cancer 314
– – lymphatic drainage 314
– folds 311
– impression
– – on liver 331
– – on spleen 346
– lymph nodes 307, 314, 361
– veins 312
Gastrocnemius 156, 180, 190, 201, 204
– bursa 187, 188
– lateral head 187, 188, 189, 190, 204
– medial head 187, 188, 189, 190, 204
Gastrocolic ligament 299, 300, 302, 303, 304, 310, 333
Gastroduodenal
– artery 312, 318, 325, 329, 334, 340, 342, 345
– ligament 302
Gastroesophageal
– junction 309
– reflux disease (GERD) 309
Gastro-omental lymph nodes 314
Gastropancreatic fold 303
Gastrophrenic ligament 300
Gastrosplenic ligament 297, 300, 302, 303, 310, 346
Gemellus
– inferior 166, 167, 168
– internus 168
– superior 166, 167, 168
Geniculate ganglion 466, 508, 510, 580, 590, 591, 592, 600
– lesions 593
Geniculocalcarine tract 500
Genioglossus 468, 469, 470, 473, 475, 476, 530, 602
Geniohyoid 468, 469, 470, 473, 474, 477, 526, 530, 547, 602
Genital
– branch of genitofemoral nerve 214, 217, 292, 356, 397, 612
– organs
– – in man 370
– – – innervation 397
– – in woman 369, 388
– – – innervation 396
– – – lymphatic drainage 395
– – – pain afferences 396
Genitofemoral nerve 214, 215, 217, 292, 296, 321, 348, 355, 356, 397
Genu
– of corpus callosum 566, 574
– of fornix 568
– valgum 156, 184
– varum 156, 184
GEROTA's fascia (renal fascia) 348, 349

GILULA arcs 123
– loss 124
GIMBERNAT's ligament (lacunar liga-ment) 292
Gingiva 455, 461
Gingival papilla 461
Glabella 426, 448
Glandular branches
– of inferior thyroid artery 547
Glans
– of clitoris 406, 407
– penis 397, 398, 403
Glaucoma 496
– optic disc 498
Glenohumeral
– joint 88, 89, 96, 97
– – dislocation 97
– – radiograph 96
– – range of motion 98
– ligament 96
Glenoid
– fossa 89, 91, 95, 96, 97
– joint, downward and upward rota-tion 100
– labrum 97
Globus pallidus 568
Glomerulus
– of olfactory bulb 582
– renal corpuscle 354
Glossopharyngeal
– nerve [CN IX] 272, 437, 438, 467, 470, 471, 478, 479, 503, 509, 530, 533, 534, 544, 563, 566, 576, 578, 579, 581, 586, 589, 590, 594, 597, 604
– – complete lesion 599
– – fiber qualities 577, 594, 595, 596
– – innervation 577
– – lesions 596
– – parasympathetic ganglion 581
– – sensory ganglion 580
– part of superior constrictor 455, 469, 532
Glottic space (glottis) 543
– enlarged view 543
Gluteal
– cleft (gluteal sulcus) 156, 157, 364
– fascia 168, 174
– fold 156
– region 4, 156, 364
– – deep muscles 168
– – intramuscular injections 174
– – muscles 167
– – sensory innervation 217
– – surface anatomy 157
– – vessels and nerves 174
– sulcus (gluteal cleft) 157
– surface of ilium 159
– tuberosity 162
Gluteus
– maximus 41, 156, 157, 166, 167, 168, 173, 174, 211, 408, 409, 411, 413, 416
– medius 166, 167, 168, 173, 174
– – paralysis 174
– minimus 166, 167, 168, 173
– – paralysis 174
Gnathion 426
Goblet cells of conjunctiva 483
Goiter 548
GOLL's tract (gracile fasciculus) 614, 615, 616, 620
Goose bumps 280
GOWERS' tract (anterior spinocerebellar tract) 614, 615, 617

Gracile
– fasciculus (GOLL's tract) 614, 615, 616, 620
– nucleus 616
Gracilis 157, 168, 169, 172, 175, 189, 413
Granular
– cells of olfactory bulb 582
– foveolae 433
GRAVES' disease 548
Gray rami communicantes 240, 360, 606, 610
Great
– auricular nerve 229, 444, 445, 502, 520, 523, 526
– cardiac vein 257, 260, 269
– cerebral vein (vein of GALEN) 499, 560, 562, 566, 573, 574
– cord syndrome 619
– radicular artery (artery of ADAMKIEWICZ) 570, 619
– radicular artery syndrome 619
– saphenous vein 175, 190, 221, 222, 286, 296
– toe 156
Greater
– curvature of stomach 302, 303, 310, 311
– horn of hyoid 469, 473, 476, 532, 536, 537, 540, 544
– occipital nerve 445, 446, 520, 523, 525, 526
– omentum 297, 299, 300, 302, 304, 305, 310, 319, 321, 333, 339
– palatine
– – artery 454, 455, 465, 466
– – block 465
– – canal 436
– – foramen 437, 455, 456
– – nerve 437, 454, 455, 461, 465, 588, 589
– pancreatic artery 329
– pelvis 365, 367
– petrosal nerve 437, 466, 479, 488, 508, 509, 510, 512, 586, 590, 592, 606
– sciatic
– – foramen 160, 161, 168, 368, 405
– – – contents 161
– – notch 158, 159
– splanchnic nerve 229, 237, 251, 252, 278, 279, 280, 315, 328, 358, 360, 605, 606, 608
– supraclavicular fossa 425
– trochanter 156, 157, 162, 163
– tubercle 92, 93
– vestibular glands (BARTHOLIN's glands) 396, 406, 407, 417, 418
– wing of sphenoid 427, 430, 435, 436, 451, 484, 485, 490
GRIDIRON incision 289
Groin (inguinal region) 175, 283
Groove/s
– for brachiocephalic vein 245, 246
– for greater petrosal nerve 434, 510
– for inferior petrosal sinus 434, 510
– for lesser petrosal nerve 434
– for middle
– – meningeal artery 433
– – temporal artery 504
– for radial nerve 93
– for sigmoid sinus 432, 434, 436, 510
– for spinal nerve 53

Groove/s
– for subclavian
– – artery 234, 245, 246
– – vein 234
– for superior sagittal sinus 433, 434
– for transverse sinus 432, 434, 436
– for vertebral artery 56
– of promontory of tympanic cavity 504
GSA (general somatic afferent) 577
– nuclei of cranial nerves 578
GSE (general somatic efferent) 577, 584
– nuclei of cranial nerves 578
Gubernaculum testis 294, 399
Gustatory
– impairment 593
– nucleus 596, 599
– system 600
Gustometry 592, 593
Gut-associated lymphoid tissue
  (GALT) 327
GUYON's canal 134, 139, 145
GVA (general visceral afferent) 577, 603
– nuclei of cranial nerves 578
GVE (general visceral efferent) 577, 603
– nuclei of cranial nerves 578
Gynecomastia 230

H

Hair 24, 25
– bulb 24, 25
– cuticle 25
– follicle 24, 25
– papilla 25
– root 24, 25
– sebaceous glands 24, 25
– shaft 24, 25
Hair cells 513, 515
– damage 514
– neural pathway 513
– synapse 513
Hallux valgus 200
Hamate 119, 122, 123, 124, 134
Hamstring/s 211
– muscles 173, 176, 180
– part of adductor magnus 172
– region 156
Hand 3, 88, 122
– arteries 139, 140
– bones 119
– deep tendons 134
– hypothenar muscles 137
– joints 124
– ligaments 124
– movements 8
– nerves 139
– radiograph 122
– superficial tendons 134, 135
– surface anatomy 118
– thenar muscles 136
Handle of malleus 505, 506, 509
Hands in pocket 78
Hard palate 452, 455, 456, 464, 507
– neurovascular supply 465
Haustra of colon 321, 322
HAVERSIAN canal 15
Head 3
– arteries 446, 447
– blood vessels 444, 445, 446, 447
– intra- and extracranial veins 562
– lateral deepest regions 447

Head
– lateral deep regions 444, 446
– lateral regions 447
– lateral superficial regions 444
– nerves 444, 445, 446, 447
– of epididymis 400, 401
– of femur 162, 163, 164
– of fibula 156, 178, 179, 181, 191, 193
– of humerus 92, 93, 97
– of malleus 506
– of mandible 457, 459, 460, 503
– of metatarsal 194
– of pancreas 342, 344
– of phalanx of foot 194
– of radius 6, 110, 121
– of rib 234
– of talus 194, 197, 198
– of ulna 120
– position during endotracheal intubation 542
– regions 4, 425
– sensory innervation 524, 526
– superficial lymph nodes and lymphatic
  vessels 550
Headache 444
HEAD's zones 284, 611
Hearing impairment, asymmetric 510
Hearing loss, unilateral 511
Heart 27, 254, 257
– anterior view 257
– autonomic innervation 272
– conducting system 268, 270
– contours 254
– cross section 255
– fibrous skeleton 258
– innervation 272
– murmurs 263
– position within the pericardium 255
– posterior view 257
– projection onto the anterior thoracic
  wall 228, 254
– silhouette, chest X-ray 254
– veins 269
Heel 4
HEGAR's sign 387
HEISTER's valve (spiral fold) 339
Helicine branches of uterine artery 394
Helicotrema 511
Helix 502
Hematocele testis 400
Hemianesthesia 620
Hemiazygos vein 239, 240, 279, 308, 337
Hemidiaphragm
– radiograph 236
Hemiplegia
– BROWN-SÉQUARD syndrome 619, 620
Hemorrhoidal knots 371, 374
Hemorrhoids 374
HENLE's layer 25
HENLE's loop 354
HENSEN's cells 512
Hepatic
– artery proper 318, 329, 331, 332, 334,
  335, 340, 345
– bile duct 335
– branches
– – of vagal trunk 315
– – of vagus nerve 307, 597, 598
– lymph nodes 314, 338, 345, 358, 361
– plexus 597, 598

Hepatic
– portal vein 273, 308, 312, 313, 316, 318,
  325, 331, 332, 334, 335, 336, 337, 340,
  342
– – tributaries 336
– veins 273, 335, 337
Hepatoduodenal ligament 300, 302, 303,
  305, 310, 332, 333, 334, 346
Hepatogastric ligament 300, 302, 303,
  310, 312, 333, 346
Hepatopancreatic
– ampulla 317, 339, 341, 344
– – arteries 341
– fold 303
Hepatorenal
– recess of omental bursa (MORRISON's
  pouch) 301, 333
Herniated intervertebral disk (slipped
  disk) 148, 610
Herpes zoster 609
– ophthalmicus 585
HESCHL's transverse convolutions
  (transverse temporal gyri) 513, 514
HESSELBACH's ligament (interfoveolar
  triangle) 290
HESSELBACH's triangle (inguinal
  triangle) 290, 295, 377
HEUBNER's recurrent artery (distal medial
  striate artery) 565, 567
Hiatal gastric hernia 309
Hiatus
– for lesser petrosal nerve 596
– saphenus 296
High endothelial venules (HEVs) 30, 287
Hilar lymph nodes (tracheobronchial
  lymph nodes) 245, 249, 252, 307
Hilum
– of kidney 349, 351
– of lung 243, 245, 246
Hindbrain 556
Hindgut
– blood supply, innervation and lymphatic
  drainage 327
Hinge joint 17
Hip 3
– abduction 9
– adduction 9
– anterior
– – deep muscles 170
– – superficial muscles 169
– bone 158, 159
– extension 7
– external/internal rotation 9
– flexion 7
– fracture 162
– impingement 164
– joint 163, 164, 167
– – abduction 166
– – adduction 166, 172
– – extension 166, 171, 173
– – external rotation 166, 168
– – flexion 166, 170
– – internal rotation 166
– – medial rotation 166
– – movements 166
– – osteoarthritis 164
– – radiograph 162, 163
– – range of motion 170
– movements 9
– posterior
– – deep muscles 168
– – muscles 167

Hippocampal sulcus 557
Hippocampus 573, 574, 600
HIS, bundle of (atrioventricular
  bundle) 258, 268, 270
Hoarseness 599
Homonymous
– hemianopsia (hemianopia) 500
– quadrantanopia (quadrantanopsia,
  quadrant anopia) 500
Hordeolum (stye) 483
Horizontal
– axis 7
– cells of retina 499
– fissure of right lung 245
–– projection onto the anterior thoracic
  wall 227
– part of duodenum 299, 317, 342, 347
– plane 6
– plate of palatine 431, 449, 450, 451,
  456
HORNER's muscle (lacrimal part of orbicularis oculi) 486
HORNER's syndrome 551, 607
Horseshoe kidney 348
HOUSTON's valves (transverse folds of
  rectum) 371
HUETER's triangle 112
Humeral axillary lymph nodes 231, 232
Humeroradial joint 88, 110, 111
Humeroulnar joint 88, 111
Humerus 6, 88, 89, 92, 93, 110, 119
– anatomical neck 92
– fractures 93
–– radiograph 93
– proximal fractures 144
– radiograph 92
– range of motion 100
Humpback 65
HUXLEY's layer 25
Hyaline cartilage 16, 18
Hydrocele testis 400
– ultrasound image 400
Hydrocephalus 574
– ex vacuo 574
Hydronephrosis 353, 381
Hymen 406
Hyoepiglottic ligament 530, 537
Hyoglossus 469, 470, 474, 529, 532, 547,
  602
Hyoid bone 441, 468, 469, 471, 473, 474,
  476, 477, 521, 528, 529, 530, 532, 536,
  537, 539, 540, 543, 546, 547, 551
Hyperacusis 508, 593
Hyperhydrosis 603
Hyperkyphosis 65
Hyperlordosis 43
Hyperopia (farsightedness) 497
Hyperthyroidism 548
Hypesthesia 567
Hypochondriac region 283
Hypochondrium 225, 283
Hypodermis 24
Hypogastric
– nerve 373, 396, 403, 421, 422, 605
– plexus 422
– region 283
Hypogastrium 299, 364
– position oft the abdominal viscera 299
Hypogeusia 600

Hypoglossal
– canal 432, 434, 437, 438, 602
– nerve [CN XII] 437, 438, 441, 447, 467,
  470, 473, 474, 475, 476, 477, 478, 520,
  524, 525, 526, 529, 533, 534, 563, 576,
  578, 579, 602
–– fiber qualities 577, 578, 602
–– innervation 577
–– palsy 468
Hyponychium 26
Hypopharynx 530
Hypophysial fossa 434, 436, 450, 564
Hypophysis 560
Hyposmia 582
Hypothalamus 32, 556, 600
Hypothenar 136
– eminence 87
– muscles 137
– region 118, 137
Hypotympanic recess 505
Hypotympanum 505
Hysterectomy 392

I

Ileal
– arteries 324, 325, 329
– branch of ileocolic artery 324
– diverticulum 320
– lymph nodes 361
– orifice 322
– papilla 322
– veins 336
Ileocecal
– fold 299
– junction 319
– valve (BAUHIN's valve) 322
Ileocolic
– artery 324, 325, 329
– lymph nodes 327, 361
– vein 336
Ileum 299, 305, 323, 325
– arterial arcades 320
– position 319
Ileus 320
– malrotation 298
Iliac
– artery 355
– crest 41, 68, 102, 157, 158, 159, 364
– fossa 159
– lymph nodes 395
– tuberosity 159
– vein 355
Iliacus 77, 80, 170, 171, 172, 296, 321, 384,
  385
Iliococcygeus 368
Iliocostalis 72
– cervicis 72
– lumborum 70, 72
– thoracis 70, 72
Iliofemoral ligament 163, 164
Iliohypogastric nerve 214, 215, 217, 284,
  300, 321, 348, 350, 356
Ilioinguinal nerve 214, 215, 217, 284, 291,
  292, 293, 300, 348, 350, 356, 411
Iliolumbar
– artery 409, 419
– ligament 160
Iliopectineal arch 160, 290, 296
Iliopsoas 166, 170, 171, 172, 211, 296, 382
Iliopubic eminence 159

Iliotibial band (ITB) 166, 167, 169, 186
Ilium 68, 74, 158, 159, 163, 365, 367
Impingement syndrome 100
Impressions of cerebral gyri 434
Inca bone (interparietal bone) 429
Incisive
– artery 454
– block 465
– bone 456
– branch of nasopalatine nerve 461
– canal 432, 448, 450, 451
– foramen 437, 449, 456, 465
– fossa 437, 448, 456
– nerve 454
– papilla 464
– suture 456
Incudomallear joint 506
Incudostapedial joint 506, 509
Incus 505, 506, 508, 509, 513, 592
Index finger 87, 118
Indirect inguinal hernia 289, 294, 295
Indirect laryngoscopy 541
Infectious meningitis 444
Inferior 5
– alveolar
–– artery 442, 446, 447, 466, 473, 478
–– block 465
–– nerve 446, 447, 460, 461, 465, 473,
  478, 585, 589
–– vein 466, 473, 478
– anal nerves 411, 414, 416
– angle of scapula 41, 91
– articular
–– process 44, 49, 55, 57, 67, 68, 69
–– surface
––– of tibia 192, 197
––– of vertebra 69
– belly of omohyoid 520, 521, 524, 526,
  528, 529, 546
– border
–– of left lung 246
–– of right lung 245
– branch/es
–– of oculomotor nerve [CN III] 492, 583,
  584
–– of transverse cervical nerve 523
– bulb of jugular vein 524, 533
– carotid artery 527
– cerebellar peduncle 617
– cervical
–– cardiac
––– branches of vagus nerve 272, 307,
  597, 598
––– nerve 272, 551, 605
–– ganglion 551, 605
– clunial nerves 217, 411, 416
– colliculus 514
– conjunctival fornix 489
– constrictor 521, 525, 532, 533, 597
– coracohumeral ligament 96
– costal facet 44, 66
– crura 486
– deep cervical lymph nodes (scalene
  lymph nodes) 249
– deep lateral cervical lymph nodes 550
– dental plexus 447, 465, 589
– duodenal fossa 299
– epigastric
–– artery 285, 286, 290, 292, 294, 295,
  359, 377, 402, 419
––– anastomoses 285
–– vein 286, 290, 292, 337, 377, 402, 420

Inferior
- extensor retinaculum 206
- eyelid 482, 488
- ganglion
-- of accessory nerve 601
-- of glossopharyngeal nerve 533, 580, 594, 595, 596, 599, 600, 603
-- of vagus nerve 533, 580, 597, 598, 599, 600, 603, 611
- gemellus 166, 167, 168
- gluteal
-- artery 161, 174, 219, 220, 394, 409, 419
-- line 159
-- nerve 161, 167, 174, 214, 216
-- vein 161, 174
- head of lateral pterygoid 459, 460
- hemorrhoidal artery 329
- horn
-- of lateral ventricle 572, 573
-- of thyroid cartilage 536, 537, 538, 540, 544
- hypogastric
-- ganglion 360
-- plexus 328, 373, 375, 396, 398, 403, 421, 422, 604, 605
- hypophysial artery 564
- ileocecal recess 299
- labial
-- branch (of facial artery) 442
-- vein 443
- lacrimal
-- canaliculus 489
-- punctum 489
- laryngeal artery 544
- lateral
-- cutaneous nerve of arm 108, 144, 147, 229
-- genicular artery 189, 212, 220
- left homonymous
-- quadrantanopia (quadrantopsia, quadrant anopia) 500
- ligament of epididymis 400
- lingular segment of left lung 247
- lobar bronchus 245
- lobe
-- of left lung 246
-- of right lung 245, 246, 265
- longitudinal muscle of tongue 468, 602
- medial genicular artery 189, 212, 220
- mediastinum 250
-- anatomical structures 250
- mesenteric
-- artery 325, 329, 359, 374, 421, 605
--- branches 326
--- course 326
-- ganglion 328, 360, 373, 421, 604
-- lymph nodes 327, 361, 375
-- plexus 328, 421, 605
-- vein 313, 337
--- course 326
--- tributaries 336
- nasal
-- concha 426, 450, 451, 452, 454, 456, 489, 531, 583
-- meatus 451, 452, 489
- nuchal line 429
- oblique 487, 489, 490, 491, 494, 583, 584
- ophthalmic vein 443, 487, 492, 562
- orbital fissure 426, 436, 437, 451, 484, 485, 488, 490
-- neurovascular structures 492

Inferior
- palpebral arch 487
- pancreatic
-- artery 329, 345
-- lymph nodes 345
- pancreaticoduodenal
-- artery 324, 325, 329, 345
--- anterior branch 324
--- posterior branch 324
-- vein 318
- parathyroid gland 532, 534, 544, 547, 548
- petrosal sinus 560
- phrenic
-- artery 237, 357, 358, 359
-- lymph nodes 307, 338
-- vein 337
- pubic
-- ligament 160, 405, 407, 413
-- ramus 158, 159, 160, 407
- pulmonary artery 256
- recess
-- of acoustic meatus 503
-- of omental bursa 302, 303, 304, 333
- rectal
-- artery 329, 374, 409, 414, 416
-- nerves 410, 411, 414, 416
-- vein 336, 337, 374, 375, 409, 420
- rectus 487, 490, 491, 583, 584
- renal polar artery 352
- root of ansa cervicalis (cervical plexus) 524, 526
- sagittal sinus 560, 562
- salivatory nucleus 477, 479, 509, 578, 579, 581, 595, 596
- superficial inguinal lymph nodes 287
- suprarenal artery 348, 357, 358
- surface of tongue 476
- tarsal plate 486
- tarsus 486, 487
- temporal
-- line of parietal bone 429, 441
-- retinal
--- arteriole 498
--- venule 498
- terminal branches of middle cerebral artery 567
- thoracic aperture 233
- thyroid
-- artery 307, 525, 533, 534, 544, 547, 551
-- notch 538
-- tubercle 538
-- vein 275, 525, 529, 547, 551
- tibiofibular joint 191
- tracheobronchial lymph nodes (carinal lymph nodes) 245, 246, 249, 253
- transverse
-- fold of rectum 375
-- scapular ligament 108
- trunk of brachial plexus 106, 141
- tympanic artery 509
- ulnar collateral artery 149
- vena cava 237, 254, 255, 256, 257, 259, 269, 273, 279, 308, 313, 323, 325, 332, 337, 343, 348
- vertebral
-- end plate 69
-- notch 54, 68
- vesical
-- artery 355, 394, 419, 420
-- vein 420
- vestibular nucleus (ROLLER's nucleus) 512, 516, 578

Inflammatory bowel disease (IBD) 327
- perianal abscess 416
Inflammatory headache 444
Inflated lung 243
Infracallosal part
- of anterior cerebral artery 563
Infraclavicular part of brachial plexus 106, 525
Infracolic compartment (hypogastrium) 299, 301
Infraglenoid tubercle 91, 96
Infrahyoid 520
- bursa 537
- muscles 521
Inframammary region 225
Infranuclear (peripheral) facial palsy 591
Infraorbital
- artery 442, 447, 466, 487, 492, 494
- block 465
- canal 451, 484, 485
- fissure 466, 485
- foramen 427, 430, 453, 484, 585
- groove 484
- margin 427
- nerve 441, 445, 446, 447, 454, 465, 487, 488, 489, 490, 494, 583, 585, 588
-- local infiltrative anesthesia 465
- region 425
- vein 487, 492
Infrapatellar
- branch of saphenous nerve 217
- cartilage 18
- fat pad 182
Infrapiriform foramen 168, 174
Infrascapular region 4, 225
Infraspinatus 104, 142
Infraspinous
- fossa of scapula 91
Infrasternal angle 226
- vertebral projection 228
Infratemporal
- crest 435
- fossa 485, 490
Infratrochlear
- artery 487
- nerve 446, 447, 487, 494, 587
- vein 487
Infundibular recess of fourth ventricle 572
Infundibulopelvic ligament (suspensory ligament of ovary) 369, 385, 388, 389, 391, 394
Infundibulum
- of pituitary gland 564
- of uterine tube 389
Inguinal
- canal 291, 292, 293
-- borders 292
-- walls and content 292
- falx (conjoint tendon) 292
- hernia 289, 295
-- congenital 400
- ligament 77, 78, 156, 157, 160, 175, 291, 292, 295, 296, 364, 397, 405
- lymph nodes 30, 327, 375, 395, 404
- nerve 292, 321, 397
- region 283, 364
-- radiating pain 356
-- sensory innervation 217
- ring 399
- triangle (HESSELBACH's triangle) 290, 377
Inion 429

Inner
- border cells 512
- ear 510, 511, 515
-- blood supply and innervation 511
-- mechano-electrical sound conduction 513
-- sensory cells 515
- hair cells 512, 513, 515
- lip of iliac crest 159
- pharyngeal cells 512
- pilar cells 512
- spiral sulcus 512
- subarachnoid spaces 572
Innermost intercostal muscle 238, 241, 242, 244
INSALL-SALVATI ration of the patellar ligament length 185
Inspiration muscles 238
Insula 556, 567, 568, 600
Insular part of middle cerebral artery 563
Integumentary system 11, 24
- functions 24
Interarticular portion
- of vertebrae, fracture 68, 69
Interarytenoid
- fold of rima glottidis 541
- notch 541, 544
Interatrial septum 259
Intercarpal joints 123
Intercartilaginous part of rima glottidis 541
Intercavernous sinuses 560, 564
Interclavicular ligament 94
Intercondylar
- eminence 178, 179, 192
- fossa 178, 179
- notch 178
Intercostal
- arteries 239, 241, 242, 248, 285
- muscles 235
- nerves 106, 147, 231, 238, 241, 242, 244, 251, 278, 279, 280, 608
-- cutaneous branches 229, 240
- neurovascular structures 241
- space
-- arteries 239
-- structures 244
- veins 241, 242
Intercostobrachial nerves 141, 147, 525
Intercrural fibers 291
Interdental
- cells 512
- (gingival) papilla 461
Interfascicular
- fasciculus
-- cervical part (SCHULTZE's comma tract) 614
-- lumbar and sacral tract (triangle of PHILIPPE-GOMBAULT) 614
Interfoveolar ligament (HESSELBACH's ligament) 290
Interganglionic branches of sympathetic trunk 606
Intergluteal cleft 405
Interlobar
- artery of kidney 354
- vein of kidney 354
Interlobular
- artery of liver 335
- bile duct 335
- vein of liver 335
Intermammary cleft 226
Intermaxillary suture 427

Intermediate
- column of spinal cord 613, 614
- cuneiform 194, 195
- dorsal cutaneous nerve 217
- hepatic vein 332, 335
- line of iliac crest 159
- nerve 479, 576, 578, 581, 590, 593
- periaqueductal gray substance 614
- sacral crest 75
- supraclavicular nerves 523, 526
- tendon of digastric 474
- tubule of kidney 354
Intermediolateral nucleus of spinal cord 614
Intermembranous part of rima glottidis 541
Intermetacarpal joints 123
Intermetaphyseal artery 82
Intermetatarsal joints 200
Intermuscular septum 22
Internal
- acoustic
-- meatus 432, 438, 510, 511, 512, 590, 593
-- opening 510
-- pore 432, 434, 438, 504, 510
- anal sphincter 371, 372, 373, 383
- auditory artery 509
- axis of eyeball 495
- branch
-- of accessory nerve [CN XI] 533, 534
-- of recurrent laryngeal nerve 544
-- of superior laryngeal nerve 533, 544, 547, 551
- capsule 567, 568, 573
- carotid
-- artery 274, 442, 446, 447, 466, 478, 487, 488, 493, 494, 499, 507, 508, 510, 520, 525, 533, 534, 563, 564, 565, 566, 567, 568, 592, 594
--- angiogram 565
-- nerve 466, 533
-- plexus 466, 488, 590, 594
-- venous plexus 507
- cerebral veins 562, 574
- female genitalia
-- blood supply 394
-- development 388
-- lymph nodes and vessels 395
-- structure/function 388
-- veins 395
- geniculum of facial nerve 593
- hernia 304
- iliac
-- artery 81, 219, 321, 329, 355, 359, 374, 392, 394, 409, 414, 419, 420, 421, 570
--- branches 419
-- lymph nodes 327, 358, 375, 395, 404
-- vein 321, 337, 355, 374, 392, 395, 420
- intercostal
-- membrane 235
-- muscles 235, 238, 241, 242, 278, 279
- jugular vein 249, 275, 361, 441, 443, 466, 470, 478, 507, 520, 524, 525, 528, 529, 533, 551, 562
- male genitalia 397
-- blood vessels 401
-- development 399
-- lymphatic drainage 404
-- lymph nodes and lymph vessels 404
- mammary
-- artery 239, 240, 286
-- vein 239, 240, 286

Internal
- nasal branches
-- of anterior ethmoid nerve 587
-- of infraorbital nerve 454, 587
- oblique 70, 77, 78, 79, 288, 289, 291, 292, 294, 295, 349
- obturator 385, 393
- occipital protuberance 434, 436
- opening of carotid canal 438, 564
- part of thyroarytenoid 540
- plate 433
- pudendal
-- artery 161, 174, 219, 374, 394, 409, 411, 413, 414, 416, 418, 419
--- branches 409
-- nerve 418
-- vein 161, 174, 409, 413, 416, 418, 420
- spermatic fascia 291, 293, 294, 295, 399, 400
- table of calvaria 425, 433
- thoracic
-- artery 231, 232, 237, 239, 240, 241, 251, 278, 285, 286, 525, 527, 551
-- vein 231, 232, 239, 241, 275, 286, 529, 551
- urethral
-- orifice 369, 378
-- sphincter 376
- vertebral venous plexus 569, 571
Internasal suture 426
Interosseous
- border
-- of fibula 193
-- of radius 121
-- of tibia 192
-- of ulna 120
- intercarpal ligaments 123, 124
- membrane 16
-- of forearm 119, 132
-- of leg 188, 191, 201
- metacarpal ligaments 123, 124
- sacroiliac ligament 160
- veins of forearm 150
Interparietal bone (inca bone) 429
Interpectoral
- lymph nodes (ROTTER's lymph nodes) 231, 232
Interphalangeal joint 194
Interpubic disc 160
Interscalene brachial plexus block 275
Intersected muscle 21
Intersigmoid recess 299
Interspinales cervicis 73
Interspinous
- ligament 50, 571, 613
- plane 283
Intertendinous connections of extensor digitorum 135
Interthalamic adhesion 572, 574
Intertragic incisure 502
Intertransversarii
- mediales lumborum 73
- thoracis 73
Intertransverse ligaments 51, 73
Intertrochanteric
- crest 158
- line 162, 163
Intertubercular
- groove or sulcus of humerus 92, 93, 96
- plane 283
- tubercle 181

Interventricular
- foramen (foramen of MONRO) 562, 572, 573, 574
- septal branches
-- of left coronary artery 267
-- of right coronary artery 267
- septum 259, 260, 273
Intervertebral
- disc 45, 47, 48, 50, 67, 234, 571, 613
-- degeneration 48
-- prolapse 48
-- space 65, 68
- fibrocartilage 48
- foramen 45, 48, 55, 68, 234
-- narrowing 45, 46, 148
- joint 53
- surface 67, 68
- vein 82
Intestinal
- branches of vagus nerve 597, 598
- loop 298
- lymphatic trunk 361
- rotation 298
- tract, autonomic innervation 330
- trunk 307, 327
- wall, gangrene 320
Intestine
- blood supply 324, 327
- innervation 327, 328
- lymphatic drainage 327
- parasympathetic nerve fibers 328
- sympathetic nerve fibers 328
Intracerebral bleeding 561
Intracranial part
- of vertebral artery 527
Intrajugular process 436, 504
Intramural
- ganglia (AUERBACH's plexus) 581
- part of ureter 355
- urethra 378
Intraocular pressure, increased 496
Intraparotid plexus 592
Intraperitoneal (subperitoneal) abdominal organs 300
Intrapulmonary
- lymph nodes 249
- lymph system 249
- peribronchial lymphatic system 249
Intraureteric crest 376
Intravenous pyelography 353
Intrinsic foot muscles 211
Introchanteric crest 162
Investing layer of cervical fascia 521
Involuntary proprioception 617
Iridocorneal angle 495, 496
- blockade 496
Iris 482, 495, 496
Irregular bones 13
Ischemic stroke 567
Ischial
- spine 158, 159
- tuberosity 157, 158, 159, 163, 168, 173, 405, 407, 413, 416
Ischioanal fossa 382, 393, 408, 413, 416, 417, 418
- borders 416
- inflammation 371
- in man 415, 416, 418
-- neurovascular structures 416
- in woman 418
Ischiocavernosus 406, 407, 408, 409, 411, 412, 413, 415, 416, 418

Ischiococcygeus (coccygeus) 367, 368, 420
Ischiofemoral ligament 163, 164
Ischiopubic ramus 159, 405, 407, 413
Ischium 158, 159, 365
Isometric contraction 20
Isthmus
- of cervix 391
- of fauces 455, 530
- of omental bursa 303
- of thyroid gland 529, 546, 547, 548
- of uterine tube 389
- of uterus 387, 388, 391

J

JACOBSON's anastomosis 509, 594, 595, 596
JACOBSON's nerve (tympanic nerve) 479, 594, 595, 596
Jejunal
- arteries 324, 325, 326, 329
- lymph nodes 361
- veins 325, 326, 336
Jejunum 299, 316, 324, 325, 343
- arterial arcades 320
- position 319
Joint
- capsule 23
- of head of rib 66, 234
Joints 12
- types 16
JONE's fracture 195
Jugular
- foramen 434, 437, 438, 510, 533, 594, 595, 596, 597, 599, 601
- fossa 504
- ganglion
-- of glossopharyngeal nerve 580
-- of vagus nerve 580
- nerve 533
- notch 226, 233, 436, 519, 528
-- of sternum 86
-- projection onto the thoracic wall 228
- process 436
- pulse 443
- (superior) ganglion of accessory nerve 601
- trunk 307
- tubercle 436
- vein 508, 524
- venous arch 529
Jugulodigastric lymph node 550
Jugulo-omohyoid lymph node 550
Juxtaesophageal lymph nodes 253
Juxtaintestinal mesenteric lymph nodes 327

K

KEITH-FLACK, node of (sinuatrial node, SA node) 259, 270
KELLGREN-LAWRENCE classification
- osteoarthritis of the knee joint 177
KERCKRING's valves (circular folds of small intestine) 317
Kidney 34, 302, 343, 347, 349, 351, 357, 358, 388, 399, 402
- angiography 34
- blood supply 351
- CT cross section 349
- functional organization 354

Kidney
- innervation 358
- lymphatic drainage 358
- malignant tumors 349
- position
-- in relation to the nerves of the lumbar plexus 350
-- in the retroperitoneal space 348
- projection onto the dorsal body wall 348
- spatial relation 348
- structural organization 353
- ultrasound image 350
KIESSELBACH's area 454
KILLIAN's dehiscence 532
KILLIAN's muscle (transverse part of inferior constrictor) 532
KILLIAN's triangle 532
Knee
- adduction 167
- anterior cruciate ligament (ACL) 183
- axes 181
- bones
-- anterior view 178
-- posterior view 179
- conventional radiograph (X-ray) 12
- joint 177, 188
-- APEX ligament 183
-- bursae 187
-- bursitis 187
-- collateral ligaments 182
-- extension 171, 181, 185
-- external rotation 173
-- flexion 173, 181
-- internal rotation 173
-- ligaments 177, 183
-- locked-out position 182
-- menisci 184
--- injuries 184
-- movements 9
-- osteoarthritis 177
-- PAIN ligament 183
-- radiograph 177, 178
-- stability 177
- ligamentous instability 180
- MRI 18
- pivot-hinge joint 181
- posterior cruciate ligament (PCL) 183
- range of motion 180
- screw home mechanism 181
- surface anatomy
-- anterior view 176
-- posterior view 176
- valgus force 167
Knee-jerk reflex (patellar tendon reflex) 612
Knock-knees (valgus deformity) 156
KOCH's triangle 259, 270
KOHLRAUSCH's fold (middle transverse fold of rectum) 371, 375
KRISTELLER, mucous plug of 387
Kyphosis 43, 65

L

Labial
- glands 596
- part of orbicularis oris 439
Labium
- majus 406
- minus 406, 407

Labyrinthine
- artery 511, 563, 565
-- thrombotic occlusion 511
- infarction 511
- veins 511
- vestibule 510
Labyrinthitis 515
Lacrimal
- apparatus 489
- artery 487, 488, 493, 494
- bone 427, 450, 451, 484, 485
- canaliculi 489
- caruncle 482, 489
- fold 489
- gland 466, 479, 483, 487, 488, 493, 494, 593, 604
-- excretory ducts 489
-- innervation 488
-- sympathetic and parasympathetic innervation 488
- groove 449
- lake 489
- nerve 466, 487, 488, 492, 493, 494, 583, 587
- nucleus 488
- papilla 482, 489
- part of orbicularis oculi (HORNER's muscle) 486
- punctum 482, 489
- sac 489
Lacrimomaxillary suture 428
Lactiferous
- duct 230
- sinus 230
Lacunae 15
Lacunar ligament (GIMBERNAT's ligament) 292, 296
Lacus lacrimalis 482, 489
Lagophthalmos 439, 591, 593
LAIMER's triangle 532
Lambda 429
Lambdoid
- border 436
- suture 428, 429, 430, 431, 432, 433
Lamina
- affixa 574
- cribrosa of sclera 495
- of cricoid cartilage 530, 538, 539
- of thyroid cartilage 546
LANZ's point 322
Laparoscopy 340
Large intestine 31, 299
- blood supply 324
- lymphatic drainage 327
- projection onto the anterior abdominal wall 321
- radiograph 322
- structural characteristics 321
Laryngeal
- cartilages 537, 539
- glands 543
- inlet 530, 544
- muscles 540, 599, 601
-- paralysis 599
- prominence (ADAM's apple) 528, 529, 536, 538, 546
- ventricle (of MORGAGNI) 541, 543
Laryngopharynx 522, 530
Laryngoscopy 541
Laryngotracheobronchitis 544

Larynx 247, 536, 539, 542, 543
- arteries and nerves 544
- compartments 543
- lymph nodes and lymphatic vessels 550
- preparation for endotracheal intubation 542
- squamous cell carcinoma 541
Lateral 5
- abdominal wall, layers 288
- angle of eye 482, 483
- aortic lymph nodes 395
- aperture of fourth ventricle (foramen of LUSCHKA) 572, 573
- arcuate ligament 237
- atlantoaxial joint 58, 59
- atlanto-occipital ligament 59
- basal segment
-- of left lung 247
-- of right lung 247
- branch/es
-- of left coronary artery (clin. term: diagonal branches) 267
-- of spinal nerve 610
-- of supraorbital nerve 445, 446, 447, 493
- canthotomy 486
- cerebral fossa 557
- cervical
-- cysts 545
-- fistulas 545
-- lymph nodes 550
-- region 4, 225, 425
--- blood vessels and nerves 523, 524, 525
- circumflex femoral
-- artery 162, 175, 219, 220
-- vein 221
- collateral ligament (LCL) 177, 181, 182, 183, 186
-- sprains 182
- collateral ligaments of hand 126
- condyle
-- of femur 162, 176, 178, 179, 181
-- of tibia 176, 178, 179, 181, 192
- cord of brachial plexus 106, 141, 145, 146
- corticospinal (pyramidal) tract 614, 615
- costotransverse ligament 51, 52
- cricoarytenoid 540
- crus
-- of major alar cartilage of nose 448
-- of superficial inguinal ring 291
- cuneiform 194, 195
- cutaneous
-- branch/es
--- of iliohypogastric nerve 217
--- of intercostal artery 240
--- of intercostal nerve 229, 240
--- of spinal nerve 229
--- of subcostal nerve 284
--- of thoracic nerve 608
--- of thoracoabdominal nerve 284
-- nerve
--- of forearm 133, 145, 147
--- of thigh 214, 217, 290, 321, 356
- dorsal cutaneous nerve 217
- epicondyle 178
-- of femur 162
-- of humerus 87, 110, 112, 118, 128
- fasciculus proprius 614
- femoral cutaneous nerve 217, 356
- frontobasal artery 563

Lateral
- funiculus of spinal cord 613
- geniculate body 497, 499, 566
- glossoepiglottic fold 467
- head
-- of gastrocnemius 176, 189, 204
-- of triceps brachii 108, 115, 128
- horn of spinal cord 614
- humeral axillary lymph nodes 232
- incisor tooth 461
- inguinal fossa 290, 294, 377
- intercondylar tubercle 178, 179, 192
- lacunae 561
- lamina of pterygoid process 532
- lemniscus 514
- ligament
-- of malleus 506
-- of temporomandibular joint 458
- longitudinal plantar arch 203, 210
- malleolar
-- arterial network 212, 213
-- branches of fibular artery 212, 220
-- facet of talus 197
-- fossa 193
- malleolus 156, 190, 191, 193, 197, 198, 199, 206
- mammary
-- arteries 231, 232
-- branch/es of intercostal artery 240
-- veins 231, 232
- margin of orbit 485
- membranous ampulla 512
- meniscus 177, 182, 183, 184
- nasal
-- cartilages 448
-- wall 452
- palpebral
-- artery 487
-- commissure 482, 483
-- ligament (lateral canthal tendon) 486, 487
- part
-- of medial pterygoid 460
-- of occipital bone 430, 431, 436
- patellar retinaculum 186
- pectoral
-- cutaneous branches of intercostal nerves 147, 231
-- nerve 106, 145, 146
- pharyngeal (parapharyngeal) space 473, 478
- plantar
-- artery 213, 220
-- nerve 213, 216
- plate of sphenoid (pterygoid process) 432, 435, 450
- process
-- of calcaneal tuberosity 194, 198
-- of malleus 506
-- of talus 194, 198
- pterygoid 459, 460
- recess of fourth ventricle 572
- rectus 490, 492, 493, 494, 583
-- paralysis 492, 583
- sacral
-- arteries 409, 414, 419
-- artery 219, 570
-- crest 75
- segment
-- of liver 330, 331
-- of right lung 247

Lateral
- semicircular
-- canal 510, 511
-- duct 510, 511, 515
- spinothalamic tract 614, 615, 616
- sulcus 557, 568
- superior olivary nucleus 513
- supraclavicular nerves 229, 523, 526
- supracondylar line 162
- suprapepicondylar ridge 110
- sural cutaneous nerve 174, 189, 217
- surface
-- of fibula 193
-- of tibia 192
-- of zygomatic 426
- talocalcaneal ligament 199
- tarsal artery 213, 220
- thoracic
-- artery 107, 149, 231, 232, 286
-- vein 231, 232, 286
- thyrohyoid ligament 536, 537, 540
- tibial condyle 178, 179
- tract, dorsal aponeurosis of hand 135
- umbilical
-- fold 290, 377, 420
-- ligament 290
- vein of lateral ventricle 562
- ventricle 568, 572, 573, 574
- vestibular nucleus (DEITERS' nucleus) 512, 516, 578
Latissimus dorsi 41, 71, 86, 102, 103, 143, 238
LE-FORT fractures 427
Left
- anterior descending artery (LAD) 267
- atrioventricular
-- orifice 260
-- valve (mitral valve) 258, 260, 261
--- auscultation site 263
--- during systole and diastole 262
--- projection onto the thoracic wall 228
--- projection onto the ventral thoracic wall 254
--- stenosis 253
- atrium 257, 260, 262, 265, 266, 269, 273
- auricle 254, 257, 258, 260, 266, 269
- bundle branch 270
- colic
-- artery 325, 326, 329
-- flexure 299, 301, 321, 322
-- vein 325, 326, 336, 337
- commissural cusp of left atrioventricular valve (mitral valve) 261
- coronary artery 257, 260, 266, 267, 268, 269
-- branches 267
- fibrous
-- ring 258, 260, 261
-- trigone of heart 258, 261
- gastric
-- artery 312, 318, 325, 329, 334
-- vein 308, 312, 313, 336, 337
- gastro-omental (gastroepiploic)
-- artery 312, 314, 325, 329, 334
-- vein 312, 313, 325, 336
- hemidiaphragm 236
- hepatic vein 332
- inferior
-- lobar bronchus 247
--- projection onto the thoracic wall 228
-- phrenic vein 351
-- pulmonary veins 246, 260

Left
- intracolic compartment 299
- lamina of thyroid cartilage 532, 536, 538
- lobe
-- of liver 302, 303, 305, 310, 330, 331, 333, 334, 339
-- of thyroid gland 532, 547, 548
- lung 246, 247
- main [principal] bronchus 246, 247, 264, 306
-- projection onto the thoracic wall 228
- marginal
-- branch
--- of left coronary artery 267
--- of right coronary artery 266
-- vein 269
- paracolic gutter 301
- pulmonary
-- artery 246, 269
-- veins 246, 269
- renal vein 337
- semilunar cusp 260
-- of aortic valve 261
-- of pulmonary valve 261
- superior
-- lobar bronchus 247
--- projection onto the thoracic wall 228
-- pulmonary veins 246, 260
- triangular ligament of liver 300, 333
- ventricle 254, 255, 257, 258, 260, 262, 265, 269, 273
-- projection onto the thoracic wall 228, 254
Leg 3
- anterior muscles 201, 202
- lateral muscles 201, 203
- posterior compartment, deep layer 205
- transverse section 201
- vessels and nerves 212
Lens 495, 496, 497
LEONARDO DA VINCI's cord (moderator band) 259, 270
Leptomeninges 558
Lesser
- curvature of stomach 302, 303, 310, 311, 333
- horn of hyoid 469, 473, 536, 537, 540
- occipital nerve 229, 444, 445, 446, 520, 523, 524, 525, 526
- omentum 297, 300, 302, 303, 304, 305, 310, 319, 333
- palatine
-- artery 465
-- canal 436
-- foramina 437, 456
-- nerves 465, 588, 589
- pelvis 365, 367
- petrosal nerve 508, 509, 589, 592, 594, 595, 606
- sciatic
-- foramen 160, 161, 168, 405
--- contents 161
-- notch 159
- splanchnic nerve 237, 252, 278, 280, 307, 315, 328, 358, 360, 605, 606
- supraclavicular fossa 425
- trochanter 158, 162, 163, 164
- tubercle 92, 93
- wing of sphenoid 427, 434, 435, 451, 484

Levator
- anguli oris 439, 441, 590
- ani 367, 368, 371, 374, 375, 382, 384, 393, 408, 409, 411, 412, 413, 416, 418
- hiatus 368
- labii superioris 439, 440, 441, 486, 590
-- alaeque nasi 439, 440, 441, 486, 590
- palpebrae superioris 486, 487, 490, 493, 494, 583, 584
-- paralysis 491
- scapulae 61, 71, 103, 142, 519, 521, 525
- veli palatini 472, 507, 532, 594, 596, 597
-- loss of function 507
-- paralysis 596
Levatores costarum 73
Ligament
- of head of femur 164
- of left vena cava 331
- of ovary 369, 388, 389, 391, 392, 394
Ligaments 12, 22, 23
- organization 23
Ligamentum(-a)
- arteriosum 252, 255, 257, 273
- flavum 50, 51, 52, 571
- venosum 273, 331
Limbic lobe 557
Limbus fossae ovalis 259
Limen nasi 452
Linea
- alba 77, 78, 288, 289, 291
- aspera 162
- semilunaris 79
- terminalis 161, 365
Linear skull fractures 433
Lingual
- aponeurosis 468
- artery 442, 446, 447, 470, 473, 475, 477, 524, 533, 547
- branch/es
-- of glossopharyngeal nerve 467, 544, 594, 595
-- of vagus nerve 597, 598
- gland 468, 477, 479
- nerve 446, 447, 460, 465, 467, 470, 473, 475, 476, 477, 479, 529, 589, 590, 600
- septum 468
- tonsil 467, 471, 530
- vein 470, 473
Lingula
- of left lung 246
- of mandible 457, 458
LISFRANC's region (tarsometatarsal joints) 194, 195, 200
Little finger 87, 118
LITTRÉ, glands of (urethral glands) 378
Liver 31, 297, 302, 303, 304, 306, 313, 316, 330, 331, 343
- acinus 335
- arteries 334
- blood flow 335
- caudal lymph drainage 338
- cirrhosis 330, 335, 337
- cranial lymph drainage 338
- intraparenchymal lymphatic system 338
- lobules 335
- lymph nodes and vessels 314, 338
- metastases 332
- peritoneal attachments 333
- segments 330, 331, 332
-- relation to the intrahepatic blood vessels 332

Liver
- sonography 335
- subperitoneal lymphatic system 338
Loading response 211
Lobectomy 248
- of thyroid gland 546
Lobes of mammary gland 230
Lobule/s
- of auricle 502
- of testis 400, 401
Local infiltrative anesthesia
- of infraorbital nerve (branches) 465
Long
- ciliary nerves 494, 496, 583, 584, 587, 607
- head
-- of biceps
--- brachii 97, 114
--- femoris 173
-- of triceps brachii 108, 115
- limb of incus 505, 506
- plantar ligament 199, 200, 209
- posterior ciliary arteries 487, 495
- thoracic nerve 105, 106, 142, 525
-- injury 142
Long bones 13
- anatomical features 15
- microstructure 15
Longissimus 72
- capitis 58, 72
- cervicis 72
- thoracis 70, 72
Longitudinal
- arch of foot
-- lateral 210
-- medial 210
- axis 7
- cerebral fissure 557, 567
Longus
- capitis 58, 62, 528, 551
- colli 62, 548, 551
Loop of HENLE 354
Lordosis of cervical spine 53
Loss
- of balance 510
- of GILULA arcs 124
LOUIS, angle of (sternal angle) 226, 228, 233, 250
- vertebral projection 228
Low back pain 170
Lower
- dental arch 461
- esophageal sphincter (LES) 309
- extremity 3
-- arteries 219, 220
-- basic movements 9
-- dermatomes 218
-- innervation 216
-- lymphatic vessels 222
-- paralysis 566
-- sensory innervation 217
-- skeletal ossification 14
-- surface anatomy 156
-- veins 221
- eyelid 482
- facial nerve palsy 439
- head of lateral pterygoid 459, 460
- jaw 457, 473
-- cross-section 473
-- deciduous teeth 463
-- floor of oral cavity 473
-- panoramic radiograph 462, 463

Lower
- leg 3
-- anterior muscles 202
-- fascia 22
-- fractures 191
-- posterior compartment, superficial layer 204
-- surface anatomy 190
-- vessels and nerves 212
- respiratory tract 247
- (supranuclear) facial palsy 591
- tracheotomy 539
Lowest splanchnic nerve 360
Low pressure system 29
Lumbar
- arteries 359, 570, 571
- cistern 613
- epidural block 396
- ganglia 605
- lordosis 43
- lymphatic trunk 361
- lymph nodes 327, 345, 358, 395, 404
- nerve plexus 606
- nerves 217, 571, 610
-- roots 608
- part
-- of diaphragm 237, 571
-- of vertebral column, MRI 613
- plexus 214, 215
-- nerves 356
- puncture 571
- region 4, 283
-- facet joints 49
- segmental arteries 81
- segments of spinal cord 608
- spine 67
-- CT image 46
-- increase in lordotic curve 170
-- radiograph 67, 68
- splanchnic nerves 328, 360, 373, 605, 606
- trunk 307, 327
- vein 571
- vertebrae 42, 44, 67, 571
-- distinguishing features 69
-- lateral radiograph 47
-- radiograph 67, 68
--- scotty dog sign 68
Lumbarization 74
Lumbocostal triangle 237
Lumbosacral
- enlargement of spinal cord 613
- plexus 214, 215
- region, arteries 81
- trunk 214, 356, 421
Lumbricals
- of foot 208, 209
- of hand 137, 138
Lumpectomy 232
Lunate 119, 122, 123, 124
- surface of acetabulum 159, 164
Lung 27, 245, 246
- alveoli 248
- blood vessels 248
- cancer
-- clinical staging 249
-- lobectomy/segmental resection 248
- collapse 242, 243
- lymphatic drainage 249
- lymph nodes 249
- lymph vessels 249
- metastases 248

Lung
- neurovascular structures 245
- projection 242
-- onto the thoracic wall 227
- pulmonary circulation 248
- segments 247
Lunule 26
Lunules of semilunar cusps 260
LUSCHKA, foramen of (lateral aperture of fourth ventricle) 572, 573
Lymphatic
- duct 30, 249
-- confluence 249
- organs 30
- system 11, 30
- vessels 30
Lymph nodes 30
- cross section 30

M

MACKENRODT's ligament (cardinal ligament, transverse cervical ligament) 391, 392
Macula
- lutea 498
- of retina 495, 498
- of saccule 511, 515
- of utricle 511, 515
Macular degeneration, age-related (AMD) 499
MAGENDIE, foramen of (median aperture of fourth ventricle) 572, 573
Major
- alar cartilage of nose 448
- circulus arteriosus of iris 495, 496
- duodenal papilla (ampulla of VATER) 317, 339, 341, 344
-- sphincter 341
- renal calyx 353
- salivary glands 477
- sublingual duct 476, 477
Malleolar
- canal 212, 213
- groove 191, 192, 193
- mortise 191
- prominence 505
- stria 505
Malleolus
- lateralis 197
- medialis 197
Malleus 505, 506, 508, 513, 592
MALT (mucosa-associated lymphoid tissue) 30, 322, 327, 531
Mamillary process 44, 69
Mammary
- carcinoma
-- frequency 232
-- lumpectomy/mastectomy 232
-- sentinel lymph node 232
- gland 230
-- aplasia 230
-- arteries 231
-- blood supply 232
-- lymphatic drainage 232
-- lymph nodes 232
-- veins 231
- region 225
- ridge (milk line) 230

Mandibular
- bone (mandible) 426, 427, 430, 431, 447, 457, 468, 469, 473, 519
-- of a five year old child 463
-- panoramic radiograph 462, 463
- canal 462
- foramen 457, 461
- fossa 459, 460, 504
- fractures, panoramic radiograph 457
- nerve [CN V/3] 437, 438, 447, 465, 470, 479, 488, 493, 494, 507, 526, 581, 583, 585, 586, 589, 594, 600
-- branches 589
- notch 457
- plane 428
- symphysis 430
Mandibulofacial dysostosis (FRANCESCHETTI's syndrome) 502
Manubriosternal
- angle 250
- joint 226, 233
-- vertebral projection 228
Manubrium of sternum 226, 233, 235, 277, 527
- vertebral projection 228
Marginal
- mandibular branch of facial nerve [CN VII] 440, 444, 590, 591
- mandibular gingiva 461
- maxillary gingiva 461
- nucleus 614
- part of orbicularis oris 439
- sinus 560
Masseter 61, 439, 441, 460, 475, 478
Masseteric
- artery 446, 447
- fascia 475, 478
- nerve 446, 447, 589
Mastectomy 232
Masticatory muscles 441, 460, 586
Mastoid
- antrum 504, 509
- artery 509
- border 436
- branch of occipital artery 442
- canaliculus 437
- cells 504, 507
-- inflammation 507
- emissary vein 443, 562
- fontanelle 430, 431
- foramen 429, 432, 434, 437, 504
- lymph nodes 550
- notch 429, 504
- process 61, 428, 429, 503, 504, 505, 508, 532, 592
- region 425
- wall 504
Mastoiditis 507
Maxillary
- artery 442, 446, 447, 466, 559
- bone (maxilla) 426, 427, 430, 431, 436, 448, 452, 456, 471, 484, 485, 489, 530
-- of a five year old child 463
-- panoramic radiograph 462, 463
- hiatus 450, 451, 453
- nerve [CN V/2] 438, 454, 465, 479, 493, 494, 526, 530, 564, 581, 583, 585, 586, 588
-- branches 588
- sinus 449, 451, 452, 453, 456, 462, 485, 489, 490, 583
-- development 452

Maxillary
- surface 435
- tuberosity 436
- vein 443, 447, 466
McBURNEY's abdominal incision 289
McBURNEY's point 322
- appendicitis 322
Mechano-electrical sound conduction of inner ear 513
MECKEL's diverticulum 298, 320
Medial 5
- angle of eye 482, 483
- antebrachial cutaneous nerve 141
- arcuate ligament 237
- basal segment of right lung 247
- border of tibia 192
- branch/es
-- of intercostal artery 240
-- of spinal nerve 610
-- of supraorbital nerve 445, 446, 447, 493
- bundle of lymph collectors
-- in the upper arm 151, 232
- circumflex femoral
-- artery 162, 174, 175, 219, 220
-- vein 221
- clear space (MCS), radiograph 197
- clunial nerves 217
- collateral
-- artery 108, 149
-- ligament (MCL) 177, 182, 183, 186
--- sprains 182
-- ligaments of hand 126
- condyle 183
-- of femur 162, 176, 178, 179, 181
-- of tibia 176, 178, 179, 181, 192
- cord of brachial plexus 106, 141, 145, 146
- cranial fossa 436
- crest of fibula 193
- crural cutaneous nerve 217
- crus
-- of major alar cartilage of nose 448
-- of superficial inguinal ring 291
- cuneiform 194, 195, 198, 200
- cutaneous nerve
-- of arm 106, 147
-- of forearm 105, 106, 147
-- of leg 217
- dorsal cutaneous nerve 217
- epicondyle
-- of femur 162, 178, 179
-- of humerus 87, 110, 112, 118, 128
- frontobasal artery 563
- geniculate body 497, 499, 514, 566
- head
-- of gastrocnemius 176, 189, 204
-- of triceps brachii 115, 128
- incisor tooth 461
- inguinal fossa (HESSELBACH's triangle) 290, 295, 377
- intercondylar tubercle 178, 179, 192
- intermuscular septum of arm 116, 146
- lemniscus 615, 616
- ligament of ankle joint 199
- longitudinal
-- fasciculus 614
-- plantar arch 210
- malleolar
-- arterial network 213
-- branches 220
-- facet of talus 197
- malleolus 156, 190, 191, 192, 197, 198, 199

Medial
- mammary
-- arteries 231, 232
-- branches
--- of intercostal artery 240
--- of intercostal nerve 231
-- veins 231, 232
- meniscus 177, 182, 183, 184
- nucleus of trapezoid body 513
- palpebral
-- artery 487
-- commissure 482
-- ligament 439, 441, 486, 487, 489
-- margin 483
- parabrachial nucleus 600
- part of medial pterygoid 460
- patellar retinaculum 186
- pectoral nerve 106, 141, 145
- plantar
-- artery 213, 220
-- nerve 213, 216
- plate of sphenoid (pterygoid process) 432, 435, 450
- process of calcaneal tuberosity 194
- pterygoid 460, 532
- rectus 490, 491, 494, 583, 584
- segment
-- of liver 330, 331
-- of right lung 247
- superior olivary nucleus 513
- supraclavicular nerves 523, 526
- supracondylar line 162
- supraepicondylar ridge 110
- sural cutaneous nerve 174, 189
- surface
-- of fibula 193
-- of tibia 192
- talocalcaneal ligament 199
- tarsal arteries 213, 220
- temporal artery 446
- thigh
-- muscles 172
-- sensory innervation 217
- tibial condyle 178
- tigh 4
- tract, dorsal aponeurosis of hand 135
- umbilical
-- fold 290, 377, 389
-- ligaments 273
- vestibular nucleus (SCHWALBE's nucleus) 512, 516, 578
- vestibulospinal tract 614
Median
- abdominal incision 289
- antebrachial vein 109, 118, 150
- aperture of fourth ventricle (foramen of MAGENDIE) 572, 573
- arcuate ligament 237
- artery 133, 149
- atlantoaxial joint 58
- cervical line 520
- cricothyroid ligament 528, 530, 536, 537, 539, 540, 546, 547
- cubital vein 150
- eminence of hypthalmus 575
- episiotomy 412
- glossoepiglottic fold 467
- nerve 105, 106, 108, 116, 117, 129, 133, 134, 139, 141, 146, 147
-- compression 134
-- entrapment 139
- palatine suture 456, 465

Median
- plane 6
- sacral
-- artery 359
-- crest 74, 75
-- vein 374
-- vessels 394
- sulcus of fourth ventricle 572
- thyrohyoid ligament 528, 530, 536, 537, 539, 540
- umbilical
-- fold 290, 377
-- ligament 294, 376, 380
Mediastinal
- branches of thoracic aorta 278
- fascia 243
- pleura 243, 244
- surface of left lung 246
Mediastinum 251, 252
- of testis 400
- partitions 250
Mediolateral episiotomy 412
Medulla
- oblongata 512, 556, 557, 566, 568, 572, 605
- of suprarenal gland 357
Medullary
- bone of femur 162
- cavity 15
- straight
-- arteries of kidney 354
-- veins of kidney 354
- stria of fourth ventricle 572
MEIBOMIAN glands (tarsal glands) 483
- granulomatous inflammation 483
MEISSNER's plexus (submucosal plexus) 320, 581
Membranous
- labyrinth 510, 511
- lamina of auditory tube 507
- part of urethra 378, 398
MENIERE's disease 511
Meningeal
- arteries 559
- branch/es
-- of ascending pharyngeal artery 559
-- of internal carotid artery 564
-- of mandibular nerve [CN V/3] 437, 438, 589
-- of maxillary nerve [CN V/2] 588
-- of occipital artery 559
-- of spinal nerve 569, 606, 608, 610
-- of vagus nerve [CN X] 438, 597, 598
-- of vertebral artery 559
Meninges 558, 561
- of spinal cord 569
Meningocele 558, 569
Meningoencephalocele 558
Meningohydroencephalocele 558
Meningomyelocele 569
Menisci, knee joint 184
- injuries 184
Meniscus 183
Mental
- artery 446
- branch (of facial artery) 442
- foramen 427, 430, 439, 457, 461, 585
- nerve 445, 446, 447, 461, 465, 585, 589
- protuberance 427, 457
- region 425
- spine 457
- tubercle 457

Mentalis 439, 440, 441, 590
Mesencephalic
- nucleus of trigeminal nerve 578, 579, 586
Mesencephalon 499, 514, 556, 557, 568
Mesentery 299, 300, 305, 319
- position of the root 319
Mesoappendix 305
Mesocolic
- lymph nodes 327
- taenia 321, 322
Mesocolon 298
Mesoderm 300
Mesoduodenum 298
Mesogastrium 297, 298
Mesonephric duct (WOLFFIAN duct) 388, 399
Mesopharynx 530
Mesorchium 399
Mesorectal
- fascia (visceral pelvic fascia) 375
-- MRI 375
- space, MRI 375
Mesorectum 375
Mesosalpinx 389, 391
Mesotympanum 505
Mesovarium 389, 391
Metacarpal
- ligaments 124
- region 88
Metacarpals 88, 119, 122
Metacarpophalangeal joints (MCP) 88, 118, 126
- abduction 138
- adduction 138
- flexion 138
- range of motion 127
Metanephros 348
Metaphyseal anastomosing artery 82
Metaphysis 15
Metatarsals 194, 195
- transverse fracture, radiograph 195
Metatarsophalangeal joints 200
- range of motion 200
Metencephalon 556, 557
MEYER's loop 499, 500
MEYNERT's axis 556
Midaxillary line 227
Midbrain 556, 568
Midcarpal joint 88, 123
Midclavicular
- line 226
- plane 283
Middle
- abdominal incision 289
- cardiac vein (posterior interventricular vein) 257, 269
- cerebral artery 527, 563, 564, 565, 566, 567, 568
-- clinical segments 563
- cervical
-- cardiac nerve 272, 525, 533, 551, 605
-- ganglion 272, 280, 525, 533, 534, 551, 605
- colic
-- artery 324, 325, 326, 329
-- lymph nodes 327
-- vein 325, 326, 336
- constrictor 469, 532, 533, 594, 597
- coracohumeral ligament 96
- cranial fossa 434, 485
- cuneiform 194
- duodenal artery 334

Middle
- ear
-- arteries 509
-- auditory ossicles 506
-- autonomic and sensory innervation 509
-- infection 592
-- neighboring structures 508
-- pharyngotympanic (auditory) tube 507
-- tympanic membrane 505
- finger 87, 118
- genicular artery 189, 220
- gluteal artery 394
- hemorrhoidal artery 329
- inferior mediastinum 250
- lobar bronchus 245
- lobe of right lung 245, 246
- mediastinum 250
-- anatomical structures 250
- meningeal artery 442, 446, 447, 493, 559
- nasal
-- concha 427, 450, 451, 452, 453, 454, 489
-- meatus 451
- phalanx 88
-- of foot 194, 195
-- of hand 118, 119, 122
- rectal
-- artery 355, 374, 375, 394, 402, 409, 419
-- vein 336, 374, 394, 420
- sacral artery 219
- scalene 61, 62, 141, 235, 238, 521, 528, 551
- superior alveolar
-- block 465
-- nerve 461, 465
- suprarenal artery 348, 357, 358, 359
- temporal
-- artery 442, 446, 447
-- branch of middle cerebral artery 567
-- vein 446, 447
- thyroid vein 529, 547
- transverse fold of rectum (KOHLRAUSCH's fold) 371, 375
- trunk of brachial plexus 106, 141
Midface, central fractures 427
Midgut
- arteries 318
- blood supply, innervation and lymphatic drainage 327
Midinguinal point 291
Midline groove of tongue 467
Migraine 444
Milk line (mammary ridge) 230
Milk teeth 463
Mimic (facial) muscles 439, 440, 441
- paralysis 593
Minor
- alar cartilages of nose 448
- circulus arteriosus of iris 495, 496
- duodenal papilla 341, 344
- renal calyx 353
- sublingual ducts 476, 477
Miosis (myosis) 496, 607
Mitral
- cells of olfactory bulb 582
- valve (left atrioventricular valve) 258, 260, 261
-- auscultation 254, 263
-- during systole and diastole 262
-- projection onto the anterior thoracic wall 254
-- stenosis 253

Moderator band (LEONARDO DA VINCI's cord) 259, 270
Molar tooth/teeth 451, 453, 461
Monoplegia 619
Monosynaptic
– reflex arc 611, 612
– spinal reflexes 612
MONRO, foramen of (interventricular foramen) 562, 572, 573
Mons pubis 379, 405, 406
MORGAGNI ventricle (laryngeal ventricle) 543
MORRISON's pouch (hepatorenal recess of omental bursa) 301, 333
Motoneuron 606
α-motoneurons 618
Motor
– nucleus/i
– – of abducens nerve 578
– – of cranial nerves 618
– – of facial nerve 578, 579, 591, 593
– – of trigeminal nerve 578, 579, 586
– root of trigeminal nerve 586
Mouth 306
MR angiogram
– of arterial supply to brain 564
MTP see Metatarsophalangeal joints 200
Mucosa-associated lymphoid tissue (MALT) 30, 322, 327, 531
Mucous
– membrane of tongue 468
– plug of KRISTELLER 387
MÜLLERIAN ducts (paramesonephric ducts) 388, 399
Multifidus 70, 73
Multipennate muscle 21
Multipolar cells 514
Mumps (epidemic parotitis) 475
Muscle
– architecture 21
– contraction 20
– levers 21
– types of 19
Muscular
– branch/es of tibial nerve 174, 189
– layer
– – of esophagus 311, 532
– – of stomach 311
– process of arytenoid 538, 539
– triangle 425, 528
Musculocutaneous nerve 105, 106, 108, 114, 141, 145, 147, 612
Musculophrenic artery 237, 239, 285
Musculoskeletal system 11, 12, 21
Musculotubal canal 504
Musculus uvulae 455, 534
Mydriasis 496
Myelencephalon 556, 557
Myeloschisis 569
Myenteric nerve plexus (AUERBACH's plexus) 320
Mylohyoid 460, 468, 470, 473, 474, 475, 477, 521, 524, 525, 528, 529, 530, 586
– groove 457, 458
– line 457
– raphe 474
Mylopharyngeal part of superior constrictor 532
Myocardial
– infarction (MI) 263, 267
– – bypass 285
– – patent foramen ovale 259

Myocardial infarction (MI)
– – referred pain 611
– perfusion in CAD 267
Myocardium 255, 258, 259, 260
Myofibril 20
Myometrium 386, 388, 390, 391
Myopia (nearsightedness) 497
Myositis ossificans 171
Myotomes 609
Myringotomy 506

N

Nail 26
– bed 26
– dystrophy 26
– matrix 26
– wall 26
Narrowing (stenosis) of the vertebral canal 148
Nasal
– apex 448
– balloon tamponade 454
– bone 426, 427, 430, 448, 450, 452, 485
– – fractures 448
– cavity 247, 436, 451, 453, 485, 507, 583
– – anterolateral bony demarcation 449
– – arteries 454
– – innervation 454
– – lateral wall 450, 451
– – topographic relationships 530
– crest 426, 432, 456
– glands 479, 593
– hemiretina 500
– region 425
– septal branch of superior labial branch 454
– septum 448, 452, 531, 583
– – bony part 450
– skeleton 448
– surface 449
– vestibule 247, 452
Nasalis 439, 440, 441, 590
Nasion 426, 448
Nasociliary
– nerve 492, 493, 494, 583, 587, 607
– (sensory) root of ciliary ganglion 583, 584, 587
Nasofrontal vein 443, 487
Nasolabial
– angle 448
– fold 448
Nasolacrimal
– canal 456, 485
– duct 485, 489
Nasomaxillary suture 427, 428, 448
Nasopalatine
– artery 454
– block 465
– nerve 437, 454, 465, 588
Nasopharynx 505, 530
– endoscopy 531
Nausea 515
Navicular 194, 195, 198, 200, 210
– articular surface of talus 197
– fossa 378
Nearsightedness (myopia) 497
Neck 3
– anterior
– – and lateral regions 520
– – and posterior triangles 520

Neck
– blood vessels and nerves 529
– cross-sectional anatomy 522
– deep muscles 62
– flexion 61
– movements 10
– MRI 522
– muscles 61, 62, 521
– neurovascular structures 529
– of femur 158, 162, 163
– of fibula 178, 179, 181, 193
– of gallbladder 339
– of mandible 457
– of radius 110, 121
– of rib 234
– of talus 197, 198
– of tooth 462
– posterior muscles 63
– regions 425
– rotation 7, 61
– sensory innervation 524, 526
– spread of infections 522
– structures 551
– suboccipital muscles 64
– superficial lymph nodes and lymphatic vessels 550
– superficial muscles 61, 63, 519
– superficial veins 529
– surface anatomy 519, 528, 546
– triangles 528
NEER classification of humeral fractures 93
Nephrectomy 349, 350
Nephrolithiasis 356
Nephron 354
– organization 354
Nerve
– of pterygoid canal (VIDIAN nerve) 466, 488, 590
– to external acoustic meatus 447, 589
– to lateral pterygoid 447, 589
– to medial pterygoid 589
– to mylohyoid 446, 447, 474, 520, 524, 525, 589
– to obturator internus 161
– to quadratus femoris 161
– to stapedius 508, 590, 592, 593
– to tensor
– – tympani 589
– – veli palatini 472, 589
Nervous system 11, 35
– organization 35
Neural foramina 45
Neurocranium 426
Neurohypophysis 564, 575
Neuronal layer of retina 495
Nipple 230
– absence 230
Nodding the head 64
Nodose (inferior) ganglion
– of vagus nerve 580, 601, 603, 611
Nodules of semilunar cusp 260
Non-communicating hydrocephalus 574
Non-homonymous hemianopsia (hemianopia) 500
Norepinephrine 357
Nose
– bleeding (epistaxis) 454
– bony septum 450
– lateral wall 452
– shape 448
Notch of ligamentum teres 331

Nuchal groove 41
Nucleus/i
- ambiguus 578, 579, 581, 595, 596, 597, 598, 599, 601
- of abducens nerve 492, 578, 579, 584
- of accessory nerve 578
- of BEKHTEREV/BECHTEREW (superior vestibular nucleus) 512, 516
- of facial nerve 590
- of hypoglossal nerve 578, 579, 602
- of lateral lemnisci 514
- of lens 497
- of oculomotor nerve 491, 578, 579, 584
- of solitary tract 272, 578, 579, 590, 593, 595, 596, 597, 598, 599, 600, 611
- of spinal accessory nerve 578, 579
- of trigeminal nerve 595, 616
- of trochlear nerve 578, 579
- proprius of medulla spinalis 614
- pulposus 45, 47, 48
NUEL's space 512
Nutrient artery 82
Nystagmus 515, 516
- test 516

O

Oblique
- abdominal incision GRIDIRON (McBURNEY) 289
- arytenoid 534
- cord of interosseous membrane of fore-arm 119
- diameter of pelvis 365
- fissure of lung 245, 246
-- projection onto the thoracic walls 227
- head of adductor hallucis 209
- line of thyroid cartilage 538, 540
- part
-- of arytenoid 540, 544
-- of cricothyroid 532, 540
- pericardial sinus 256, 257
- popliteal ligament 188
- vein of left atrium 269
Obliquus capitis
- inferior 63, 64, 73
- superior 58, 63, 64, 73
Oblong fovea of arytenoid 538
Obstetric conjugate 365
Obstructive uropathy 353
Obturator
- artery 162, 175, 219, 290, 368, 394, 409, 419, 421
- canal 163, 164, 175, 296, 368
- crest 159
- externus 166, 167, 168, 416
- fascia 413, 416
- foramen 158, 159, 161, 163
- groove 159
- internus 166, 167, 168, 367, 368, 382, 384, 392, 408, 416, 418
- membrane 163, 164, 296
- nerve 161, 172, 175, 214, 215, 217, 290, 321, 356, 368, 382, 394, 421
- neurovascular bundle 392
- vein 175, 290, 368, 394, 420
Occipital
- artery 442, 446, 447, 520, 523, 524, 525, 534, 559
- belly of occipitofrontalis 440, 441, 523, 590

Occipital
- bone 429, 431, 432, 434, 435, 436, 450
- branch/es
-- of occipital artery 442
-- of posterior auricular artery 442
-- of posterior auricular nerve 590
- condyle 56, 428
- diploic veins 443, 561
- emissary vein 562
- horn of lateral ventricle 572, 573, 574
- lobe 36, 556, 557, 572
- lymph nodes 550
- margin of temporal bone 504
- pole 557
- region 425
- sinus 560
- vein 443, 523, 524, 529, 562
Occipitofrontalis 439, 440, 441, 486, 523, 590
Occipitomastoid suture 428, 429, 434
Occiput 429
Occluded auditory tube 506
Occlusal plane 428
Ocular fundus 498
- fluorescence angiography 498
Oculomotor
- nerve [CN III] 438, 479, 490, 491, 492, 493, 494, 497, 516, 556, 563, 564, 568, 576, 578, 579, 581, 583, 586, 607
-- complete paresis 583
-- fiber qualities 491, 577, 584
-- innervation 577
-- palsy 491
-- parasympathetic ganglion 581
- (parasympathetic) root of ciliary ganglion 479, 583, 584
Oculosympathetic palsy 607
ODDI, sphincter of (sphincter of ampulla) 317, 339, 341
Odontoid process 58
Oily spots on nails 26
Olecranon 6, 87, 109, 110, 111, 112, 120, 128
- bursa 120
- bursitis 120
- fossa 110
Olfactory
- bulb 454, 563, 582
- cells 582
- epithelium 582
- mucosa 582
- nerve [CN I] 438, 454, 576, 579, 582
-- fiber qualities 577
-- innervation 577
- sensory cells 582
- tract 563, 582
Olivocochlear tract 514
Olivospinal
- fibers 614
- tract 615
Omental
- appendices (epiploic appendices) 299
- branches
-- of gastro-omental (gastroepiploic)
--- artery 312
--- vein 312
- bursa 297, 302, 303, 304, 346, 347
-- boundaries 304
-- development 297
- foramen (epiploic foramen, foramen of WINSLOW) 302, 303, 310, 333
- taenia 321, 322
- tuberosity of liver 342

Omoclavicular triangle 425
Omohyoid 521, 524, 525, 526, 528, 529, 546, 602
Omotracheal triangle 425
Omphalocele 298
Omphaloentric cyst 320
Open-angle glaucoma 496
Opening/s
- of auditory tube 531
- of cervical fistulas 545
- of cochlear canaliculus 504
- of frontal sinus 451
- of sinus coronarius 259
- of smallest cardiac veins 259
- of sphenoid sinus 435, 451
- of vestibular canaliculus 504
Open kinetic chain movements 9
Opercular part of middle cerebral artery 563
Ophthalmic
- artery 487, 492, 493, 499, 527, 563, 564, 565, 566
- herpes zoster 585
- nerve [CN V/1] 438, 465, 479, 488, 492, 493, 494, 564, 581, 583, 584, 585, 586, 587
-- branches 587
-- neuralgia 585
Ophthalmoplegia (ophthalmoparesis) 492
Opponens
- digiti minimi
-- of foot 209
-- of hand 137
- pollicis 136, 146
Optic
- axis 490, 495
- canal 434, 436, 438, 484, 485, 493, 494
-- neurovascular structures 492
- chiasm 499, 500, 564, 566, 568, 572
- cup 556
- disc 490, 495, 498
- nerve [CN II] 438, 487, 488, 490, 492, 493, 494, 497, 499, 500, 563, 564, 576, 579, 583
-- fiber qualities 577
-- innervation 577
- part of retina 495
- radiation 497, 499
- tract 499, 500
Optical reflex 587
Oral
- cavity 471
-- anterior view 455
-- frontal view 455
-- topographic relationships 530
- mucosa 461
- part of pharynx (oropharynx) 455
- region 425
- vestibule 306, 455
Ora serrata 495
Orbicularis
- oculi 439, 441, 486, 489, 590
-- paralysis 593
- oris 439, 440, 441, 590
Orbit 426, 436, 452, 453, 484
- arteries and nerves 487, 493, 494
- bones 484
- lateral wall 485
- medial wall 485
- neurovascular structures 492
- roof 484
- veins 487

Orbital
- apex syndrome 492
- bone 436
- cavity 484
- fractures, coronal computed tomography (CT) 15
- hernia 485
- part
-- of frontal bone 426, 451, 485
-- of lacrimal gland 488, 493, 494
-- of orbicularis oculi 439, 440, 441, 486
- plate of ethmoid bone 451, 452, 484, 485
- process of palatine 484
- region 425
- septum 486, 487
- surface
-- of frontal bone 485
-- of maxilla 485
-- of sphenoid bone 427, 435, 451
-- of zygomatic bone 426, 484
Orchis see Testis
Oropharyngeal region
- muscles 472
Oropharynx 306, 455, 530
Osseous spiral lamina 512
Osteoarthritis 122
- of the knee joint 177
Osteocyte 15
Osteon 15
Osteoporosis 66
- COLLES' fracture 121
Otic ganglion 477, 479, 509, 581, 586, 589, 594, 595, 596, 604
Otitis media 506, 507, 592, 593
Otolithic membrane 515
Otoliths 515
Otosclerosis 506
Otoscopy 503, 505
Outer
- border cells 512
- hair cells 512, 513, 515
- lip of iliac crest 159
- phalangeal cells 512
- pilar cells 512
- sheath of optic nerve [CN II] 495
- subarachnoid space 573
- tunnel 512
Oval window 504, 508, 510, 513
Ovarian
- artery 321, 347, 351, 355, 359, 389, 391, 394, 396
- branches of uterine artery 394
- fimbria 391
- follicle 391
- ligament 389
- nerve plexus 396
- vein 321, 337, 347, 351, 355, 389, 391, 394, 395
Ovary 32, 33, 347, 369, 385, 388, 389, 390, 391, 394, 396
- peritoneal duplications 369, 391

P

PACCHIONIAN granulations (arachnoid granulations) 561, 573
Palatal plane 428
Palate
- defects in formation 464
- development 464

Palatine
- bone 431, 432, 435, 449, 450, 451, 456, 484, 485
- glands 455, 479, 593
- grooves 456
- muscles 596, 599
- process of maxilla 431, 432, 448, 449, 450, 451, 456
- raphe 455, 464
- rugae 464
- spines 456
- tonsil 455, 467, 471, 478, 530, 531, 534, 544, 594
-- blood and nerve supply 471
-- recurrent infections 471
- tonsillitis 530
Palatoglossal arch 455, 464, 467
Palatoglossus 455, 469, 471, 472, 478, 507, 596, 597
- paralysis 596
Palatopharyngeal arch 455, 464, 467, 530, 534
Palatopharyngeus 455, 471, 472, 478, 534, 596, 597
- paralysis 596
Palm 4, 87
- central compartment, muscles 138
- thenar muscles 136
Palmar 5
- aponeurosis 134, 136
- branch
-- of median nerve 139, 146, 147
-- of ulnar nerve 147
- carpal
-- branch
--- of radial artery 140, 149
--- of ulnar artery 140, 149
-- ligament 134, 145
- carpometacarpal ligament 124, 134
- digital
-- arteries 139, 149
-- veins 150
- intercarpal ligament 124
- interossei 137, 138
- ligaments 126
- metacarpal
-- arteries 140, 149
-- ligaments 124
-- veins 150
- radiocarpal ligament 124
- ulnocarpal ligament 124
Palmaris
- brevis 137
- longus 116, 128, 129, 134, 136, 137, 146
Palpebral
- commissure 482
- conjunctiva 482, 483
- fissure 483
- part of orbicularis oculi (muscle of RIOLAN) 439, 440, 441, 483, 486
Pampiniform plexus 292, 293, 397, 399, 400, 401, 402
PANCOAST's tumor 551, 607
Pancreas 31, 32, 303, 304, 305, 306, 316, 343
- arteries 345
- excretory duct system 344
- imaging 344
- lymphatic drainage 345
- posterior view 342
- projection onto the body surface 317
- spatial relations in the retroperitoneal space 342

Pancreatic
- branches of splenic artery 345
- carcinomas 341
- duct (duct of WIRSUNG) 317, 339, 341, 342, 344
-- sphincter 341
-- variations 344
- lymph nodes 361
- veins 336
Pancreaticoduodenal
- lymph nodes 345, 361
- veins 336
Papilla of parotid duct 478
Papillary muscles
- of left ventricle 262
Para-aortic lymph nodes 327, 404
Paracolic
- gutters 301
- lymph nodes 327
Paracortical zone of lymph node 30, 287
Parafollicular C-cells of thyroid gland 549
Parageusia 600
Parahippocampal gyrus 557, 573
Paralysis 620
Paramammary lymph nodes 231, 232
Paramedian abdominal incision 289
Paramesonephric ducts (MÜLLERIAN ducts) 388, 399
Paranasal sinuses 247, 452, 453
- CT 453
Paranephric fat 349
Parapharyngeal space 473, 478, 530
- blood vessels and nerves 533, 534
Paraplegia 619, 620
Pararectal
- abdominal incision 289
- lymph nodes 375
Pararenal adipose tissue 349
Parasternal lymph nodes 231, 232
Parasympathetic
- ganglia of cranial nerves 581
- nerve fibers
-- of abdominal viscera 360
-- of esophagus 307
-- of female genitalia 396
-- of intestine 328
-- of middle ear 509
-- of pelvis 422
- nervous system 603, 604, 606
- nuclei 604
- (oculomotor) root of ciliary ganglion 479, 583, 584
- postganglionic fibers 607
- preganglionic fibers 607
- root
-- of ciliary ganglion 479, 583, 584
-- of pterygopalatine ganglion 590, 592
Parathyroid glands 32, 532, 549
- carcinoma 549
- hyperplasia or adenoma 549
Parathyroid hormone (PTH) 549
Paratracheal lymph nodes 249, 307, 550
Paraumbilical veins 286, 336, 337
Paravertebral line 227
Paravesical space 392
Paredrine test, HORNER's syndrome 607
Parietal
- bone 427, 430, 431, 432, 434, 441
- branch of superficial temporal artery 442, 444, 446, 447
- emissary vein 443, 561, 562
- foramen 432

Parietal
- lobe 36, 556, 557, 572
- margin 435
- notch 504
- operculum 556, 557
- pelvic fascia 375
- peritoneum 288, 292, 300, 349
-- somatic nerves 300
- pleura 242, 243, 245, 246, 251, 252, 255, 256
- region 425
- serous pericardium 255
- tuber 428, 429, 430, 431
Parietomastoid suture 428, 429
Parieto-occipital sulcus 557, 566, 568
Parotid
- branch/es of auriculotemporal nerve 479, 589
- duct (STENSON's duct) 439, 441, 444, 475, 478
- fascia 440, 475, 478
- gland 439, 441, 444, 475, 478, 479, 519, 523, 528, 529, 532, 594, 596
-- innervation 509
-- tumors 440
- papilla 478
- plexus of facial nerve [CN VII] 445
- region 425
- tumor 475, 592, 593
Parotitis 475
PARROT's beak meniscal tear 184
Pars
- flaccida of tympanic membrane (SHRAPNELL's membrane) 505
- tensa of tympanic membrane 505
PASSAVANT's ridge, failure 596
Patella 12, 156, 169, 171, 176, 177, 178, 181, 182, 185, 186
- alta 185
- baja 185
- infera 185
- sesamoid bone 185, 186
Patellar
- anastomosis 175
- ligament 169, 171, 176, 182, 184, 185, 186
- surface of femur 162
- tendon reflex (Knee-jerk reflex) 612
Patellofemoral joint (PFJ) 178, 186
Patent
- ductus arteriosus 273
- foramen ovale 259, 273
PCL (posterior cruciate ligament) 183, 184
- injury 180
Pecten pubis 159, 365, 367
Pectinate
- line (dentate line) 371, 373, 375
- muscles 259
Pectineal
- ligament 296
- line of femur 162
Pectineus 166, 172, 175, 296
Pectoral
- axillary lymph nodes 231, 232
- fascia 230
- girdle 89
- lymph nodes 151, 287
- nerves 105, 145, 146
- region 4, 225
Pectoralis
- major 78, 86, 101, 108, 145, 146, 230, 289, 529
- minor 101, 105, 145, 146

Pedicle of vertebral arch 44, 66, 69
Pelvic
- arteries, angiogram 219
- cavity 367
-- laparoscopic view 389
- diameters 365
- diaphragm 367, 368, 376, 416
- fascia 366, 375, 389, 392, 417
- floor 367, 370, 376
-- insufficiency 367, 386
-- in woman 368
-- muscles 367, 368
- ganglia 373, 396, 403
- inlet 158, 365, 367
- kidney 348
- lymph nodes 30, 395
- organ plexus 403
- outlet 365, 367, 405
-- bones and ligaments 405
- pain line 396
- part of ureter 355
- plexus 422
- splanchnic nerves 360, 373, 396, 403, 421, 606
- surface of sacrum 75
- viscera
-- in man 370, 380
--- blood drainage 420
-- in woman 385
--- cross-section 393
--- MRI 393
Pelvis 3, 158, 367
- avulsion type fracture 158
- body regions 364
- 3-D CT angiography 28
- CT cross-section 349
- differences between female and male 365
- fractures 158
- in man 366, 370
-- autonomic and somatic nerves 421
-- coronal plane 384
-- cross-section 382
-- MRI 382, 383, 384
-- parasagittal section 383
- in woman 366, 369, 379
-- cross-section 390
-- frontal section 417
-- MRI 385, 386, 390, 393
- joints 160
- ligaments 160
- malpositions 158
- metastases 158
- osteoarthritis 158
- parasympathetic nerves 422
- radiograph 158
- supporting ligaments 161
- surface anatomy 157, 364
- surface landmarks 364
Pelvitrochanteric muscles 168
Pelviureteric junction 355
Penile
- carcinoma 404
- erection 403
Penis 33, 397, 398, 399
- arterial and venous blood supply 398, 399
- cross-section 398
- innervation 398
Peptic ulcers 315

Perforating
- arteries 174, 219, 220
- branch/es
-- of fibular artery 220
-- of posterior auricular artery 502
Perianal abscess
- inflammatory bowel disease (IBD) 416
Peribronchial lymphatic vessels 249
Pericallosal
- artery 566
- cistern 573
Pericardiacophrenic
- artery 237, 251, 252, 256, 551
- vein 251, 252, 256
Pericardiac trigone 254
Pericardial
- branches of phrenic nerve 236
- cavity 255
- effusion 256
-- tamponade 256
Pericarditis 256
Pericardium 236, 244, 255, 257, 306
- layers 255
- position of the heart 255
Perichoroidal space 495
Pericranium 425, 441
Peridental branches
- of posterior superior alveolar artery 446
Peridural anesthesia 571
Periglomerular cells of olfactory bulb 582
Perilymph 512
Perilymphatic space 511
Perimetrium 391
Perimysium 20
Perineal
- artery 409, 414, 416
- body 368, 406, 412
- branches (posterior cutaneous nerve of thigh) 411
- fascia 417
- flexure (anorectal flexure) 368, 371
- membrane (urogenital diaphragm) 406, 407, 413, 416, 417, 418
- muscles
-- in man 413
-- in woman 407
- nerve 411, 416
- raphe 406, 413
- region 417, 418
-- in man 413
-- in woman 406, 418
- spaces
-- in man 418
-- in woman 417, 418
- structures, surface projection 405
Perinephric fat (perirenal adipose capsule) 348, 349, 351
Perineum
- in man 413, 415
-- blood supply 414
-- MRI 415
- in woman 411
-- blood supply 409
-- branches of the pudendal nerve 411
-- cross-section 408
-- MRI 408
-- sensory innervation 411
Periodontium 462
Periolivary nuclei 513
Periorbita 490

Periorbital region
- arteries 487
- nerves 487
- veins 487
Periorchium 399
Periosteum 15
Peripheral
- facial nerve palsy 439, 591
- nervous system (PNS) 35
-- neuronal connectivities 603
- zone of prostate 380, 384
Perirenal adipose capsule (perinephric fat) 348, 349, 351
Peritoneal
- carcinosis 304
- cavity 297, 300, 301
-- compartments 301
-- development 297
-- of pelvis 366, 417, 418
-- posterior wall 347
- duplicatures 369
- folds 300
- ligaments 300, 391
- space, CT cross-section 349
Peritoneum 417
Peritonitis 304
Periurethral zone of prostate 380
Perivisceral space 521
Permanent teeth 461, 462
- lower jaw 462
- upper jaw 462
Peroneal (fibular)
- brevis 207
- retinaculum 203, 204, 206
Peroneus (fibularis)
- brevis 201, 203, 206
- longus 190, 201, 203, 208, 209
- tertius 201, 202, 207
Perpendicular plate 484
- of ethmoid 432, 448, 449, 450, 451
- of palatine 435, 436, 449, 450, 451
Persistent vaginal process of peritoneum 294
Pes
- anserinus 169, 172
-- bursa 187
- cavus (high arched foot) 210
- hippocampi 573
- planus (flatfoot) 210
Petro-occipital
- fissure 434
- synchondrosis 510, 532
Petrosal
- fossula 504
- ganglion of glossopharyngeal nerve 580
Petrosphenoidal fissure 508, 592
Petrosquamous fissure 434
Petrotympanic fissure 504
Petrous part
- of internal carotid artery 563, 564
- of temporal bone 430, 431, 434, 504, 507, 510
PEYER's patches 322, 327
PFANNENSTIEL incision 289
Phalanx/Phalanges, of foot 194
Pharyngeal
- arches 579, 590
- artery 466
- branch/es
-- of descending palatine artery 471
-- of glossopharyngeal nerve [CN IX] 533, 594, 595

Pharyngeal branch/es
-- of inferior thyroid artery 533
-- of vagus nerve [CN X] 307, 533, 594, 597, 598
- constrictors 507, 596
- gag reflex 596
- gland 532
- muscles 532, 596, 599, 601
- nerve 589
- opening of auditory tube 471, 530, 531, 534, 594
- plexus 588, 594, 597, 598
-- branches of glossopharyngeal and vagus nerves [CN IX + CN X] 467, 472
-- sensory and sympathetic nerve fibers 530
- pouch, remnants 545
- raphe 532
- recess (fossa of ROSENMÜLLER) 507, 534
- tonsil 471, 507, 530, 531, 534
-- enlargement 507
-- hyperplasia 531
- veins 443, 533
Pharyngitis 531
Pharyngobasilar fascia 532, 534
Pharyngoesophageal
- (cervical) constriction of esophagus 306
- diverticulum 532
Pharyngotympanic tube (auditory tube, EUSTACHIAN tube) 503, 505, 507, 508, 509, 592, 594
- occlusion 506
Pharynx 247, 306, 471, 530, 537
- arteries 533
- blood vessels and nerves 534
- levels 530
- nerves 533
- veins 533
PHILIPPE-GOMBAULT, triangle of (interfascicular fasciculus, lumbar and sacral tract) 614
Phimosis 397
Phlebitis of sinus venosus 443
Phrenic nerve 106, 141, 236, 238, 244, 251, 252, 256, 278, 280, 358, 524, 525, 526, 529, 551
Phrenicoabdominal
- artery 237
- branch/es
-- of internal thoracic artery 237
-- of phrenic nerve 236, 358
Phrenicocolic ligament 301, 302, 310, 333
Phrenicoesophageal ligament 309
Phrenicopleural fascia 242
Physiological umbilical hernia 298
Pial part of filum terminale 613
Pia mater 558, 569
Pigmented layer of retina 495, 499
Pineal
- body 556
- gland 568, 574, 575, 578
- recess of third ventricle 572, 573
Piriform
- aperture 426, 456
- fossa 534, 541
- recess 543
Piriformis 161, 166, 167, 168, 174, 368, 419, 420
Pisiform 119, 122, 124, 139
Pisohamate ligament 124
Pisometacarpal ligament 124
Pituitary gland 32, 556, 564

Pivot-hinge joint
- knee joint 181
Pivot joint 17, 123
Placenta 273, 387
Plane
- joint 17
- of ADDISON (transpyloric plane) 283, 310
Plantar 5
- aponeurosis 208, 209
- arch of foot 210
- calcaneocuboid ligament 200
- calcaneonavicular ligament 199, 200
- cuboideonavicular ligament 200
- cuneonavicular ligament 200
- interossei 208, 209
- ligaments 200
- metatarsal
-- arteries 213
-- ligaments 200
- tarsal ligaments 200
- tarsometatarsal ligaments 199, 200
Plantarflexion 196
Plantaris 204, 205
Plantar reflex 612
Platysma 439, 440, 444, 455, 473, 519, 523, 590
- bands 523
Pleura
- function 244
- innervation 244
- projection 242
-- onto the thoracic wall 227
- sensory innervation 244
Pleural
- cavity 242, 243, 250, 251, 252
- effusion 244
- fluids 244
- movements during respiration 244
Pneumothorax 242, 243
Polar arteries of kidney 352
Polymastia 230
Polysynaptic
- inhibitory neuron 612
- reflex arc 611, 612
Polythelia 230
Pons 514, 556, 557, 566, 568, 572, 578, 605
Pontine
- arteries 565, 566
- nuclei 618
- nucleus of trigeminal nerve 578, 579
Pontocerebellar
- cistern 573
- fibers 618
Popeye deformity 114
Popliteal 187
- artery 174, 175, 189, 212, 220
- fossa 4, 156, 176, 190
-- neurovascular structures 189
- lymphatic vessels 189
- lymph nodes 189
- pulse 28
- surface of femur 179, 188
- vein 174, 189, 221
Popliteofibular ligament 181
Popliteus 180, 181, 188, 205
- bursa 187
Porta hepatis 331, 335
Portal
- hypertension 308, 337
- lobule 335
- triad 332

Portal-systemic collateral pathways 337
Portocaval anastomoses 308, 313, 337, 374
Postcentral gyrus 600, 616
Postcommunicating part
– of anterior cerebral artery 563, 566
– of middle cerebral artery 563
– of posterior cerebral artery 563
Posterior 5
– abdominal wall 80, 305
– – muscles 80
– alveolar foramina 436
– arch of atlas 56
– arm 4
– – triceps region 115
– articular facet of dens 57
– atlanto-occipital membrane 59
– auricular
– – artery 442, 446, 447, 502, 524
– – nerve 446, 447, 508, 523, 524, 590, 591, 592
– – vein 523, 524
– axillary
– – fold 86, 105
– – line 227
– basal segment
– – of left lung 247
– – of right lung 247
– belly of digastric 441, 474, 475, 508, 521, 524, 528, 532, 533, 590, 592
– bony ampulla 510
– border
– – of fibula 193
– – of left lung 246
– – of right lung 245
– branch/es
– – of great auricular nerve 523
– – of intercostal nerve 229, 240
– – of medial cutaneous nerve of forearm 147
– – of spinal nerve 526, 608, 610
– cerebellomedullary cistern 573
– cerebral artery 499, 527, 563, 565, 566, 568
– – clinical segments 563
– cervical region 4, 225, 425, 520
– – blood vessels and nerves 524
– – muscles 524
– – superficial blood vessels and nerves 523
– – superficial layer 523
– chamber of eyeball 495, 496
– choroidal arteries 565
– circumflex humeral artery 107, 108, 149
– clinoid process 434, 435, 436
– cochlear nucleus 512, 514
– column of spinal cord 613, 614
– commissure 497
– communicating artery 527, 563, 564, 566
– compartment of forearm 128
– – deep muscles 132
– – superficial muscles 131
– cord of brachial plexus 106, 141, 144
– cord syndrome 620
– cranial fossa 434, 560
– cricoarytenoid 534, 540, 544
– – ligament 538
– cruciate ligament (PCL) 177, 183, 184, 187
– – injury 180
– crural artery 509

Posterior
– cusp
– – of left atrioventricular valve (mitral valve) 260
– – of right atrioventricular valve (tricuspid valve) 259, 261
– cutaneous
– – branch/es of thoracic nerves 147
– – nerve
– – – of arm 108, 144, 147, 229
– – – of forearm 108, 144, 147
– – – of thigh 214, 217, 411
– deep temporal artery 442, 446, 447
– elastic nodule 540, 541
– elbow 4
– ethmoid
– – artery 454, 487, 494
– – cells 452, 453
– – foramen 484, 485
– – nerve 494, 583, 587
– external vertebral venous plexus 82
– fasciculus proprius 614
– femoral cutaneous nerve 161, 174, 217
– fold of malleus 505
– fontanelle 430, 431
– forearm 4
– funiculus of spinal cord 613, 614
– gastric
– – artery 312
– – veins 313
– gluteal line 159
– horn
– – of lateral ventricle 572, 573
– – of spinal cord 613, 614
– inferior
– – cerebellar artery 563, 565, 566, 568
– – iliac spine 158, 159
– – mediastinum 250
– – nasal nerves 454
– intercondylar area 179, 192
– intercostal
– – arteries 239, 240, 241, 251, 252, 278, 279, 285, 527, 570
– – veins 239, 240, 241, 251, 252, 279
– intermediate sulcus of spinal cord 613
– intermuscular septum of leg 201
– internal vertebral venous plexus 82
– interosseous
– – artery 133, 149
– – nerve 133
– – – of arm 144
– – – of forearm 139, 144
– interventricular
– – branch of right coronary artery 257, 266, 267
– – sinus 257
– – sulcus (groove) 257, 258, 269
– – vein (middle interventricular artery) 257, 269
– labial
– – artery 409
– – branches of perineal artery 409
– – nerves 396, 410, 411, 414
– lacrimal crest 484
– lateral
– – choroidal branches of posterior cerebral artery 566
– – nasal arteries 454
– left ventricular branch of left coronary artery 267
– ligament of incus 506

Posterior
– limb
– – of internal capsule 568
– – of stapes 506
– limiting lamina of cornea (DESCEMET's membrane) 495
– longitudinal ligament 50, 571, 610, 613
– lower leg 4
– marginal branch of right coronary artery 266
– medial choroidal branches of posterior cerebral artery 566
– median sulcus of spinal cord 613
– mediastinal lymph nodes 253, 307
– mediastinum 250
– – anatomical structures 250
– – lymph nodes 253
– – nerves 280
– – veins 279
– membranous ampulla 512
– meningeal artery 533, 559
– meniscofemoral ligament 184
– meniscotibial ligament 184
– myocardial infarction (PMI) 268
– nasal spine 449, 450, 451, 456
– palpebral margin 482, 483
– papillary muscle
– – of left ventricle 260, 261
– – of right ventricle 259
– parietal artery 567
– part of tongue 467, 534
– pole
– – of eyeball 495
– – of lens 495, 497
– process
– – of septal nasal cartilage 448
– – of talus 198
– radicular artery 570
– ramus of spinal nerve 240
– region
– – of arm 87
– – of forearm 87
– – of knee 156
– root of spinal nerve 229, 569, 570
– sacral foramina 75
– sacroiliac ligament 160
– scalene 61, 62, 235, 238, 520, 521, 551
– scrotal
– – artery 414
– – nerves 414, 416
– segment
– – of liver 330, 331
– – of right lung 247
– semicircular
– – canal 510, 511
– – duct 510, 511
– semilunar cusp of aortic valve 260, 261
– septal branch of sphenopalatine artery 454
– sinus of tympanic cavity 504
– spinal
– – artery 565, 566, 569, 570
– – vein 569
– spinocerebellar tract (FLECHSIG's tract) 614, 615, 617
– spinous line 53
– sternoclavicular ligament 94
– superior
– – alveolar
– – – artery 442, 466
– – – block 465

Posterior superior alveolar
– – – branches 446, 447
– – – nerves 461, 465
– – iliac spine 157, 158, 159, 364, 405
– – lateral nasal branches of maxillary
   nerve 454, 588
– – medial nasal branches of maxillary
   nerve 588
– – pancreaticoduodenal artery 329, 345
– – pancreaticoduodenal vein 336
– superior iliac spine 41
– surface
– – of eyelid 482
– – of fibula 193
– – of petrous part of temporal bone 504
– – of tibia 192
– talofibular ligament 199
– temporal
– – branch/es of middle cerebral
   artery 567
– – diploic veins 443, 561
– thigh 4
– – muscles 173
– thoracic nucleus (CLARKE's
   column) 614, 617
– thoracic wall
– – cutaneous nerves 229
– – muscles 235
– – projections of the borders of lung and
   pleura 227
– – segmental innervation 229
– tibial
– – artery 189, 212, 213, 220
– – pulse 28
– – recurrent artery 220
– – veins 221
– tibiofibular ligament 199
– tibiotalar part (of medial ligament of
   ankle joint) 199
– triangle
– – of cervical region 528
– – of neck 520
– tubercle
– – of atlas 56
– – of transverse process 55
– tympanic
– – artery 506, 509
– – branch of stylomastoid artery 509
– vagal trunk 280, 307, 315, 328, 358,
   597, 598
– vein of left ventricle 269
– ventral nucleus 600
– vertebral line 53
– wall
– – of stomach 310
– – of trunk, arteries 278
Posterolateral
– central arteries 565
– sulcus of spinal cord 613
Posteromedial central arteries 565
Postganglionic
– neuron 606
– parasympathetic nerve fibers 272
– – lacrimal apparatus 488
– sympathetic nerve fibers 272, 280
– – lacrimal apparatus 488
– – of stomach 315
Postnatal circulation 273
Postremal [vitreous] chamber of eyeball 495
Post-zoster neuralgia 585
Preaortic lymph nodes 395

Precallosal part of anterior cerebral
   artery 563
Precentral gyrus 591, 618
Prechiasmatic sulcus 436
Precommunicating part
– of anterior cerebral artery 563
– of middle cerebral artery 563
– of posterior cerebral artery 563
Pre-epiglottic fat body 530, 537
Prefrontal artery 567
Preganglionic
– autonomic fibers 606
– neurons 272
– parasympathetic cardiac fibers 272
– parasympathetic nerve fibers
– – lacrimal apparatus 488
– sympathetic nerve fibers
– – of stomach 315
Prelaryngeal lymph nodes 550
Premolar tooth/teeth 461
Prenatal circulation 273
Preoccipital notch 557
Prepatellar
– bursa 187
– bursitis 187
Prepuce
– of clitoris 406, 407
– of penis 397
Presacral fasica (WALDEYER's fascia) 375
Presbyopia 497
Presternal region 225
Pretectal area 497
Pretracheal
– fascia 522
– layer of cervical fascia 521, 530
– lymph nodes 550
Prevertebral
– layer of cervical fascia 478, 521, 522,
   530, 548
– muscles of neck 478
– part of vertebral artery 81, 525, 527
– plexus 606
Primary
– auditory cortex 513
– brain vesicles 556
– intestinal loop 298
– retroperitoneal organs 300
Primordial gut 297
Princeps pollicis artery 140, 149
Principal
– posterior nucleus 578
– sensory nucleus of trigeminal
   nerve 578, 586
Procerus 439, 440, 441, 590
Processus
– cochleariformis 504
– vaginalis of peritoneum 294, 295
Proctodeal glands (anal glands) 371
Proctodeum
– blood supply, innervation and lymphatic
   drainage 327
Profunda
– brachii artery 107, 108, 149
– femoris vein 175, 221
Progesterone 388
Prolapse
– of urinary bladder 386
– of uterus 386
Prominence
– of facial canal 504, 508
– of lateral semicircular canal 504, 508

Promontory 68
– of sacrum 43, 75, 365
– – palpation 387
– of tympanic cavity 504, 509
Pronator
– quadratus 130, 134, 146
– teres 116, 117, 118, 128, 129, 130, 146
Proper
– hepatic artery 312
– palmar digital
– – arteries 139, 140
– – nerves 139
– – – of median nerve 147
– – – of ulnar nerve 147
– plantar digital nerves 213
Proprioception 586, 617
Proptosis 564
Prosencephalon 556
Prostate 33, 366, 370, 371, 375, 376, 378,
   380, 381, 382, 383, 384, 398, 399, 403,
   418
– adenoma 381
– carcinoma 370, 381
– – digital rectal examination 370
– – vertebral metastases 420
– central zone 380
– digital rectal examination (DRE) 381
– enlargement and clinical
   consequences 381
– hyperplasia 381
– peripheral zone 380, 384
– transition zone 380, 384
Prostatic
– ducts 376, 378
– plexus 403, 421
– sinus 376
– urethra 378, 380
– utricle 376
– venous plexus 402, 420
Protopathic sensibility 585, 586, 615, 616
Proximal 5
– femur 162
– humerus 93
– – fractures 144
– interphalangeal joints (PIP) 88, 118, 126
– – dislocation 126
– – radiograph 126
– – range of motion 127
– phalanx
– – of foot 194, 195
– – of hand 118, 119, 122
– radioulnar joint 88, 110, 111, 119, 123
– tibiofibular joint 178
– tubule of kidney 354
PSIS (posterior superior iliac spine) 157,
   158, 159, 364
Psoas
– major 70, 77, 80, 170, 171, 172, 237,
   296, 321, 385
– minor 80, 296, 385
Psoriasis, nail dystrophy 26
Pterygoid
– canal 435, 436
– – nerves 466
– fossa 432, 435, 448
– hamulus 432, 435, 448, 450, 455, 458,
   465, 532
– notch 435
– plexus 443, 447, 466, 562
– process 431, 432, 435, 436, 450, 456,
   458, 465, 485, 532

Pterygoid
- tuberosity 457, 458
- venous plexus 487
Pterygomandibular raphe 455, 478, 532
Pterygomaxillary fissure 485
Pterygopalatine
- fossa 436, 466, 485
-- bony demarcations 436
- ganglion 466, 479, 488, 581, 583, 586,
  588, 590, 593, 594, 604
-- branches 588
-- parasympathetic root 512
Pterygospinous ligament 458
Pteryopharyngeal part of superior
  constrictor 532
Ptosis (drooping eyelid) 491, 607
Pubic
- arch 365
- bone 383
- hair 397
- ligament 405
- region 4, 283, 364
- symphysis 157, 158, 160, 296, 364, 365,
  367, 368, 383, 384, 405, 407, 413
-- joint 160
- tubercle 157, 158, 159, 364, 407
Pubis 158, 159, 365, 367, 383
Pubococcygeus 368, 371
Pubofemoral ligament 163, 164
Puboprostatic ligaments 376
Puborectalis 368, 372, 373
Pubovesical ligament 392
Pudendal
- canal (ALCOCK's canal) 409, 411, 413,
  414, 416, 417
- nerve 161, 214, 216, 327, 373, 379, 396,
  403, 411, 413, 414, 416, 418, 421
-- block 387, 396, 410
-- branches 411
-- in man 414
-- in woman 410
- neurovascular bundle 392
Pulmonary
- artery 28, 245, 248, 251, 252, 255, 256,
  257, 264, 273
- branches
-- of thoracic ganglia 606
-- of vagus nerve 606
- circulation 248
- embolism 249
- (intrapulmonary) lymph nodes 249
- ligament 245, 246, 251
- nerve plexus 581, 597, 598, 606
- plexus 251, 252, 307
- ring 258
- trunk 254, 255, 256, 257, 258, 260, 264,
  266, 273
- valve 261
-- auscultation 254, 263
-- projection onto the anterior thoracic
  wall 254
-- projection onto the thoracic wall 228
- vasculature 248
- veins 245, 248, 251, 252, 255, 257, 260,
  262, 269, 273, 275
Pulp cavity of tooth 462
Pump handle movement of rib cage during
  respiration 238
Pupil 482, 496
Pupillary
- dilator muscle 496

Pupillary
- light reflex (PLR) 496
-- neuronal pathways 497
- margin of iris 496
- motor functions 496
- muscles 496
- reflexes 497
- sphincter muscle 496
Putamen 567, 568
Pyelography, intravenous 353
Pyelonephritis 356
Pyloric
- antrum 311
- canal 311
- lymph nodes 314
- part of stomach 305, 310, 311, 317, 319
- sphincter 311, 344
-- malfunction 315
Pylorus 310, 311, 316
Pyramidal
- (anterior corticospinal) tract 614
- eminence 504
- lobe of thyroid gland 546
- process 508, 592
- process of palatine 456, 485
- tract 618
- tracts of spinal cord 615
Pyramidalis 79

Q

Q angle 186
- measurement 186
Quadrangular
- axillary space (QAS) 108, 144
- membrane 543
Quadrate lobe of liver 331
Quadratus
- femoris 166, 167, 168, 415
- lumborum 70, 77, 80, 237, 348
- plantae 208
Quadriceps femoris 156, 171, 180, 182,
  185, 211
- tendon 186
Quadrigeminal part of posterior cerebral
  artery 563
Quadriparesis 619

R

Rachischisis 569
Radial
- artery 116, 117, 133, 135, 139, 140, 149
-- branches 149
- collateral
-- artery 108, 117, 133, 149
-- ligament
--- of elbow joint 111
--- of wrist joint 123, 124
- deviation 8, 125, 129, 131
- fovea 135
- groove of humerus 93
- nerve 106, 108, 115, 116, 117, 131, 133,
  139, 141, 144, 147, 229, 612
- notch 110, 120
- pulse 28
- recurrent artery 117, 133, 149
- styloid process 87, 121, 123
- tuberosity 110, 119, 121

Radial
- tunnel 117, 144
- vein 150
Radialis indicis artery 140, 149
Radiate
- carpal ligament 124
- ligament of head of rib 50, 51, 52
Radiculopathy 48
Radiocarpal joint 123
Radius 6, 12, 88, 110, 119, 121, 122
- distal fracture 121
Ramus
- communicans 608, 610
- of ischium 159
- of mandible 427, 441, 457, 459
Raphe of scrotum 293, 399
Rebound tenderness 322
Recess of EISLER 486
Rectal
- ampulla 370, 371, 375, 383, 384
- arteries 374
- cavernous bodies 374
-- bleedings 374
- plexus 373, 421
- venous plexus 374, 375, 420
Rectocele 386
Rectoprostatic fascia (DENONVILLIER's
  fascia) 366, 370, 375, 381
Rectorectal space 366
Rectouterine
- fold 391
- ligament (uterosacral ligament) 391, 392
- pouch (DOUGLAS, pouch of) 301, 319,
  347, 366, 369, 387, 389, 392
Rectovaginal septum 366
Rectovesical space (pouch) 305, 319, 366,
  370, 376
Rectum 31, 305, 322, 326, 369, 370, 371,
  375, 376, 381, 382, 383, 384, 385, 386,
  392, 393, 408, 417, 418
- innervation 373
- lymphatic drainage 375
- projection onto the body surface 371
Rectus
- abdominis 70, 77, 78, 79, 288, 289,
  290, 294
- capitis 62
-- anterior 58, 62
-- lateralis 58, 62
-- posterior 64
--- major 58, 63, 64, 73
--- minor 58, 63, 64, 73
- femoris 157, 164, 166, 171, 175, 180, 211
-- tendon 163
- sheath 77, 78, 79, 288
Recurrent
- branch
-- of anterior tibial artery 212, 220
-- of posterior tibial artery 189, 220
- interosseous artery 117, 149
- laryngeal nerve 251, 252, 255, 256, 272,
  278, 280, 307, 520, 525, 529, 534, 544,
  547, 548, 551, 597, 598
- meningeal branch
-- of ophthalmic artery 487
-- of ophthalmic nerve 587
Red nucleus 578, 618
Referred pain 611
Reflected inguinal ligament 291, 292
Reflux
- esophagitis 309
- of urine 355, 376, 381

REINKE's
– edema 543
– space 543
REISSNER's membrane (vestibular
  membrane) 512
Renal
– artery 348, 349, 351, 352, 354, 355, 357,
  358, 359, 605
– calyx 34, 354
– columns 353
– concrements 356
– corpuscle (glomerulus) 354
– cortex 353
– cysts 350
– fascia (GEROTA's fascia) 348, 349
– impression
– – on liver 331
– – on spleen 346
– infarction 354
– medulla 353
– nerve plexus 597, 598
– papillae 353
– pelvis 34, 349, 351, 353, 354
– plexus 360, 605
– pyramids 34, 353
– sinus 353
– system 34
– transplantation 350
– vein 337, 348, 349, 351, 354, 357
Renin 354
Renin-angiotensin pathways 352
Reproductive system 11
– in man 33
– in woman 33
Respiration
– muscles 238
– pump handle and bucket handle
  movements of rib cage 238
Respiratory
– bronchioles 248
– movements of thorax 238
– muscles 238
– reflexes 603
– system 27
Rete testis 400
Reticulospinal tract 614, 615, 618
Retina 495, 497
– blood vessels 495
– capillary lamina 495
– neuronal network 499
– vascular lamina 495
Retinal
– ablation 498
– – laser therapy 498
– ganglion 499
Retrobulbar
– fat 493
– hemorrhage 486
Retroflexion of the uterus 386
Retroinguinal, space, muscular and
  vascularcompartment 296
Retromandibular vein 443, 446, 447, 466,
  478, 520, 523, 524, 525, 529, 562
Retromolar
– fossa 457
– triangle 457
Retro-orbital edema, GRAVES' disease 548
Retropatellar pain 185
Retroperitoneal
– abdominal organs 305
– space 347
– – somatic nerves 356

Retropharyngeal
– recess (fossa of ROSENMÜLLER) 534
– space 521, 522, 530
Retropubic space (RETZIUS' space) 366,
  377, 387
Retrorectal (presacral) space 366
Retroversion of the uterus 386
RETZIUS' space (retropubic space) 366,
  377, 387
REXED laminae 614, 616
Rhombencephalon 556, 557
Rhomboid
– major 71, 72, 102, 103, 108, 142
– minor 71, 103, 142
Rib cage
– bucket handle movement during
  respiration 238
– projections onto the thoracic wall 226
– pump handle movement during respiration 238
Rib/s 226, 233, 234
Right
– anterior ventricular vein 269
– atrioventricular valve (tricuspid
  valve) 258, 259, 261
– – auscultation 254, 263
– – projection onto the anterior thoracic
  wall 228
– – projection onto the ventral thoracic
  wall 254
– atrium 255, 257, 258, 259, 265, 266,
  269, 270, 273
– – projection onto the anterior thoracic
  wall 254
– – projection onto the thoracic wall 228
– auricle 257, 259, 260
– bronchial branch of intercostal
  artery 248
– bundle branch 270
– colic
– – artery 324, 325, 326, 329
– – flexure 299, 301, 321, 322
– – lymph nodes 361
– – vein 325, 336
– commissural cusp of left atrioventricular
  valve (mitral valve) 261
– coronary artery 257, 259, 260, 266, 267,
  268
– – branches 267
– fibrous
– – ring of heart 258, 261
– – trigone of heart 258, 261
– gastric
– – artery 312, 314, 318, 329, 334
– – vein 308, 312, 313, 336
– gastro-omental (gastroepiploic)
– – artery 312, 314, 318, 325, 329, 334
– – vein 312, 313, 325, 336
– hemidiaphragm 236
– hepatic vein 332, 335
– inferior lobar bronchus 247
– – projection onto the thoracic wall 228
– intracolic compartment 299
– lamina of thyroid cartilage 532, 536,
  537, 538
– lobe
– – of liver 302, 303, 305, 310, 330, 331,
  333, 339
– – of thyroid gland 532, 547
– lung 245, 247

Right
– lymphatic duct 30, 232
– main (principal) bronchus 245, 247,
  264, 306
– – projection onto the thoracic wall 228
– marginal
– – branch of right coronary artery 266,
  267
– – vein 269
– middle lobar bronchus 247
– – projection onto the thoracic wall 228
– paracolic gutter 301
– posterolateral branch of right coronary
  artery 267
– pulmonary
– – artery 245, 257, 264, 269
– – veins 245, 260
– semilunar
– – cusp of aortic valve 260, 261
– – cusp of pulmonary valve 261
– superior lobar bronchus 245, 247
– – projection onto the thoracic wall 228
– triangular ligament of liver 333
– ventricle 255, 257, 258, 259, 265, 273
– – projection onto the anterior thoracic
  wall 254
Rima glottidis 541
Rim of tympanic membrane 505
Ring finger 87, 118
RIOLAN, muscle of (orbicularis oculi,
  palpebral part) 483, 486
RIOLAN's anastomosis 324, 325, 326, 329
Risorius 439, 440, 441
ROLLER's nucleus (inferior vestibular
  nucleus) 512, 516
ROMBERG test 516
Roof of shoulder 96
Root
– apex of tooth 462
– canal of tooth 462
– of mesentery 347
– of tongue 467, 468
– of tooth 462
– pulp of tooth 462
ROSENMUELLER's or CLOQUET's lymph
  node (deep inguinal lymph node) 296
ROSENMÜLLER's fossa (retropharyngeal
  recess) 534
ROSENTHAL's vein (basal vein) 562
Rostral part
– of mesencephalon 514
– of pons 514
Rostrum of corpus callosum 574
Rotational axis
– of cricothyroid joint 540
– of the upper arm 88
Rotator cuff 104
– muscles 96, 104
Rotatores 70, 73
Rots of retina 499
ROTTER's lymph nodes (interpectoral
  lymph nodes) 231, 232
Round
– ligament
– – of liver 273, 297, 302, 303, 305, 319,
  330, 331, 332, 333, 334
– – of uterus 291, 369, 388, 389, 390,
  391, 392, 395
– window 508, 510, 511, 513
Rubrospinal tract 614, 615, 618
Rubrothalamic tract 618

S

Saccule 511, 512, 515
Sacral
- canal 75
- flexure 371
- foramina 74, 75
- ganglia 605
- hiatus 75
- horn 74
- kyphosis 43
- lymph nodes 395, 404
- nerves 217
- - roots 608
- plexus 214, 216, 373, 396, 414, 421, 606
- preganglionic parasympathetic nerve fibers 328
- region 364
- segments of spinal cord 608
- splanchnic nerves 396, 605, 606
- tuberosity 75
Sacralization 74
Sacrococcygeal
- joint 75
- ligament 405
Sacroiliac joint 67, 74, 158, 160, 367
Sacropelvic surface (of ilium) 159
Sacrospinous ligament 160, 161, 163, 365, 405, 416, 419
Sacrotuberous ligament 160, 161, 163, 168, 365, 368, 405, 413, 416, 419
Sacrum 42, 68, 74, 156, 157, 158, 365, 367, 368
- distinguishing features 75
- radiograph 67, 74
Saddle anesthesia 613
Saddle joint 17
Sagittal
- plane 6
- septum 478
- suture 429, 431, 561
Sail sign 110
Salivary glands 31
- parasympathetic innervation 479
- stones 476
Salpingitis 369, 389, 391
Salpingopalatine fold 530
Salpingopharyngeal fold 467, 530, 534
Salpingopharyngeus 472, 507, 534, 597
SA nodal artery 268
SA node (sinuatrial node, node of KEITH-FLACK) 259, 270
SANTORINI's (corniculate) cartilage 540
SANTORINI's duct (accessory pancreatic duct) 341, 344
Saphenous
- branch of descending genicular artery 220
- nerve 175, 217
- opening 296
Sarcomere 20
Sartorius 156, 157, 166, 169, 170, 171, 172, 175
Scala
- media 512
- tympani 511, 512, 513
- vestibuli 511, 512, 513
Scalene
- lymph nodes (inferior deep cervical lymph nodes) 249
- tubercle 234

Scalenus
- anterior 61, 62, 141, 235, 238, 521, 524, 525, 528, 551
- medius 61, 62, 141, 235, 238, 521, 528, 551
- posterior 61, 62, 235, 238, 520, 521, 551
Scalenus anticus syndrome 275
Scalp 425
- injuries 562
- soft tissue layers 425
Scapha 502
Scaphoid 119, 123, 124
- fossa 435
- fracture 122
Scapholunate ligamentous complex, radiograph 124
Scapula 88, 89, 91
- upward rotation 100
Scapular
- line 227
- nerves 106
- region 4, 225
Scapularis 115
Scapulohumeral motion 100
- impairment 100
SCARPA's fascia 288, 290, 294
SCARPA's vestibular ganglion 580
SCHEUERMANN's disease (adolescent kyphosis) 65
SCHIRMER's test 489, 593
SCHLEMM, canal of (scleral venous sinus) 495, 496
SCHULTZE's comma tract (interfascicular fasciculus, cervical part) 614
SCHWALBE's nucleus (medial vestibular nucleus) 512, 516
SCHWANN's cells
- tumor 510, 591
Sciatica 46
Sciatic nerve 161, 173, 174, 214, 216, 217, 382, 408, 415
Scintigraphy of thyroid gland 32
Sclera 495, 496
Scleral venous sinus (canal of SCHLEMM) 495, 496
Scoliosis 43
Scooty dog sign
- radiograph of lumbar vertebrae 68
Screw home mechanism
- knee joint 181
Scrotum 33, 397, 399, 405
Secondary
- brain vesicles 556
- follicle (B cell zone) of lymph nodes 30
- retroperitoneal abdominal organs 300, 305
Segmental
- arteries 82
- medullary artery 570
- spinal artery 570
Segmental resection
- lung cancer or metastases 248
Selective proximal vagotomy (SPV) 315
Sella-nasion (SN) plane 428
Sella turcica 432, 436, 564
Semicircular canals 505, 511, 515
Semilunar
- cusp of aortic valve 260
- fold of conjunctiva 482, 489
- folds of colon 322
- ganglion (GASSERIAN or trigeminal ganglion) 580, 607

Semilunar
- hernia (SPIEGELian hernia) 289
- hiatus 451, 452, 453
- line (SPIEGEL's line) 289
- valves 261
- - stenosis 263
Semimembranosus 166, 167, 173, 176, 180, 187, 188, 189
- bursa 187, 188
Seminal
- colliculus (verumontanum) 376, 378
- gland/vesicle 33, 370, 380, 381, 382, 383, 384, 398, 399, 403, 418
Semispinalis
- capitis 58, 63, 73, 440, 520, 521
- cervicis 63, 73
- thoracis 63, 70, 73
Semitendinosus 166, 167, 168, 169, 173, 176, 180, 189
Senile cataract 497
Senile kyphosis 65
Sensorineural hearing impairment 515
Sensory
- ganglia 581
- receptors 24
- root
- - of ciliary ganglion 583, 584, 587
- - of trigeminal nerve [CN V] 494, 586
Sentinel lymph node 287
- breast cancer 232
Septal
- branch
- - of anterior ethmoid nerve 454
- - of posterior ethmoid artery 454
- cusp of right atrioventricular valve [tricuspid valve] 259, 261
- lymphatic vessels 249
- nasal cartilage (cartilaginous part of nasal septum) 448
- papillary muscle 259
Septa testis 400
Septate uterus 388
Septomarginal
- fasciculus (FLECHSIG, oval bundle of) 614
- trabecula 259, 270
Septum
- of musculotubal canal 504
- of scrotum 293, 294, 399
- pellucidum 574
- transversum 297
Serotonin
- antagonists 575
- receptors 575
Serous pericardium 256, 257, 259, 260
Serratus
- anterior 78, 86, 101, 103, 230, 242, 520
- posterior 71
- - inferior 70, 71, 103
- - superior 71, 103
Sesamoid bone 13
- of foot 194, 195
- of hand 119, 122, 124
- patella 185, 186
Shaft
- axis of humerus 88
- of fibula 191
- of fifth metatarsal 194
- of radius 121
- of tibia 191
- of ulna 120
Shaking the head 64

Shingles, varicella-zoster virus
  infection 229, 609
Short
– ciliary nerves 479, 494, 496, 497, 583,
  587
– gastric
– – arteries 312, 325, 329, 334
– – veins 308, 312, 313, 336
– head of biceps
– – brachii 114
– – femoris 173
– limb of incus 506
– posterior ciliary arteries 487, 495
Short bones 13
Shoulder
– abduction/adduction 7, 98
– anterior muscles 101
– arteries 107
– axillary region 105
– blade 91
– deep posterior muscles 103
– depression 99
– elevation 99
– extension/flexion 98
– external/internal rotation 98
– girdle 88, 89
– – acromioclavicular joint 95
– – glenohumeral joint 96, 97
– – radiograph 89
– – range of motion 99
– – sternoclavicular joint 94
– horizontal
– – abduction/addduction 99
– – extension/flexion 99
– impingement 100
– innervation 142, 144
– – infraclavicular branches 143
– – supraclavicular branches 142
– – terminal branches
– – – of lateral cord 145
– – – of medial cord 145
– – – of posterior cord 144
– joint 97
– movements 8
– nerves 106
– posterior muscles 102
– protraction 99
– range of motion 98
– region, surface anatomy 86
– retraction 99
– rotator cuff 104
– separation, radiograph 95
– superficial muscles 102
– tendinitis/tendinopathy 114
Sialoliths 476
Sigmoid
– arteries 326, 329, 374
– colon 299, 305, 319, 321, 322, 325, 326,
  347, 384
– lymph nodes 361
– mesocolon 347
– sinus 507, 508, 560, 562
– veins 326, 336, 337, 374
SILVIUS, aqueduct of (aqueduct of midbrain, cerebral aqueduct) 572, 573, 574
Simple bony limb 510
Singer's nodules 541
Sinuatrial
– nodal branch
– – of left coronary artery 267
– – of right coronary artery 266, 267

Sinuatrial
– node (SA node, node of
  KEITH-FLACK) 259, 270
– – blood supply 268
Sinus
– of pulmonary trunk 258
– of venae cavae 269
– tympani 504
– venosus 259
– – phlebitis 443
– – thrombosis 443
Sinuses 560
Situs inversus 298
Skeletal
– muscle 19
– – architecture and function 20, 21
– – fast twitch and slow twitch fibers 19
– – organization 20, 21
– ossification of the upper and lower
  extremities 14
Skeleton
– bony landmarks 41
– types of bones 13
Skin 24
Skull
– fractures 433
– inner aspect 434
– of a newborn 430, 431
– reference lines 428
– x-ray image 432
Sliding hiatal hernia 309
Slit lamp examination 497
Small
– cardiac vein 257, 269
– intestine 31, 299, 304, 306
– – arterial arcades 320
– – blood supply 324
– – layers of the wall 320
– – lymphatic drainage 327
– pits on nails 26
– saphenous vein 174, 189, 221, 222
Smallest cardiac veins (THEBESIAN
  veins) 269
SMA syndrome (superior mesenteric artery
  syndrome) 318
Smooth muscle 19
Snuff box 118, 135
SOELDER's lines/zones 585
Soft palate 455, 464, 465, 467, 471, 530
– muscles 472
– neurovascular supply 465
Soleal line 191, 192
Sole (of foot) 4
– nerves and vessels 213
Soleus 190, 201, 204, 205
Solitary liver metastases 332
Solitary nucleus see Nucleus/i of solitary
  tract
Somatic
– nervous system 35, 611
– plexus 606
Somatic nerve fibers 606
– of female genitalia 396
– of parietal peritoneum 300
Somatomotor system 603
Somatostatin 575
Spermatic cord 79, 291, 292, 293, 296,
  382, 397, 399
– borders 292
– coverings 293, 294
Sphenofrontal suture 427, 428, 434

Sphenoid 435
– bone 427, 430, 431, 432, 434, 435, 436,
  450, 451, 484, 485, 490
– concha 435
– crest 435, 450
– fontanelle 430
– lingula 435, 436
– margin of temporal bone 504
– part of middle cerebral artery 563
– rostrum 435
– sinus 432, 448, 450, 451, 452, 453, 507,
  564
– yoke 436
Sphenomandibular ligament 458, 460,
  532
Sphenopalatine
– artery 442, 447, 454, 466
– foramen 436, 450, 451, 454, 485
– ganglion 581
Sphenoparietal
– sinus 560
– suture 427
Sphenopetrosal
– fissure 437, 438, 507
– synchondrosis 510
Sphenosquamous suture 428, 434
Sphenozygomatic suture 427, 428
Sphincter
– of ampulla (sphincter of ODDI) 317, 339,
  341
– of bile duct 341
– of ODDI 317, 339, 341
– of pancreatic duct 341
– pupillae 479, 491, 495, 496, 583, 607
SPIEGELian hernia (semilunar hernia) 289
SPIEGEL's line (semilunar line) 289
Spina bifida 569
– aperta 569
– cystica 569
– occulta 569
Spinal
– accessory nerve [CN XI] 437, 444, 523,
  524, 525, 526, 529, 533, 534, 563, 578,
  579, 594, 601
– – motor fibers 601
– accessory nucleus 597
– anesthesia 396, 571
– arachnoid mater 569
– artery 82
– branch of inercostal artery 240
– canal, veins 569
– cord 35, 556, 557, 607, 608, 613
– – injury 218
– – laminar organization 614
– – lesions 619, 620
– – major ascending and descending
    white matter tracts 615
– – meninges 569
– – metastasis, MRI 613
– – organization
– – – of the gray matter 614
– – – of the white matter 614
– – pathways
– – – of involuntary proprioception 617
– – – of motor system 618
– – positional information and organiza-
    tion 556
– – position within the vertebral canal 571
– – schematic representation 37
– – segmental
– – – arterial blood supply 570
– – – organization 613

Spinal segmental
– – segments 608
– dura mater 530, 569, 571
– nerve 37, 608, 616, 617
– – injury 218
– – nomenclature 608
– – schematic representation 37
– nucleus/i
– – of accessory nerve 601
– – of trigeminal nerve 578, 579, 585, 586, 590, 593, 596, 599
– part of deltoid 86
– pia mater 569
– reflexes, monosynaptic 612
– root
– – ganglia 569
– – of accessory nerve 601
– – – fiber qualities 601
– sensory ganglion 569, 610, 616, 617
– stenosis 46
– tract of trigeminal nerve 595
Spinalis 72
– capitis 72, 73
– cervicis 72
– thoracis 72
Spine
– curvatures 43
– lateral view 47
– motion segment 47
– of scapula 41, 91
– of sphenoid 435, 458
Spinocerebellar tract 615
Spinolaminar line 53
Spino-olivary tract 614, 615, 616, 617
Spinoreticular tract 616
Spinotectal tract 614
Spinothalamic tract 615, 620
Spinous process 41, 44, 45, 55, 57, 66, 67, 68
Spiral
– fold (valve of HEISTER) 339
– ganglion 512, 513, 514, 515, 580
– ligament 512
– limbus 512
– organ (organ of CORTI) 511, 512, 513
Splanchnic nerves 315, 360, 606
Spleen 297, 302, 303, 310, 313, 316, 334, 343, 346, 347
– attachment to the posterior abdominal wall 346
– infarction 346
– rupture 346
– segments 346
Splenic
– artery 302, 312, 314, 316, 318, 325, 329, 334, 342, 346
– branch/es of splenic artery 325
– hilum 346
– lymph nodes 314, 345, 361
– nerve plexus 597, 598
– niche 346
– recess of omental bursa 303, 304
– vein 313, 316, 325, 326, 336, 337, 342, 343, 346
– – tributaries 336
Splenium of corpus callosum 566
Splenius
– capitis 58, 63, 72, 73, 440, 444, 520, 521, 523, 524, 525
– cervicis 61, 63, 72
Splenomegaly 337
Splenorenal ligament 297, 300, 302, 346

Spondylolisthesis 69
Spondylolysis 68, 69
Spondylophytes 45
Spongy
– trabeculae 15
– urethra 378
Sprained ankle 199
Squamosal margin sphenoid bone 435, 436
Squamous
– cell carcinoma of larynx 541
– part
– – of frontal bone 426, 431, 449, 450, 485
– – of occipital bone 429, 430, 431, 432, 436
– – of temporal bone 428, 431, 432, 434, 451, 504
– suture 428, 429, 432
SSA (specific somatic efferent) 577, 578
Stalk of epiglottis 537, 538, 539
Stapedial
– branch of posterior tympanic artery 509
– ligament 506
– membrane 506
Stapedius 506, 508, 590, 592, 593
– paralysis 508
– reflex test 592, 593
Stapes 505, 506, 508, 511, 513, 592
Statoacoustic nerve 510
Stellate
– (cervicothoracic) ganglion 272, 280, 533, 534, 604, 605, 607
– – block 605, 612
– veins of kidney 354
Stenosis of the vertebral canal 148
STENSON's duct (parotid duct) 439, 441, 444, 475, 478
Sternal
– angle (angle of LOUIS) 226, 228, 233, 250
– – vertebral projection 228
– end of clavicle 90
– head
– – of pectoralis major 86, 101
– – of sternocleidomastoid 61
– part of diaphragm 237
– region 4
Sternoclavicular
– joint 86, 89, 94
– – dislocation, radiograph 94
– – radiograph 94
– part of pectoralis major 101
Sternocleidomastoid 58, 61, 439, 440, 441, 445, 446, 475, 478, 519, 520, 521, 523, 524, 525, 526, 528, 529, 545, 601
– artery 442
– branch of superior thyroid artery 442
– region 225, 425
Sternocostal
– surface of heart 257
– triangle 237
Sternohyoid 235, 521, 526, 528, 529, 546, 548, 602
Sternothyroid 521, 524, 525, 526, 528, 530, 546, 548, 602
Sternum 86, 233, 310
Stomach 31, 280, 302, 304, 305, 306, 310, 311, 312, 314, 316, 334, 339, 346
– arteries 312
– autonomic innervation 315
– lymphatic drainage 314
– lymph nodes and vessels 314
– muscular layers 311

Stomach
– parasympathetic innervation 315
– projection onto the ventral abdominal wall 310
– regional lymph nodes 314
– spatial relations 310
– vascular supply 312
– veins 313
Straight
– cortical artery of kidney 354
– part
– – of cricothyroid 532, 540
– – of distal tubulus 354
– – of proximal tubulus 354
– sinus 560, 562, 573
Stratified squamous nonkeratinized epithelium of conjunctiva and cornea 483
Streptococcal pharyngitis 531
Stretch reflexes 612
Stria
– terminalis 574
– vascularis of cochlear duct 512
Striate area 497, 499
Stridor 544
Stroke 495
– patent foramen ovale 259
Stye (hordeolum) 483
Styloglossus 469, 470, 478, 532
Stylohyoid 441, 474, 475, 478, 508, 521, 524, 528, 529, 532, 546, 590, 592, 593
– branch of facial nerve [CN VII] 446, 474, 508, 592
– ligament 532
– process of temporal bone 508
Styloid process
– of radius 87, 119, 121, 123
– of temporal bone 428, 429, 432, 441, 458, 478, 503, 504, 505, 532
– of ulna 87, 119, 120, 122, 123
Stylomandibular ligament 458, 532
Stylomastoid
– artery 442, 509
– foramen 437, 504, 508, 590, 592
Stylopharyngeal
– aponeurosis 478
– branch of glossopharyngeal nerve 594, 595
– ligament 470
Stylopharyngeus 470, 478, 532, 533, 594, 596, 597
Subacromial
– bursa 97
– space, alterations 100
Subarachnoid
– bleedings 565
– space 495, 558, 561, 569, 572, 573, 613
Subarcuate
– artery 509
– fossa 434, 504
Subchondral bone 16
Subclavian
– artery 81, 107, 141, 231, 236, 239, 240, 248, 253, 257, 274, 275, 276, 278, 280, 306, 520, 524, 525, 527, 529, 534, 547, 551, 564, 570, 597, 605
– – branches 527
– – compression 234
– groove of clavicle 90
– lymphatic trunk 232, 249, 551
– nerve 106, 142
– vein 150, 231, 232, 236, 249, 274, 275, 276, 279, 361, 520, 524, 529, 534, 551

Subclavius 101, 142
Subcommissural organ 575
Subcostal
– angle 226
– artery 278, 279, 285, 359
– incision 289
– muscle 235
– nerve 214, 284, 300, 321, 348, 350, 356
– plane 283
– vein 279
Subcostales 238
Subdural
– hematoma 561
– space 558
Subendocardial branches of
   atrioventricular bundle 270
Subepicardial adipose tissue 255
Subepithelial venous plexus of
   tongue 470
Subfornical organ 575
Subgaleotic layer 425
Subglottic space (subglottis) 543
Subhepatic recess of omental bursa 333
Subiculum of promontory 504
Sublingual
– artery 447, 470, 477, 524
– caruncle 476, 477
– fold 476, 477
– fossa 457
– ganglion 479
– gland 447, 470, 473, 475, 476, 477,
   479, 590, 593
– nerve 470, 477, 589
– space 473
– vein 470, 475
Sublobar vein of liver 335
Submandibular
– duct (WHARTON's duct) 475, 476, 477
– fossa 457
– ganglion 447, 470, 475, 477, 479, 581,
   586, 589, 590, 593, 604
– gland 441, 473, 475, 476, 477, 479, 524,
   528, 529, 532, 546, 590, 593
– lymph nodes 475, 550
– space 473
– triangle 425, 528
Submental
– artery 442, 446, 447, 475, 524, 525
– lymph nodes 550
– triangle 425, 528
– vein 443, 446, 447, 475, 524, 529
Submucous
– plexus (MEISSNER's plexus) 320, 581
– venous plexus of esophagus 308
Suboccipital
– muscles 64
– triangle 64
Subperitoneal
– (infraperitoneal) abdominal organs 300
– pelvic
– – fascia 417
– – space 366, 370
– – viscera 393
– space 418
Subphrenic recess of omental bursa 301,
   333
Subpleural
– fascia 242
– lymphatic vessels 249
Subpubic angle 158

Subscapular
– artery 149
– axillary lymph nodes 231, 232
– fossa 91
– nerves 106, 143
Subscapularis 104, 143
Substantia nigra 618
Subtalar joint 198
– radiograph 198
– range of motion 196
SUDECK's point 374
Sulcus
– of auditory tube 435
– sclerae 482
– terminalis
– – cordis 257
– – of tongue 534
Superciliary arch 426
Superficial
– abdominal veins 286
– anastomoses between SVC and IVC 286
– ansa cervicalis 445
– axillary lymph nodes 232
– branch
– – of lateral plantar nerve 213
– – of medial circumflex femoral
     artery 174, 175
– – of radial nerve 117, 133, 135, 144
– – of transverse cervical artery 524
– – of ulnar nerve 139, 145
– cervical
– – artery 525, 527
– – vein 529
– circumflex iliac
– – artery 285, 286
– – vein 221, 286, 296
– dorsal
– – artery of penis 398
– – vein of penis 397, 398
– epigastric
– – artery 285
– – vein 221, 296, 337
– facial muscles 441
– fascia of penis 397
– femoral artery 219
– fibular nerve 212, 216, 217
– infrapatellar bursa 187
– inguinal
– – lymph nodes 222, 287, 375, 395, 404
– – ring 39, 79, 289, 291, 292, 293, 294,
     295, 399
– lateral cervical lymph nodes 550
– layer of cervical fascia 475, 521, 530
– lymphatic vessels of arm 150
– lymph collectors of mammary gland 232
– palmar
– – arch 139, 140, 149
– – branch of radial artery 139, 140, 149
– parotid lymph nodes 550
– part
– – of masseter 441, 460
– – of parotid gland 475, 478
– perineal
– – fascia 417
– – nerve 410, 411, 414
– – space (pouch)
– – – in man 413, 418
– – – in woman 406, 416, 417, 418
– petrosal artery 509
– popliteal lymph nodes 222
– posterior sacrococcygeal ligament 160,
     405

Superficial
– prepatellar bursa 187
– temporal
– – artery 441, 442, 444, 445, 446, 447,
     487, 502
– – branches of auriculotemporal
     nerve 587, 589
– – nerves 589
– – vein 443, 447, 487
– thyroid
– – artery 530
– – vein 530
– transverse
– – metacarpal ligament 134, 136, 137
– – perineal muscle 406, 408, 409, 411,
     412, 413, 415, 416
– venous
– – palmar arch 150
– – system 29
Superior 5
– alveolar nerves 446, 454, 465, 588
– angle of scapula 91
– anterior pancreaticoduodenal
   artery 318, 334
– arcuate line 543
– articular
– – process 44, 49, 55, 57, 67, 68, 69, 74
– – surface
– – – of tibia 192
– – – of vertebra 69
– belly of omohyoid 520, 521, 524, 526,
   528, 546, 602
– border of petrous part of temporal
   bone 434, 504
– branch/es
– – of oculomotor nerve [CN III] 494, 583,
     584
– – of transverse cervical nerve 523
– bulb of jugular vein 533, 534, 560, 562
– cerebellar
– – artery 563, 565, 566, 568
– – peduncle 617
– cerebral veins 560, 562
– cervical
– – cardiac
– – – branches of vagus nerve [CN X] 307,
       525, 533, 534, 551, 597, 598
– – – nerve 272, 525, 533, 605
– – ganglion 272, 466, 497, 525, 533, 594,
     605
– choroid vein 562
– clunial nerves 217
– colliculus 499
– conjunctival fornix 489
– constrictor 455, 469, 470, 471, 478,
   532, 533, 534, 594, 596, 597
– – paralysis 596
– coracohumeral ligament 96
– costal facet 44, 66
– costotransverse ligament 51
– crura 486
– deep lateral cervical lymph nodes 550
– dental plexus 465
– duodenal
– – artery 334
– – fossa 299
– epigastric
– – artery 231, 239, 285, 286
– – – anastomoses 285
– – vein 231, 286
– eyelid 482, 483, 488
– fold of malleus 505

Superior
- ganglion
-- of accessory nerve 601
-- of glossopharyngeal nerve 580, 594, 595, 596
-- of vagus nerve 580, 597, 598, 599
- gemellus 166, 167, 168
- gluteal
-- artery 161, 162, 174, 219, 409, 419
-- nerve 161, 167, 170, 174, 214, 216
--- injury 167
--- lesions 174
-- vein 161, 174
- head of lateral pterygoid 459, 460
- hemorrhoidal (rectal) artery 326, 329, 374
- horn of thyroid cartilage 536, 537, 538, 539, 544
- hypogastric
-- ganglion 360
-- plexus 328, 373, 396, 403, 421, 604, 605
- hypophysial artery 564, 565
- ileocecal recess 299
- intercostal vein 239
- labial
-- artery 454
-- branch of facial artery 442, 454
-- vein 443
- lacrimal
-- canaliculus 489
-- punctum 489
- laryngeal
-- artery 524, 525, 532, 534, 544, 546, 547, 551
-- branch of vagus nerve [CN X] 467
-- nerve 307, 467, 525, 532, 533, 534, 544, 546, 547, 551, 597, 598
-- vein 532, 534, 546
- lateral
-- cutaneous nerve of arm 144, 147, 229
-- genicular artery 189, 212, 220
- left homonymous
-- quadrantanopia (quadrantopsia, quadrant anopia) 500
- ligament
-- of epididymis 400
-- of incus 506
-- of malleus 506
- lingular segment of left lung 247
- lobar bronchus 245
- lobe
-- of left lung 246
-- of right lung 245
- longitudinal muscle of tongue 468, 602
- medial genicular artery 174, 189, 212, 220
- mediastinum 250
-- anatomical structures 250
-- arteries 274
-- blood vessels, surface projection 274
-- veins 274
- mesenteric
-- artery 318, 324, 325, 326, 329, 334, 342, 343, 345, 358, 359, 374, 421, 605
--- branches 324
--- course within the mesentery 325
--- origin 325
--- SMA syndrome 318
-- ganglion 328, 358, 360, 421, 597, 598, 604
-- lymph nodes 318, 327, 345, 361
-- plexus 328, 421, 605

Superior mesenteric
-- vein 313, 318, 325, 342, 343
--- course within the mesentery 325
--- tributaries 336
- nasal concha 450, 451, 452, 454
- nuchal line 429
- oblique 487, 490, 491, 493, 494, 583
-- paralysis 491
- olivary nuclei 513, 514, 515
- ophthalmic vein 443, 487, 492, 560, 562, 583
- orbital fissure 426, 434, 435, 436, 438, 451, 484, 485, 491, 492, 586
-- fractures 492
-- neurovascular structures 492
- palpebral arch 487
- pancreatic lymph nodes 345
- pancreaticoduodenal
-- artery 329, 345
-- vein 318
- parathyroid glands 532, 547
- part of duodenum 305, 317, 347
- pelvic aperture 161
- petrosal sinus 560
- phrenic
-- arteries 237
-- artery 278
-- lymph nodes 338
- posterior
-- alveolar branch of facial artery 442
-- pancreaticoduodenal artery 318, 334, 341
- pubic
-- ligament 160
-- ramus 158, 159, 160, 407
- pulmonary vein 255, 256
- quadrantanopia 499
- recess
-- of omental bursa 303, 304, 333
-- of tympanic membrane 505
- rectal
-- artery (superior hemorrhoidal artery) 326, 329, 374, 394
-- lymph nodes 361, 375
-- vein 326, 336, 337, 374, 420
- rectus 487, 490, 491, 494, 583, 584
- renal polar artery 352
- root of ansa cervicalis (cervical plexus) 524, 525, 526, 529
- sagittal sinus 560, 561, 562, 573
- salivatory nucleus 477, 479, 578, 579, 581, 590, 593
- segment
-- of left lung 247
-- of right lung 247
- suprarenal arteries 357, 358, 359
- tarsal
-- muscle 607
-- plate 486
- tarsus 486, 487
- temporal
-- line (of parietal bone) 428, 429
-- retinal
--- arteriole 498
--- venule 498
- terminal branches of middle cerebral artery 567
- thalamostriate vein 562, 574
- thoracic
-- aperture 233, 235
--- blood vessels and nerves 275, 529

Superior thoracic aperture
--- cross-section 276
--- structures 551
-- artery 107, 149
- thyroid
-- artery 442, 524, 525, 529, 533, 547, 551
-- notch 536, 538, 539, 540
-- tubercle 538
-- vein 443, 524, 525, 529, 547
- tibiofibular joint 191
- tracheobronchial lymph nodes 249, 253
- transverse
-- fold of rectum 375
-- scapular ligament 108
- trunk of brachial plexus 106, 141, 524, 601
- tympanic artery 509
- ulnar collateral artery 108, 149
- vena cava 236, 251, 254, 255, 256, 257, 258, 259, 264, 269, 273, 275, 277, 279, 529, 534
-- projection onto the thoracic wall 228
- vertebral
-- arch 68
-- endplate 69
-- notch 54, 68
- vesical
-- artery 355, 394, 402, 409, 419
-- vein 420
- vestibular nucleus (nucleus of BEKHTEREV/BECHTEREW) 512, 516, 578
Supermedial superficial inguinal lymph nodes 287
Superolateral superficial inguinal lymph nodes 287
Supinator 132
- canal 117
Supracallosal part
- of anterior cerebral artery 563
Supraclavicular
- nerves 147, 445, 520, 523
- part of brachial plexus 106, 525, 529
Supracolic compartment (epigastrium) 299, 301
Supracristal plane 283
Supraduodenal artery 329
Supraglenoid tubercle 91, 96
Supraglottic space (supraglottis) 543
Suprahyoid 520
- muscles 474
Supramastoid crest 504
Suprameatal triangle 504
Supranuclear (central) facial palsy 591
Supraoptic
- recess of fourth ventricle 572
Supraorbital
- artery 445, 487, 493, 494
- foramen 426, 430, 484, 585
- horizontal line 559
- margin 426, 449, 484
- nerve 444, 446, 447, 488, 493, 585, 587
- notch 449, 484
- vein 487
Suprapatellar bursa 187
Suprapineal recess of third ventricle 572, 573
Suprapiriform foramen 168, 174
Suprapleural fascia 243
Suprapubic
- angle 365
- cystostomy 377
- incision 289
- region 283, 364

Suprarenal
– arteries 357
– gland 32, 342, 343, 347, 348, 351, 357, 402
–– arteries 357
–– innervation 358
–– lymphatic drainage 358
–– position in the retroperitoneal space 348
–– stress response 357
–– veins 357
– impression on liver 331
– plexus 597, 598
– veins 348, 351, 357
Suprascapular
– artery 108, 520, 524, 525, 527, 551
– nerve 106, 108, 141, 142, 520, 525
– notch 91
– region 4
Suprascapularis 108
Supraspinatus 104, 142
– tendon, compression 100
Supraspinous
– fossa of scapula 91
– ligament 41, 50, 51, 160, 571
Suprasternal
– notch 86
–– projection onto the thoracic wall 228
–– vertebral projection 228
– space 521, 548
Supratonsillar fossa 455
Supratrochlear
– artery 446, 487, 494
– nerve 445, 446, 487, 493, 587
– vein 443, 487
Supravaginal part of cervix 391
Supravesical fossa 290, 294, 377
Supreme intercostal artery 81, 239, 240, 278, 527, 551
Sural
– artery 189, 220
– nerve 174, 217
Surface anatomy of man and woman 3
Surgical neck of humerus 93
Suspensory
– ligament
–– of clitoris 407
–– of duodenum (ligament of TREITZ) 317
–– of ovary (infundibulopelvic ligament) 369, 385, 388, 389, 391, 394
–– of penis 293, 397, 399
– ligaments of breast (COOPER's ligaments) 230
– muscle of duodenum (muscle of TREITZ) 317
Sustentaculum tali 194, 195, 198, 200
Sutural
– bones 13, 429
– joints 16
SVA (specific visceral afferent) 577, 578
SVE (specific visceral efferent) 577, 578
Swallowing 535
– difficulties 596
Sweat glands, innervation 603
SYLVIUS, aqueduct of (aqueduct of midbrain, cerebral aqueduct) 572
Sympathetic
– central fibers 607
– ganglia 279, 328, 606, 608
–– of cranial nerves 581

Sympathetic
– nerve fibers
–– of abdominal viscera 360
–– of esophagus 307
–– of female genitalia 396
–– of intestine 328
–– of kidney 358
– nervous system 603, 604, 605, 606
– nuclei 604
– postganglionic fibers 607
– preganglionic fibers 607
– root
–– of ciliary ganglion 583, 584
–– of pterygopalatine ganglion 590, 594
– trunk 251, 252, 278, 279, 280, 307, 358, 421, 478, 525, 533, 534, 551, 594, 605
Symphysial
– cavity 160
– surface 159
Symphysis 16
Synchondrosis 16
Syndesmosis 16
Synovial
– bursae of knee joint 187
– fluid 16
– folds 16
– joints 16, 17
– membrane 16
Systemic arteries 28
Systemic circulation
– arteries 28
– veins 29
Systole 262
– blood flow and valve position 262
– ventricular action 261, 262
Systolic murmur 263

T

Tachycardia 272, 599
– electrocardiography (ECG) 271
– pulmonary embolism 249
Tachypnea, pulmonary embolism 249
Taenia
– coli 301
– thalami 574
Tail
– of epididymis 400, 401
– of pancreas 305, 321, 342, 344, 347
Tail bone 76
– injuries 76
Talocalcaneal joint 198
– radiograph 198
– range of motion 196
Talocalcaneonavicular joint 198
Talocrural joint 197
– radiograph 197
– range of motion 196
Talonavicular joint 200
Talotarsal joint, range of motion 196
Talus 194, 195, 197, 198, 199, 210
Tanycytes 575
Tarsal
– bones 195
– glands (MEIBOMIAN glands) 483
–– granulomatous inflammation 483
– sinus 195, 198
Tarsometatarsal
– joints (LISFRANC's region) 194, 195, 200
– ligaments 200
Tarsus 483

Taste
– perception 600
– receptors 593
TAWARA, node of (atrioventricular node, AV-node) 259, 270
T cell zone of lymph node 287
Tear film, components 483
Tectorial membrane 513
Tectospinal tract 614, 618
Tectum of midbrain 499, 566
Teeth/Tooth 31
– blood supply 466
– innervation 465
– structure and support system 462
Tegmen tympani 508, 509
Tela choroidea
– of third ventricle 566, 574
Telencephalon 514, 556, 557
Temporal
– bone 428, 430, 431, 432, 434, 451, 503, 504, 505, 507
– branch/es
–– of facial nerve [CN VII] 440, 444, 590, 591
–– of middle cerebral artery 567
–– of posterior cerebral artery 566
– fascia 441
– hemiretina 500
– horn of lateral ventricle 572, 573, 574
– line
–– of frontal bone 441
–– of parietal bone 428
– lobe 36, 556, 557, 572, 573
–– hernia 559
– operculum 556
– pole 557
– pulse 28
– region 425
– surface
–– of sphenoid bone 435
–– of temporal bone 504
Temporalis 441, 460
Temporofacial branch of facial nerve [CN VII] 440
Temporomandibular joint 428, 458, 459
– capsule 441
– lateral ligament 441, 458
– radiograph 459
– range of motion 459
Temporoparietalis 439, 440, 441
Temporozygomatic suture 428
Tendinous
– arch of levator ani 368
– intersections of rectus abdominis 77, 78, 79
– sheath
–– of extensor
––– digitorum longus 206
––– hallucis longus 206
–– of flexor
––– digitorum longus 206
––– hallucis longus 206
–– of tibialis
––– anterior 206
––– posterior 206
Tendons 22, 23
– insertion to bone 23
– organization 23
Tension headache 444
Tensor
– fasciae latae 166, 169, 170, 382
–– paralysis 174

Tensor
- tympani 505, 506, 507, 508, 509, 586, 592
- veli palatini 472, 507, 534, 586
-- loss of function 507
Tentorial
- branch of ophthalmic nerve 587
- nerve 493, 587
- notch 560
Tentorium cerebelli 560
Teres
- major 41, 86, 102, 108, 143
- minor 104, 144
Terminal
- arteries 320
- hair (long hair) 25
- ileum 322
- line (linea terminalis) 161, 365
- part of middle cerebral artery 563
- sulcus of tongue 467, 534
Testicular
- artery 292, 293, 321, 351, 359, 397, 399, 400, 401, 402, 403
- cancer 401, 404
-- cryptorchidism 399
- descent 294, 399
- plexus 293, 403, 421
- torsion 401
- vein 292, 321, 337, 351, 397, 401, 402
Testis 32, 33, 294, 370, 400, 403
- blood vessels 401
Tetraparesis 619
Tetraplegia 619
Thalamoparietal fibers 616
Thalamus 36, 556, 557, 562, 566, 568, 574, 600, 616, 618
THEBESIAN veins (smallest cardiac veins) 269
Thenar
- eminence 87
- muscles 136
- region 136
Thermoregulation 280
Thigh
- anterior muscles 171
- anterior view 157
- medial muscles 172
- posterior
-- muscles 173
-- vessels and nerves 174
- vessels and nerves 175
Third ventricle 556, 566, 572, 573, 574
Thoracic
- aorta 237, 239, 240, 248, 252, 253, 256, 273, 274, 278, 280, 306, 307, 570, 605
-- branches 278
- aortic nerve plexus 252, 280
- arteries 570
- (bronchoaortic) constriction of esophagus 306
- cardiac branches of vagus nerve 251, 252, 272, 307, 597, 598
- cavity 242
- duct 30, 232, 249, 252, 278, 279, 327, 335, 361, 550, 551
-- confluence 249
- fascia 244
- ganglion 251, 252, 605
- joints 234
- kyphosis 43
- nerves 147, 231, 251, 278, 279, 280, 286, 608
-- roots 608

Thoracic
- outlet (superior thoracic aperture) 233
- outlet syndrome (TOS) 234, 275
- part of esophagus 252, 253, 280, 306, 307
- region, arteries 81
- segmental arteries 81
- segments of spinal cord 608
- skeleton 233
- spine 65
- splanchnic nerves 606
- vertebrae 42, 44, 65, 66, 233
-- distinguishing features 66
-- facet joints 49
-- radiograph 65
-- structures 66
- wall
-- anterior muscles 235
-- arteries 239
-- layers 242
-- posterior muscles 235
-- projections of heart and cardiac valves 254
-- projections of the rib cage 226
-- veins 239
Thoracoabdominal nerves 284
Thoracoacromial
- artery 107, 149, 525
- trunk 107
- vein 529
Thoracocentesis 244
Thoracodorsal
- artery 149
- nerve 106, 141, 143, 238, 525
Thoracoepigastric veins 150, 151, 231, 232, 286, 525
Thoracolumbar
- fascia 50, 71, 73, 77, 80, 102
- region, range of motion 70
Thorax 3
- cross sectional anatomy 264, 265
- CT cross-section 264, 265, 276, 277
- epifascial blood vessels 231
- excursions during respiration 238
- radiograph (X-ray) 27
- regions 225
Thrombosis
- of cavernous sinus 487, 564
- of sinus venosus 443
Thumb 87, 118
- abduction 136
- adduction 138
- flexion 136
- opposition 136
- range of motion 127, 138
Thymic veins 275, 529
Thymus 251, 252
Thyroarytenoid 540, 543
Thyrocervical trunk 240, 525, 527, 534, 547, 570
Thyroepiglottic ligament 530, 537, 539
Thyroglossal duct 545, 546
- cyst 545
- fistula 545
- persistence 545
Thyrohyoid 521, 526, 528, 529, 532, 546, 547, 602
- cartilage 537
- membrane 532, 536, 537, 539, 540, 543, 544, 546, 547, 551
Thyroid
- articular surface on cricoid 538, 539
- cancer 548

Thyroid
- cartilage 247, 528, 529, 530, 532, 536, 537, 538, 539, 540, 542, 543, 544, 545, 546, 547, 551
- gland 32, 525, 528, 529, 532, 533, 544, 545, 546, 547, 549
-- arteries 547
-- C-cells 549
-- development 545
-- laryngeal nerves 547
-- lymph nodes and lymphatic vessels 550
-- position 546
-- pyramidal lobe 546
-- scintigraphy 32
-- transverse section 548
-- veins 547
- membrane 542, 551
- plexus 275, 529
- scintigraphy 548
- surgery 546
- venous plexus 548
Thyroidectomy 546, 548
Thyropharyngeal part of inferior constrictor 532
Tibia 12, 177, 178, 179, 181, 182, 183, 184, 187, 191, 192, 194, 197, 198, 199, 201, 202
- distal end 197
- fractures 191
- medial rotation on the femur 188
Tibial
- collateral ligament 182, 188
- nerve 174, 189, 212, 214, 216, 612
- shaft 191
- tuberosity 156, 171, 176, 178, 179, 181, 182, 186, 190, 191, 192
Tibialis
- anterior 176, 190, 201, 202, 206, 207, 211
- posterior 205, 209
Tibiocalcaneal
- ligament 199
- part of deltoid ligament 199
Tibiofemoral joint 178, 179
Tibiofibular
- joint 12, 179, 191
- syndesmosis 197
- trunk 212
Tibionavicular part of deltoid ligament 199
Tigh 3
Tinnitus 511, 514
TODARO's tendon 258, 259
Tongue 31, 467
- blood vessels 470, 477
- extrinsic muscles 469
- innervation 467
- intrinsic muscles 468
- lymph nodes and lymphatic vessels 550
- muscles 468
- nerves 470, 477
- protrusion 469
- subepithelial venous plexus 470
Tonsil of cerebellum, hernia 559
Tonsillar
- branch/es
-- of ascending palatine artery 471, 544
-- of ascending pharyngeal artery 471
-- of glossopharyngeal nerve 467, 471, 544, 594, 595
-- of lesser palatine nerves 471
- crypts 467
- pits 467

Tonsillectomy 471
Tonsillitis 530
Torus
– levatorius 530, 531
– tubarius 530, 531, 534
Total
– mesorectal excision (TME) 375
– thyroidectomy 546
Trabeculae carneae 260
Trabecular
– or cancellous bone 15
– tissue of sclera 495, 496
– urinary bladder 381
Trachea 247, 253, 276, 277, 306, 525, 530, 532, 537, 544, 546, 547, 548
– lymph nodes and lymphatic vessels 550
– projection onto the thoracic wall 228
Tracheal
– bifurcation 247, 253, 306
– branch/es
– – of inferior thyroid artery 544
– – of vagus nerve 597, 598
– cartilages 247, 532, 536, 539, 540
Tracheobronchial lymph nodes (clin. term hilar nodes) 245, 246, 249, 252, 307
Tracheostomy tube 542
Tracheotomy 539, 542
Tragus 502
Tragus-ocular angle plane 428
Transglottic space 543
Transition zone of prostate 380, 384
Transpyloric plane (plane of ADDISON) 283, 310
Transtrabecular plane 283
Transumbilical plane 283, 287
Transurethral
– catheter 378, 379
– resection of the prostate (TURP) 376
Transversalis fascia 77, 79, 288, 290, 292, 294, 295
Transverse
– abdominal 77, 79, 288, 292, 294, 295, 321, 349, 356
– abdominal incision 289
– acetabular ligament 164
– arytenoid 534
– cervical
– – artery 520, 524, 525, 529
– – ligament (cardinal ligament, MACKENRODT's ligament) 391, 392
– – nerve 445, 520, 523, 524, 526
– – vein 445, 523, 529
– colon 297, 299, 301, 302, 303, 304, 305, 310, 316, 319, 321, 322, 325, 339, 343
– costal facet 66
– diameter of pelvis 365
– facial artery 442, 446, 487
– folds of rectum 371, 375
– foramen 53, 55, 56, 57
– head of adductor hallucis 209
– humeral ligament 96
– ligament
– – of atlas 58
– – of knee 183, 184
– – of WHITNAL 486
– mesocolon 301, 303, 304, 325, 347
– metatarsal arch 210
– muscle of tongue 468, 602
– occipital suture (var.) 429, 431
– palatine
– – folds 464
– – suture 448, 449, 456

Transverse
– part
– – of arytenoid 540, 544
– – of inferior constrictor (KILLIAN's muscle) 532
– – of trapezius 102
– – of vertebral artery 527
– pericardial sinus 256, 257
– perineal ligament 407, 413
– plane 6, 66
– process 44, 55, 67, 68, 158
– ridges of sacrum 75
– sinus 560
– tarsal joint (CHOPART's region) 194, 195, 198
– temporal gyri (HESCHL's transverse convolutions) 513, 514
Transversus
– abdominis 77, 79, 288, 292, 294, 295, 321, 349, 356
– tendinous arch (conjoint tendon) 292
– thoracis 235
Trapezium 119, 122, 123, 134
Trapezius 41, 58, 61, 71, 86, 102, 440, 445, 446, 519, 520, 521, 523, 524, 528, 529, 601
Trapezoid 119, 122, 123, 124, 134
– body 514
– ligament 95
– line of clavicle 90
TREITZ, ligament of (suspensory ligament of duodenum) 317
TREITZ, muscle of (suspensory muscle of duodenum) 317
TRENDELENBURG's sign 174
Triangle
– of CALOT (cystohepatic triangle) 340
– of KOCH 259
Triangular
– axillary space (TAS) 108
– fossa of auricle 502
– fovea of arytenoid 538
– ligament 300, 330
– subdivisions of cervical region 528
Triceps
– brachii 87, 108, 109, 115, 116, 118, 128, 144
– reflex 612
– slit 144
– surae 211
Tricuspid valve (right atrioventricular valve) 258, 259, 261
– auscultation 254, 263
– projection onto the anterior thoracic wall 254
Trigeminal
– ganglion (GASSERIAN or semilunar ganglion) 465, 493, 507, 580, 587, 589, 600, 607
– impression 504
– nerve [CN V] 465, 479, 488, 493, 494, 563, 566, 576, 578, 579, 581, 585, 587, 589, 616
– – fiber qualities 577, 578
– – hypersensitivity 585
– – innervation 577
– – origin 588
– – sensory ganglion 580
– – structures and functions 586
– neuralgia 585
– nucleus 600
Trigone of bladder 376
Triquetrum 119, 122, 123, 124
Triticeal cartilage 536, 537, 540

Trochanteric fossa 162
Trochlea
– of humerus 110
– of talus 194, 195, 197, 198
Trochlear
– nerve [CN IV] 438, 491, 493, 494, 516, 564, 566, 576, 578, 579, 583
– – fiber qualities 491, 577, 584
– – innervation 577
– – palsy 491
– notch 110, 111, 120, 123
TROLARD's vein 562
True
– (obstetric) conjugate 365
– ribs 233
Trunk 3
– movements 10
– of accessory nerve 601
– of spinal nerve 569, 606, 608, 610
– range of motion 70
Tubal
– artery 509
– branch/es
– – of tympanic plexus 594
– – of uterine artery 394
Tuber cinereum 499
Tuberculum sellae 434, 436
Tuberosity
– for serratus anterior 234
– of distal phalanx of foot 194
– of fifth metatarsal (bone) 194, 206
– of first metatarsal (bone) 194
– of navicular 194
– of ulna 110, 120
Tufted cells of olfactory bulb 582
Tunica
– albuginea
– – of corpora cavernosa 398
– – of testis 400
– externa 28
– intima 28
– media 28
– vaginalis 293, 294, 295, 399, 400
Tunnel of WERTHEIM 392
TURP (transurethral resection oft the prostate) 376
Tympanic
– amorphous substance 512
– branch of glossopharyngeal nerve [CN IX] 508
– canaliculus 509
– cavity 503, 505, 510, 512, 594
– – arteries 509
– – levels 505
– – medial wall 504
– – recesses 505
– – topographical relationships 508
– cells 504
– membrane 503, 505, 506, 508, 509, 511, 513, 592
– – arteries 509
– – defects 506
– – spontaneous perforation 506
– nerve (JACOBSON's nerve) 479, 509, 594, 595, 596
– opening 504
– part of temporal bone 431, 504
– plexus 509, 594, 595
– ring 431
Tympanomastoid fissure 504
Tympanotomy 506

U

Ulna 6, 12, 88, 110, 119, 120, 122
Ulnar
– artery 116, 117, 133, 134, 139, 140, 149
– – branches 149
– collateral ligament
– – of elbow joint 111
– – of wrist joint 123, 124
– deviation 8, 125, 129, 131
– head of flexor carpi ulnaris 129
– nerve 105, 106, 108, 117, 129, 133, 134, 139, 141, 145, 147
– – compression 117, 139
– notch 121
– pulse 28
– recurrent artery 117, 133, 149
– styloid process 87, 120, 122, 123
– vein 150
Umbilical
– arteries 273, 387, 394, 409, 419, 420
– cord 273
– fissure 330
– hernia 289, 298
– ligament 290
– region 77, 283
– ring 77, 286, 289, 322
– vein 273, 387
Umbilicus 78, 157
Umbo
– of malleus 506, 507
– of tympanic membrane 505
Uncinate process
– of pancreas 342, 344
– of vertebra 53, 451
Uncus of body (uncinate process) 53, 451
UNTERBERGER stepping test 516
Upper
– abdominal cavity, development 297
– arm
– – medial bundle of lymph collectors 151
– – posterolateral bundle of lymph collectors 151
– – radiograph 92
– dental arch 461
– extremity 3, 86
– – arteries 108, 149
– – basic movements 8
– – bones 88
– – cutaneous nerves 147
– – cutaneous sensory innervation 148
– – deep venous system 150
– – dermatomes 148
– – free part 88
– – innervation 141
– – joints 88
– – lymphatic vessels 150
– – lymph nodes 150
– – nerves 108
– – neurovascular supply 141
– – sensory innervation 147
– – skeletal ossification 14
– – superficial venous system 150
– – veins 150
– eyelid 482, 483, 488
– gastrointestinal bleeding (UGIB) 317
– head of lateral pterygoid 459, 460
– intervertebral surface 69
– jaw 448
– – deciduous teeth 463
– – panoramic radiograph 462, 463

Upper
– nasal meatus 452
– respiratory tract 247
– thoracic aperture, neurovascular structures 529
– tracheotomy 539
Ureter 34, 321, 347, 351, 353, 355, 358, 380, 385, 388, 389, 392, 393, 402
– blood supply 355
– course 355
– duplex 355
– lymphatic drainage 358
– position in the retroperitoneal space 348
– spatial relations 355
Ureteric
– closure mechanisms 376
– constrictions 355
– openings 376
– orifice 376, 378, 379
– – cystoscopy 376
Urethra 379, 382, 384, 385, 398, 408
– in man 33, 370, 376, 378, 415
– in woman 369, 379, 407, 418
Urethral
– artery 398
– crest 376
– glands (LITTRÉ, glands of) 378
– lacunae 378
– orifice 388
Urethrovaginal sphincter 379
Urinary
– bladder 34, 305, 347, 366, 369, 370, 377, 379, 381, 382, 383, 384, 385, 386, 388, 392, 393, 398, 399, 403, 417, 418
– – empty and filled 377
– – in man 376
– – sphincter mechanisms 376
– – voluntary sphincters 379
– continence 376
– organs
– – in man 370
– – in woman 369, 388
– system 11, 34
– tract, infections 355, 376
Urogenital
– diaphragm (perineal membrane) 406, 407, 413, 416, 417
– hiatus 368
– region 364
– sinus 399
– triangle 405, 406, 413
Uterine
– artery 355, 392, 394, 409, 419
– – ovarian branch 394
– – tubal branch 394
– cavity 386, 388, 390, 391, 418
– ostium of tube 391
– part of tube 391
– septum 388
– tube (FALLOPIAN tube) 33, 347, 369, 388, 389, 390, 391
– – peritoneal duplicatures 369
– vein 355, 395
– venous plexus 394, 395
Uterosacral
– ligament (recto-uterine ligament) 389, 391, 392
– peritoneal folds 389
Uterovaginal
– sphincter 407
– venous plexus 393, 396, 420

Uterus 33, 369, 379, 385, 388, 389, 391, 392, 417, 418
– bimanual palpation 387
– descensus 386
– duplex/didelphys 388
– extraperitoneal pelvic attachments 392
– MRI 388
– peritoneal duplicatures 369, 389, 391
– position in the pelvis 385, 386, 387
– septus/subseptus 388
– with fetus and placenta 387
Utricle 511, 512, 515
Utriculosaccular duct 511
Uvea 495
Uvula
– of palate 455, 464, 471, 507
– paralysis 596
Uvular muscle 472, 507

V

Vagal trunk 606
Vagina 33, 379, 385, 386, 387, 388, 391, 407, 408, 418
– position in the pelvis 386
Vaginal
– artery 355, 394
– branches of uterine artery 394
– distension during parturition 387
– nerve 394, 396
– orifice 379, 406, 407, 418
– part of cervix 387, 391
– process
– – of peritoneum 295
– – of sphenoid 435
– vein 395
– venous plexus 395
Vagus nerve [CN X] 251, 252, 255, 272, 278, 280, 328, 360, 437, 438, 441, 447, 467, 478, 502, 520, 524, 525, 529, 530, 533, 534, 547, 551, 563, 566, 576, 578, 579, 594, 597, 598, 604, 606, 611
– abdominal part 307
– complete lesion 599
– fiber qualities 577, 599
– innervation 577
– parasympathetic ganglion 581
– sensory ganglion 580
Valgus
– deformity (knock-knee) 156
– force 167
Vallate papillae 467, 544
Valve
– of coronary sinus 259, 270
– of foramen ovale 260
– of HEISTER (spiral fold) 339
– of inferior vena cava 259, 270
Valvular insufficiencies 263
Varicella zoster 609
Varicella zoster virus 585
– shingles 229
Varicocele 401
Varus deformity (bowleg) 156
Vascular
– fold of cecum 299
– lamina of choroid 495
– organ of lamina terminalis 575
– space 160
Vas deferens 33, 293, 294, 295, 370, 380, 383, 397, 399, 400, 401, 402, 403
Vasovagal reflex arc 611

Vastus
- intermedius 171, 180
- lateralis 157, 171, 176, 180, 186
- medialis 157, 171, 175, 176, 180, 186
VATER, ampulla of (major duodenal papilla) 317, 339, 341, 344
Vein/s 27, 29
- of bulb
-- of penis 398
-- of vestibule 409
- of cochlear aqueduct 511
- of GALEN 562, 566
- of LABBÉ 562
- of scala tympani 511
- of scala vestibuli 511
- of vestibular aqueduct 511
Vellus hair (fluffy hair) 25
Vena comitans of hypoglossal nerve 443, 477
Venous
- duct 273
- plexus of foramen ovale 560, 562
- sinus thrombosis 443
- valves 29
Ventral 5
- abdominal wall
-- folds and fossae 290
-- inside view 377
-- structure 294
- column of spinal cord 614
- hepaticum 297
- horn of spinal cord 614, 617
- mesogastrium 297, 300, 333
- pancreatic bud 342
- ramus of spinal nerve 610
Ventricles 572, 573, 574
Ventricular
- action 262
- blood flow 262
Ventromedial collecting system 222
Vermis of cerebellum 568, 617
Vertebra/e 44
- prominens 41, 53, 55
Vertebral
- arch 44, 45, 57, 68
-- connections 52
- artery 81, 274, 525, 527, 551, 563, 564, 565, 566, 568, 570
-- atlantic part 64
-- branches 527
-- variations of entry level 527
- body 44, 45, 57, 67
- canal 45
-- position of the spinal cord 571
-- stenosis 148
-- veins 82, 569
- column 42
-- arteries 81, 82
-- curvatures 43
-- ligaments 50, 51
-- lumbar part, MRI 613
-- nerves 610
-- segmental motion 47
-- veins 82
- foramen 44, 45, 69
- ligaments 52
- region 4, 225
- subluxation 53
- tributary of cerebral arteries 563
- vein 525, 551
Vertex 429

Vertical
- axes 7
- muscle of tongue 468, 602
Vertigo 511
Verumontanum (seminal colliculus) 376, 378
Vesical
- nerve 421
- venous plexus 402, 418, 420, 421
Vesicoureteric junction 355
Vesicourethral angle 376
Vesicouterine pouch 347, 366, 369, 387, 389, 418
Vesicovaginal septum 366
Vesicular appendices of epoophoron 388
Vestibular
- aqueduct 510
- fold 530, 541, 543
- ganglion 512, 515
- labyrinth 503, 505, 511, 515
- ligament 537, 543
- membrane (REISSNER's membrane) 512
- nerve 510, 511, 512, 515
- nuclei 515, 516, 578, 579
- schwannoma, MRI 510
- veins 511
Vestibule
- of omental bursa 303
- of vagina 379, 385, 406, 407
Vestibulocerebellar tract 516
Vestibulocochlear nerve [CN VIII] 438, 510, 511, 512, 513, 515, 563, 566, 576, 578, 579
- central auditory and vestibular pathways 515
- fiber qualities 577
- innervation 577
- sensory ganglion 580
Vestibulospinal tract 516, 615, 618
Vestibulothalamic tract 516
VIDIAN nerve (nerve to pterygoid canal) 590
Visceral
- efferent fibers 606
- pain 360
- pain fibers of female genitalia 396
- pelvic fascia (mesorectal fascia) 375
- peritoneum 300
- pleura 242, 243, 244
- plexus 606
- referred pain 284
- serous pericardium 255
- surface
-- of liver 310, 331
-- of spleen 346
Viscerocranium 426, 451
Visual
- axis 490
- pathway 499, 500
-- blood supply 499
Vitelline duct, remnants 298
Vitrectomy 499
Vitreous
- body 495
- chamber of eyeball 495
Vocal
- fold 530, 541
-- benign tumors (polyps) 541
- ligament 537, 538, 539, 540, 542, 543
- process of arytenoid 538, 539, 540
- tendon 540
Vocalis 540, 543
VOLKMANN's canal 15

Vomer 426, 427, 431, 432, 448, 450, 451, 465
Vortex of heart 258
Vorticose veins 443, 487, 495
Vulva 379
Vulvar carcinoma, metastases 395

W

WALDEYER's fascia (presacral fascia) 375
WALDEYER's lymphatic ring 467, 531
WERNICKE's area 514
WERTHEIM tunnel 392
WHARTON's duct (submandibular duct) 475, 476, 477
White
- ramus communicans 240, 606, 610
- spots on nails 26
WHITNAL's ligament (transverse ligament) 486
WILLIS, circle of (cerebral arterial circle) 527, 563, 565
Winging scapula 142
WINSLOW, foramen of (omental foramen, epiploic foramen) 302, 303, 333
WIRSUNG, duct of (pancreatic duct) 317, 341, 344
- sphincter 341
- variations 344
WOLFFIAN duct (mesonephric duct) 388, 399
WOLFF-PARKINSON-WHITE syndrome 271
Wrist
- arteries 139
- bones 119
- crease 118
- deep tendons 134
- drop deformity 93
- extensor retinaculum 135
- fractures 122
- joint 88, 123
-- extension 125
-- flexion 125
-- range of motion 125
- ligaments 124
- movements 8
- nerves 139
- superficial tendons 134, 135
- surface anatomy 118

X

Xiphisternal joint 226, 233
Xiphoid process 226, 233, 310

Z

ZENKER's diverticulum 532
ZINN, anulus of (common tendinous ring) 490, 492, 583
Z-line (border of mucous of stomach) 309
Zona columnalis 375
Zonular fibers 496
Zygapophysial joints 49
Zygomatic
- arch 426, 428, 441, 453
- bone 426, 430, 436, 451, 484, 485
- branches of facial nerve [CN VII] 440, 444, 486, 590, 591

Zygomatic
– margin of sphenoid 435
– nerve 446, 466, 488, 492, 583, 588
– process 484
–– of frontal bone 426
–– of maxilla 456
–– of temporal bone 504
– region 425

Zygomaticofacial
– branch
–– of maxillary nerve 588
–– of zygomatic nerve 446
– foramen 426, 484
– suture 484
Zygomaticomaxillary suture 428, 451, 484
Zygomatico-orbital
– artery 442, 446
– foramen 485, 488

Zygomaticotemporal
– branch
–– of maxillary nerve 588
–– of zygomatic nerve 446, 466
– nerve 488
Zygomaticus
– major 439, 440, 441, 486, 590
– minor 439, 440, 441, 486, 590